Retinal Glia

Colloquium
Digital Library of Life Sciences

This e-book is an original work commissioned for the *Colloquium Digital Library of Life Sciences*, a curated collection of time-saving pedagogical resources for researchers and students who want to quickly get up to speed in a new area of life science/biomedical research. Each e-book available in *Colloquium* is an in-depth overview of a fast-moving or fundamental area of research, authored by a prominent contributor to the field. We call these resources 'Lectures' because authors are asked to provide an authoritative, state-of-the-art overview of their area of expertise, in a manner that is accessible to a broad, diverse audience of scientists (similar to a plenary or keynote lecture at a symposium/meeting/colloquium). Readers are invited to keep current with advances in various disciplines, gain insight into fields other than their own, and refresh their understanding of core concepts in cell & molecular biology.

For the full list of available Lectures, please visit:
http://www.morganclaypool.com/page/LSindex

All Lectures available as PDFs on our website. Access is free for readers at institutions that license Colloquium. Please e-mail info@morganclaypool.com for more information.

Colloquium Series on Neuroglia in Biology and Medicine: From Physiology to Disease

Editors

Alexei Verkhratsky, M.D., Ph.D., D.Sc., M.A.E., M.L., M.R.A.N.F.

The University of Manchester, Manchester, U.K.; IKERBASQUE, Basque Foundation for Science, Bilbao, Spain

Vladimir Parpura, M.D., Ph.D., M.A.E.

Department of Neurobiology, Center for Glial Biology in Medicine, Atomic Force Microscopy & Nano-technology Laboratories, Civitan International Research Center, Evelyn F. McKnight Brain Institute, University of Alabama, Birmingham, AL, U.S.A.; Department of Biotechnology, University of Rijeka, Croatia

This series of e-books is dedicated to physiology and pathophysiology of neuroglia. It will be valuable for the researchers and workers in the field of neurobiology and medicine in general. Illustrations provided will be suitable for professional presentations and instructional materials by researchers, physicians, teachers and members of the pharmaceutical industry. As the topic of neuroglia is generally overlooked in the majority of neuroscience curricula, this series could fill a need for materials to be used in courses and/or seminars aimed at exploring the role of glia in the brain in health and disease.

Published titles

For titles please see the website, www.morganclaypool.com/toc/ngl/1/1.

Retinal Glia

Andreas Reichenbach and Andreas Bringmann

www.morganclaypool.com

ISBN: 9781615046706 paper
ISBN: 9781615046713 ebook
DOI: 10.4199/C00122ED1V01Y201412NGL003

A Publication in the

COLLOQUIUM SERIES ON NEUROGLIA IN BIOLOGY AND MEDICINE: FROM PHYSIOLOGY TO DISEASE

Series Editors: Alexei Verkhratsky, University of Manchester; IKERBASQUE, Basque Foundation for Science; Department of Neurosciences, University of the Basque Country. Vladimir Parpura, Department of Neurobiology, Center for Glial Biology in Medicine, Atomic Force Microscopy & Nanotechnology Laboratories, Civitan International Research Center, Evelyn F. McKnight Brain Institute, University of Alabama, Birmingham; Department of Biotechnology, University of Rijeka, Croatia

Series ISSN
ISSN 2375-9917   electronic
ISSN 2375-9933   print

Retinal Glia

Andreas Reichenbach
Paul Flechsig Institute for Brain Research, University of Leipzig

Andreas Bringmann
Department of Ophthalmology and Eye Hospital, University of Leipzig

*COLLOQUIUM SERIES ON NEUROGLIA IN BIOLOGY AND MEDICINE:
FROM PHYSIOLOGY TO DISEASE*

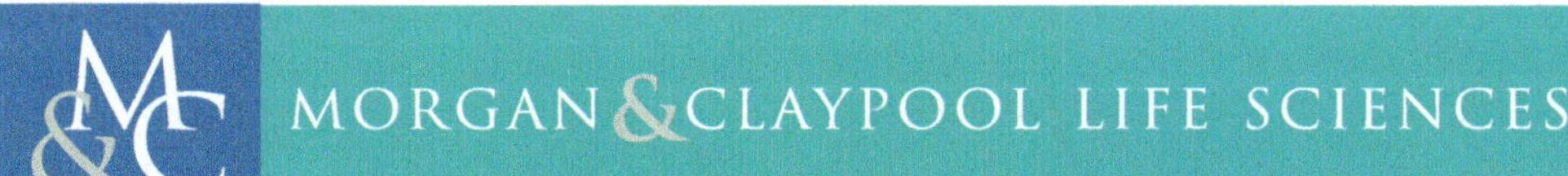

ABSTRACT

In 1851, Heinrich Müller discovered what he called "radial fibers" and what we now call Müller cells, as the principal glial cells of the vertebrate retina. Later on, other glial cell types were found in the retina, including astrocytes, microglia, and even oligodendrocytes. It turned out that retinal glial cells are essential constituents of the tissue. For instance, Müller cells appear to constitute the "core" of columnar units of clonally and functionally related groups of neurons. Their primary function is to support neuronal functioning by guiding the light towards the photoreceptor cells, removing excess neurotransmitter molecules from extracellular space, and performing efficient clearance of excess extracellular potassium ions. The latter two functions are also crucial for neuronal survival and are coupled to water clearance which is also essential. Müller cells are capable of "sensing" neuronal activity and modifying it by the release of signal substances (gliotransmitters). In cases of retinal injuries the Müller cells become reactive, and all above-mentioned functions are impaired. However, such de-differentiated Müller cells may proliferate, and may even serve as stem cells for the regeneration of a damaged retina. As well as the Müller cells, retinal astrocytes and microglial cells are important players in retinal development and function. This book gives a comprehensive survey of the present knowledge on retinal glia.

KEYWORDS

retina, microglia, oligodendroglia, astrocyte, Müller glia, potassium homeostasis, water homeostasis, neurotransmitter recycling, gliotransmitter, receptor, gliosis, Müller stem cell

Contents

1. Retinal Structure 1

2. Retinal Astrocytes and Blood Vessels 11
    2.1 Retinal Vasculature 24
    2.2 Development of Retinal Vasculature 30
    2.3 Astrocytic Functions in the Normal Retina 40
    2.4 Astrocytes in the Aging Retina 47
    2.5 Astrocytes in the Diseased Retina 47
        2.5.1 Glaucoma 48
        2.5.2 Diabetic Retinopathy 50
        2.5.3 Retinal Neovascularization 53
        2.5.4 Bacterial and Viral Infections 54
        2.5.5 Neuroprotective Effects of Astrogliosis 55

3. Retinal Microglia 57
    3.1 Microglia Precursors 57
    3.2 Resting Microglia 59
    3.3 Microglia Activation 62
        3.3.1 Trigger of Microglia Activation 64
        3.3.2 Characteristics of Activated Microglia 66
    3.4 Migration of Microglia 68
    3.5 Microglial Contribution to Neuronal Degeneration............... 68
    3.6 Microglial Contribution to Neuronal Survival 70
    3.7 Suppression of Microglia Activation 71
    3.8 Microglia in the Aging Retina.. 73

4. Retinal Oligodendroglia 77
    4.1 Development of Optic Nerve and Retinal Myelination 78
    4.2 Oligodendroglia in Optic Nerve Injury 80

5.   Müller Cells **83**

5.1   Morphology of Müller Cells 83

5.2   Ultrastructure of Müller Cells 88

5.3   Müller Cells as Cores of Retinal Columns 96

5.4   Light Guidance through Müller Cells 98

    5.4.1   Light Scattering in the Retinal Tissue 98

    5.4.2   Light-Guiding Properties of Müller Cells 101

5.5   Homeostatic and Metabolic Support of Retinal Neurons 103

    5.5.1   Mechanical Tissue Homeostasis 103

        5.5.1.1   Mechanical Forces in the Retinal Tissue 103

        5.5.1.2   Viscoelastic Properties of Müller Cells 108

        5.5.1.3   Increased Stiffness of Reactive Müller Cells 109

        5.5.1.4   Sensing Mechanical Tissue Deformations 110

    5.5.2   Neurotransmitter Recycling 112

        5.5.2.1   Glutamate Uptake and Metabolism 115

            5.5.2.1.1   Functional Role of the Glial Glutamate Uptake 115

            5.5.2.1.2   Glial Glutamate Transporters 117

            5.5.2.1.3   Ion Dependency of the Glial Electrogenic Glutamate Transport 118

            5.5.2.1.4   Regulation of GLAST 121

            5.5.2.1.5   Glutamate Uptake in Retinal Development 125

            5.5.2.1.6   Glutamate Uptake Under Pathological Conditions 127

            5.5.2.1.7   Uptake of Ammonia 130

            5.5.2.1.8   Removal of N-acetylaspartylglutamate 131

            5.5.2.1.9   Production of Glutamine 131

            5.5.2.1.10   Glutamine Transport 134

            5.5.2.1.11   Regulation of Glutamine Synthetase Expression in Retinal Development 135

            5.5.2.1.12   Regulation of the Glutamine Synthetase Under Pathological Conditions 137

            5.5.2.1.13   Regulation of Glutamine Synthetase by Soluble Factors 142

5.5.2.1.14 Ammonia-Dependent Regulation of the Glutamine Synthetase—Hepatic Retinopathy ... 143

5.5.2.1.15 Production of Glutathione ... 145

5.5.2.2 GABA Uptake and Metabolism ... 148

5.5.2.2.1 GABA Uptake ... 148

5.5.2.2.2 GABA Release ... 149

5.5.2.2.3 Expression of GABA Transporters ... 149

5.5.2.2.4 GABA Metabolism ... 150

5.5.2.3 Uptake of Glycine and Arginine ... 151

5.5.2.4 Uptake of Dopamine and Anandamide ... 152

5.5.3 Retinal Potassium Homeostasis ... 152

5.5.3.1 Kir Channels ... 157

5.5.3.2 Whole-Cell Kir Currents ... 158

5.5.3.3 Subcellular Distribution of the Potassium Conductance ... 160

5.5.3.4 Increase of Kir Currents in Developing Müller Cells ... 163

5.5.3.5 Kir Currents in Gliotic Müller Cells ... 164

5.5.3.6 BK Channels ... 169

5.5.3.7 Decrease of the BK Channel Activity in Developing Müller Cells ... 176

5.5.3.8 Whole-Cell BK Currents ... 178

5.5.3.9 K_A Currents ... 179

5.5.3.10 Other Types of Potassium Channels ... 181

5.5.4 Retinal Water Homeostasis ... 182

5.5.4.1 Retinal Water Transport ... 182

5.5.4.2 Retinal Water Channels ... 184

5.5.4.3 Glial Expression of AQP1 ... 187

5.5.4.4 Glial Expression of AQP4 and AQP6 ... 191

5.5.4.5 Possible Coupling of Glial Water and Potassium Transport ... 193

5.5.4.6 AQP4-Mediated Support of Synaptic Activity ... 195

5.5.4.7 AQP4-Mediated Suppression of Retinal Inflammation ... 196

5.5.5   Müller Cell Volume Regulation 197
       5.5.5.1   Kir4.1-Dependent Cell Volume Regulation 198
       5.5.5.2   AQP4-Dependent Cell Volume Regulation 199
       5.5.5.3   Receptor-Dependent Cell Volume Regulation 201
              5.5.5.3.1   Receptor-Dependent Cell Volume
                           Regulation During Ontogenetic
                           Development 206
              5.5.5.3.2   Receptor-Dependent Cell Volume
                           Regulation Under Pathological Conditions 207
              5.5.5.3.3   Involvement of Ecto-Nucleotidases in
                           Cell Volume Regulation 208
       5.5.5.4   Cell Volume Regulation By the Release of Organic
                  Osmolytes 210
       5.5.5.5   Müller Cell-Mediated Volume Regulation of
                  Bipolar Cells 211
5.5.6   Removal of Carbon Dioxide and Regulation of Extracellular pH.... 211
5.5.7   Metabolic Support of Photoreceptors and Neurons 213
       5.5.7.1   Glucose Metabolism 213
       5.5.7.2   Supply of Monocarboxylates 214
       5.5.7.3   Glycogen and Creatine Metabolism 216
       5.5.7.4   Lipid Metabolism 217
       5.5.7.5   Metabolism of Toxic Compounds 218
5.5.8   Support of Photoreceptor Function and Viability 218
       5.5.8.1   Recycling of Photopigments 219
       5.5.8.2   Circadian Protection of Photoreceptors 221
5.6   Regulation of Neuronal Activity by Gliotransmitters 222
5.6.1   Glial Release of Glutamate 222
       5.6.1.1   Non-Vesicular Release of Glutamate 222
       5.6.1.2   Vesicular Release of Glutamate 223
       5.6.1.3   Neuronal Effects of Glial Glutamate 226
5.6.2   Release of D-Serine 227
5.6.3   Glial release of Purinergic Receptor Agonists 228
       5.6.3.1   Release of ATP 228
       5.6.3.2   Release of Adenosine 229

5.6.3.3   Propagation of Glial Calcium Waves by Extracellular ATP Signaling 230

5.6.3.4   Neuronal Effects of Glial ATP and Adenosine 232

5.6.4   Release of ACBP and Retinoic Acid................................... 234

5.6.5   Production of NO, Carbon Monoxide, and Hydrogen Sulfide 234

5.7   Glial Forward and Feedback Regulation of the Neuronal Activity.................. 236

5.8   Neurovascular Coupling 238

5.9   Further Ion Channels of Müller Cells 239

5.9.1   Voltage-Gated Calcium Channels................................... 239

5.9.2   Voltage-Gated Sodium Channels.................................... 242

5.9.3   Epithelial Sodium Channels 244

5.9.4   Cation Channels... 244

5.9.5   Chloride Channels 245

5.10   Receptor Expression by Müller Cells 245

5.10.1   Glutamate Receptors... 246

5.10.1.1   iGluRs 246

5.10.1.2   mGluRs 248

5.10.2   Purinergic Receptors 250

5.10.2.1   Adenosine Receptors 251

5.10.2.2   Ionotropic P2X Receptors 251

5.10.2.3   Metabotropic P2Y Receptors............................ 252

5.10.2.4   Involvement of Purinergic Receptors in the Ontogenetic Development................................. 255

5.10.2.5   Increase of Purinergic Calcium Responses Under Pathological Conditions................................ 257

5.10.3   GABA Receptors 258

5.10.4   Glycinergic Receptors.. 261

5.10.5   Cholinergic Receptors 261

5.10.6   Catecholaminergic Receptors 262

5.10.7   Dopaminergic and Histaminergic Receptors....................... 262

5.10.8   VEGF Receptors 263

5.10.9   Thrombin Receptors 263

5.10.10   Further Peptidergic Receptors 264

5.10.11   Steroid Hormone Receptors 266

5.10.12   Receptors for Extracellular Matrix Components 267
5.10.13   Other Receptors of Müller Cells 268
5.11 Müller Cell Gliosis 270
5.11.1   The "Janus Face" of Müller Cell Gliosis 270
5.11.1.1   Protective Effects of Müller Cell Gliosis 270
5.11.1.2   Detrimental Effects of Müller Cell Gliosis 271
5.11.2   Characteristics of Müller Cell Gliosis 274
5.11.2.1   Unspecific and Specific Müller Cell Responses 274
5.11.2.2   Heterogeneity of Müller Cell Responses 275
5.11.2.3   "Conservative" and Massive Gliosis 275
5.11.2.4   Resistance and Susceptibility of Müller Cells to
            Pathogenic Stimuli 277
5.11.2.5   Primary Müller Cell Injuries 279
5.11.2.6   Glial Scar Formation 280
5.11.2.7   Prevention of Retinal Regeneration 281
5.11.2.8   Promotion of Retinal Remodeling 282
5.11.3   Upregulation of Intermediate Filaments 283
5.11.3.1   Intermediate Filaments are Crucial for Glial Scarring 286
5.11.3.2   Cellular Signaling Involved in Upregulation of
            Intermediate Filaments 286
5.11.3.3   Cellular Signaling Mediated by Intermediate
            Filaments 287
5.11.4   Network of Reactive Gliosis 288
5.11.5   Müller Cell-Mediated Spread of Retinal Degeneration—
         Retinal Detachment 288
5.11.6   Immunomodulatory Role of Müller Cells 296
5.11.6.1   Antigen Presentation 297
5.11.6.2   Müller Cell-Derived Inflammatory and Immune
            Response-Related Factors 297
5.11.7   Müller Cell-Derived Neuroprotective Factors 299
5.11.7.1   BDNF and Neurotrophin-3 301
5.11.7.2   NGF 302
5.11.7.3   GDNF and Neurturin 303
5.11.7.4   Osteopontin 304

5.11.7.5   CNTF 304

5.11.7.6   Endothelin-2 and LIF 305

5.11.7.7   bFGF 306

5.11.7.8   Prostaglandins 307

5.11.7.9   Other Neuroprotective Factors 307

5.11.7.10 Neurotrophic Signaling 309

5.11.8   Glial Regulation of Retinal Neovascularization 309

5.11.9   Retinal Edema 313

5.11.9.1   Vasogenic Edema 315

5.11.9.1.1 Glial Regulation of the Blood-Retinal
                    Barrier 316

5.11.9.1.2 Impairment of the Fluid Clearance 319

5.11.9.2   Cytotoxic Edema 320

5.11.9.2.1 Neuronal Cell Swelling 321

5.11.9.2.2 Glial Cell Swelling 323

5.11.9.2.3 Mechanisms of Osmotic Müller Cell
                    Swelling 324

5.11.9.3   Link between Vasogenic and Cytotoxic Edema 327

5.11.9.4   Resolution of Edema 328

5.11.10   Müller Cell Proliferation 332

5.11.10.1 Cellular Signaling involved in Müller Cell
                 Proliferation 333

5.11.10.2 Membrane Conductance of Proliferating Müller
                 Cells 335

5.11.10.3 Purinergic Stimulation of Müller Cell
                 Proliferation 337

5.11.10.4 Growth Factor Stimulation of Müller Cell
                 Proliferation 340

5.11.10.4.1   FGFs 341

5.11.10.4.2   PDGF 341

5.11.10.4.3   EGF, HB-EGF 342

5.11.10.4.4   HGF 343

5.11.10.5 Other Proliferative Factors and Conditions 344

5.11.10.6 Antiproliferative Factors 345

5.11.11 Glial Cell Involvement in Epiretinal Membrane Formation 347
 5.11.11.1 Composition of Epiretinal Membranes 348
 5.11.11.2 Transdifferentiation to Myofibrocytes 348
 5.11.11.3 Pathogenic Mechanisms of Early Epiretinal
  Membrane Formation 349
 5.11.11.4. Peeling of Epiretinal Membranes 352
5.11.12 Müller Stem Cells 354
 5.11.12.1 Retinas of Cold-Blooded Vertebrates 354
 5.11.12.2 Avian Retina 358
 5.11.12.3 Mammalian Retina 359
5.11.13 Müller Cells in Therapeutic Approaches 361

References 365

Author Biographies 367

Abbreviations

ACBP	acyl coenzyme A-binding protein
ADP	adenosine 5'-diphosphate
AGE	advanced glycation end product
Akt	protein kinase B
ALE	advanced lipoxidation end product
AMD	age-related macular degeneration
AMP	adenosine 5'-monophosphate
AMPA	α-amino-3-hydroxy-5-methyl-4-isoxazolepropionic acid
ANP	atrial natriuretic peptide
AP	activator protein
Apo	apolipoprotein
AQP	aquaporin
Ascl1	achaete-scute homologue 1
ATP	adenosine 5'-triphosphate
BDNF	brain-derived neurotrophic factor
bFGF	basic fibroblast growth factor
BK	big-conductance potassium
BMP	bone morphogenetic protein
cAMP	adenosine 5'-monophosphate
CDK	cyclin-dependent kinase
cGMP	cyclic guanosine monophosphate
Chx10	Ceh-10 homeodomain-containing homologue
CNS	central nervous system
CNTF	ciliary neurotrophic factor
CRALBP	cellular retinal binding protein
CREB	cAMP-responsive element-binding protein
Crx	cone-rod homeobox
CTGF	connective tissue growth factor
CX3CR	fractalkine receptor

Dkk	Dickkopf
DLL	delta-like ligand
EAAC	excitatory amino acid carrier
EAAT	excitatory amino acid transporter
EGF	epidermal growth factor
EnaCα	α-epithelial sodium channel
ERK	extracellular signal-regulated kinase
GABA	γ-aminobutyric acid
GAT	GABA transporter
GDNF	glial cell line-derived neurotrophic factor
GFAP	glial fibrillary acidic protein
GLAST	glutamate-aspartate transporter
GLT	glutamate transporter
GM-CSF	granulocyte-macrophage colony-stimulating factor
gp130	glycoprotein-130
GSSG	glutathione disulfide
HB-EGF	heparin-binding epidermal growth factor-like growth factor
HGF	hepatocyte growth factor
HIF	hypoxia-inducible factor
HVA	high threshold voltage-activated
ICAM	intercellular adhesion molecule
IGF	insulin-like growth factor
IGFBP	insulin-like growth factor binding protein
iGluR	ionotropic glutamate receptor
IFN	interferon
IL	interleukin
IP$_3$	inositol 1,4,5-triphosphate
IP$_3$R	IP$_3$ receptor
JAK	Janus kinase
JNK	c-Jun N-terminal kinase
KA	kainate
K$_A$	transient (A-type) potassium
K$_{DR}$	delayed rectifying potassium
Kir	inwardly rectifying potassium
L	long-lasting

LDL	low-density lipoprotein
LIF	leukemia inhibitory factor
LRP	lipoprotein-related protein
LVA	low threshold voltage-activated
MAPK	mitogen-activated protein kinase
MCP	monocyte chemoattractant protein
M-CSF	macrophage colony-stimulating factor
mGluR	metabotropic glutamate receptor
MHC	major histocompatibility
MIP	macrophage inflammatory protein
MMP	matrix metalloproteinase
MT1-MMP	membrane-type 1 matrix metalloproteinase
NADPH	nicotinamide adenine dinucleotide phosphate
NF	nuclear factor
NGF	nerve growth factor
NMDA	N-methyl-D-aspartate
NO	nitric oxide
NOD	nucleotide-binding oligomerization domain
NPY	neuropeptide Y
NTPDase	nucleoside triphosphate diphosphohydrolase
P2Y	metabotropic purinergic
P2X	ionotropic purinergic
p75^{NTR}	p75 neurotrophin receptor
PACAP	pituitary adenylyl cyclase activating polypeptide
Pax	paired box
PDGF	platelet-derived growth factor
PDR	proliferative diabetic retinopathy
PEDF	pigment epithelium-derived growth factor
PGE$_2$	prostaglandin E$_2$
PI3K	phosphatidylinositol-3 kinase
PKA	protein kinase A
PKC	protein kinase C
PLA$_2$	phospholipases A$_2$
PLC	phospholipase C
PVR	proliferative vitreoretinopathy

RAGE	receptor for advanced glycation endproducts
RCS	Royal College of Surgeons
Shh	sonic hedgehog
Sox2	sex-determining region Y-related box 2
Src	sarcoma
STAT	signal transducers and activators of transcription
T	transient
TASK	two-pore domain
TGF	transforming growth factor
TIMP	tissue inhibitor of matrix metalloproteinases
TLR	toll-like receptor
TNF	tumor necrosis factor
Trk	tropomyosin-related kinase
TRPC	transient receptor potential canonical
TRPV	transient receptor potential vanilloid
UDP	uridine 5'-diphosphate
UTP	uridine 5'-triphosphate
VEGF	vascular endothelial growth factor
VIP	vasoactive intestinal peptide
Wnt	wingless-type MMTV integration site family

CHAPTER 1

Retinal Structure

The vertebrate sensory retina, a highly specialized extension of the brain, is a thin (~0.25 mm thick in the human eye), multi-layered photosensitive tissue coating the inner back of the eyeball (Fig. 1A). The retina is responsible for photoreception and transduction of light energy into neuronal activity, and for the initial stages of visual processing and integration according to the environmental light conditions (Reichenbach and Bringmann, 2012). The visual information is transferred through the optic nerve to the brain. The sensory retina is composed of two main layered structures, the neural retina (or neuroretina) which contains, among others, photoreceptors and other neurons, and the retinal pigment epithelium which is a cellular monolayer. The interface between these structures is the subretinal space; it contains a fluid compartment and the interphotoreceptor matrix. The outer (basal) side of the pigment epithelium has contact to the Bruch's membrane (Fig. 1B), a multi-layered basement membrane. The pigment epithelium and the outer neuroretina are supplied with oxygen and nutrients by the choriocapillaris. The choriocapillaris is the innermost part of the choroidea which finally borders on the sclera, the outer capsule of the eye (Fig. 1A, B).

The neural retina has a well-organized structure with seven main layers (Figs. 1B, 2A, G). Three layers contain the cell bodies with the cell nuclei (outer nuclear layer, ONL; inner nuclear layer, INL; ganglion cell layer, GCL), two layers contain (in addition to cell processes) neuronal synapses (the outer plexiform layer, OPL, which is primarily composed of ribbon synapses, and the inner plexiform layer, IPL, which mainly contains conventional synapses), one layer contains the nerve fibers that draw to the optic nerve head (nerve fiber layer, NFL), and the outermost layer is formed by the photoreceptor segments (PRS). The neural retina is divided into an inner and outer part. The inner half includes the NFL, GCL, IPL, and INL, and the outer part consisted of the OPL, ONL, and PRS. The inner surface of the neural retina is covered by a basal lamina; the basement membrane together with the vitreal surface of Müller cell endfeet constitute the inner limiting membrane (ILM) (Fig. 1B). The outer limiting membrane (OLM) is the border between the neural retina and the subretinal space. This thin, eosinophilic structure is made by adherens and tight junctions between Müller glial and photoreceptor cells (Omri et al., 2010).

The neural retina is composed of at least 60 different cell (sub-) types (Kolb et al., 2001); most cells represent two kinds of cells: neurons (including photoreceptor cells) and glial cells. A

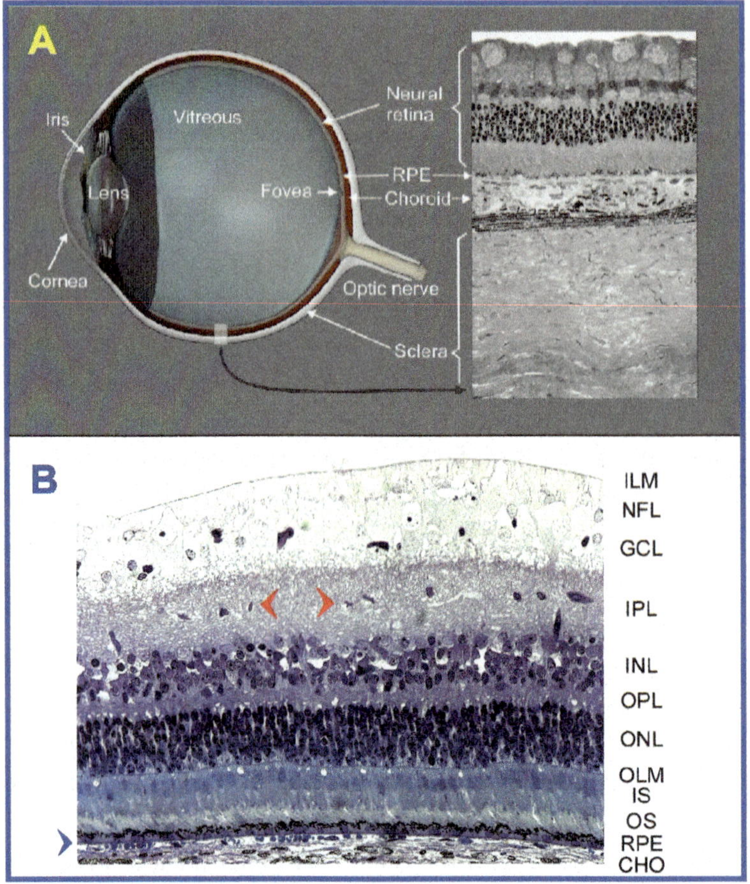

FIGURE 1: Retinal histology. **A.** Section through the back wall of the eye (*right*). **B.** Toluidin blue-stained semithin sections of the porcine retina. *Blue arrowhead*, Bruch's membrane. *Red arrowheads*, blood vessels in the mid of the inner plexiform layer (IPL). CHO, choriocapillaris; GCL, ganglion cell layer; ILM, inner limiting membrane; INL, inner nuclear layer; IS, inner photoreceptor segments; NFL, nerve fiber layer; OLM, outer limiting membrane; ONL, outer nuclear layer; OPL, outer plexiform layer; OS, outer photoreceptor segments; RPE, retinal pigment epithelium. Modified from Reichenbach and Bringmann (2012).

third constituent, blood vessels, is present in vascularized retinas (i.e., in many but not all mammalian retinas and in some fish retinas such as that of the eel). Three types of neurons lie in series and transfer the visual signal through the retina, from the photoreceptor outer segments (where light is absorbed by the photopigments) at the outer surface of the neuroretina to the axons at the inner surface of the retina running towards the optic nerve: photoreceptor cells (rods and cones, the first-order neurons of the retina), bipolar cells (the major second-order neurons), and ganglion cells (the third-order neurons) (Fig. 2A). The interneurons of the retina—horizontal and amacrine cells—perform the processing of visual information. A subtype of amacrine cells—the interplexiform cell—performs information processing between the two plexiform (synaptic) layers.

Vascularized neuroretinas contains three main types of glial cells: microglial cells and two types of neuron-supporting macroglial cells: astrocytes and Müller glial cells (Fig. 2A) (Schnitzer, 1987, 1988d; Holländer et al., 1991 ; Bringmann et al., 2006). In addition, oligodendroglia, the myelin-forming glia of the central nervous system (CNS), is present in the retinas of some fish, birds, rabbits, and hares (see 4.). Microglial cells are the primary resident innate immune cells of the retina. They play (in close relationship to other types of glial cells; see 5.11.4.) important roles in the host defense against microorganisms, the initiation of inflammatory processes, and tissue repair (see Ch. 2). Astrocytes are present only in mammalian species with completely or locally vascularized retinas (see Ch. 3). Avascular retinas/retinal areas do not contain astrocytes (Stone and Dreher, 1987; Reichenbach, 1987; Won et al., 2000; Fischer et al., 2010b); here, Müller cells are the only main type of neuron-supporting macroglial cells. In addition to the conventional types of glia, novel types of glial cells, such as the peripapillary radial glial cells in the avian retina (Schuck et al., 2000; Quesada et al., 2004; Stanke et al., 2010; Kim et al., 2011a), perivascular glial cells in the murine retina which express neural stem cell markers (Trost et al., 2014), diacytes in the retinas of various vertebrates (see below), and further glial cell types (Lin et al., 2013a) were described. Furthermore, dendritic cells (which are antigen-presenting cells distinct from microglia) are present in the retina, tightly associated with retinal ganglion cell axons (Eter et al., 2008; Lehmann et al., 2010; Heuss et al., 2012; Gregerson and Yang, 2003; Forrester et al., 2010).

Diacytes (or non-astrocytic inner retinal glial [NIRG] cells) are scattered across the inner layers of the avian retina and the retinas of dogs and non-human primates, but not in the retinas of rodents (Fischer et al., 2010a,b; Rompani and Cepko, 2010; Cebulla et al., 2012). Diacytes show features intermediate between those of astrocytes and oligodendrocytes (Rompani and Cepko, 2010). These cells express the intermediate filaments vimentin and transitin (the avian homologue of nestin; see 5.11.3.), similar to Müller cells and retinal progenitors (Fischer et al., 2010a). Diacytes express sex-determining region Y-related box 2 (Sox2), Sox9, Nkx2.2, transitin, and vimentin, but arc negative for the intermediate filament glial fibrillary acidic protein (GFAP) and paired box 2 (Pax2), and do not upregulate GFAP in response to acute retinal damage (Fischer et al., 2010a). The functions of diacytes in the retina remain unclear. In the developing avian retina, insulin-like growth factor (IGF)-1 stimulates the proliferation of diacytes, the migration of the cells into the retina, and upregulation of transitin (Fischer et al., 2010a; Zelinka et al., 2012). Diacytes accumulate at sites of retinal cell death (Fischer et al., 2010a; Zelinka et al., 2012). After focal retinal detachment, diacytes accumulate in the inner retina and in subretinal scars, along with Müller cell-derived cells

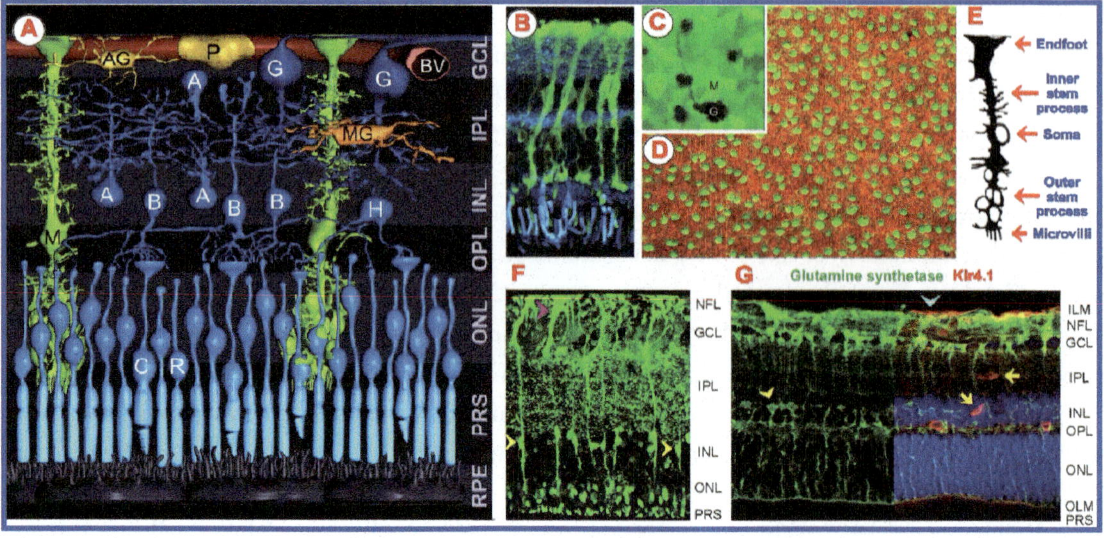

FIGURE 2: Müller cells (M) span the entire thickness of the neuroretina and are arranged in a regular pattern. **A.** Schematic drawing of the cellular constituents of a human retina. The inner retina contact the vitreal cavity (*top*) and contains the following retinal layers: nerve fiber layer, ganglion cell layer (GCL), inner plexiform layers (IPL), and inner nuclear layer (INL). The outer retina is directed to the outer surface of the eye and contains the following retinal layers: outer plexiform layer (OPL), outer nuclear layer (ONL), the subretinal space containing the photoreceptor segments (PRS), and the retinal pigment epithelium (RPE). The outer retina is supplied with oxygen and nutrients by the choriocapillaris, while the inner retina is supplied by intraretinal blood vessels (BV). Astrocytes (AG) are localized in the nerve fiber/ganglion cell layers. Both astrocytes and Müller cells contact the superficial blood vessels and the inner surface of the retina. The perikarya of Müller cells (M) are localized in the INL. From the perikaryon, two stem processes of Müller cells extend towards both surfaces of the neuroretina. The funnel-shaped endfeet of Müller cells form (in association with a basement membrane) the inner surface of the retina. In the IPL and OPL, side branches which form perisynaptic membrane sheets originate at the stem processes. In the ONL, the stem process of Müller cells forms membrane sheaths which envelop the perikarya of rods (R) and cones (C). Microvilli of Müller cells extend into the subretinal. Microglial (MG) cells are located in both plexiform layers and GCL. A, amacrine cell; B, bipolar cell; G, ganglion cell; H, horizontal cell; P, pericyte. **B-D.** Confocal images of living guinea-pig retina preparations. **B.** Radial section, illustrating the tight package of the cellular elements shown in **A.** The Müller cells are labeled with the vital dye, Mitotracker Orange (*green*); synapses and the outer segments of photoreceptor cells are counter-labeled with another vital dye, FM-43 (*blue*). **C, D.** Optical "horizontal sections" through a flat-mounted retina, illustrating the regular pattern of Müller cell stem processes (*green*) in the IPL (**D**) and the almost total occupation of the GCL by Müller cell endfeet (*green*; M); only the

somata of the ganglion cells (G) appear "empty" (**C**). **E.** A Golgi-stained human Müller cell. The main subcellular compartments are indicated. **F, G.** Müller cells in the porcine retina. **F.** A freshly isolated retinal slice was stained with the vital dye Mitotracker Orange which is predominantly taken up by Müller cells (Uckermann et al., 2004a). The somata of Müller cells lie in the mid portion of the INL (*yellow arrowheads*). *Red arrowhead*, Müller cell endfoot. **G.** A retinal slice was immunostained against the glial marker glutamine synthetase (*green*) and the glial potassium channel Kir4.1 (*red*). Cell nuclei are *blue* stained. The somata of Müller cells lie in the mid portion of the INL (*yellow arrowhead*). *Arrows*, perivascular Kir4.1. *Blue arrowhead*, Kir4.1 localized to vitreous-abutting enfeet membranes of Müller cells. Note that Kir4.1 is also localized to the microvilli extending into the subretinal space *in situ*. ILM, inner limiting membrane; NFL, nerve fiber layer.

(see 5.11.2.6.) (Cebulla et al., 2012). The survival of diacytes seems to be dependent on the presence of microglial cells (Zelinka et al., 2012).

The most abundant type of glial cells in the retina is the Müller cell. One turtle retina contains ~54,000 Müller cells and virtually no astrocytes, one rabbit retina contains ~4,200,000 Müller cells but only a few thousand astrocytes, and a human retina contains 4-5 millions of Müller cells (Gaur et al., 1988; Robinson and Dreher, 1990; Reichenbach et al., 1991b). Müller cells are specialized radial glial cells which span the entire thickness of the retina, from the inner to the outer limiting membrane (Fig. 2A, B, F, G). Their somata are localized in the mid of the inner nuclear layer (Fig. 2A). Two stem (trunk) processes radiate from the soma in opposite directions (Fig. 2E). The outer stem process draws towards the subretinal space into which it projects microvilli which run in between the photoreceptor inner segments. The inner stem process projects towards the vitreous chamber; the end of this process is expanded like a cup and forms the so-called endfoot (Fig. 2E) that lies adjacent to the basement membrane at the inner surface of the retina (Fig. 2C). Lateral processes expand into the plexiform layers of the tissue and form extensive sheaths that surround synaptic structures, as well as into the inner and outer nulear layers where they form a honey-comb-like, velate "embedding" of the neuronal somata. The Müller cell population forms a dense, regular pattern (Figs. 2D, 3B, C, 4C); each of these cells can be considered as the core of a columnar 'micro-unit' of retinal neurons (Fig. 5; see 5.3.). The processes of Müller cells contact the extracellular clefts around virtually each retinal neuron and ensheath neuronal somata and processes, and blood vessels.

Müller cells were firstly described by Heinrich Müller in 1851 (Müller, 1851). These cells have long been assumed to be 'functionally inert' support fibers, i.e., Müller cells are electrically inexcitable elements whose passive properties serve to maintain the constancy of the extracellular milieu, to prevent the electrotonic propagation of neuronal depolarizations, and to provide the mechanical/structural support of the retinal tissue. However, investigations in the last 35 years reversed

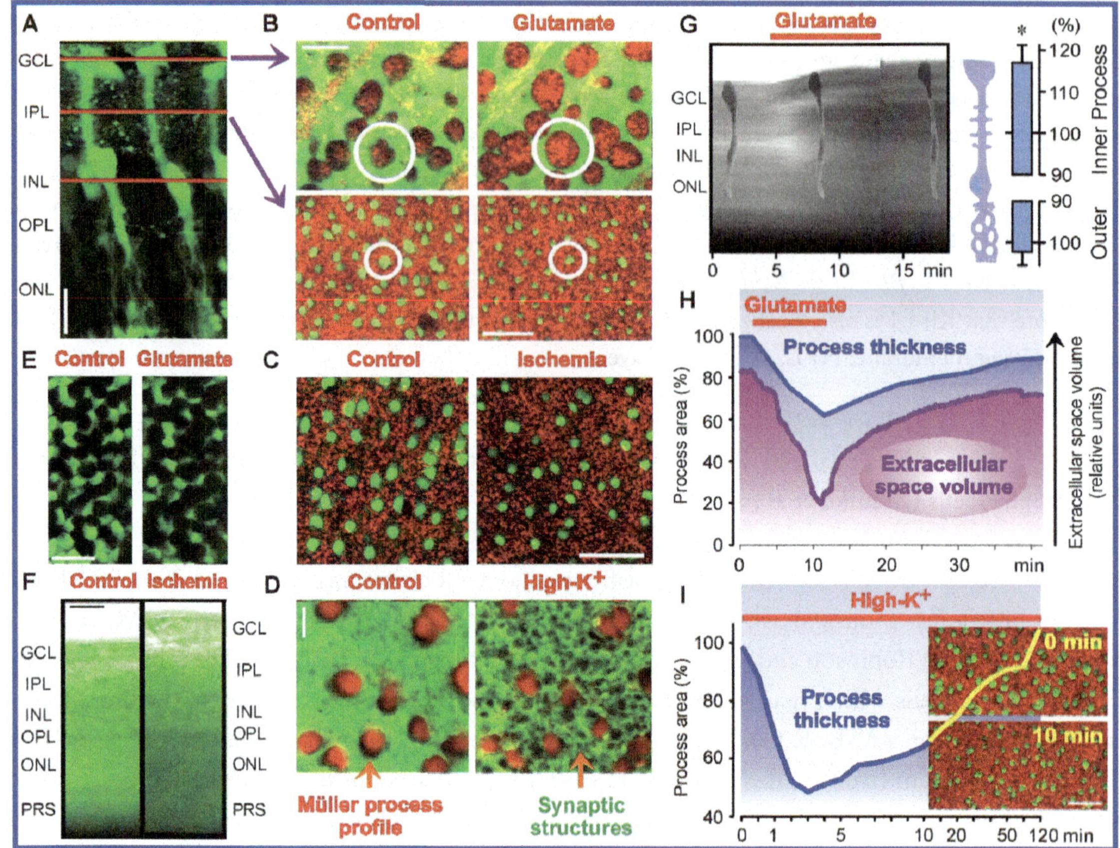

FIGURE 3: Glutamate induces morphological alterations of neurons and Müller cells in the guinea-pig retina. **A.** The retinal slice displays *green* Müller cells and the optical planes in the ganglion cell layer (GCL), inner plexiform layer (IPL), and inner nuclear layer (INL) which were used to record the morphological alterations of the cells. Müller cells were selectively *green* stained with a vital dye, while neuronal structures remained dark. **B-E.** The images were taken from a freshly isolated retinal whole-mounts. **B.** The tissue was exposed to glutamate (1 mM) for 10 min. *Above:* Glutamate exposure results in a swelling of the neuronal cell bodies in the GCL (*red*). The *elongated structures* are nerve fiber bundles. *Below:* Glutamate causes a reduction in the thickness of Müller cell stem processes that traverse the IPL (*green*) resulting from a swelling of the synapses between the Müller cell processes (*red*). **C.** A decrease of the thickness of Müller cell processes (and an increase of the size of neuronal cell bodies; not shown) was also observed shortly after a 1-h ischemia of the retina. **D.** A decrease of the thickness of Müller cell processes (*red*) was also observed in the presence of high (50 mM) potassium which induces a release of endogenous glutamate. Note the appearance of bullous structures between the Müller cell processes (*green*), probably reflecting swollen synapses. **E.** Glutamate (1 mM for 10 min) induces a swelling of

the neuronal cell bodies in the INL (*black*). This results in a decreased size of the Müller cell somata between the neuronal cell bodies (*green*). Note that the Müller cells somata are irregularly shaped because they are impressed by the stiffer neuronal somata. **F.** Freshly isolated retinas isolated shortly after a 1-h retinal ischemia display a thickening of the inner retinal layers compared to control. **G.** Superfusion of a retinal slice with glutamate (1 mM) induces a swelling of the inner but not outer retina (*left*). This is associated with an elongation of the inner stem process of Müller cells (*right*). **H.** Glutamate (1 mM) induces a decrease of the extracellular space volume in the IPL. This is associated with a decrease of the cross-sectional area of Müller cell processes that traverse the IPL. **I.** Time-dependence of the effect of high (50 mM) potassium on the cross-sectional area of Müller cell processes in the IPL. When the high potassium solution was applied longer than 3 min, the thickness of the Müller cell processes returned slowly to the control value, and a full recovery was observed after 120 min. ONL, outer nuclear layer; OPL, outer plexiform layer; PRS, photoreceptor segments. Scale bars, 20 μm (A-C, E, F, I) and 5 μm (D). Modified from Uckermann et al. (2004b).

---

the picture of passive cells. It becomes more and more clear that Müller cells are active players in the normal retinal function and in virtually all forms of retinal injuries and diseases where they play positive and negative roles (Reichenbach et al., 1993a; Newman and Reichenbach, 1996; Sarthy and Ripps, 2001; Bringmann et al., 2006; Reichenbach and Bringmann, 2010, 2013; see 5.11.). Müller cells interact with most, if not all neurons in the retina, resembling a symbiotic relationship. They constitute an anatomical and functional link between neurons and the compartments with which they need to exchange molecules (blood vessels, vitreous chamber, and subretinal space). Most nutrients, waste products, ions, water, and other molecules are transported through Müller cells between retinal vessels and neurons. Müller cells act as living optical fibers which guide the light through the inner retinal layers towards the photoreceptors (see 5.4.). Müller cell processes function as a soft, compliant embedding for neurons which supports synaptic plasticity and activity-dependent morphological alterations of retinal neurons (see 5.5.1.). They provide trophic substances to neurons (see 5.5.7.) and remove metabolic waste (see 5.5.6.). Müller cells regenerate the chromophores of cone photopigments (see 5.5.8.1.), mediate the retinal potassium (see 5.5.3.), water (see 5.5.4.), and acid-base homeostasis (see 5.5.6.), regulate the extracellular space volume (see 5.5.5.), maintain the inner blood-retinal barrier (see 5.11.9.1.1.), and regulate the retinal blood flow (see 5.8.). Müller cells support the synaptic activity by neurotransmitter recycling that involves the supply of neurons with precursors of neurotransmitters (see 5.5.2.). By the uptake of neurotransmitters, Müller cells are involved in the regulation of the synaptic activity in particular in the inner retina. In addition to their homeostatic functions, Müller cells play a more active role in the control of neurotransmission

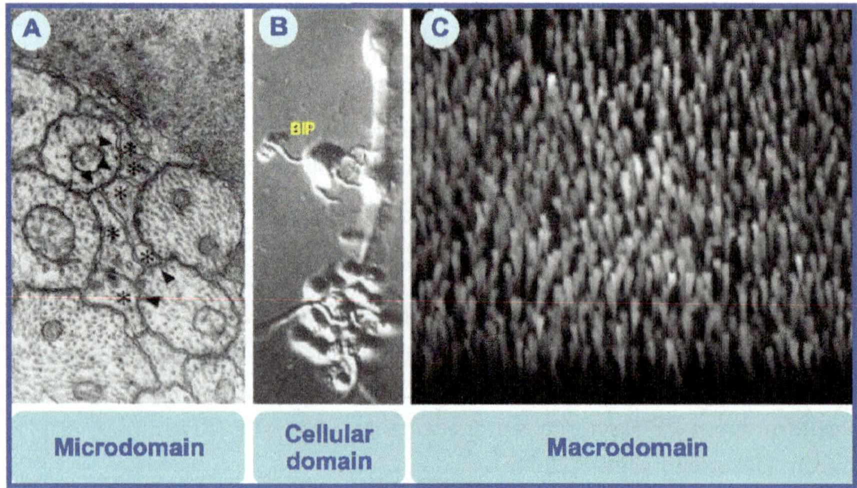

FIGURE 4: Ascending hierarchic levels of glial domains involved in glia-neuron interactions. **A.** Example of a microdomain, consisting of a few finger-like end branches which interact with the node-like specialization of a ganglion cell axon. **B.** Cellular domain, consisting of an entire Müller cell interacting with the neurons of "its" columnar unit. **C.** A macrodomain, consisting of a large population of Müller cells, together interacting with the (light-stimulated) neurons and the intraretinal blood vessels of a given retinal area. **A.** Transmission electron micrograph of a tree shrew retina. Modified from Reichenbach et al. (1995a). **B.** Group of unstained cells enzymatically dissociated from guinea-pig retina. BIP, bipolar cell. Original (courtesy of J. Grosche, Leipzig). **C.** 3D reconstruction of a series of confocal images of a guinea-pig retina. Müller cells are visualized by vimentin immunohistochemistry. Original courtesy of J. Grosche, Leipzig.

and synaptic activity by the release of gliotransmitters (see 5.6.). Müller cells support the survival of photoreceptors and neurons (see 5.11.7.), are responsible for the structural stabilization of the retina (Willbold and Layer, 1998; Willbold et al., 2000; Byrne et al., 2013), and modulate immune and inflammatory responses (see 5.11.6.). All of the functions of Müller cells directly or indirectly modify the neuronal information processing. The Müller cell-mediated homeostasis of the extracellular space composition and volume have a great impact for the setting of the signal-to-noise ratio of the synaptic transmission and the spatial distribution of light-induced signaling. The importance of Müller cells for the maintenance of the retinal structure and function is elucidated by the fact that selective Müller cell destruction causes retinal dysplasia, photoreceptor cell death, breakdown of the blood-retinal barrier, intraretinal neovascularization and, eventually, retinal degeneration and proliferation of retinal pigment epithelial cells (Dubois-Dauphin et al., 2000; Shen et al., 2010a, 2012, 2014a; Byrne et al., 2013).

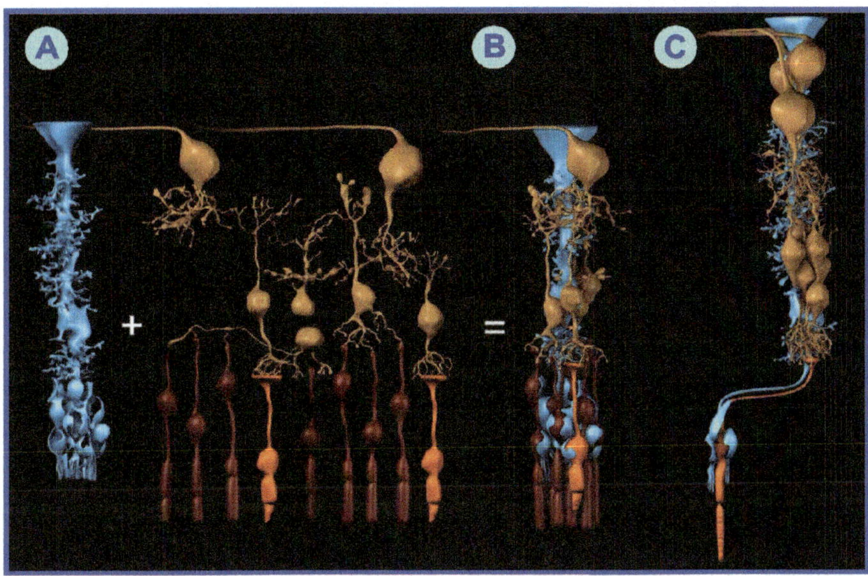

FIGURE 5: Müller cells form the cores of radial units of retinal neurons. Every Müller cell is surrounded by a distinct group of retinal neurons (**a**) with which it interacts specifically during development, mature functioning, and injury of the retina. These repetitive radial units are almost identical throughout most regions of the retina (**b**) but differ in the (peri-)fovea (**c**) by the lack of rods, an increased number of neurons of the inner nuclear and ganglion cell layers, and by an elongation and a z-shaped course of the outer processes of Müller cells. *Blue*, Müller cells; *yellow*, retinal neurons; *orange*, cones; *brown*, rods.

Müller cells become activated upon virtually all pathogenic stimuli. Reactive Müller cells are neuroprotective and support the survival of photoreceptors and neurons, but may also quit the support of neurons and rather contribute to neuronal degeneration (see 5.11.1.). A subpopulation of Müller cells in the mature retina represents latent neural progenitor/stem cells which may, upon retinal injury, transdifferentiate into new photoreceptors and neurons, at least in retinas of lower vertebrates (see 5.11.12.). Currently, the many roles of Müller cells in the regulation of retinal function are still not resolved and are subject of intensive research.

Müller cells have functional roles that are carried out by the concerted action of astrocytes, oligodendroglia, and ependymal cells in other regions of the CNS. The retina is a part of the brain (Reichenbach and Bringmann, 2012) and is easily accessible by non-invasive diagnostic methods such as optical coherence tomography (Drexler and Fujimoto, 2008). This together with the relatively simple, well-layered structure of the retina and the well-defined sensory function make the retina and Müller cells versatile model systems for studies on brain development and function.

CHAPTER 2

Retinal Astrocytes and Blood Vessels

In the retina, two main types of astrocytes are present: (1) "fibrous" type I astrocytes (Raff et al., 1983) that express GFAP and connexin 43, and (2) type II astrocytes that express GFAP, but not connexin 43. Type I astrocytes are further divided into type Ia and type Ib. Type Ia astrocytes are present in the optic nerve head, while type Ib astrocytes are present in the nerve fiber/ganglion cell layers of the retina. In addition, a small population of GFAP-negative astrocytes is present in the retina (Pérez-Alvarez et al., 2008; Mansour et al., 2008).

Astrocytes are present only in mammalian species with completely or locally vascularized retinas, and in some fish retinas such as that of the eel. Non-vascularized neural retinas (of lower vertebrates, birds, and some mammals such as echidna and horse) or retinal areas (e.g., rabbit [with the exception of the medullary rays; Fig. 6C], hare, the peripheral retina of the cat, the "pseudangiotic retina" of the guinea pig which lack intraretinal blood vessels [Fig. 7G] with the exception of a narrow rim around the optic nerve head) do not contain astrocytes (Schnitzer, 1985, 1987, 1988d; Stone and Dreher, 1987; Reichenbach, 1987; Gábriel et al., 1993; Distler and Kopatz, 1996; Triviño et al., 1997). The presence of intraretinal blood vessels is correlated with the retinal thickness; vascularized retinaa are ~60% thicker than avascular retinas (Chase, 1982; Buttery et al., 1991; Dreher et al., 1992). When present, retinal blood vessels are restricted to the inner neuroretina (Figs. 2G, 7G, 8C, 9A, 10C, 11B, 12A); photoreceptor cells in the outer retina consume most of the oxygen delivered by the choriocapillaris (Yu and Cringle, 2001).

In vascularized retinas/retinal areas, astrocytes are located to the nerve fiber and ganglion cell layers (Figs. 2A, 13A-C, 14C, D, 15A). Astrocytes may also send processes towards the inner plexiform layer which surround the blood vessels in the inner portion of this layer (Ramirez et al., 1994). Astrocytic processes run parallel to and between the axons of the nerve fiber bundles (Fig. 6A) (Büssow, 1980). Both astrocytes and Müller cells are in contact with: (i) the superficial blood vessels of the retina via processes that wrap the vessels and form ("*en passant*"-) perivascular endfeet (Figs. 6B, 13B); (ii) bundles of ganglion cell axons which they loosely ensheath; (iii) the initial segments and node-like structures of these axons where they form coronae of finger-like processes (Figs. 4A, 16A, B); and (iv) the basal lamina at the inner surface of the retina (Stone and Dreher, 1987; Reichenbach et al., 1988c; Holländer et al., 1991; Rungger-Brändle et al., 1993;

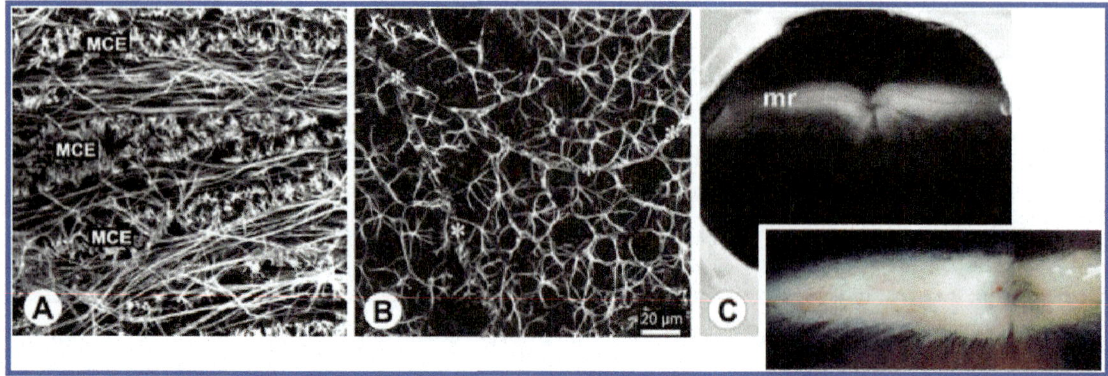

FIGURE 6: Astrocytes and oligodendrocytes in mammalian retinas. **A, B.** (Fibrous) astrocytes are present in vascularized retinas. **A.** In the central murine retina, the processes of many astrocytes run rather parallel to the bundles of ganglion cell axons, and form (together with the Müller cell endfeet, MCE) perivascular endfeet (mostly of the "en passant" type). **B.** In the periphery of the same murine retina, the density of nerve fibers is low; accordingly, the pattern of astrocytic processes is rather irregular but still these processes form endfeet at the blood vessels (*asterisk*). Immunohistochemical staining of GFAP; modified from Reichenbach and Wolburg (2005). **C.** In the rabbit retina, a horizontal stripe contains blood vessels, astrocytes, and oligodendrocytes which myelinate the central portions of the ganglion cell axons. These myelinated fibers are macroscopically visible as so-called "medullary rays" (mr). Native, unstained eyecup from an adult rabbit, after removal of cornea, lens, and most of the vitreous body (courtesy of Mike Francke, Leipzig). *Inset*, medullary rays at higher magnification.

Distler et al., 1993; Stone et al., 1995b; Makarov et al., 1999; Reichenbach and Wolburg, 2005). The glial sheaths that surround the somatas of retinal ganglion cells are formed predominantly by Müller cells, while the glial processes that attach the node-like specialisations of their axons are formed mainly by astrocytes (Stone and Dreher, 1987; Dreher et al., 1988; Holländer et al., 1991; Distler et al., 1993; Makarov et al., 1999). The inner rim of the superficial retinal vessels is surrounded by astrocytic processes while the outer rim is surrounded by Müller cell membranes (Uga and Ikui, 1974; Iandiev et al., 2007a). In avascular retinas/retinal areas, nerve fibers and superficial vessels are only surrounded by Müller cell processes (Hildebrand and Waxman, 1983).

The density of retinal astrocytes is proportional to the thickness of the nerve fiber layer. Astrocytes are found at high spatial densities in the central retina and around blood vessels, while they are sparsely distributed in the peripheral retina (Ogden, 1978; Büssow, 1980; Karschin et al., 1986a, b; Lewis et al., 1988; Davidson et al., 1990; Distler et al., 1993). The central primate fovea does not contain astrocytes, and the central retinal areas of various other mammals display a local minimum of astrocyte density (Karschin et al., 1986a,b; Distler et al., 2000). Morphologically, there are at least three subclasses of astrocytes in the retina: intervascular stellate astrocytes, which are located between the major arterioles and which have rare contacts to vessels or axons, perivascular astrocytes, which have an intricate relationship with the retinal vasculature (Fig. 13B), and elongated bipolar astrocytes which are associated with axon bundles (Ogden, 1978; Karschin et al., 1986a,b; Schnitzer and Karschin, 1986; Robinson and Dreher, 1989; Chan-Ling et al., 1991; Ramirez et al., 1994; Triviño et al., 2000; Zahs and Wu, 2001). A loss of retinal ganglion cell axons results in a shift of the astrocyte morphology from bipolar to stellate and in a decrease of the density of astrocytes (Karschin et al., 1986b). The distribution of stellate astrocytes is not influenced by the surrounding neurons but is caused by interaction between astrocytes; astrocytes maintain contact with their neighbours through their processes, but keep their somas apart (Chan-Ling and Stone, 1991a). The association of astrocytes with axon bundles is caused by axon-derived, but not vessel-derived factors (Chan-Ling and Stone, 1991a). In the rat retina, astrocytes show no affinity for axons, and the distribution of astrocytes is uniform (Chan-Ling and Stone, 1991a). Retinal ganglion cells attract astrocytic processes towards their initial segments and the node-like structures of the axon membrane (Figs. 4A, 16A, B) and induces an alteration of the astrocyte morphology to a bipolar shape by the activity-dependent release of soluble factors (Gargini et al., 1998).

Retinal astrocytes are immigrants from the brain and do not arise from retinal progenitor cells; astrocytes (as well as vascular endothelial cells, pericytes, and microglia) enter the retina via the optic nerve head during the embryonic and postnatal development (Kondo et al., 1984; Ling and Stone, 1988; Watanabe and Raff, 1988; Ling et al., 1989; Huxlin et al., 1992; Provis, 2001; Li et al., 2007c). (The only glial cell that develops from retinal progenitors is the Müller cell.) As the retinal development proceeds, migrating astrocytes gradually increase in number and spread toward the ora serrata (the transition zone between the retina and the ciliary body) along the inner surface of the retina (Kondo et al., 1984). Astrocyte precursor cells arise from multipotent neuroepithelial stem cells or astrocytic stem cells (Steindler and Laywell, 2003; Ransom and Chan-Ling, 2004). These astrocyte precursor cells (which are $Pax2^+/vimentin^+/GFAP^-/S100^-$) give rise to immature perinatal astrocytes (which are $Pax2^+/vimentin^{+/-}/GFAP^+/S100^+$, and which have proliferative and migratory potential) and finally to adult type I astrocytes ($Pax2^-/GFAP^+/S100^+$) (Schnitzer, 1988b; Mi and Barres, 1999; Chu et al., 2001; Sarthy et al., 1991). Both immature $Pax2^+$ and mature $Pax2^-$ astrocytes are present in adult rodent and human retinas (Chu et al., 2001; Mansour et al., 2008). In human retinas, immature $Pax2^+$ astrocytes are restricted to a limited region around the optic nerve head (Chu et al., 2001) while in the rat retina, immature astrocytes are scattered throughout the tissue (Mansour et al., 2008). This suggests that a small subpopulation of astrocyte precursor cells is retained in the retina throughout adult life and that immigration of astrocytes into the retina may

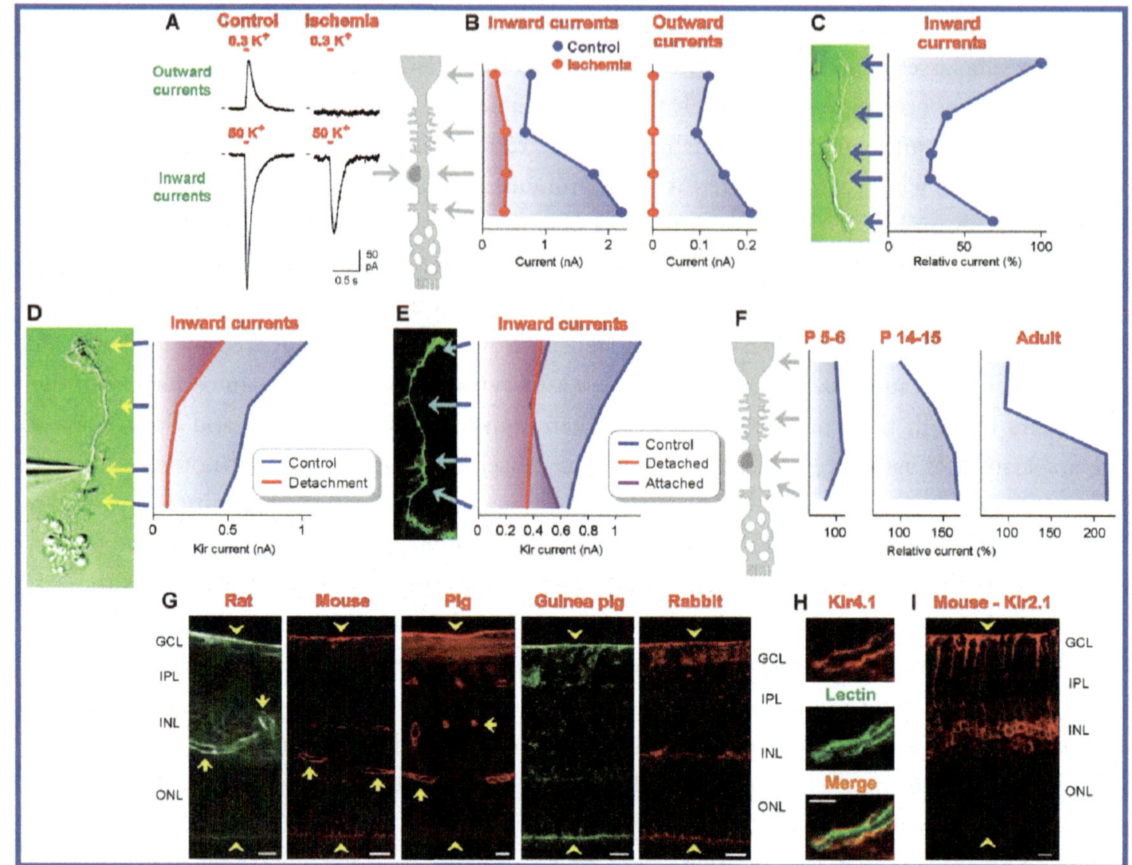

FIGURE 7: The potassium conductance displays a non-uniform distribution across the surface of Müller cells and decreases under pathological conditions. The subcellular distribution of the potassium conductance was determined by focal ejections of a high- (10 or 50 mM) and a low-potassium (0.3 mM) solution, respectively, onto different membrane domains of isolated Müller cells (endfoot, inner stem process, soma, inner part, and end of the outer stem process). The solutions induced inward and outward potassium currents, respectively. The control potassium concentration was 3 mM. **A.** Current traces induced in the soma membrane of rat Müller cells. The cells were isolated from a control retina and a retina obtained 3 days after transient ischemia. Retinal ischemia-reperfusion was induced by a 1-h elevation of the intraocular pressure above the systolic blood pressure. Note the decrease of the amplitude of the inward current and the almost complete absence of outward currents in the cell of the postischemic retina in comparison to the control cell. **B.** Subcellular distribution of the inward and outward potassium conductance in rat Müller cells from control and postischemic retinas. **C.** Subcellular distribution of the inward potassium conductance in Müller cells of the guinea pig. The cell endfoot is *above*. **D.** Alteration of the

subcellular distribution of the inward potassium conductance in rabbit Müller cells after experimental retinal detachment. The cells were derived from control retinas and from retinas that were detached from the pigment epithelium for 3 days. The cell endfoot is *above*. **E.** Alteration of the subcellular distribution of the inward potassium conductance in porcine Müller cells after local retinal detachment. The cells were isolated from un-operated control and detached retinas, and from non-detached retinal areas that surrounded the local detachment *in situ*, and were investigated 7 days after surgery. The cell endfoot is *above*. **F.** Developmental alteration in the subcellular distribution of the inward potassium conductance in Müller cells of the rat. The prominent inward conductance in the middle portion of the cells develops relatively late. Relative currents (normalized to the currents at the endfoot region, 100%) are shown. **G.** Distribution of the Kir4.1 protein in slices of vascularized (rat, mouse, pig) and avascular retinas (guinea pig, rabbit). In the vascularized retinas, the Kir4.1 protein is prominently located around the vessels within the inner nuclear (INL; *arrows*) and at the limiting membranes of the retina (*arrowheads*). In the avascular retinas, the Kir4.1 protein is located predominantly at the limiting membranes (*arrowheads*). **H.** Perivascular glial Kir4.1 in the rat retina at higher magnification. The vessel of the deep vascular plexus was stained with lectin (*green*). **I.** Distribution of the Kir2.1 protein in a slice of the mouse retina. GCL, ganglion cell layer; IPL, inner plexiform layer; ONL, outer nuclear layer. P, postnatal day. Scale bars, 10 and 5 (H) μm. Modified from Kofuji et al. (2002), Pannicke et al. (2004, 2006), Iandiev et al. (2006b), and Wurm et al. (2006b).

---

occur as the retina and eyeball grow in adult life, in rats at least until 9 months of age (Mansour et al., 2008). Immigration of astrocytes may accompany expansion of the vascular tree in the growing retina (Mansour et al., 2008). In the avascular avian retina, the immigration of astrocytes from the optic nerve head into the retina is prevented by αB-crystallin-expressing peripapillary glial cells which wrap the optic nerve head and which are densely located at the junction between the optic nerve head and retina (Kim et al., 2011b).

In the embryonic rabbit retina (which contains a vascularized myelinated streak; Fig. 6C), the first glial cells that invade the tissue via the optic nerve are vimentin-expressing astrocytes which replace vimentin by GFAP around the time of birth (Morcos and Chan-Ling, 1997). Shortly after birth, oligodendrocyte precursor cells and immature oligodendrocytes invade the retina from the optic nerve head (Schnitzer, 1988b; Morcos and Chan-Ling, 1997).

2.1   RETINAL VASCULATURE

In mammalian species that have vascularized neuroretinas ("euangiotic retinas", e.g., man, monkey, pig, cat, dog, rat, mouse), the third major constituent of the neural retina (in addition to neurons and glial cells) are blood vessels. The human retinal vasculature is comprised of the central retinal

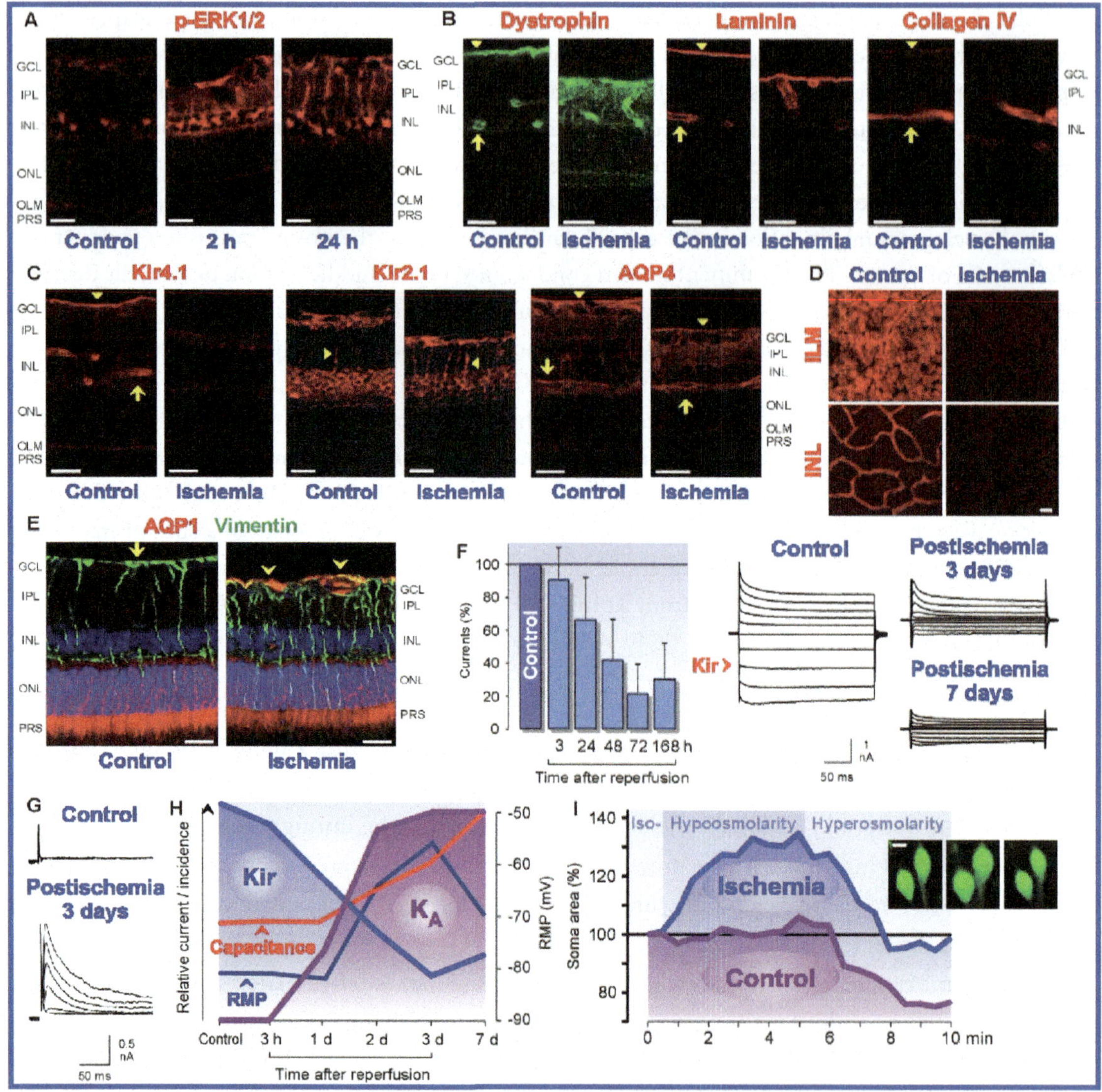

FIGURE 8: Ischemia-induced alterations of the potassium conductance of rat Müller cells are associated with altered cell swelling characteristics. The tissues and cells were isolated at different time periods after a 1-h transient retinal ischemia induced by elevation of the intraocular pressure above the systolic blood pressure. **A.** After ischemia, Müller cells display increased expression of the activated (phosphorylated) extracellular signal-regulated kinases 1 and 2 (p-ERK1/2) in their somata and inner processes. Slices of a control and of postischemic retinas (2 and 24 h after reperfusion) were immunostained against ERK1/2. **B.** Immunolocalization of extracellular matrix proteins in slices of a control and a 7-days

postischemic retina. The ischemia-induced mislocation of Kir4.1 is accompanied by a more diffuse location of the dystrophin protein which is implicated in the membrane clustering of Kir4.1 channels. The distributions of laminin and type IV collagen were not altered after ischemia. **C.** Immunolocalization of glial Kir channels and aquaporin-4 (AQP4) in a normal and a 7-days postischemic retina. The Kir4.1 protein is predominantly localized at the limiting membranes of the neuroretina (*arrowheads*) and around the blood vessels (*arrow*). The Kir2.1 protein is localized in the inner retina in membrane domains of Müller cells that abut on neuron compartments, e.g. in the processes that traverse the inner plexiform layer (IPL) (*arrowheads*). The AQP4 protein is localized in membrane domains through which Müller cells absorb and release potassium ions in periods of neuronal activity. The *arrows* indicate perivascular staining, the *arrowheads* mark labeling at the limiting membranes. Seven days after ischemia, the expression of Kir4.1 protein is largely downregulated whereas the localization of Kir2.1 and AQP4 proteins are unaltered. Note the decrease in the thickness of the inner retina reflecting the ischemia-induced neuronal degeneration. **D.** Views onto the inner limiting membrane (*above*) and the inner nuclear layer (INL; *below*) in wholemounts of a control (*left*) and a 7 days-postischemic retina (*right*) which were stained for Kir4.1, displaying the protein expression in the vitreous-facing Müller cell endfeet (*above*) and around intraretinal vessels (*below*). Note the absence of Kir4.1 in the postischemic retina. **E.** Immunolocalization of aquaporin-1 (AQP1) and vimentin in slices of a control and a 4 weeks-postischemic retina. Note that ischemia-reperfusion induces expression of AQP1 in glial cells in the nerve fiber/ganglion cell layers (*arrowheads*). *Arrow*, AQP1-positive erythrocyte within a vessel. **F.** Mean decrease in the Kir currents in dependence on the time of reperfusion after ischemia. The *right side* displays examples of whole-cell potassium currents of Müller cells from control retina and postischemic retinas. **G.** Fast transient (A-type) potassium (K_A) currents are absent in a cell of a control retina and present in a cell from a postischemic retina. **H.** The expression levels of Kir and K_A currents are counter-regulated in the course of retinal ischemia-reperfusion injury. The following parameters are shown in dependence on the time period of reperfusion (3 h to 7 days) after transient ischemia: relative amplitude of the Kir currents, incidence of Müller cells that display K_A currents (from 0–100%), relative whole-cell capacitance that is proportional to the cell membrane area, and the resting membrane potential of the cells (RMP). **I.** Müller cells in slices of 3 days-postischemic retinas swell rapidly during exposure to a hypoosmotic extracellular solution (60% osmolarity) whereas cells in control retinas do not alter their size. Cells of both populations shrink in the presence of a hyperosmotic extracellular solution (140% osmolarity). The *insets* show Müller cell somata before, during, and after hypoosmotic exposure. GCL, ganglion cell layer; INL, inner nuclear layer; OLM, outer limiting membrane; ONL, outer nuclear layer; PRS, photoreceptor segments. Scale bars, 20 μm. Modified from Pannicke et al. (2004, 2005a) and Iandiev et al. (2006a,c), and unpublished results (I. Iandiev, Leipzig).

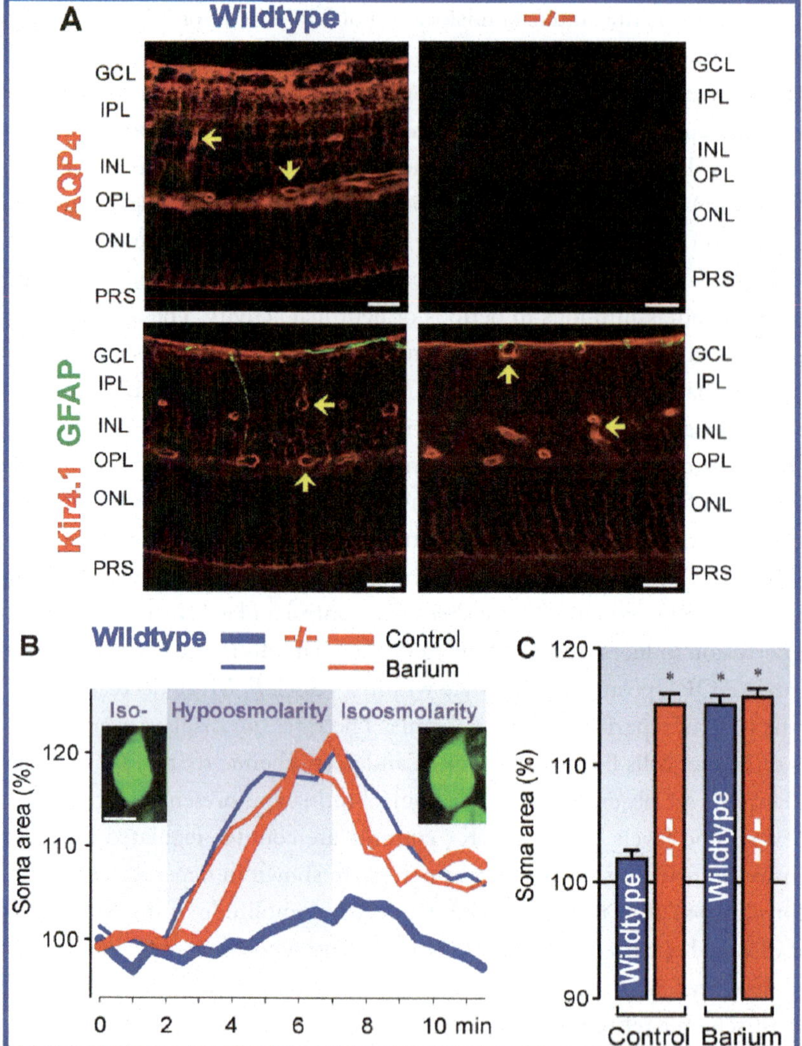

FIGURE 9: Deletion of AQP4 alters the osmotic swelling properties of Müller cells. **A.** Immunolabeling of retinal slices from wildtype and AQP4 null (−/−) mice against AQP4, Kir4.1, and glial fibrillary acidic protein (GFAP). The *arrows* point to perivascular staining. Note the absence of specific AQP4 immunolabeling in the slice from the AQP4 null animal. Bars, 20 μm. **B.** Osmotic swelling properties of Müller glial cells from wildtype and AQP4 null (−/−) mice. The *traces* show time-dependent alterations of the cross-sectional area of Müller cell somata in freshly isolated retinal slices. The slices were superfused with a hypoosmotic solution (60% of control osmolarity) in the absence (control) and presence of barium chloride (1 mM), respectively. Hypoosmotic challenge induced a swelling of Müller cell bodies

in retinal slices from AQP4 null animals but not in slices from wildtype animals. Müller cell bodies in slices from both wildtype and AQP4 null mice swelled in the presence of barium. The *insets* show an example of a Müller cell soma in a slice from an AQP4 null mouse recorded before (*left*) and during (*right*) superfusion with the hypoosmotic solution. Bar, 5 μm. **C.** Mean cross-sectional area of Müller cell somata measured after a 4-min superfusion with a hypoosmotic solution. Data are expressed in percent of the soma size recorded before hypoosmotic challenge (100%). *$P<0.001$. GCL, ganglion cell layer; INL, inner nuclear layer; IPL, innner plexiform layer; ONL, outer nuclear layer; OPL, outer plexiform layer; PRS, photoreceptor segments. Bars, 20 μm. Modified from Pannicke et al. (2010).

---

artery which enters the optic disc through the lamina cribrosa where it branches into four principal intraretinal arteries. (The lamina cribrosa is a sieve-like structure continuous with the sclera which distinguishes the extra- and intraocular portions of the optic nerve and through which the bundles of optic nerve axons pass.) The arteries bifurcate to form smaller arteriole branches and terminal arterioles which feed into a capillary bed as they extend toward the peripheral retina.

Intraretinal blood vessels, which supply cells of the inner and middle layers of the retina with oxygen and nutrients, are distributed in a trilaminar pattern (Michaelson, 1954; Schnitzer, 1988a). During the ontogenetic development, the vessels grow from the optic nerve head along the inner surface of the retina where they form the superficial (primary) vascular plexus; the principal (lobular) arteries are located at the nerve fibre layer/ganglion cell layer interface while the arteriole branches and capillaries are located deep in the ganglion cell layer (Figs. 13A-E, 17E). In the further course of development, two deeper vascular plexi are formed (Figs. 8D, 15B). In the rodent retina, the intermediate and deepest (outer) vascular plexi are localized at the inner and outer edges of the inner nuclear layer (Figs. 7G, 8C, 9A, 18B, 19). In the porcine retina, the intermediate and deepest vascular plexi are localized in the middle portions of the inner plexiform and inner nuclear layers (Figs. 1B, 7G, 10C, 11B, 12A, 20A). The superficial plexus contains arterioles, venules, and capillaries, while the deeper vascular plexi consist predominantly of capillaries. A third intraretinal plexus, reported in the cat and human retina and known as the radial peripapillary capillaries, is located in the nerve fiber layer in a small rim surrounding the optic nerve head (Chan-Ling et al., 1990; Hughes et al., 2000). The primate retina also contains avascular zones: the fovea and the peripheral margin of the retina (Stone and Dreher, 1987; Schnitzer, 1987, 1988d; Distler et al., 2000). The thinness of the fovea permits adequate oxygenation of the photoreceptors via the choroidal circulation (Ahmed et al., 1993).

Retinal capillaries are endowed with vascular endothelial cells and pericytes which are covered by a basement membrane, and are ensheathed by glial cell processes arising from astrocytes and Müller cells. Retinal arteries also contain smooth muscle cells (Pournaras et al., 2008). Astrocytes

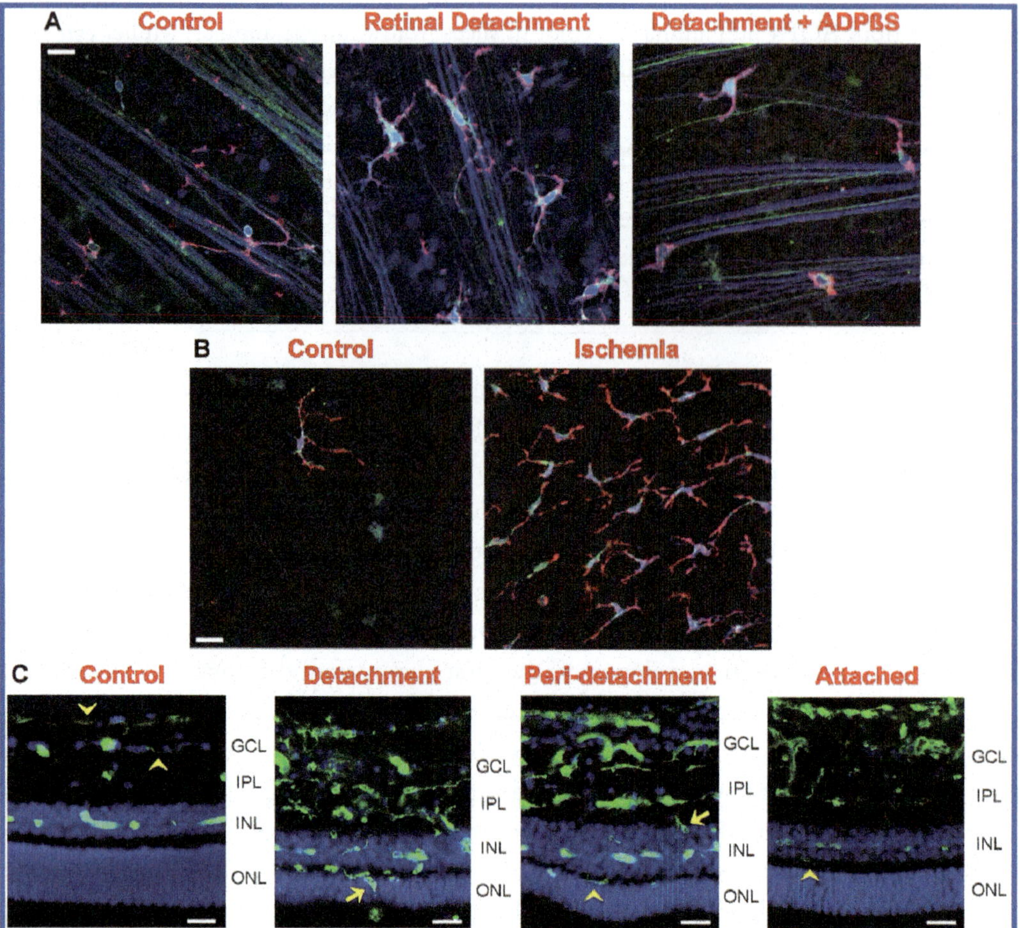

FIGURE 10: Retinal microglia activation. **A.** In the avascular regions of the rabbit retina (retinal areas outside the medullary rays), microglial cells are located in the innermost retinal layers. Acutely isolated wholemounts of a control retina (*left*) and a retina obtained 2 days after experimental retinal detachment (*middle*) are viewed at the vitreal surface (i.e., the nerve fiber/ganglion cell layers). Intravitreal application of ADPßS (2 mM), a non-hydrolyzable ADP analogue and an agonist of P2Y$_1$ receptors, accelerated the process retraction of microglial cells and induced a decreased density of microglial glial in the detached retina (*right*). Microglial cells are *red* stained; cell nuclei are *blue* stained. *Elongated structures* are light reflections on nerve fibers. **B.** Microglia cells at the vitreal surface of a control rabbit retina (*left*) and a retina obtained 8 days after a transient retinal ischemia of 1 h (*right*). **C.** Microglia migration in the porcine retina after local retinal detachment. The retinal slices were derived from an attached control retina, from a detached retina 7 days after surgery, and from peri-detached and attached retinal areas

that surrounded the detached retina. The slices were labeled with isolectin to stain blood vessels and microglial/immune cells (*green*). Cell nuclei are *blue* stained. The *arrows* and *arrowheads* mark microglial cell bodies and processes, respectively. Note the thinner outer nuclear layer (ONL) in the detached retina compared to the control retina, reflecting the degeneration of photoreceptor cells. GCL, ganglion cell layer; INL, inner nuclear layer; IPL, inner plexiform layer. Scale bars, 20 µm. Modified from Uhlmann et al. (2003), Uckermann et al., (2005a, d), and Iandiev et al. (2006b).

---

and Müller cells have contact to the vessels of the superficial plexus; the capillaries of the deeper vascular plexi are ensheathed by Müller cell processes (Uga and Ikui, 1974; Kondo et al., 1984). Whereas the astrocytes mainly form true endfeet at the vessels, the pericvascular Müller cell sheaths are called '*en passant* endfeet' because they arise from side branches of the stem processes (Holländer et al., 1991). The capillaries of the deepest vascular plexus are in contact to Müller and horizontal

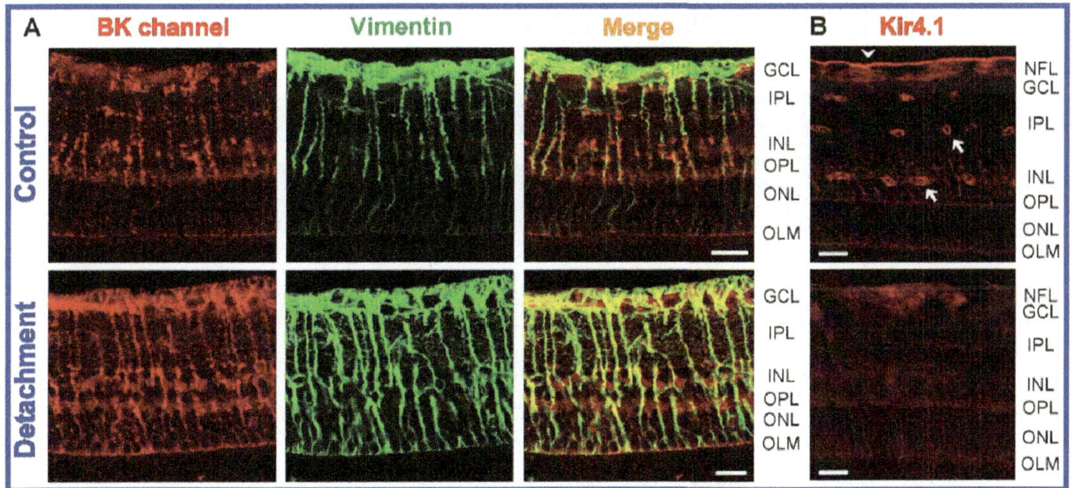

FIGURE 11: Porcine Müller cells express BK channel **(A)** and Kir4.1 proteins **(B)**. **A.** Slices of a a control retina (*above*) and a retina which was experimentally detached from the retinal pigment epithelium for 7 days (*below*) were immunostained for the α-subunit of BK channels (*red*) and vimentin (*green*). Co-localization of both proteins yields a *yellow* merge signal. Note the increase in BK channel immunoreactivity in the slice of the detached retina compared to control. **B.** Immunoreactivity for Kir4.1. The *arrowhead* indicates the inner limiting membrane; the *arrows* mark perivascular staining. Note the absence of the prominent Kir4.1 staining around the vessels and at the inner limiting membrane in the slice of the detached retina compared to control. GCL, ganglion cell layer; INL, inner nuclear layer; IPL, inner plexiform layer; NFL, nerve fiber layer; OLM, inner limiting membrane; ONL, outer nuclear layer; OPL, outer plexiform layer. Scale bars, 20 µm. Modified from Bringmann et al. (2007).

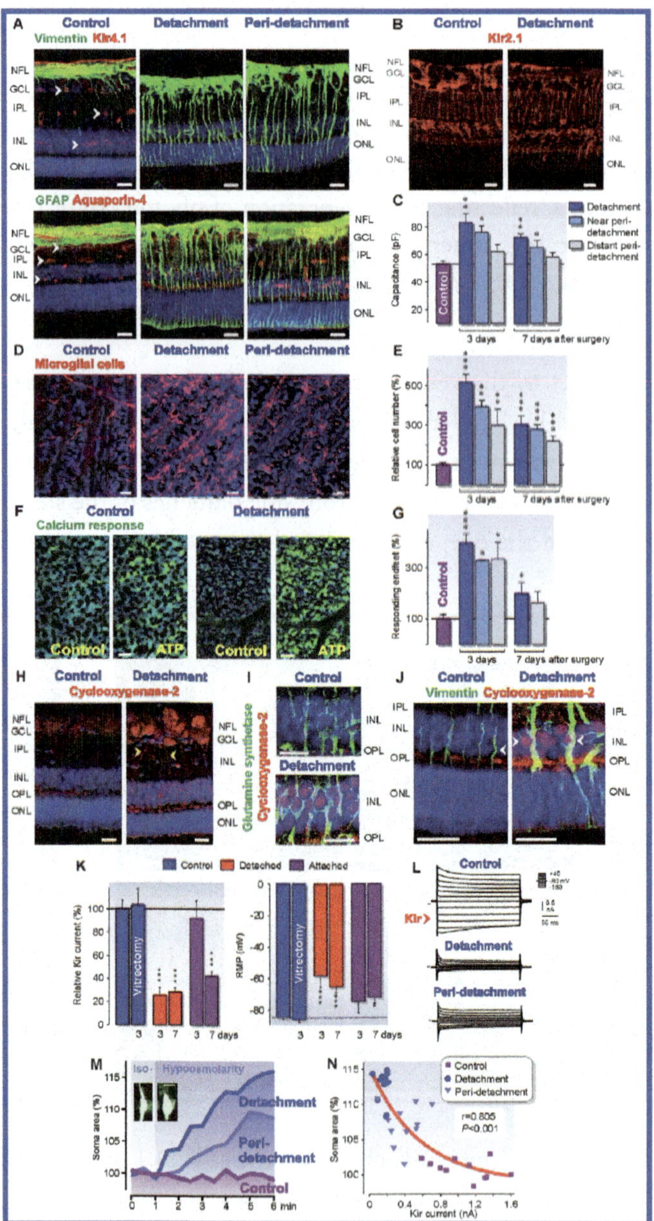

FIGURE 12: Gliosis in the porcine retina in response to local retinal detachment. **A.** Retinal slices were immunostained against vimentin and Kir4.1 protein (*above*), and GFAP and aquaporin-4 protein (*below*). Cell nuclei are *blue* stained. The slices were derived from a control retina, a retina which was detached for 7 days, and from a non-detached retinal tissue that was localized distant to the detached retina *in situ* (peri-detachment). Note the upregulation of the intermediate filaments in the detached and peri-detached tissues compared to the control retina, and the decrease in the Kir4.1 protein labeling. In contrast, aquaporin-4 labeling remained unaltered after detachment. *Arrowheads*, blood vessels.

B. The retinal distribution of Kir2.1 protein does not alter after detachment compared to control. **C.** Müller cell hypertrophy is indicated by the increase in the membrane capacitance of the cells which is proportional to the cell membrane area. Hypertrophy of Müller cells is also observed in the near and distant peri-detached retinal areas, suggesting a spread of Müller cell gliosis in a declining wave from the locally detached retina into the surrounding non-detached tissue. Müller cells of the porcine retina were investigated 3 and 7 days after local retinal detachment. **D.** Staining of microglial cells in the nerve fiber (NFL)/ganglion cell layers (GCL) in wholemounts of the porcine retina. The wholemounts were derived from a control retina, a retina which was detached for 3 days, and from a non-detached retinal tissue distant to the detached retina *in situ* (peri-detachment). **E.** Relative number of microglial cells at the vitreal surface of the porcine retina. **F.** Retinal detachment increases the calcium responsiveness upon P2Y receptor stimulation in the endfeet of Müller cells. The calcium imaging records were obtained from the NFL/GCL of retinal wholemounts before (*control*) and during administration of ATP (200 µM). The wholemounts were derived from a control retina and a 7 days-detached retina. In the control retina, single endfeet of Müller cells showed a calcium response (*green*) while in the detached retina, the majority of Müller cell endfeet displayed responses. **G.** Relative number of Müller cell endfeet that showed calcium responses upon administration of ATP (200 µM). **H.** Cyclooxygenase-2 protein in slices of a control retina and a 7 days-detached retina. The *arrowheads* point to Müller cell fibers that pass through the inner plexiform layer (IPL). **I.** Cyclooxygenase-2 and glutamine synthetase proteins in in the inner nuclear layer (INL) of a control retina and a 7 days-detached retina. Note that most cell somata in the INL express Cyclooxygenase-2 protein after retinal detachment. **J.** Vimentin and cyclooxygenase-2 proteins in slices of a control and a 7 days-detached retina. Vimentin-expressing Müller cell fibers are thicker in the detached retina compared to the control retina, reflecting a hypertrophy of Müller cells. The retinal staining of the inflammatory enzyme cyclooxygenase-2 increased after detachment, for example in the somata of Müller cells (*arrowheads*). **K.** Kir currents (*left*) and resting membrane potential (RMP; *right*) of Müller cells derived from control (un-operated and vitrectomized), 3 days-detached, 7 days-detached, and attached retinal areas. Note the time-dependent decrease of the Kir currents in the cells of the attached retinal area. **L.** Examples of whole-cell potassium currents of Müller cells isolated from a control retina, a retina which was detached for 7 days, and a peri-detached retinal area of an operated eye. **M.** Local retinal detachment causes an alteration in the osmotic swelling properties of Müller cells in the detached and peri-detached retinal areas. The cross-sectional area of Müller cell somata was measured in retinal slices. Acute exposure of retinal slices to a hypoosmolar solution (60% of normal osmolarity) induced a time-dependent swelling of Müller cell bodies in detached and peri-detached retinal areas, and had no effect on the size of Müller cell bodies in control retinas. The *images* display original records of a dye-filled Müller cell body in a slice of a detached retina, obtained before (*left*) and during (*right*) hypoosmotic exposure. **N.** Relation between the amplitude of the Kir currents and the severity of osmotic cell swelling in Müller cells derived from control, 7 days-detached, and peri-detached retinas. *$P<0.05$; **$P<0.01$, ***$P<0.001$, *vs.* control. ONL, outer nuclear layer; OPL, outer plexiform layer. Scale bars, 20 (**A, B, D, F, H-J**) and 5 µm (**M**). Modified from Iandiev et al. (2006b) and Wurm et al. (2006a).

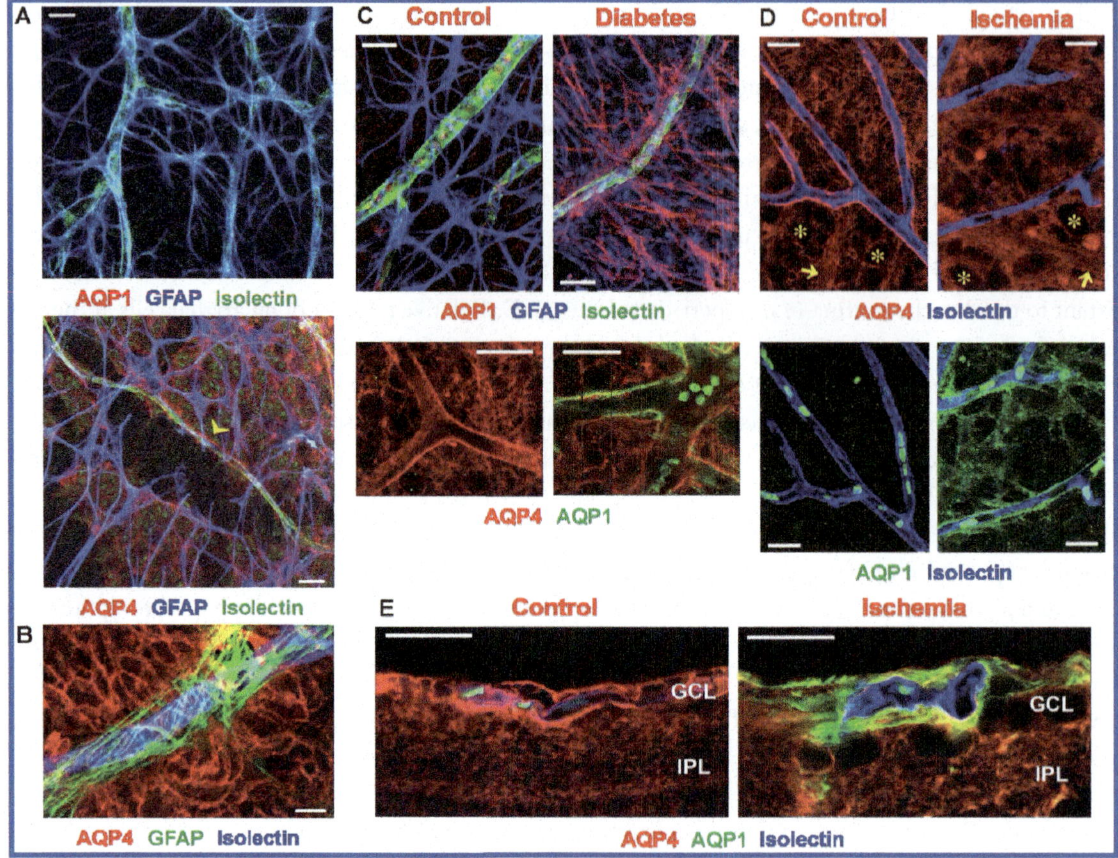

FIGURE 13: The type of glial aquaporins (AQPs) that surround the superficial vessels of the retina alters in diabetes (**C**) and after ischemia (**D, E**). **A.** Views onto the nerve fiber/ganglion cell layers of rat retinal wholemounts. Astrocytes were immunostained for GFAP (*blue*). The vessels are *green* labeled with isolectin. *Above:* In the normal rat retina, AQP1 (*red*) is not expressed in the nerve fiber/ganglion cell layers. *Below:* Müller cells express AQP4 (*red*) in their endfeet and in perivascular membranes (*arrowhead*). **B.** Views onto the ganglion cell layer of a porcine retinal wholemount. GFAP (*green*)-expressing astrocytes surround a large blood vessel (*blue*). Note the expression of AQP4 (*red*) in the lateral membranes of Müller cell endfeet. **C.** Views onto the nerve fiber/ganglion cell layers of retinal wholemounts derived from control and 6 months-diabetic rats. *Above:* Astrocytic processes are in contact with the blood vessels in the nerve fiber/ganglion cell layers. Astrocytes were immunostained for GFAP (*blue*). The wholemounts were also stained for AQP1 (*red*). The vessels are *green* labeled with isolectin. Note the co-localization of GFAP and AQP1 in the tissue from the diabetic animal, but not from the control animal. Red blood cells within the vessels also express AQP1. *Below:* The superficial vessels of the retina

are surrounded by AQP4 (*red*) in the control retina, and by both AQP4 and AQP1 (*green*) in the diabetic retina. In addition, red blood cells express AQP1. **D.** Views onto the nerve fiber/ganglion cell layers of retinal wholemounts derived from a control rat and a rat 7 days after a 1-h transient retinal ischemia. The superficial vessels of the retina are surrounded by AQP4 immunoreactivity (*red*) in the control retina, and by AQP1 immunoreactivity (*green*) in the postischemic retina. Blood vessels are labeled with isolectin (*blue*). In the control tissue, only red blood cells were labeled for AQP1. *, AQP4 labeling which encircles ganglion cell bodies. *Arrows*, AQP4 labeling around nerve fibers. **E.** Sections through the ganglion cell (GCL) and inner plexiform layers (IPL) of a control and a 14 days-postischemic rat retina. The vessels in the GCL are surrounded by AQP4 in the control tissue, and by AQP1 and AQP4 in the postischemic retina. Bars, 20 μm. Modified from Iandiev et al. (2006a, 2007a) and Wurm et al. (2011a).

---

cell processes; other cell types which have sparse contacts to retinal capillaries are microglial and amacrine cells (Knabe and Kuhn, 2000; Ochs et al., 2000). At branching sites of the vessels, pericytes are located between the vascular endothelial cells and the basement membrane. α-Smooth muscle actin-expressing pericytes are contractile cells and regulate the local blood flow (Pfister et al., 2013). Non-vascularized neural retinas/retinal areas receive oxygen and nutrients predominantly from the choroidea (across the pigment epithelium) and (to a much lower level) from the vitreous fluid. The retinal parenchyma is isolated from the blood by blood-retinal barriers. The inner blood retinal barrier is formed by tight junctions between the non-fenestrated vascular endothelial cells (Raviola, 1977; Morcos et al., 2001; Provis, 2001; Klaassen et al., 2013); this barrier is also characterized by a low level of vesicular transport across the vascular endothelium (Cunha-Vaz, 1979). The outer blood-retinal barrier is formed by tight junctions between the retinal pigment epithelial cells (the choroidal capillaries themselfes are fenestrated and thus 'leaky') (Morcos et al., 2001; Strauss, 2005). Because astrocytes and Müller cells encapsulate virtually all neuronal somata, dendrites, and axons in the retina, many molecules supplied from the blood reach retinal neurons (with the exception of photoreceptor segments that extend into the subretinal space) when they are transported into glial cells and then rereleased either in their original molecular form or after metabolism.

2.2 DEVELOPMENT OF RETINAL VASCULATURE

In humans, the innermost plexus arises the retina at gestational age, while the deeper vascular plexi are formed at around 24 weeks of gestation and continue developing after birth (Gariano et al., 1994). In the rat, retinal vessels are first distributed in the nerve fiber layer from postnatal day 3; afterward, the vascular branches sprout and penetrate deeply into the retina (Lee et al., 2012a). In the

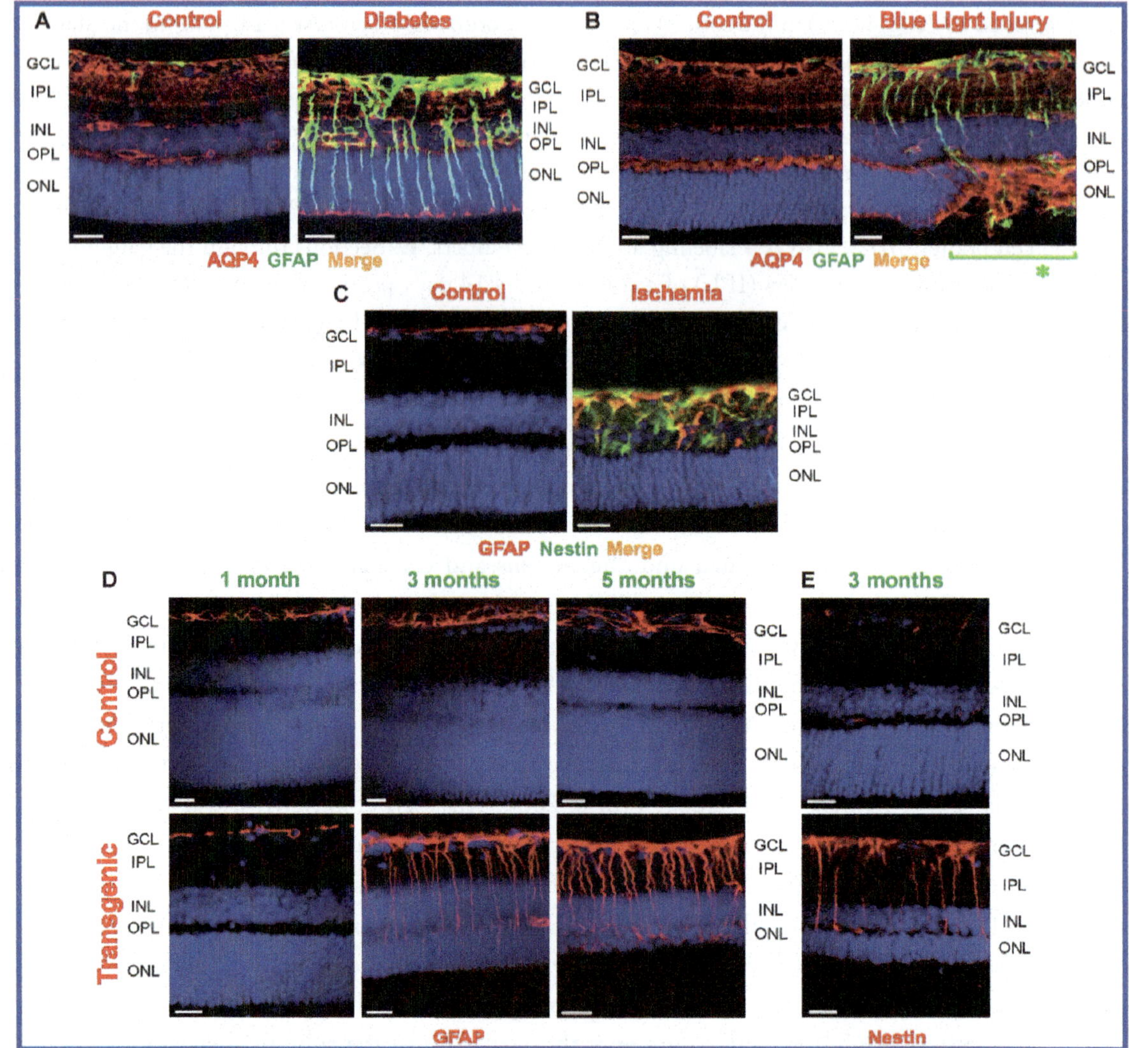

FIGURE 14: Upregulation of intermediate filaments such as glial fibrillary acidic protein (GFAP) and nestin is a characteristic event of Müller cell gliosis under pathological conditions. **A.** Retinal slices of a 6 months-diabetic (*right*) and an age-matched control rat (*left*) were immunostained against GFAP (*green*) and the glial water channel, aquaporin-4 (AQP4; *red*). Cell nuclei are *blue* stained. In the control retina, only astrocytes at the inner margin of the retina contained GFAP. In the retina of the diabetic animal, hypertrophied Müller cell fibers which traverse the whole retinal tissue display strong labeling for GFAP. **B.** Retinal slices of a rat were stained 3 days after treatment of a circumscribed area of the retina with excessive blue light which resulted in apoptotic death of photoreceptor cells. The light-injured retinal area

is shown *right* (*), the uninjured area is shown *left*. The strong upregulation of AQP4 in Müller cell processes within the outer nuclear layer (ONL) is likely a response to the outer retinal edema which develops due to the light-induced injury of the retinal pigment epithelium (resulting in increased permeability of the outer blood-retinal barrier) and the volume decrease of apoptotic cells which is mediated by an efflux of osmolytes (especially potassium and chloride ions) and water. **C.** Retinal slices of a rat were stained 7 days after a 1-h transient retinal ischemia against GFAP and nestin. Co-labeling yielded a *yellow-orange* merge signal. **D, E.** Age-dependent upregulation of GFAP (**D**) and nestin (**E**) in a transgenic rat model of slow primary photoreceptor degeneration due to the expression of a mutant polycystin-2 gene. The retinal degeneration in the transgenic rats is characterized by initial photoreceptor degeneration and glial activation, followed by vasoregression and neuronal degeneration (Feng et al., 2009). Retinal slices were derived from 1 month, 3 months, and 5 months old control (*above*) and transgenic rats (*below*). GCL, ganglion cell layer; INL, inner nuclear layer; IPL, inner plexiform layer; OPL, outer plexiform layer. Bars, 20 µm. Modified from Iandiev et al. (2007a, 2008a), Vogler et al. (2013b), and unpublished results (I. Iandiev, Leipzig).

---

mouse, the superficial vasculature develops during the first postnatal week; between postnatal days 7 and 10, these superficial retinal vessels dive into the retina to form the deeper vascular plexi (Dorrell et al., 2002). The deepest vascular plexus is complete by postnatal day 14 while the intermediate plexus is complete by postnatal day 21 (Dorrell et al., 2002). During retinal vascular development, nutrients are supplied by hyaloid vessels which arise from the optic nerve head, extend through the vitreous, and surround the developing lens. In the growing eye, the development of the retinal vasculature coincides with the macrophage-mediated regression of the hyaloid vasculature (Latker and Kuwabara, 1981; Lang and Bishop, 1993; Lang et al., 1994; Zhu et al., 2000; Hose et al., 2005). The hyaloid vascular system is regressed before birth in humans and during the first three postnatal weeks in rodents (Ito and Yoshioka, 1999).

Retinal vessels in rodents are formed by angiogenesis, i.e., budding from preexisting vessels, while in dogs and man, the vessels are also formed by vasculogenesis via assembly of dispersed vascular endothelial precursor cells (angioblasts) that spread across the retina (Ashton, 1970; Flower et al., 1985; McLeod et al., 1987a, 2006; Chan-Ling, 1997; Dorrell et al., 2002; Fruttiger, 2002; Stahl et al., 2010). The superficial vessels of the central one-third of the human retina are formed by vasculogenesis while the remaining vessels including the deeper vascular plexi are formed by angiogenesis (Hughes et al., 2000; Kur et al., 2012). Thus, the outer two-thirds of the retina, the entire deep vascular plexi, and the increasing capillary density in the central one-third of the human retina are

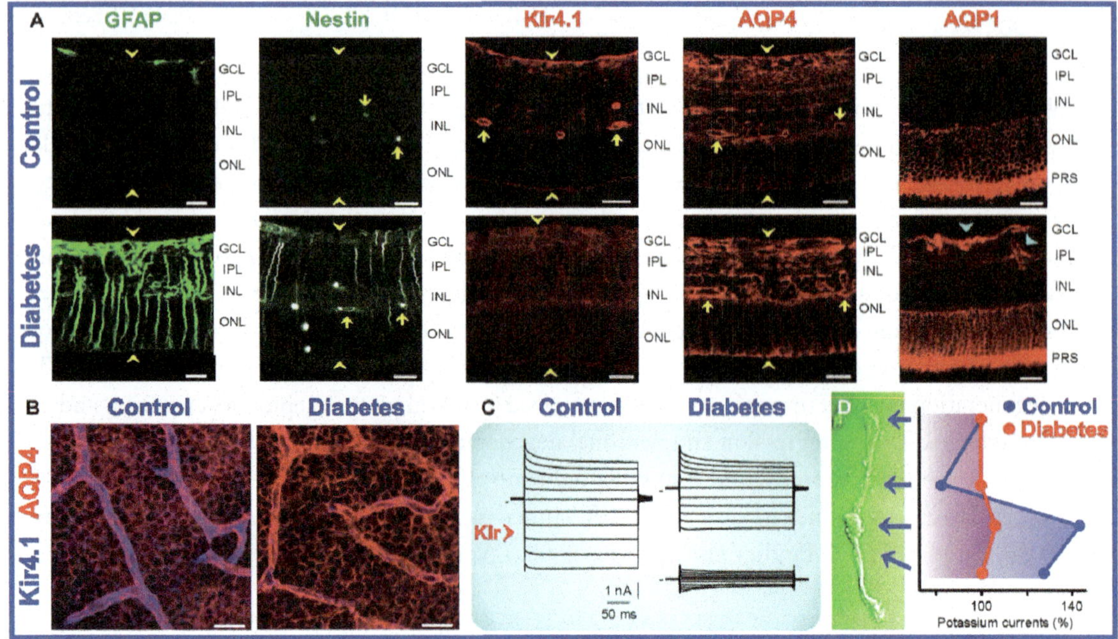

FIGURE 15: Müller cell gliosis in experimental diabetes. Retinal slices and Müller cells from 6 months-diabetic rats and age-matched control rats were investigated. **A.** Immunostaining of retinal slices from control (*above*) and diabetic animals (*below*). Müller cell gliosis is indicated by the upregulation of the intermediate filaments GFAP and nestin. In control tissues, GFAP is largely restricted to the astrocytes in the ganglion cell layer (GCL), and nestin is localized solely to blood cells within the vessels (*arrows*). In the diabetic retina, nestin is also expressed by Müller cell fibers that traverse the inner retina, and by blood-derived leukocytes infiltrated in the outer nuclear layer (ONL). In control retinas, the Kir4.1 protein displays a prominent localization around the blood vessels (arrows) and at both limiting membranes of the retina (*yellow arrowheads*). In retinas of diabetic animals, the Kir4.1 protein is redistributed from these prominent expression sites and is localized diffusely to Müller cells. In contrast, the distribution of the glial water channel protein AQP4 remains largely unaltered in the course of diabetes. In tissues of control and diabetic animals, AQP1 is expressed by photoreceptor cells. In the course of diabetes, glial cells in the GCL and inner plexiform layer (IPL) also express AQP1 protein (*blue arrowheads*). **B.** AQP4 (*red*) and Kir4.1 (*blue*) in retinal wholemounts. The images were obtained at the plane of the blood vessels within the inner nuclear layer (INL). In the control retina, both AQP4 and Kir4.1 are localized to Müller cell membranes that surround vessels. In the diabetic retina, perivascular Kir4.1 is downregulated. **C.** Examples of whole-cell potassium currents of Müller cells. Müller cells from diabetic animals display a reduction in the potassium conductance when compared to control, with a substantial variation in the current amplitude in different cells. **D.** Subcellular distribution of the potassium conductance in Müller cells. Cells of control animals display their largest conductance in the middle portion of their cell bodies whereas cells from diabetic animals display a uniform distribution of their potassium conductance across the whole plasma membrane. PRS, photoreceptor segments. Scale bars, 20 µm. Modified Pannicke et al. (2006) and Iandiev et al. (2007a).

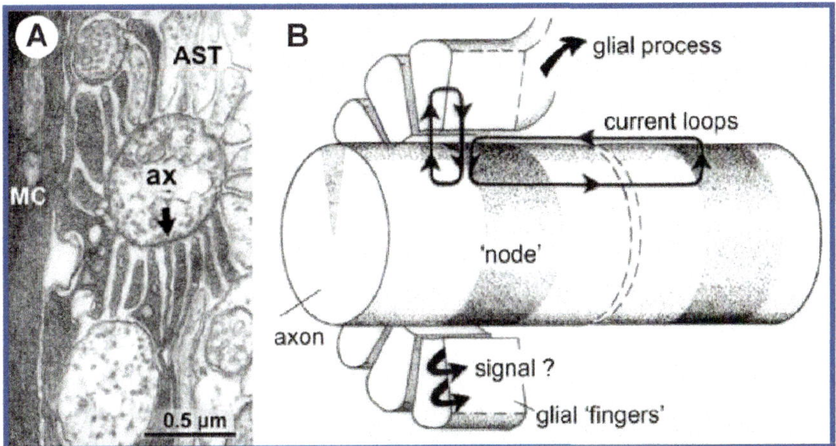

FIGURE 16: Periaxonal processes extending from Müller cells and astrocytes. **A.** Transmission electron microphotograph of a part of the nerve fiber layer of a cat retina. The axons of the retinal ganglion cells (ax) display local "node-like" specializations (*arrow*) probably representing sites of high sodium channel density, for saltatory action potential propagation. Both the astrocyte (AST) and the Müller cell (MC) extend fine, finger-like processes towards this axolemmal area; together they form a corona of such fine processes. **B.** Semi-schematic view of such a corona of finger-like Müller cell processes at the "node" of a ganglion cell axon, together with the proposed flux of transmembraneous ion currents. Modified from Holländer et al. (1991) and Chao et al. (1994b).

formed by angiogenesis (Hughes et al., 2000; Kur et al., 2012). Retinal angioblasts are in advance of the forming vasculature (Hasegawa et al., 2008). Endothelial cell development concomitant with pericyte differentiation is the primary process of vessel formation (Hughes and Chan-Ling, 2004; Kur et al., 2012). Subsequent events consist of vessel guidance, branching, and recruitment of vascular-associated cells, including astrocytes and microglial precursors (Kur et al., 2012).

Both astrocytes and microglial cells play crucial roles in the retinal vascularization (Stone et al., 1995a; Provis, 2001; Checchin et al., 2006). "Physiological hypoxia" is suggested to be an essential stimulus for the ingrowth of blood vessels into the retina (Chan-Ling et al., 1990, 1995; Zhang et al., 1999). Intraretinal blood vessels develop relatively late, around the birth in many mammals. In the embryonic retina, all immature cells have a glycolytic metabolism which is sufficiently supported by the glucose delivery from the choroid. However, because active neurons consume vast amounts of oxygen and nutrients (Cringle et al., 2006), the energy demands of retinal neurons increase

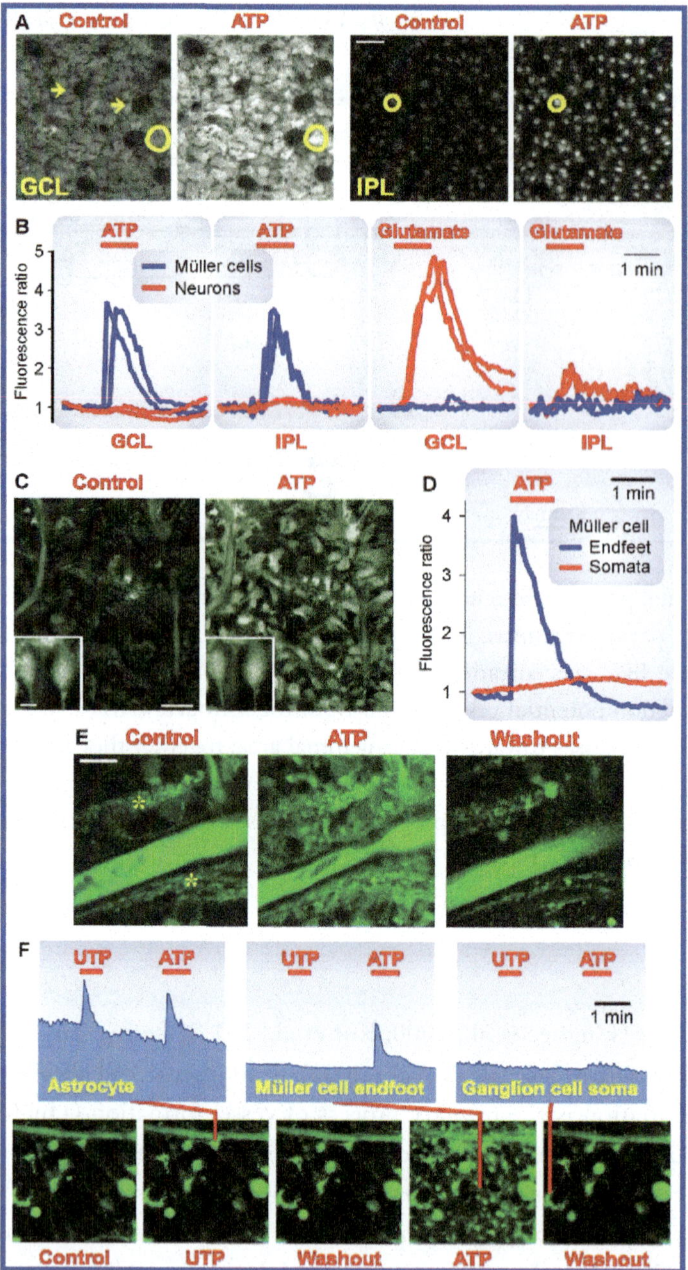

FIGURE 17: Glutamate- and ATP-induced intracellular calcium responses in tissue preparations of the rat and guinea-pig retina. **A, B.** In the guinea-pig retina, ATP evokes intracellular calcium responses in Müller cells while glutamate induces calcium responses in neurons. **A.** Views onto the ganglion cell layer (GCL) (*left*) and inner plexiform layer (IPL) (*right*). The images were recorded before (*control*) and at the peak calcium responses upon application of ATP (200 µM). Examples of Müller cell endfeet (in the

GCL) and profiles (in the IPL) are encircled. *Arrows*, ganglion cell bodies. Note that almost all Müller cells respond to exogenous ATP with an intracellular calcium rise. **B.** Time-dependent calcium responses in Müller cell and neuronal cell structures. Upon administration of ATP, Müller cell endfeet in the GCL and Müller cell profiles in the IPL respond with a transient calcium rise (*grey traces*) whereas neuronal cell bodies and synaptic structures in the IPL are non-responsive (*black traces*). Upon administration of glutamate (1 mM), neuronal cell bodies and synaptic structures display calcium responses (*black traces*) whereas Müller cell endfeet and profiles are non-responsive (*grey traces*). A fluorescence ratio of one means no change in the cytosolic calcium level. **C, D.** ATP (200 μM) evokes calcium responses in the endfeet but not in the somata of Müller cells in tissue preparations of the rat retina. **C.** View onto the nerve fiber/ganglion cell layers of a retinal wholemount and (*insets*) onto Müller cell somata within the inner nuclear layer of a retinal slice. The *elongated structures* are blood vessels. The images were taken before (*control*) and during the peak calcium response. **D.** Mean calcium responses in rat Müller cell endfeet and somata. **E.** Peak calcium response in Müller cell endfeet on the vitreal surface of a rat retina induced by ATP (500 μM). Note the constriction of the arteriole in response to ATP. The Müller cell endfeet fill the spaces between the arteriole and nerve fiber bundles (*). **F.** Calcium responses induced by UTP and ATP (both 250 μM) in the ganglion cell layer of a freshly isolated wholemount of the rat retina. The traces *above* show calcium responses recorded in an astrocyte, a Müller cell endfoot, and a ganglion cell soma. Scale bars, 20 and 5 (*insets*) μm. Modified from Uckermann et al. (2004b, 2006) and Wurm et al. (2011b).

---

dramatically in the course of neuronal differentiation. One way to satisfy these demands is to 'switch' to the more efficient oxidative metabolism. At this time, the choroidal oxygen supply is insufficient to support an oxidative metabolism of the differentiating postnatal neurons. Thus, the cells are enforced to maintain the inefficient glycolytic metabolism with a very high rate of glucose consumption. The resulting glucose deficiency in association with hypoxia was suggested to stimulate immigrating astrocyte precursors to secrete vascular endothelial growth factor (VEGF)-A (Pierce et al., 1995; Stone et al., 1995a, 1996; Provis et al., 1997; Yi et al., 1998; Zhang et al., 1999; Provis, 2001; Stalmans et al., 2002). Further factors such as nerve growth factor (NGF) also induce VEGF in astrocytes (Kim et al., 2013). VEGF derived from the network of spindle-shaped astrocyte precursors that precedes the vascular front was suggested to induce retinal vascularization by acting at VEGF receptor-2 expressed by angioblasts (Yamaguchi et al., 1993; Millauer et al., 1993). Activation of VEGF receptor-2 promotes the proliferation, migration, differentiation, and survival of vascular endothelial cells and is thus implicated in both the vasculogeneic and angiogenic mechanisms of vascular development (Alon et al., 1995; Stone and Maslim, 1997; Provis et al., 1997; Neufeld et al., 1999; Provis, 2001; Gerhardt et al., 2003; Uemura et al., 2006). When newborn animals (or

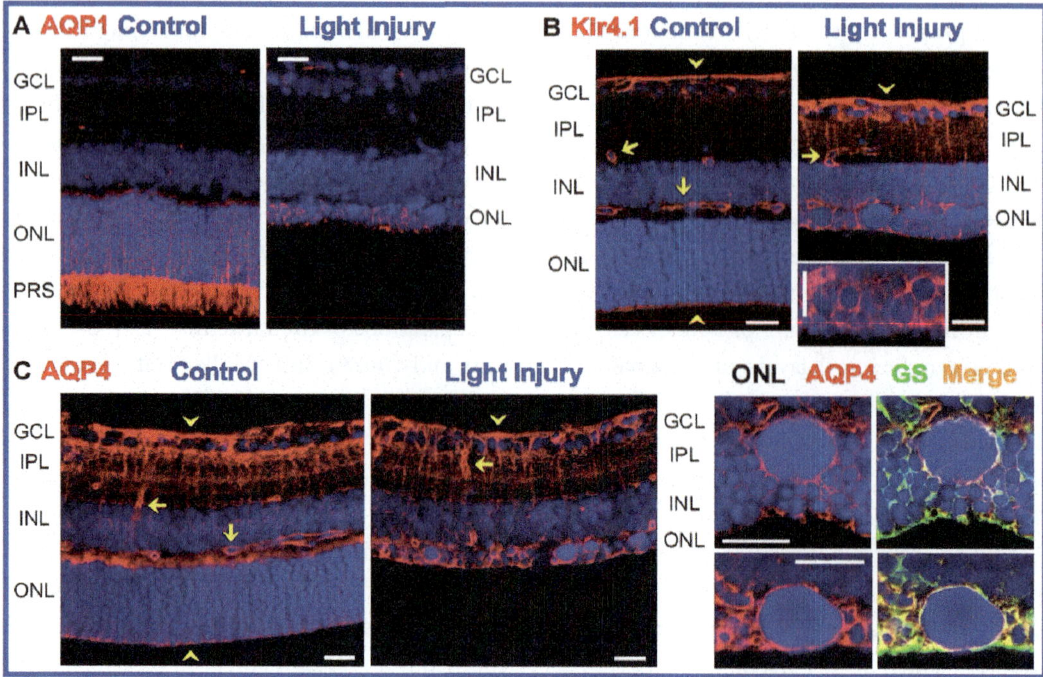

FIGURE 18: Müller cell reactivity in a mouse model of retinal bright white light damage. Retinal slices were immunostained 10 days after exposure of one eye of an animal to white light (15,000 lux; 2 h). Cell nuclei are *blue* stained. **A.** Aquaporin-1 (AQP1) protein is predominantly expressed in the outer retina by the photoreceptor cells and segments. In the inner retina, AQP1 is present in erythrocytes within the vessels. The light-induced degeneration of photoreceptors is reflected by the decrease of the AQP1 staining. **B.** Staining of Kir4.1 protein. The *arrows* point to perivascular labeling, and the *arrowheads* indicate the inner and outer limiting membranes of the retina. The *inset* displays the outer nuclear layer (ONL) at higher magnification. Note the presence of the strong Kir4.1 staining around the remaining photoreceptor nuclei. **C.** Distribution of AQP4 protein. The *right side* displays staining of the ONL against AQP4 and co-staining of AQP4 and the glial cell marker glutamine synthetase (GS) in the outer retina. The *yellow* merge signal indicates that Müller cells express AQP4 around the degnerating photoreceptor cells. Note the presence of large spherical bodies in the ONL of the degenerating retinas that are *blue* stained and thus represent photoreceptor nuclei which are fused together. INL, inner nuclear layer; IPL, inner plexiform layer. PRS, photoreceptor segments. Bars, 20 μm. Modified from Iandiev et al. (2008b).

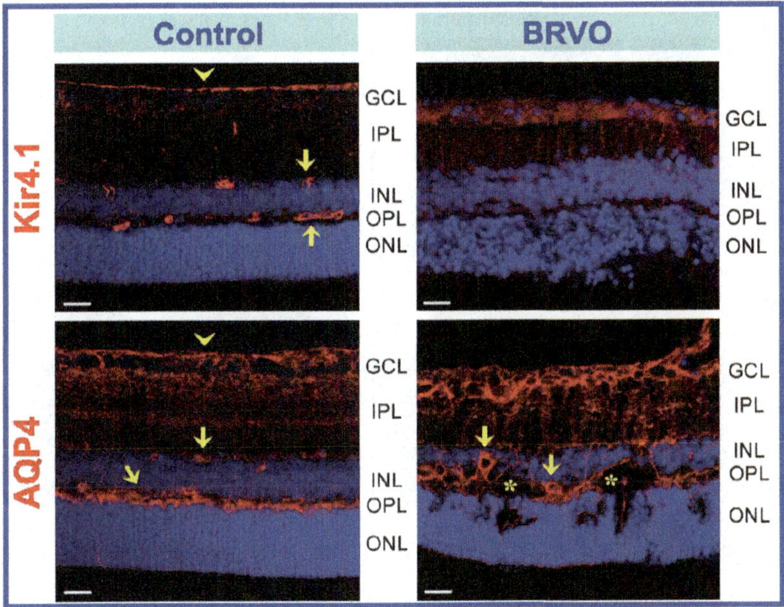

FIGURE 19: Müller cell reactivity in experimental branch retinal vein occlusion (BRVO) is associated with a cystoid degeneration of the outer plexiform layer (OPL) and the outer nuclear layer (ONL). Slices of a control rat retina (*left*) and a retina obtained 3 days after laser photocoagulation of branch retinal veins (*right*) were immunostained against Kir4.1 (*above*) and AQP4 (*below*). In the control tissue, Kir4.1 protein is enriched at the inner limiting membrane (*arrowhead*) and around the blood vessels (*arrows*). This prominent localization is lost within 3 days of BRVO. The localization of AQP4 remained unaltered within 3 days of BRVO, with the exception of the sites of cystoid degeneration (*asterisks*). Cell nuclei are *blue* stained. GCL, ganglion cell layer; INL, inner nuclear layer; IPL, inner plexiform layer. Bars, 20 μm. Modified from Rehak et al. (2009).

premature infants) are exposed to hyperoxia, retinal astrocytes stop the production of VEGF (but not their proliferation and migration) which results in a decreased proliferation of endothelial cells and even death of the newly formed blood vessels (Chan-Ling and Stone, 1991b; Alon et al., 1995; Chan-Ling, 1997). When the animals return to normal air, which has much less oxygen, astrocytes produce large amounts of VEGF (Alon et al., 1995). The sudden increase of the VEGF level stimulates the growth of new blood vessels which are abnormally weak and leaky (because VEGF also induces vascular permeability; see 5.11.9.1.); the overstimulation of the vessel growth results in a

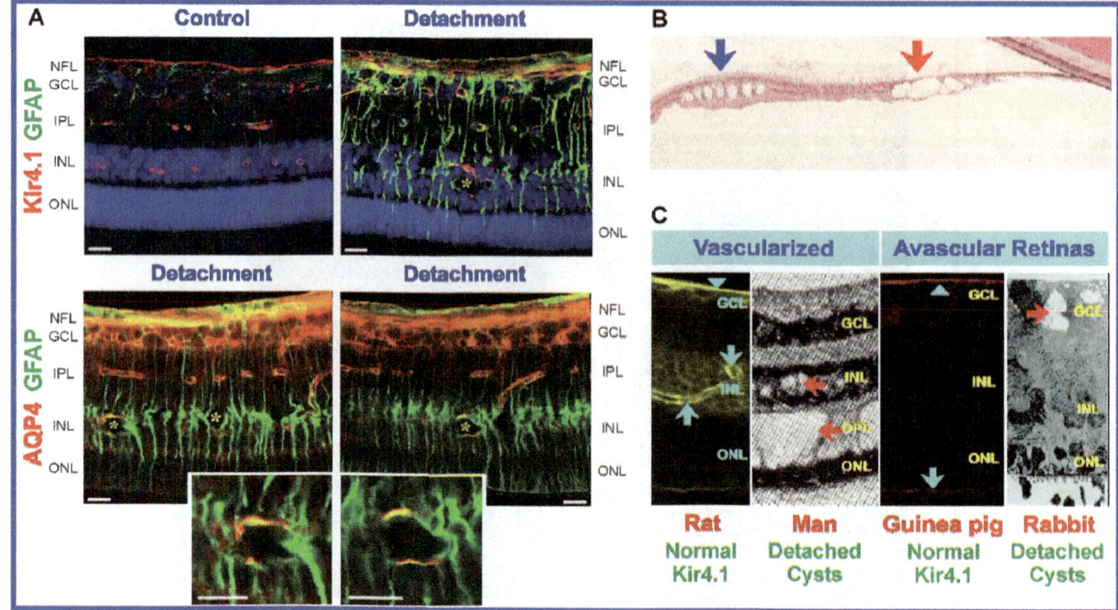

FIGURE 20: Müller cell reactivity after retinal detachment is frequently associated with a cystoid degeneration of the retina. **A.** Slices of a control porcine retina and a retina obtained after 7 days of experimental retinal detachment were immunostained against Kir4.1 (*above*) and AQP4 (*below*), and were co-stained against GFAP (*green*). Cell nuclei are *blue*. Edematous cysts (*) in the inner nuclear layer (INL) are localized beside or near the blood vessels. The *small images below* show the INL at higher magnification. **B.** Cystoid degeneration of a detached human retina (*blue arrow*). The cysts in the proximity of the ora serrata (*red arrow*) reflect physiological senile cystoid degeneration (Fischer et al., 2001). **C.** The subcellular distribution of Kir4.1 correlates with the distribution of edematous cysts in detached retinas. In vascularized retinas, the Kir4.1 protein is predominantly expressed in Müller cell membranes which abut the vitreous body (*arrowhead*) and which surround the retinal vessels (*arrows*), beside a small expression at the outer limiting membrane. In non-vascularized retinas, the Kir4.1 protein is mainly expressed at the inner limiting membrane (*arrowhead*), beside a smaller expression at the outer limiting membrane (*arrow*). The downregulation of functional Kir4.1 channels by Müller cells after detachment impairs the resolution of osmotic gradients between extra-retinal spaces and the retinal tissue at sites where Müller cells predominantly extrude potassium (i.e., in vascularized retinas into the retinal vessels, in non-vascularized retinas into the vitreous). Accumulation of potassium within Müller cells results in a higher osmotic pressure at these sites which may cause a water influx from the blood into the INL in the case of vascularized retinas (which may underlie cyst formation within the INL and outer plexiform layer, OPL) and a water influx from the vitreous in the case of non-vascularized retinas which may cause cyst formation in the ganglion cell layer (GCL). IPL, inner plexiform layer; NFL, nerve fiber layer; ONL, outer nuclear layer. Bars, 20 μm. Modified from Arruga (1936) and Francke et al. (2005), and unpublished results (I. Iandiev, Leipzig).

disruption of the retinal architecture and a loss of vision (retinopathy of prematurity) (Alon et al., 1995; Stone et al., 1996).

The developing superficial retinal vessels follow the network of retinal astrocytes (Cogan and Kuwabara, 1986; Jiang et al., 1995). After the superficial vascular network has spread across the entire retina, the vessels start to sprout downward, towards the inner plexiform and nuclear layers, where they establish the deeper vascular plexi (Engerman and Meyer, 1965; Connolly et al., 1988; Stone et al., 1995a). The vessels that branch from the superficial vascular layer to form the deeper plexi are not accompanied by astrocytes (Provis, 2001). Instead, VEGF-expressing Müller cells (and possibly amacrine and horizonzal cells) may direct the developing vessels to form the deeper capillary plexi (Stone and Maslim, 1997; Yi et al., 1998; Sandercoe et al., 2003).

In the developing human retina, neither retinal vessels nor their accompanying astrocytes grow into the incipient avascular fovea (Provis et al., 2000; Provis, 2001). In the macaque retina, the incipient fovea is transiently occupied by astrocytes which then disappear during the first postnatal weeks at least in part through apoptosis (Distler and Kopatz, 1996; Distler and Kirby, 1996; Distler et al., 2000; Gariano et al., 1996). It has been suggested that the formation of the fovea occurs as a result of the lack of intraretinal blood supply in this region (Provis, 2001). The antiangiogenic factors which inhibit the growth of retinal vessels towards the incipient fovea remain to be determined.

VEGF induces the directed extension of filopodia in endothelial tip cells (Fruttiger, 2002; Gerhardt et al., 2003). The delta-like ligand (DLL)-Notch1 signaling pathway, a downstream event of VEGF signaling, regulates the tip cell activity and thus ensures the proper vascular patterning in the retina (Hellström et al., 2007; Lobov et al., 2007; Suchting et al., 2007). Hypoxia upregulates the hypoxia-inducible factor (HIF)-1α that regulates the transcription of hypoxia-responsive genes including VEGF. Deletion of HIF-1α results in impaired vascular development characterized by decreased tip cell filopodia and reduced vessel branching (Nakamura-Ishizu et al., 2012). Removal of the VEGF gradient in the retina by VEGF-sequestering antibodies or increased expression of VEGF in transgenic mice inhibits the endothelial cell migration and delays the formation of the superficial vascular plexus (Gerhardt et al., 2003; Uemura et al., 2006; Mitchell et al., 2006). In the developing mouse retina, astrocytes transiently express fibronectin (Stenzel et al., 2011). VEGF binding to astrocytic fibronectin and heparan sulfate promotes the directional endothelial tip cell migration, while integrin binding to astrocytic fibronectin supports the filopodia adhesion to the astrocytic migration template (Stenzel et al., 2011). The blood flow in the developing vessel network delivers oxygen to the migrating astrocytes, causing them to progressively downregulate VEGF expression (West et al., 2005; Uemura et al., 2006). However, although hypoxia-driven VEGF is assumed essential for retinal vascular development (Gerhardt et al., 2003; West et al., 2005), mice in which the hypoxia response element is deleted from the VEGF promoter show slightly delayed but otherwise normal phenotypes in their retinal vascular development (Vinores et al., 2006). Furthermore, specific ablation of VEGF in astrocytes does not prevent vessel formation (Weidemann et al., 2010; Scott et al., 2010), suggesting that other cell types (such as retinal ganglion cells, Müller cells, and pericytes; Darland et al., 2003) and proteins are also involved in this process. Müller cell-derived VEGF contributes to the pathological but not to the physiological development of superficial retinal vessels (Bai et al., 2009).

The first stage of retinal vascular development is suggested to be the formation of a template by astrocytes that migrate ahead of the developing vasculature; the astrocytic template provides guidance for the growing vessels (Kopatz and Distler, 2000; Dorrell et al., 2002; Fruttiger, 2002; Gariano, 2003). Astrocytes are present in two separate layers in the developing human retina—the optic axon layer, and the developing vessel layer (Provis et al., 1997)—whereas in the rabbit and mouse retinas they are situated in the nerve fiber layer (Schnitzer, 1988c; Zhuo et al., 1997). At the leading edge of vascular sprouts, endothelial tip cells extend numerous long filopodia along the preexisting astrocyte template but not along the neural filaments (Kubota and Suda, 2009). In the mouse, astrocytes enter the retina from the optic disc beginning around embryonic day 15 (Dorrell et al., 2002). The migration of spindle-shaped immature astrocytes from the optic nerve to the retinal periphery via the axons of retinal ganglion cells in association with the inner limiting membrane (Gariano et al., 1996; Gnanaguru et al., 2013; Chan-Ling and Stone, 1991b) is followed by or associated with the formation of the primary (superficial) vascular network by endothelial cells which begins around postnatal day 1 in the mouse (Dorrell et al., 2002). The directed movement of endothelial cells begins 4 to 5 days prior to the emergence of the first angiogenic sprouts (Fruttiger, 2002; Gariano, 2003). Astrocytes express a variety of chemotactic and haptotactic proteins that subsequently induce endothelial cell sprouting and modulate the growth of the superficial vascular plexus. However, the precise role of astrocytes in the vessel guidance is still unclear.

During the development of the superficial vascular layer, large numbers of proliferating GFAP-negative astrocyte precursor cells or (in dependence on the species investigated) GFAP-expressing immature astrocytes are in advance of the vascular front by up to 100–200 µm; non-proliferating GFAP-expressing immature astrocytes are in association with the developing vessels (McLeod et al., 1987a, 2006; Chan-Ling and Stone, 1991b; Provis et al., 1997; Sandercoe et al., 1999; Provis, 2001; Fruttiger, 2002; Dorrell et al., 2002; Chan-Ling et al., 2004, 2009; Hasegawa et al. 2008). Apparently, GFAP-negative astrocyte precursor cells differentiate into GFAP-expressing immature astrocytes in the presence of invading endothelial cells (Provis, 2001). In addition to proliferating astrocyte precursor cells, a population of non-proliferating microglial cells precedes the growing blood vessels (Sanyal and De Ruiter, 1985; Diaz-Araya et al., 1995a; Provis et al., 1997;

Sandercoe et al., 1999; Provis, 2001). Migrating microglial cells are present near the endothelial tip cells and precede the microvessels in the neuroblast layer during vascular sprouting and extension, suggesting that vasculogenesis also occurs along microglia migrating routes (Lee et al., 2012a). The endothelial tip cells control adjacent endothelial cells in a hierarchical manner to form the stalk of the sprouting vessel, by using, for example, the VEGF-DLL-Notch signaling pathway, and recruit pericytes (Siemerink et al., 2013). Vascular areas which are devoid of VEGF, e.g., along the developing retinal arteries and around the optic nerve head, develop to capillary-free zones of the retina (Claxton and Fruttiger, 2003). Microglia induce vessel sprouting in the developing retina by the release of angiogenic factors distinct from VEGF-A, likely platelet-derived growth factor (PDGF) (Forsberg-Nilsson et al., 2003; Rymo et al., 2011). Retinal glial cells also stimulate the proliferation of pericytes, via the release of growth factors such as acidic fibroblast growth factor, basic fibroblast growth factor (bFGF), and PDGF (Ikuno et al., 2002a). Once becoming overlaid with vascular endothelial cells, the proangiogenic activity of retinal astrocytes ceases and they (in addition to pericytes) inhibit endothelial cell proliferation, maintain vascular stability, among others by the release of VEGF (Jiang et al., 1994; West et al., 2005; Kubota et al., 2008; Scott et al., 2010), and mediate the vascular remodeling process required to form capillary-like structures by basement membrane formation (Laterra et al., 1990; Laterra and Goldstein, 1991; Sinha et al., 2008). In the rat retina, the glial investment of retinal blood vessels becomes complete by the 18th postnatal day (Kondo et al., 1984).

In addition to astrocytes and microglia, Müller glial, retinal ganglion, and vascular endothelial cells, as well as components of the extracellular matrix and the internal limiting membrane, regulate the retinal vascularization by the release of soluble factors (Fruttiger, 2007). Retinal ganglion cells differentiate before the blood vessel formation. Succinate as intermediate of the Krebs cycle accumulates in the hypoxic developing retina of rodents; succinate activates the cognate receptor G protein-coupled receptor-91 (GPR91) in retinal ganglion cells which then regulate the production of numerous angiogenic factors including VEGF in a HIF-1-independent manner (Sapieha et al., 2008). bFGF released from retinal ganglion cell axons stimulates the proliferation of astrocytes in the optic nerve (Burne and Raff, 1997) while PDGF-A released from retinal ganglion cells stimulates the proliferation of astrocytes in the retinal parenchyma (Fruttiger et al., 1996, 2000; Yamada et al., 2000). This suggests that retinal ganglion cells control the development of astrocytes in the retina and the optic nerve by different mechanisms. The migration of astrocytes in the developing murine retina is directed by a chemotactic gradient of PDGF-A produced by retinal ganglion cells (Fruttiger et al., 1996, 2000) which in turn promotes the vascular growth by secreting VEGF (West et al., 2005). Transgenic overexpression of PDGF-A in retinal ganglion cells (Fruttiger et al., 1996) or astrocytes (West et al., 2005) reduces the extent of astrocyte migration supporting the hypothesis that astrocyte migration is dependent on a gradient of PDGF-A. Because PDGF-A also stimulates astrocyte proliferation (Fruttiger et al., 1996, 2000; Yamada et al., 2000), this results in a large increase in the number of retinal astrocytes and subsequent overproduction of capillaries in the retina. Overexpression of PDGF-A also results in the formation of an abnormal vessel network (astrocytes and blood vessels penetrate into the deeper layers of the retina which is not observed in normal animals), a delay in the regression of the hyaloid vessels, and a defective lamination of the retina (Fruttiger et al., 1996; Edqvist et al., 2012). Sonic hedgehog (Shh) expressed by retinal ganglion cells is required for the specification of astrocyte lineage cells at the optic disc and stimulates the proliferation of astrocyte precursor cells (Wallace and Raff, 1999; Dakubo et al., 2003, 2008). When the number of retinal ganglion cell axons increases, the numbers of astrocytes, microglial cells, and oligodendrocytes increase proportionally (Burne et al., 1996).

In the primate retina, the migration of astrocytes and the development of the retinal vasculature are guided by gradients of Eph-A6 expressed by retinal ganglion cells, with the ligands for Eph-A6 (ephrin-A1 and -A4) expressed by astrocytes (Kozulin et al., 2009). There is a complete absence of a retinal vascular plexus in mice deficient in retinal ganglion cells despite the presence of an astrocytic framework regarded as a substrate for vascular growth (Sapieha et al., 2008); however, branches of the hyaloid vasculature grow into the retina and form the inner retinal capillary networks (Edwards et al., 2012). In addition, processes of Müller cells extend through the disrupted inner limiting membrane and wrapp around the hyaloid vessels (Edwards et al., 2012). A similar absence of a retinal vascular plexus, formation of inner retinal vessels by the hyaloid vasculature, and sustained proliferation of astrocytes within the vitreous was found in mouse lines with mutations in Lama1, a component of the internal limiting membrane (Edwards et al., 2011). In cases of inner limiting membrane disruption and persistence of the hyaloid vasculature, astrocytes abnormally migrate into the vitreous, ensheath the hyaloid artery, and impede the normal macrophage-mediated regression of the hyaloid system (Zhang et al., 2005d, 2011a; Edwards et al., 2010). A lack of type XV and XVIII collagens, normally localized to the inner limiting membrane, is associated with a delayed regression of the hyaloid vessels, which are covered by retinal astrocytes, while the retina becomes vascularized by anomalous anastomoses from the persistent hyaloid vasculature (Fukai et al., 2002; Ylikärppä et al., 2003; Hurskainen et al., 2005). Type XV collagen is a regulator of the recruitment of astrocytes around vessels while type XVIII collagen inhibits their proliferation (Hurskainen et al., 2005). Laminins of the inner limiting membrane induce astrocyte migration and promote astrocyte differentiation (Gnanaguru et al., 2013). Impairment of the extracellular assembly of fibronectin matrices, and of astrocyte generation and maturation, in Tlx-deficient mice results in a dramatic delay of retinal vascularization (Miyawaki et al., 2004; Uemura et al., 2006). Connective tissue growth factor (CTGF) derived from endothelial cells and pericytes stimulates the migration of astrocytes and vascular cells (Pi et al., 2011). Water flux through aquaporin (AQP)-4 water channels and the activity of the casein kinase II are important for astrocyte cell shape alterations and migration (Saadoun et al., 2005; Auguste et al., 2007; Kramerov et al., 2008, 2011; Zhang et al., 2011a).

Müller cells secrete Norrin (Ye et al., 2011), a signaling molecule which binds to Frizzled-4 to activate canonical Wnt (wingless-type MMTV integration site family)/β-catenin signaling. In the absence of this signaling cascade, the development of the superficial vessels is attenuated and deeper intraretinal capillaries are not formed (Xu et al., 2004; Ye et al., 2009; Ohlmann and Tamm, 2012). Another frizzled receptor, Frizzled-5, is involved in limiting the numbers of astrocyte precursors and mature astrocytes in the retina, and in mediating the regression of the hyaloid vasculature (Liu and Nathans, 2008). Müller cells may also inhibit retinal angiogenesis by producing diols of docosahexenoic acid that inhibit the Notch signaling pathway (Hu et al., 2014) which normally stimulates the angiogenesis via inducing tip cell and filopodia formation. Astrocytes, Müller cells, and retinal ganglion cells also release transforming growth factor (TGF)-β1, e.g., upon hypoxia or stimulation with αvβ8 integrins; TGF-β1 acts at endothelial cells and inhibits the formation of the superficial vascular plexus, while it stimulates the formation of the deeper vascular plexi (Arnold et al., 2012). Active TGF-β, which is formed under hypoxic conditions, induces the expression of VEGF in Müller cells (Behzadian et al., 1998). Glia-derived TGF-β as well as a direct contact of astrocytes or Müller cells stimulate the release of the matrix metalloproteinase (MMP)-9 from retinal capillary endothelial cells (Behzadian et al., 2001). The MMP-mediated extracellular matrix turnover allows endothelial cells to penetrate their underlying basement membrane which generates leaky vessels and eliminates the contact inhibition that otherwise blocks endothelial cell proliferation (Matrisian, 1990; Castilla et al., 1999). The expression of MMPs in vascular endothelial cells is also upregulated by angiogenic factors such as VEGF (Unemori et al., 1992; Lamoreaux et al., 1998). In another study, deletion of astrocyte-expressed αvβ8 integrin results in a diminished release of soluble TGF-β and a defective TGF-β signaling in vascular endothelial cells but not astrocytes (Hirota et al., 2011). The formation of the superficial vascular plexus may be also supported by osteonectin which disrupts cell-matrix interactions and is produced by astrocytes and retinal ganglion cells (Yan et al., 1998). The formation of the deeper vascular plexi is also stimulated by angiotensin-2 and neuropilin-1, and in mice with defective Jagged1/Dll4/Notch signaling (Hackett et al., 2002; Pan et al., 2007; Benedito et al., 2009). Jagged1 is known to be released from retinal ganglion cells (Wang et al., 1998).

The proliferation and maturation of astrocytes mainly occurs at the ventricular surface of the retina surrounding the optic nerve head (Chan-Ling, 1997; Chu et al., 2001; Mansour et al., 2008). Astrocyte maturation is induced by factors released from vascular endothelial cells, in particular

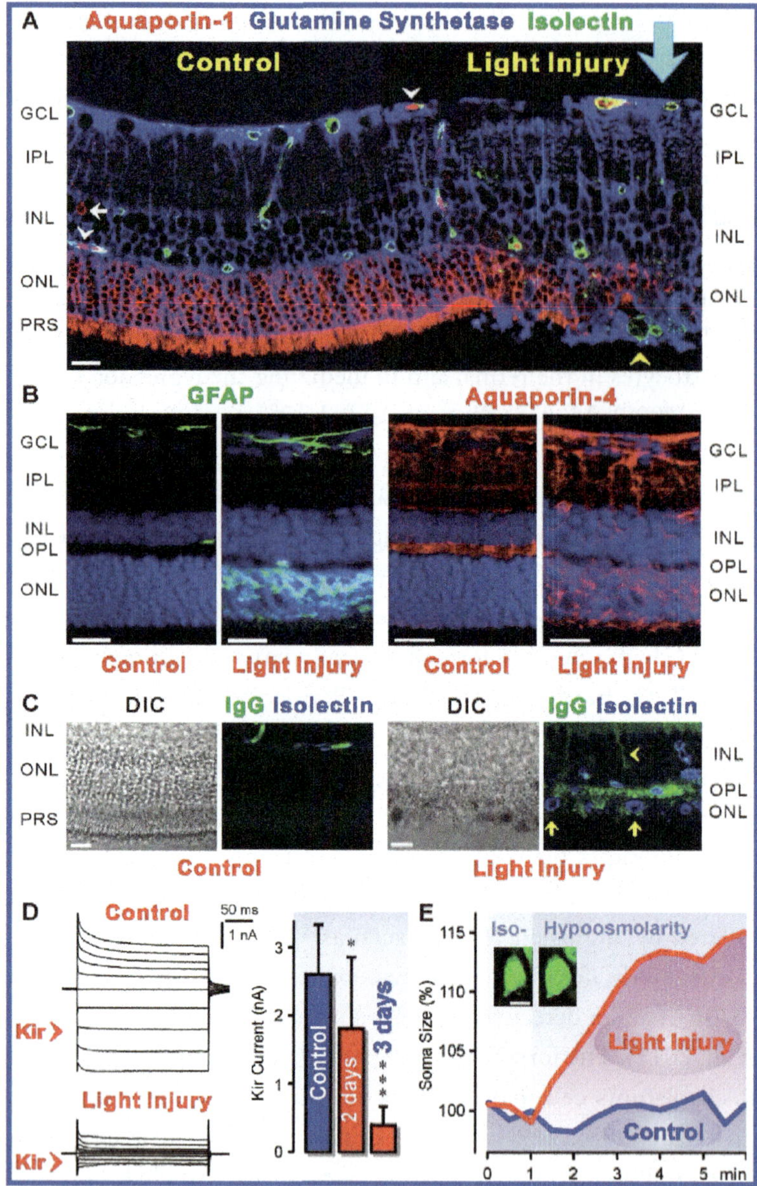

FIGURE 21: Müller cell reactivity in the blue light-injured neuroretina of the rat. **A.** Focal illumination of the rat retina with excessive blue light results in apoptotic degeneration of photoreceptor cells, as indicated by the disappearance of aquaporin-1 immunoreactivity in the photoreceptor segment (PRS) layer and outer nuclear layer (ONL; *right*). Slices of a control retina (*left*) and a retina obtained 3 days after light treatment (*right*) were immunostained against aquaporin-1 (*red*) and the Müller cell marker

glutamine synthetase (*blue*). Blood vessels and activated immune cells were labeled with isolectin (*green*). Usually, aquaporin-1 is localized to photoreceptor cells, a class of glycinergic amacrine cells (*white arrow*), and erythrocytes within the vessels (*white arrowheads*). *Yellow arrowhead*, isolectin-stained invading monocyte/macrophage. **B.** Localization of GFAP (*green*) and aquaporin-4 (*red*) immunoreactivities in slices of a control retina and a retina 2 days after light treatment. Note that both immunoreactivities are largely absent from the ONL under control conditions, and present after light treatment. Note also the diappearance of aquaporin-4 immunoreactivity in the outer plexiform layer (OPL) indicating an early loss of ribbon synapses after light treatment. Cell nuclei are *blue* stained. **C.** Blue light injury is associated with a disruption of the outer blood-retinal barrier, resulting in extravasation of blood proteins such as IgG and invasion of macrophages into the ONL which phagocytize the debris of degenerated photoreceptors. Slices of a control retina (*left*) and a retina 3 days after blue light treatment were stained against IgG (*green*) and with isolectin (*blue*) which labels blood vessels and activated immune cells including macrophages (*arrows*). The presence of IgG-labeled Müller cell fibers (*arrowhead*) indicates that Müller cells phagocytize blood-derived proteins. The *left images* show differential interference contrast (DIC) images of the slices. **D.** Potassium currents of two Müller cells isolated from a control retina and a retina 3 days after light treatment (*left*). Note the decrease of the Kir currents after light treatment. The *bar diagram* at the *right side* displays the time-dependent decrease in the mean Kir currents of Müller cells after blue light-treatment of the retina. **E.** Blue light injury causes an alteration in the osmotic swelling properties of Müller cells. The cross-sectional area of Müller cell somata was measured in slices of untreated (*control*) retinas and of retinas isolated 3 days after light exposure. Acute exposure of the slices to a hypoosmolar solution (60% of normal osmolarity) induced a time-dependent swelling of Müller cell bodies in light-injured retinas, and had no effect on the size of Müller cell bodies in control retinas. The *insets* display original records of a dye-filled Müller cell soma in a slice of a light-injured retina, obtained before (*left*) and during (*right*) hypoosmotic exposure. Bar, 5 µm. GCL, ganglion cell layer; INL, inner nuclear layer; IPL, inner plexiform layer. Scale bars, 20 µm and 5 µm (*insets*). Modified from Iandiev et al. (2008a).

---

leukemia inhibitory factor (LIF) (Kubota and Suda, 2009). LIF inhibits the normal vascular development but not the pathological angiogenesis in the retina, and causes persistence of the hyaloid vasculature (Ash et al., 2005). The vasostatic action of LIF is the result of its effects on both endothelial cells and astrocytes. LIF inhibits the hypoxia-induced VEGF expression and proliferation of astrocytes, and induces GFAP expression in astrocytes (Mi et al., 2001; Kubota et al., 2008). LIF also inhibits the VEGF- and bFGF-induced proliferation and migration of vascular endothelial cells, decreases the proteolytic activity of endothelial cells, and increases the expression of plasminogen activator inhibitor-1 in endothelial cells (Pepper et al., 1995). The production of LIF by vascular endothelial cells is stimulated by apelin; transgenic deletion of this pathway results in increased

VEGF expression by astrocytes in the vascularized area, and an aberrant overgrowth of endothelial networks in association with an overgrowth of immature astrocytes (Kubota et al., 2008; Sakimoto et al., 2012). Interleukin (IL)-6 family cytokines, whose signal transduction requires the cytokine receptor glycoprotein-130 (gp130), promote astrocyte differentiation in the retina (Fukushima et al., 2009). LIF and bone morphogenetic protein (BMP)-2 synergistically promote astrocyte differentiation (Fukushima et al., 2009). In contrast, BMP-4, expressed in the developing retina, inhibits astrocyte cell differentiation (Du et al., 2010).

Both astrocytes and Müller cells, as well as pericytes, also contribute to endothelial cell differentiation and the formation of the blood-retinal barrier (Gardner, 1995; Gardner et al., 1997; Choi and Kim, 2008a; Kim et al., 2009; Wisniewska-Kruk et al., 2012; see 5.11.9.1.1.). In rodents, the blood-retinal barrier is established between postnatal days 11 and 13 (Zeng et al., 2000a). Astrocyte-derived soluble factors induce a decrease of VEGF and an increase of thrombospondin-1 levels in vascular endothelial cells, resulting in reduced vascular permeability, decreased endothelial cell migration, and upregulation of tight junction proteins (Choi et al., 2007; Choi and Kim, 2008b). Microglia contribute to the establishment of the blood-retinal barrier via increasing the capacity of astrocytes and Müller glial cells to increase the endothelial cell resistivity (Diaz et al., 1998). Retinal micro- and macroglia also contribute to the blood-retinal barrier by phagocytosis of serum-derived substances (Fig. 21C) (Vinores et al., 1993; Zeng et al., 2000; Zou et al., 2009).

2.3 ASTROCYTIC FUNCTIONS IN THE NORMAL RETINA

In addition to the stimulatory effects of astrocytes on the development of the retinal vasculature, retinal astrocytes and Müller cells are implicated in the maturation of retinal neurons, i.e., synaptogenesis and synaptic maturation, dendritic development, and axon growth; the glial effects are mediated by direct cell contact-mediated mechanisms and the release of soluble factors (Armson et al., 1987; Le Roux and Reh, 1995; Dreyer et al., 1995; Steinbach and Schlosshauer, 2000; Belmonte et al., 2000; Nägler et al., 2001; Ullian et al., 2001; Nishiwaki et al., 2001). Müller cell-derived VEGF also stimulates the development of photoreceptor cells (Yourey et al., 2000).

Glial cells regulate the expression of genes that influence the development of dendrites and synapses, and the cholesterol and fatty acid metabolism, in neurons (Göritz et al., 2007). Astrocytes promote synapse development and axon growth by providing cholesterol complexed to apolipoprotein (Apo) E-containing lipoproteins (Mauch et al., 2001; Hayashi et al., 2004; Lorber et al., 2009). The direct contact with astrocytes induces in retinal ganglion cells the capability to receive synapses; the astrocyte contact alters the localization of the synaptic adhesion molecule neurexin away from dendrites (Barker et al., 2008). Astrocyte-secreted thrombospondins induce the formation of synapses and enhance the efficacy of presynaptic transmitter release; however, the synapses are postsynaptically silent (Christopherson et al., 2005). Astrocyte-derived glypican 4 and 6 induce postsynaptic reactivity of retinal ganglion cells (Allen et al., 2012). Glypican 4 increases the postsynaptic glutamatergic signaling by recruitment of α-amino-3-hydroxy-5-methyl-4-isoxazolepropionic acid (AMPA) receptors to synapses (Allen et al., 2012). The surface of immature astrocytes (but not of mature astrocytes; see 4.2.) is also a strong promoter of the survival of retinal ganglion cells and the outgrowth of retinal ganglion cell axons in the embryonic mammalian retina which is mediated by both diffusible and contact-mediated factors (McCaffery et al., 1984; Schwab and Caroni, 1988; Fawcett et al., 1989; Baehr and Bunge, 1990; Ard et al., 1991; Bähr et al., 1995; Lucius et al., 1996). (In contrast, astrocytes of the adult fish retina, which show a lifelong growth [see 5.11.12.1.], permit the growth of retinal ganglion cell axons; Bähr et al., 1995.) Endfeet of immature Müller cells promote the growth of retinal ganglion cell axons while the somata of the cells promote the growth of dendrites (Stier and Schlosshauer, 1995, 1998, 1999; Bauch et al., 1998). The inhibitory action of astrocytes in the mature retina on axonal outgrowth is neuron type-specific, i.e., retinal astrocytes inhibit the growth of retinal ganglion cell axons, but not the axon growth of dorsal root ganglia neurons (Steinbach et al., 2001).

Astrocytes are also implicated in the pruning of synapses during retinal development and in the adult retina under pathological conditions. Immature astrocytes induce the expression of the complement factor C1q (the initiating protein in the classical complement cascade) in postnatal neurons; C1q is localized to synapses throughout the postnatal retina (Stevens et al., 2007). In the mature retina, neuronal C1q is normally downregulated; however, it becomes upregulated and synaptically relocalized early in glaucoma where it plays a role in synapse loss (Stevens et al., 2007).

In the normal retina of higher vertebrates, the expression of the intermediate filament GFAP is restricted to astrocytes (Figs. 13A-C, 14C, D, 15A) (Dixon and Eng, 1980; Dahl and Bignami, 1982; Molnar et al., 1984; Shaw and Weber, 1984; Eisenfeld et al., 1984; Schnitzer, 1985, 1988b; Penn et al., 1988; Davidson et al., 1990; Scherer and Schnitzer, 1989, 1991; Osborne et al., 1991; Sarthy et al., 1991; Chien and Liem, 1995; Osborne and Larsen, 1996; Barber et al., 2000; Li et al., 2002a; Powner et al., 2010; Zayit-Soudry et al., 2010). In the human retina, three populations of astrocytes are distinguishable: vimentin$^+$/GFAP$^+$, vimentin$^-$/GFAP$^+$, and vimentin$^+$/GFAP$^-$ (Pérez-Alvarez et al., 2008).

Retinal astrocytes contribute to the removal of carbon dioxide and the regulation of the extracellular pH via sodium-bicarbonate cotransport (Newman, 1999). Retinal astrocytes also contribute to the clearance of the extracellular space from neuron-derived glutamate and the production of glutamine. They express multiple subtypes of excitatory amino acid transporters (EAATs) (see 5.5.2.1.2.) and glutamine synthetase (see 5.5.2.1.9.). Astrocytes may also redistribute excess

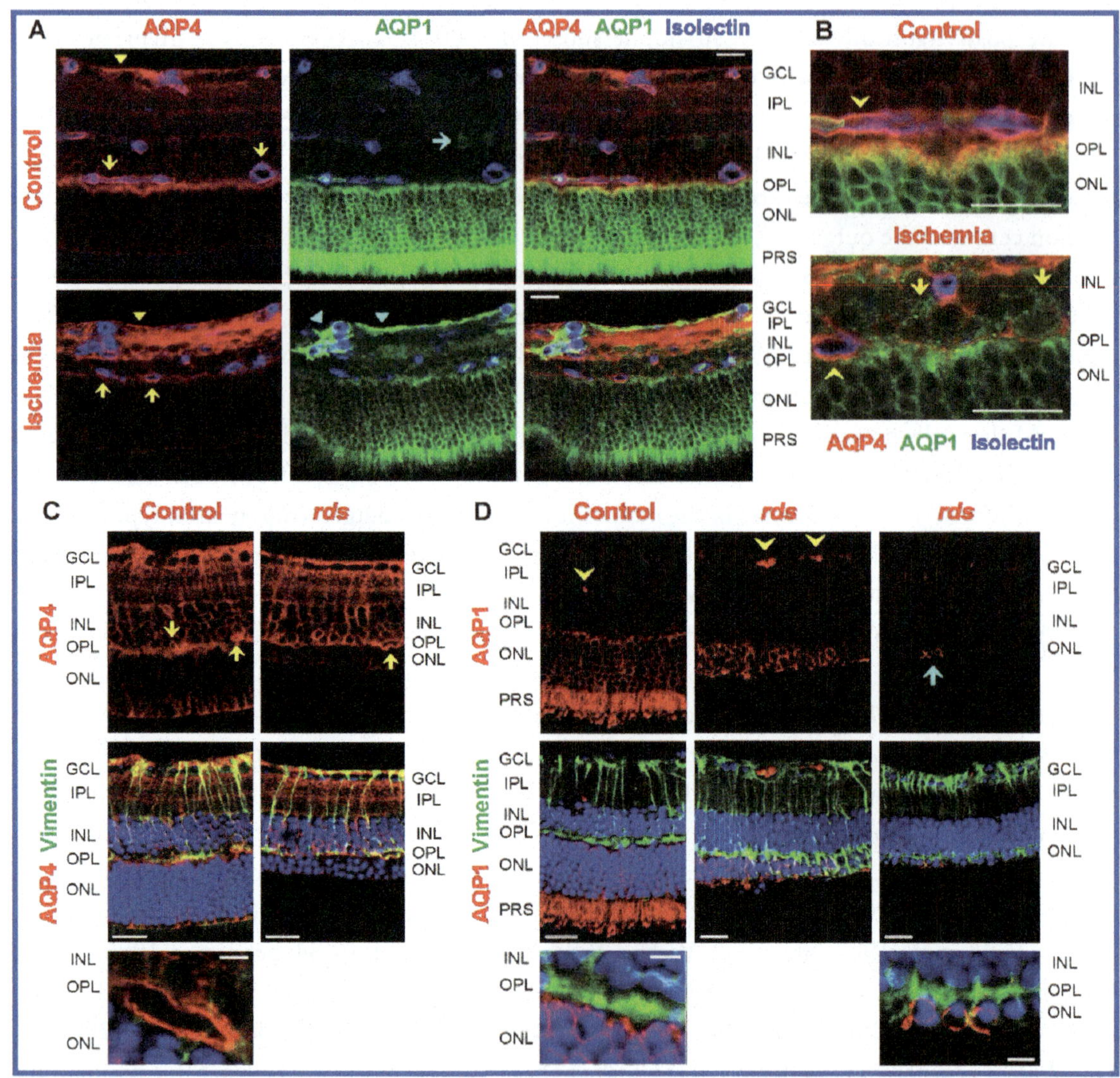

FIGURE 22: The water homeostasis of the outer neuroretina is mainly mediated by AQP1 localized to photoreceptor cells while the water homeostasis of the inner retinal tissue is mainly mediated by glial AQP4 in the normal retina and by AQP4 and AQP1 in the postischemic retina. **A, B.** Rat retinal slices were immunostained against AQP1 (*green*) and AQP4 (*red*). Blood vessels were labeled with isolectin (*blue*). **A.** The tissues were derived from a control animal (*above*), and from an animal 7 days after transient retinal ischemia induced by elevation of the intraocular pressure for 1 h (*below*). AQP4 is strongly expressed by Müller cells in the inner retina and the outer plexiform layer (OPL) while the expression of the protein in the outer nuclear layer (ONL) is faint. AQP4 is enriched in Müller cell membranes

that surround the vessels (*yellow arrows*) and in the vitreous-abutting endfeet membranes (*yellow arrowheads*). Photoreceptor cells express AQP1. In the inner retina, AQP1 is expressed by subpopulations of glycinergic and GABAergic amacrine cells under normal conditions (*blue arrow*) and additionally by glial processes around the vessels and at the inner retinal surface after ischemia (*blue arrowheads*). In addition, erythrocytes within the retinal vessels express AQP1. **B.** The OPL at higher magnification. Ribbon synapses are surrounded by AQP4-containing glial membranes in the control retina (*yellow* merge signal). After ischemia, ribbon synapses are largely absent. However, there is a punctate AQP1 labeling in the inner nuclear layer (INL) after ischemia (*arrows*) which was not observed in the control retina. The perivascular AQP4 labeling (*arrowheads*) did not alter after ischemia. **C, D.** AQP4 (**C**) and AQP1 (**D**) immunoreactivities (*red*) in retinas of control mice and mice carrying the *rds* (*Prph2^{Rd2}*) mutation. The slices were co-stained against vimentin (*green*). Double labeling yielded a *yellow–orange* merge signal. Cell nuclei are *blue* stained. The *Prph2* gene encodes the structural protein peripherin/rds which is essential for the formation of photoreceptor outer segments (Connell et al., 1991). The mice display a degeneration of photoreceptor cells of early-onset and slow progression (Sanyal et al., 1980) and are used as a model of retinitis pigmentosa. **C.** The slices were derived from 5 months-old control and *rds* mice. The *arrows* indicate perivascular AQP4. The *small image below* shows AQP4 around a vessel at the border between the innner plexiform layer (IPL) and INL at higher magnification. The retinal distribution of AQP4 remains largely unaltered in the course of the degeneration of the *rds* retina. **D.** The slices were derived from a control mouse (*left*), and a 5 months- (*middle*) and a 12 months-old *rds* mouse (*right*), respectively. Note that the AQP1 immunoreactivity disappears along with the degeneration of the photoreceptor cells in the *rds* retina. In the retina of the 5 months-old *rds* mouse (*middle*) the receptor segments are missing while a certain number of AQP1-expressing photoreceptor cell bodies is still present. Note also that there is no overlay of AQP1 and vimentin immunoreactivities. The *small images below* show the OPL (*left*) and single AQP1-expressing photoreceptor cell bodies (*right*) at higher magnification. The arrow indicates single photoreceptor nuclei which are surrounded by AQP1 immunoreactivity. The *arrowheads* point to AQP1 expressed by red blood cells. GCL, ganglion cell layer; PRS, photoreceptor segments. Bars, 20 and 5 (*small images*) μm. Modified from Iandiev et al. (2005a, 2006a).

---

extracellular potassium released from retinal ganglion cell axons via the inwardly rectifying potassium (Kir) channel Kir4.1 (Bay and Butt, 2012). However, it was suggested that the coupling between retinal astrocytes is too weak to carry significant potassium spatial buffering currents (Ceelen et al., 2001). After photoreceptor degeneration induced by urethane treatment, Müller cells withdraw from the inner limiting membrane; astrocytes hypertrophy and occupy the vitread surface of the inner limiting membrane (Burns and Tyler, 1990). The morphological alterations are associated with an increased gap junctional coupling of astrocytes which may increase the lateral spatial potassium buffering by the cells (Burns and Tyler, 1990). The homeostatic functions of retinal astrocytes is regulated by neuron-derived transmitters. Astrocytes express various neurotransmitter receptors including γ-aminobutyric acid (GABA) and glutamatergic AMPA/kainate (KA) receptors (Clark and Mobbs, 1992). The expression of voltage-gated sodium channels in astrocytes depends on the neuronal activity (Minturn et al., 1992).

Retinal astrocytes are coupled by gap junctions (Holländer et al., 1991; Ramírez et al., 1996). A gap junctional coupling is also regularly found between Müller cells of fish, amphibians, and reptiles (Uga and Smelser, 1973; Conner et al., 1985; Mobbs et al., 1988; Giblin et al., 1997; Ball and McReynolds, 1998). In contrast, avian and mammalian Müller glial cells are normally not coupled (with the exception of rabbit Müller cells) (Wolburg et al., 1990; Holländer et al., 1991; Nishizono et al., 1993; Robinson et al., 1993; Ball and McReynolds, 1998; Johansson et al., 1999; Zahs and Ceelen, 2006). The gap junctional coupling of astrocytes creates a functional syncytium which allows the intercellular propagation of intracellular signals, the control of ionic and metabolic homeostasis of retinal ganglion cell somata and axons, and the neurovascular coupling (see 5.8.). Rat (but not cat) astrocytes are also coupled to Müller cells; one astrocyte is coupled to 13–88 astrocytes and to >100 Müller cells (Holländer et al., 1991; Robinson et al., 1993; Zahs and Newman, 1997; Ceelen et al., 2001). While the gap junctional coupling between astrocytes is symmetric, the coupling between astrocytes and Müller cells is asymmetric, allowing only a unidirectional transfer of small intracellular molecules from astrocytes to Müller cells (Robinson et al., 1993; Zahs and Newman, 1997). The diffusion of internal messengers, presumably inositol 1,4,5-triphosphate (IP_3), through gap junctions mediate the propagation of intercellular calcium waves between astrocytes (but not between astrocytes and Müller cells). Retinal type I astrocytes have IP_3 receptor (IP_3R) type 1 and 3 (Kuo et al., 2008) and gap junctions composed of various types of connexins, in particular connexin-43 (Janssen-Bienhold et al., 1998; Schütte et al., 1998; Johansson et al., 1999; Söhl et al., 2000; Zahs et al., 2003; Kuo et al., 2008; Kerr et al., 2010, 2011, 2012; Danesh-Meyer et al., 2012; Mansour et al., 2013). The calcium waves between astrocytes and Müller cells are propagated by paracrine extracellular adenosine 5'-triphosphate (ATP) signaling (Fig. 17F; see 5.6.3.3.).

Adherent junctions are present among astrocytes and Müller cells, and between adjacent astrocytes and Müller cells, but not between glial cells and neurons, or among neurons (with the exception of the junctional coupling between Müller and photoreceptor cells at the level of the outer limiting membrane) (Holländer et al., 1991; Ramírez et al., 1996). This suggests that the glial cell network constitutes the mechanical stability of the retina.

2.4 ASTROCYTES IN THE AGING RETINA

The density and number of astrocytes in the retina display age-dependent alterations. In the rat retina, the number of astrocytes increases between 3 and 9 months (with a doubling of the total number of parenchymal astrocytes in the retina) and decreases between 9 and 12 months of age (Mansour et al., 2008). Proliferation of astrocytes (and of the small population of resident astrocyte precursor cells) occurs up to 6 months of age while the proportion of astrocytes that undergo apoptotic cell death increases progressively with aging (Mansour et al., 2008). A possible contribution of an astrocytic differentiation of bone marrow-derived hematopoietic stem cells to the age-related increase in the number of astrocytes (as observed under pathological conditions; Chan-Ling et al., 2006) remains to be determined (Mansour et al., 2008). In aged retinas, retinal glial cells suffer from lipid peroxidation due to an increased retinal oxidative stress level (Nag et al., 2011). During aging, astrocytes undergo hypertrophy, an increase in the density of packing of their processes, and other reactive gliosis-like changes (Mansour et al., 2008). A similar age-related decrease in astrocyte number and gliotic changes of retinal astrocytes were observed in the human retina and in age-related macular degeneration (AMD), the most common cause of blindness in the elderly (Madigan et al., 1994; Ramírez et al., 2001; Cavallotti et al., 2003). The reduction in the number of astrocytes in aged retinas and the gliotic changes will impair the capacity of astrocytes to maintain homeostasis and support neuronal function in old age, and will predispose the retina to age-related diseases such as glaucoma and AMD (Mansour et al., 2008). The age-related degeneration of astrocytes is associated with a breakdown of the blood-retinal barrier and inflammation (Chan-Ling et al., 2007). On the other hand, astrogliosis seems to be required for the survival of retinal ganglion cells in the aged and diseased retina. Normally, there is no decrease in the number of retinal ganglion cells during aging (Harman et al., 2003; Feng et al., 2007); neuronal cell loss is only seen in age-related diseases like vascular diseases and Alzheimer's disease (Munari et al., 1989; Blanks et al., 1996). Genetic inactivation of the transcription factor nuclear factor (NF)-κB, a key regulator of inflammatory responses, is associated with an age-dependent decrease in the number of retinal ganglion cells and an increased damage of the ganglion cells under excitotoxic conditions in young animals (Takahashi et al., 2007b). In addition, autoantibodies against retinal ganglion cells are produced in these animals (Takahashi et al., 2007b).

2.5   ASTROCYTES IN THE DISEASED RETINA

After retinal injury, retinal astrocytes become activated, proliferate, migrate, exhibit enlarged soma and thickened processes, and upregulate intermediate filaments such as GFAP, nestin, and synemin, but often to a lesser extent than Müller glial cells (Barron et al., 1986; Eddleston and Mucke, 1993; Wen et al., 1995; Tezel et al., 2001; Vazquez-Chona et al., 2004; Panagis et al., 2005; Anderson et al., 2008; Wohl et al., 2009; Chang et al., 2007; Luna et al., 2010). Nestin is a marker of neural, vascular endothelial, and pericyte progenitors (Walcott and Provis, 2003; Fischer and Omar, 2005; Xue et al., 2006b; Lee et al., 2012a). The upregulation of nestin and the early neuronal marker doublecortin (Chang et al., 2007) could point to a transdifferentiation potential of retinal astrocytes into neuron-like cells after injury similar to that of Müller cells (see 5.11.12.). After retinal injury, hematopoietic stem cells can differentiate into retinal astrocytes (Chan-Ling et al., 2006). In the adult mouse retina, increased expression of insulin-like growth factor binding protein (IGFBP)-3 in vascular endothelial cells results in increased differentiation of bone marrow-derived hematopoietic stem cells into pericytes and astrocytes (Kielczewski et al., 2011).

2.5.1   GLAUCOMA

Glaucoma, one of the leading causes of irreversible blindness, is characterized by a progressive loss of retinal ganglion cells. Apoptotic death of of retinal ganglion cells resulting from the degeneration of their axons is the final common pathway of glaucoma. Although elevated intraocular pressure is a major risk factor of the glaucomatous degeneration of retinal ganglion cells, an elevation of the intraocular pressure is not detected in a significant subset of patients. Further risk factors of the ganglion cell death involve glutamate-, reactive oxygen species-, and nitric oxide (NO)-mediated toxicity (Dreyer et al., 1996; Neufeld, 1999; Al-Gayyar et al., 2010). Elevation of the intraocular pressure results in deleterious changes of astrocytes in the optic nerve head and in the retina (Ganesh and Chintala, 2011). Activation of astrocytes may initially represent a cellular attempt to limit the extent of neuronal injury and to promote tissue repair, but reactive astrocytes and Müller cells may also have noxious effects on optic nerve axons by creating mechanical injury and changing the neuronal microenvironment, resulting in activation of the autonomous self-destruction of ganglion cell axons and somata (Nickells, 2007; Calandrella et al., 2007; Grieshaber et al., 2007). Dying ganglion cells may adversely affect their neighboring cells in a wave of secondary degeneration which involves gap junctions, glutamate exposure, and the release of intracellular tissue plasminogen activator (Mali et al., 2005; Nickells, 2007; Akopian et al., 2014). These alterations are associated with a damage to capillaries in the nerve fiber/ganglion cell layers, suggesting that ischemia is a further secondary pathogenic factor in glaucoma (Maeda-Yajima et al., 2001; Grieshaber et al., 2007). Astrocytes were suggested to contribute to the secondary death of retinal ganglion cells via a spread of oxidative stress through the astrocytic network from the injured axons to the ganglion cell somata (Fitzgerald et al., 2010). The lost ganglion cells and nerve fibers are replaced by Müller cell processes which form a glial scar (Maeda-Yajima et al., 2001; Nickells, 2007). The inflammatory responses of astrocytes in experimental glaucoma involve the upregulation of a number of immune mediators and regulators linked to tumor necrosis factor (TNF)-α/TNF receptor signaling, activation of the redox-sensitive transcription factor NF-κB, autophagy regulation, and inflammasome assembly (Tezel et al., 2012; Abdul et al., 2013). Suppression of the activity of astrocytic NF-κB is associated with an increased survival of retinal ganglion cells following ischemic injury (Dvoriantchikova et al., 2009). Reactive astrocytes express various inflammatory cytokines, including TNFα, IL-1β, monocyte chemoattractant protein-1 (MCP-1; Ccl2), interferon-γ (IFN-γ)-induced protein 10, and endothelin-1, the cell adhesion molecules intercellular adhesion molecule (ICAM)-1 and vascular cell adhesion molecule-1, and upregulate the expression of nicotinamide adenine dinucleotide phosphate (NADPH) oxidases, NO synthases, and cyclooxygenase-2; these proinflammatory pathways are thought to mediate the glial toxicity in retinal ganglion cells (Neufeld et al., 1997; Neufeld, 1999; Yuan and Neufeld, 2000; Cuff et al., 2000; Liu and Neufeld, 2001; Ripodas et al., 2001; Yorio et al., 2002; Prasanna et al., 2002; Desai et al., 2004; Zou et al., 2009; Dvoriantchikova et al., 2009).

Reactive astrogliosis is driven by soluble factors. Inflammatory factors such as IFN-γ and IL-1β induce the expression of the inducible NO synthase in astrocytes (Liu and Neufeld, 2000). Astroglia-derived NO increases the hypoxic and excitotoxic death of retinal ganglion cells (Morgan et al., 1999a). Epidermal growth factor (EGF) stimulates quiescent astrocytes to become reactive astrocytes, stimulates cell motility of the reactive astrocytes (but not the cell proliferation), and induces the expression of the inducible NO synthase and the cyclooxygenase-2 (Liu and Neufeld, 2003; Zhang and Neufeld, 2005, 2007; Liu et al., 2006). The inducible cyclooxygenase-2 is an immediate, early response, proinflammatory gene and is rapidly induced in diabetic retinopathy and following ischemia-hypoxia (Fig. 12H-J) (Sennlaub et al., 2003; Ju et al., 2003; Wurm et al., 2006a). The reaction products of cyclooxygenase-2, prostaglandin E_2 (PGE_2) and reactive oxygen species, are chemotactic and cytotoxic, leading to secondary neuronal injury (Dubois et al., 1998). EGF also induces a loss of the gap junctional coupling of retinal astrocytes via tyrosine phosphorylation of connexin 43; this will impair the homeostasis of retinal ganglion cells in glaucomatous eyes (Malone et al., 2007). Astrocytes also contribute to the degeneration of retinal ganglion cells by the release of a riboflavin-related substance that induces oxidative stress (Lucius et al., 1998). Upregulation of amyloid-β in retinal astrocytes may also play a pathogenic role in glaucoma (Ito et al., 2012).

TNFα contributes to the death of retinal ganglion cells, but enhances the survival of astrocytes (Stevenson et al., 2010; Dvoriantchikova and Ivanov, 2014). TNFα also stimulates the expression of neurotoxic proinflammatory factors in astrocytes (Dvoriantchikova and Ivanov, 2014). Reactive astrocytes synthesize elevated levels of MMPs 1, 2, and 9, membrane-type 1 MMP (MT1-MMP), and urokinase plasminogen activator, and promote the death of retinal ganglion cells by degrading the extracellular matrix present in the ganglion cell layer (Agapova et al., 2003; Zhang et al., 2003c, 2004b,c; Mali et al., 2005; Ganesh and Chintala, 2011). TNFα and other inflammatory cytokines stimulate the secretion of MMP-1 and -3 from astrocytes (Crosson et al., 2010). Upon injury, retinal astrocytes increase the expression of endothelin-1 and endothelin receptors (Rogers et al., 1997; Ripodas et al., 2001; Prasanna et al., 2005; Torbidoni et al., 2005). The release of endothelin-1 from astrocytes is also triggered by hypoxia and TNFα (Desai et al., 2004). Endothelin-1 stimulates the expression and activity of MMP-2 and tissue inhibitor of MMPs (TIMP)-1 and -2 (which are activators of MMP-2) in astrocytes (He et al., 2007). TNFα and endothelin-1 also stimulate the proliferation of astrocytes (Desai et al., 2004; Murphy et al., 2010); activation of endothelin receptors in astrocytes was implicated in the development of proliferative vitreoretinopathy (PVR) (Iribarne et al., 2008).

2.5.2 DIABETIC RETINOPATHY

Because astrocytes are predominantly localized to spaces around the inner vascular plexus, they are activated especially under conditions of vascular injury and retinal neovascularization. Dysfunctional astrocytes may play an early and key role in vascular degeneration (Friedlander et al., 2007) and retinal dysfunction in diabetic retinopathy, induced by the increased glucose level, inflammatory cytokines such as TNFα, and oxidative-nitrosative stress (Bressler and Goldstein, 1992; Al-Gayyar et al., 2010; Shin et al., 2014; Dorfman et al., 2014). After 4 weeks of experimental diabetes, astrocytes undergo hyperplasia and become dysfunctional as indicated by the decreased expression of connexins (Kumar and Zhuo, 2010; Ly et al., 2011). At the same time, the retina becomes hypoxic in the ganglion cell layer (Ly et al., 2011). This coincides with a decrease in the ganglion cell function (Ly et al., 2011). After 6 weeks of diabetes, Müller cell gliosis becomes more evident, simultaneously with additional functional deficits in photoreceptors and amacrine cells (Ly et al., 2011). Apparently, astrocytic dysfunction precedes Müller cell gliosis and is coincident with inner retinal hypoxia and ganglion cell dysfunction, whereas Müller cell gliosis and more extensive decreases in neuronal function occur later (Ly et al., 2011).

Diabetic retinopathy is associated with a reduction of the number of astrocytes and of their expression of GFAP whereas Müller cells proliferate and increase their expression of GFAP (Figs. 14A, 15A) (Rungger-Brändle et al., 2000; Barber et al., 2000; Lo et al., 2001; Li et al., 2002a; Asnaghi et al., 2003; Dorfman et al., 2014). Activation of the polyol pathway (which metabolizes excess glucose to sorbitol and fructose) plays a causative role in the induction of GFAP changes (and of early neuroretinal apoptosis) in the diabetic retina (Asnaghi et al., 2003). In diabetic retinopathy, astrocytes may play also a more direct role in the induction of apoptosis in retinal ganglion cells (Abu-El-Asrar et al., 2004a). Retinal ganglion cells of diabetic patients express proapoptotic molecules such as caspase-3, Fas, and Bax, while astrocytes express the cytotoxic effector molecule Fas ligand (Abu-El-Asrar et al., 2004a).

Normally, astrocytes increase the tightness of the blood-retinal barrier by the secretion of soluble factors which increase the expression of tight junction proteins in vascular endothelial cells

(Gardner, 1995). Under ischemic-hypoxic conditions, the upregulation of VEGF and TGF-β in astrocytes and Müller cells, and the downregulation of antipermeability factors like atrial natriuretic peptide (ANP) in retinal astrocytes, contribute to the breakdown of the blood-retinal barrier and the development of retinal edema (Behzadian et al., 2001; Rollín et al., 2005; Zou et al., 2009; see 5.11.9.1.). VEGF and TGF-β induce upregulation of MMPs in endothelial cells which results in a downregulation of tight junction proteins and an increased permeability of vascular endothelial cells (Unemori et al., 1992; Lamoreaux et al., 1998; Behzadian et al., 2001). In experimental autoimmune uveoretinitis, the migration of leukocytes through the blood-retinal barrier of retinal venules is associated with a loss of tight junction proteins in endothelial cells and a loss of the venules-ensheathing astrocyte processes (Xu et al., 2005). A loss of astrocyte processes which contact retinal vessels is also observed in other diseases associated with vascular inflammation and disruption of the blood-retinal barrier, e.g., cerebral malaria (Medana et al., 1996). A malfunction of astrocytes in glaucoma and diabetic retinopathy may lead to an impairment of the neurovascular coupling, i.e., the hyperemia in response to neuronal activity (see 5.8.), and may thus contribute to hypoxic conditions (Gugleta et al., 2007).

The contacts of astrocytes with the vessels of the superficial vascular plexus change in the course of experimental diabetes. Whereas astrocytic processes have contact only to the inner rim of the vessel walls in control retinas, they fully surround these vessels in the retina of diabetic rats (Iandiev et al., 2007a). In addition, the perivascular processes of astrocytes express the water channel AQP1 in diabetic and ischemic retinas (Fig. 8E, 13C-E, 15A, 22A) which is not observed in control retinal tissues (Fig. 13A, C-E, 22A) (Iandiev et al., 2006a; 2007a). A similar upregulation of AQP1 was observed in a transgenic rat model of slow primary photoreceptor degeneration due to the expression of a mutant polycystin-2 gene (Fig. 23C) (Vogler et al., 2013b). The retinal degeneration in the transgenic rats is characterized by initial photoreceptor degeneration and glial activation, followed by vasoregression and neuronal degeneration (Feng et al., 2009). The upregulation of AQP1 in perivascular astrocytic membranes was suggested to represent a response to the osmotic gradient across the glio-vascular interface (Iandiev et al., 2006a; 2007a). However, the upregulation of AQP1 in the transgenic model of photoreceptor degeneration may suggest that alteration of the AQP1 expression is a more general characteristic of astrogliosis in the retina. The functional consequences of the elevated AQP1 expression and of the altered vascular contacts remain to be determined.

Experimental Alzheimer's disease is associated with activation of astrocytes and Müller cells; hypertrophied processes of astrocytes and Müller cells envelop amyloid plaques in the retina (Edwards et al., 2014). Although amyloid plaques were also observed in the normal aged murine retina (albeit at lower level), the plaques are not associated with glial activation in the normal retina (Edwards et al., 2014). It has been suggested that the vessel degeneration observed in Alzheimer's

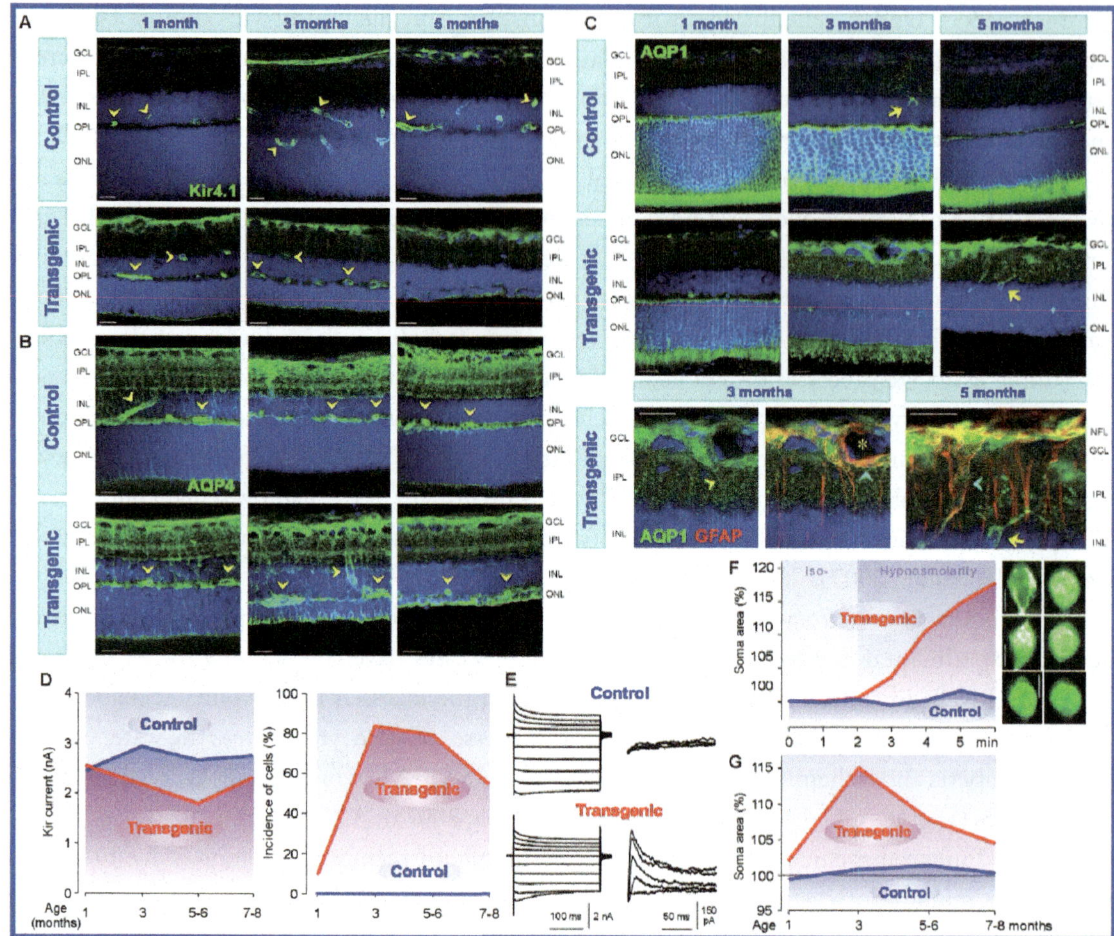

FIGURE 23: Müller cell reactivity in a transgenic rat model of slow primary photoreceptor degeneration due to the expression of a mutant polycystin-2 gene. The retinal degeneration in the transgenic rats is characterized by initial photoreceptor degeneration and glial activation, followed by vasoregression and neuronal degeneration (Feng et al., 2009). **A.** Age-dependent alterations in the retinal localization of the Kir4.1 protein. Retinal slices were derived from 1 month, 3 months, and 5 months old control (*above*) and transgenic rats (*below*). Cell nuclei are *blue* stained. *Arrowheads*, perivascular labeling. **B.** Age-dependent alterations in the retinal localization of AQP4. **C.** Age-dependent alterations in the retinal localization of AQP1. The images *below* display co-labeling against AQP1 (*green*) and GFAP (*red*). Double labeling of both proteins yielded a *yellow-orange* merge signal. *Arrows*, AQP1-positive amacrine cells. *Yellow arrowheads*, AQP1-positive Müller cell fiber. *Blue arrowheads*, GFAP- and AQP1-positive glial processes that surround large vessels. *, large vessel. **D.** Age-dependent alterations in the Kir current

amplitude (*left*) and the incidence of cells that display fast transient K_A currents (*right*). Note that the greatest alterations were found at ages of 3 (K_A currents) and 5-6 months (Kir currents), respectively. The Kir currents are only slightly decreased in Müller cells of transgenic rats compared to control. The slight decrease of the Kir currents is not associated with a depolarization of Müller cells from transgenic animals. **E.** Examples of whole-cell potassium current traces (*left*) and of the K_A currents (*right*) of cells from 3-months animals. Note that the cell of the control animal does not display K_A currents. **F.** Müller cells of transgenic 3-months animals, but not of control animals, display a rapid swelling of their somata when retinal slices are superfused with a hypoosmotic extracellular solution (60% osmolarity). The *images* display Müller cell somata in slices of 3-months transgenic rats obtained before (*left*) and during (*right*) superfusion with the hypoosmotic solution. **G.** Age-dependent alterations of the hypoosmotic swelling swelling properties of Müller cells from control and transgenic rats. Note that cells of control animals does not display a swelling under hypoosmotic conditions, and that the severity of the hypoosmotic swelling of cells from transgenic animals displays a peak after 3 months of age which coincides with the level of the photoreceptor apoptosis in this model (apoptosis occurs since the first month, peaks in the third month, and declines thereafter; Feng et al., 2009). It was suggested that inflammatory factors and reactive oxygen species released from dying photoreceptors and/or activated microglia (Feng et al., 2011) induce gliotic alterations of Müller cells. GCL, ganglion cell layer; IPL, inner plexiform layer; INL, inner nuclear layer; ONL, outer nuclear layer; OPL, outer plexiform layer. Scale bars, 20 and 5 (**F**) μm. Modified from Vogler et al. (2013b).

---

disease is associated with an activation of astrocytes around the vessels of the superficial vascular network which accumulate amyloid-β and high-mobility group box-1, an endogenous ligand of the receptor for advanced glycation endproducts (RAGE) and the Toll-like receptor (TLR)-4 (Busch et al., 2012).

2.5.3   RETINAL NEOVASCULARIZATION

Astrocytes also regulate the development of retinal neovascularization. In glaucoma, astrocytes provide an antiangiogenic environment via an increased expression of antiangiogenic factors (type XVIII collagen and ADAMTSL-3) and a decreased expression of proangiogenic factors (VEGF-C and PDGF-A) (Rudzinski et al., 2008). Exosomes released from retinal astrocytes containing antiangiogenic factors suppress vascular leakage and inhibit neovascularization (Hajrasouliha et al., 2013). Meteorin is highly expressed in astrocytes of the retina during the late embryonic and postnatal stages of mouse development (Park et al., 2008). Meteorin induces the expression and secretion of thrombospondins 1 and 2 from astrocytes; thrombospondins attenuate the angiogenic activity of vascular endothelial cells (Park et al., 2008). TGF-β also induces the production of thrombospondins in astrocytes (Fuchshofer et al., 2005). On the other hand, in response to excessive light and under diabetic and hypoxic conditions, retinal astrocytes overexpress proangiogenic growth factors such as VEGF, PDGF-BB, placenta growth factor, IGF-1, NO synthases, and cyclooxygenase-2 (Dorey et al., 1996; Sennlaub et al., 2003; Kernt et al., 2010; Foulds et al., 2010), and downregulate antiangiogenic factors such as ANP (Rollín et al., 2005); the astrocytic shift from an antiangiogenic to a proangiogenic state contributes to the development of retinal neovascularization (see 5.11.8.). Angiogenic factors such as VEGF induce upregulation of MMPs in vascular endothelial cells (Unemori et al., 1992; Lamoreaux et al., 1998); the MMP-mediated entracellular matrix turnover supports the migration of vascular endothelial cells (Matrisian, 1990; Castilla et al., 1999). In addition, PGE_2 produced by the astrocytic cyclooxygenase-2 exacerbates retinal neovascularization (Sennlaub et al., 2003).

2.5.4 BACTERIAL AND VIRAL INFECTIONS

Bacterial and viral infections are cofactors implicated in the initiation and persistence of autoimmune diseases (Wucherpfennig, 2001). Autoimmune uveitis is frequently associated with previous bacterial infections (Rosenbaum et al., 2008). In the course of autoimmune uveitis, peripheral autoreactive T cells induce a breakdown of the blood-retinal barrier and infiltrate the retinal tissue (Hu et al., 2000). In the retina, T cells are reactivated to gain pathogenic activity by antigen-presenting cells. In addition to infiltrating and resident microglia/macrophages and dendritic cells, retinal astrocytes have the potential to act as antigen-presenting cells, especially when they are activated (Jiang et al., 2008, 2009a).

Oxidative stress, hypoxia, elevated intraocular pressure, and inflammatory factors like IL-10, TNFα, and IFN-γ stimulate the antigen presentation by astrocytes, via upregulation of major histocompatibility (MHC) class I and II molecules (El-Asrar et al., 1991; Yang et al., 2001; Villarroya et al., 2001; Tezel et al., 2007b; Gallego et al., 2012). Ligands of the pattern recognition receptors of the TLR family, commonly provided by pathogens, activate retinal astrocytes, allowing them to express acute inflammatory molecules like the serine protease inhibitor 3 and to present antigen for T cell reactivation (Takamiya et al., 2001; Jiang et al., 2009a). Like TLRs, intracellular nucleotide-binding oligomerization domain (NOD)-like receptors belong to the family of pathogen recognition receptors. The combined action of TLR and NOD ligands triggers alterations in retinal astrocytes required to reactivate T cells (Jiang et al., 2012a). Retinal astrocytes express the IL-17 receptor; T cell-derived IL-17 induces increased production of proinflammatory cytokines and chemokines in retinal astrocytes which stimulate the migration of granulocytes (Ke et al., 2009). Astrocytes and

Müller cells may also stimulate acute immune responses by the macrophage migration inhibitory factor (Matsuda et al., 1997). Viral infections result in a decreased production of antiinflammatory cytokines like thrombospondin-1 in retinal glial cells (Cinatl et al., 2000).

2.5.5 NEUROPROTECTIVE EFFECTS OF ASTROGLIOSIS

Activation of astrocytes can also have neuroprotective and regenerative effects. Astrocytes protect neurons from injury by various mechanisms including the uptake of excess glutamate which is neurotoxic especially in the inner retina (see 5.5.2.1.), direct cell contact (McCaffery et al., 1985), the production of neurotrophic factors, the restoration of the blood-brain barrier, and the inhibition of neovascularization. In addition to microglia (see 3.3.) and Müller cells (see 5.11.1.1.), astrocytes contribute to the removal of harmful substances derived from damaged neurons by phagocytosis of dead cell debris (Jo et al., 1998; Wang et al., 2002c; Romero-Alemán et al., 2013). Astrocytes protect retinal ganglion cells against injury caused by oxidative stress by the release of soluble neurotrophic factors (Lucius and Sievers, 1996). Lens injury, intravitreal administration of zymosan (which activates TLR2 and the complement system), or excessive light exposure resulting in retinal inflammation induce upregulation of neuroprotective factors in retinal astrocytes including bFGF and ciliary neurotrophic factor (CNTF) (Walsh et al., 2001; Müller et al., 2007; Xiao et al., 1998; Leibinger et al., 2009). CNTF activates the Janus kinase (JAK)/signal transducers and activators of transcription 3 (STAT3) and phosphatidylinositol-3 kinase (PI3K)/protein kinase B (Akt) signaling pathways in retinal ganglion cells which stimulate the axon regeneration after optic nerve injury (Müller et al., 2007, 2009; Leibinger et al., 2009). Hypoxia induces the expression of erythropoietin and hemoglobin in retinal astrocytes; glial erythropoietin induces the expression of hemoglobin in retinal ganglion cells which increases the hypoxic survival of the neurons (Tezel et al., 2010). Hemoglobin facilitates the cellular oxygenation and may also provide free radical scavenging. Astrocyte-derived neurotrophins such as brain-derived neurotrophic factor (BDNF), NGF, and neurotrophin-3 stimulate the growth of retinal ganglion cell axons by the induction of the intramembraneous proteolysis of the low-affinity p75 neurotrophin receptor (p75[NTR]), and inactivation of Rho and EGF receptor signaling (Berry et al., 2008; Douglas et al., 2009). In addition, ApoE derived from astrocytes and Müller cells (Amaratunga et al., 1996) stimulates the outgrowth of retinal ganglion cell axons (Lorber et al., 2009). Metallothioneins, which act via intracellular free radical scavenging and heavy metal regulation, are intercellularly transferred from astrocytes to retinal ganglion cells after optic nerve transection and promote axonal regeneration (Chung et al., 2008).

CHAPTER 3

Retinal Microglia

The eye is a immunologically privileged site (Streilein, 2003; Buschini et al., 2011), a property previously attributed to the lack of a lymphatic circulation. The privileged status of the eye, however, is relative, as it is susceptible to immune-mediated infectious and autoimmune inflammatory diseases (Forrester et al., 2010; Buschini et al., 2011). Various studies confirm that the eye has a good communication through classical site-specific lymph nodes, as well as direct connection through the blood circulation with the spleen (Grüntzig et al., 1979; Forrester et al., 2010; see 3.8.). Under normal conditions, the retina contains various types of immunocompetent cells: few dendritic cells, occasional perivascular macrophages, and parenchymal microglia as the most numerous population (Provis et al., 1996; Cuff et al., 1996; Yang et al., 2002; Gregerson and Yang, 2003; Eter et al., 2008; Mendes-Jorge et al., 2009; Lehmann et al., 2010; Heuss et al., 2012). Microglial cells are the primary resident cells of the innate immunity in the retina and represent blood-borne mononuclear phagocytes and antigen-presenting cells.

3.1   MICROGLIA PRECURSORS

Microglial precursors derived from mesodermal (hemopoietic) stem cells (Herbomel et al., 2001; Ginhoux et al., 2010; Schulz et al., 2012), that are MHC class I- and II-positive and express the CD45 marker, but lack specific macrophage markers, invade the embryonic retina from the ciliary body vasculature, in part via the subretinal space, and from the vitreous via the hyaloid vasculature at the optic nerve head and the pecten in birds, respectively (Ashwell et al., 1989; McMenamin and Loeffler, 1990; Navascués et al., 1995; Diaz-Araya et al., 1995a, b; Provis et al., 1996; Marín-Teva et al., 1999a; McMenamin, 1999; Chen et al., 2002; Langmann, 2007; Santos et al., 2008). In avascular retinas, microglial precursors migrate tangentially on Müller cell endfeet before they invade the retinal parenchyma (Navascués et al., 1995; Marín-Teva et al., 1998). Microglial cells are present throughout the thickness of the early postnatal neuroretina, but as the layers of the retina differentiate, they are increasingly restricted to the inner half of the neuroretina (Ashwell et al., 1989). A second category of precursors, which express specific macrophage markers, migrate into the retina along with vascular precursors and differentiate to perivascular microglia/macrophages (Diaz-Araya et al., 1995a; Provis et al., 1996; Chen et al., 2002). Inhibition of the microglial precursor migration into the zebrafish retina, which requires signaling by the macrophage colony-stimulating factor (M-CSF) (Herbomel et al., 2001), results in microphthalmia, a delay in cell cycle withdrawal among retinal progenitors, and the absence of neuronal differentiation, suggesting that microglia are required for normal retinal growth and neurogenesis (Huang et al., 2012).

Migrating microglial precursors proliferate in the retinal parenchyma (Marín-Teva et al., 1999b) and differentiate into ramified parenchymal microglia in the adult retina. Numbers of microglia increase steadily throughout the fetal life; in the rabbit retina, the numbers of microglia increases from approximately 400 at embryonic day 14 to a peak of 28,600 at embryonic day 30, then drops to 17,150 at postnatal day 9, and increases again to about 23,800 at postnatal day 130 (Ashwell, 1989). In the rat retina, the numbers of microglia rise from about 700 at embryonic day 14 to a peak of about 27,000 at postnatal day 7, and fell to about 19,600 at postnatal day 12 (Ashwell et al., 1989).

It is unclear how microglia in the adult uninjured retina are replenished. Some studies showed that, in the normal adult mouse retina, there is a nearly complete turnover of the microglia within 6 months by recruitment of bone marrow-derived monocytic precursor cells that migrate across the blood-retinal barrier while the *in situ* proliferation of microglia is very limited (Xu et al., 2007a; Chen et al., 2012). Other studies did not describe a significant role of bone marrow-derived precursors in the maintenance of the microglia cell pool in the adult retina; infiltration of bone marrow-derived microglial precursors was only found after retinal injury (Albini et al., 2005; Caicedo et al., 2005a; Chan-Ling et al., 2006; Kaneko et al., 2008a; Boettcher et al., 2008; Kezic and McMenamin, 2008; Müther et al., 2010). Erythropoietin stimulates the infiltration of bone marrow-derived microglial precursors and the retinal expression of VEGF (Shen et al., 2014b). Under pathological conditions, VEGF induces microglia conversion of bone-marrow-derived stem cells in the presence of granulocyte-macrophage colony-stimulating factor (GM-CSF) (Avraham-Lubin et al., 2012). In addition, dendritic cells may be recruited into the retina under pathological conditions (Gregerson and Kawashima, 2004; Lehmann et al., 2010; Forrester et al., 2010; Eter et al., 2008).

Microglial cells contribute to the retinal development by inducing programmed neuronal cell death (Frade and Barde, 1998; see 3.4.) and (in cooperation with astrocytes and Müller cells) by removing neuronal cell debris (Hume et al., 1983; Thanos, 1991; Egensperger et al., 1996; Bodeutsch and Thanos, 2000; Wang et al., 2002c). In addition, microglial activity is involved in synaptic pruning in the developing retina, in dependence on the neuronal activity and complement factor C3 (Schafer et al., 2012). Whether microglia also contribute to synapse elimination in the adult retina by complement factor C3-dependent phagocytosis of synapses in response to complement factor C1q produced by retinal ganglion cells (Bialas and Stevens, 2013) remains to be determined.

3.2   RESTING MICROGLIA

In the normal, uninjured retina, microglial cells are localized to the inner retinal layers and the outer plexiform layer; the outer nuclear layer does not contain microglia (Ling, 1982; Kalinina, 1983; Roque et al., 1996; Zeng et al., 2000b, 2008; Ng and Streilein, 2001; Lewis et al., 2005; Combadière et al., 2007; Xu et al., 2009). In fish, avian, and vascularized mammalian retinas, resting microglial cells are located in the plexiform (synaptic) and nerve fiber/ganglion cell layers (Figs. 10C, 12D), and around the vessels (Hume et al., 1983; Navascués et al., 1994, 1995; Diaz-Araya et al., 1995b; Velasco et al., 1999; Yang et al., 2000; Salvador-Silva et al., 2000; Garcia-Valenzuela et al., 2005; Sobrado-Calvo et al., 2007; Santos et al., 2008; Cebulla et al., 2012). In non-vascularized mammalian retinas, microglial cells are localized to the innermost retinal layers (nerve fiber, ganglion cell, and inner plexiform layers) (Figs. 10A, B, 24, 25) (Schnitzer, 1989; Humphrey and Moore, 1995). In the rat retina, there are heterogeneous microglial populations as characterized by their differences in morphology, antigen expression, and distribution; OX42$^+$ cells have delicate processes and are located in the inner layers of the retina, while 5D4$^+$ cells are highly ramified and mostly scattered in the plexiform layers (Zhang et al., 2005b).

Resting microglia display a ramified morphology (Figs. 10A, B, 12D, 25) and act as highly motile patrolling cells that constantly survey their microenvironment with highly motile protrusions to clear metabolic products and cellular debris (Nimmerjahn et al., 2005; Lee et al., 2008). Microglia sense their microenvironment through receptors for complement, cytokines, chemokines, antibodies, and adhesion molecules (Streit, 2002). Once a pathogenic stimulus is detected, microglia become activated, proliferate (Figs. 10A, B, 12D, E), and migrate towards the region of damage (Figs. 10C, 24) where they kill bacteria, release cytotoxic agents, and phagocytize cellular debris. However, while activated microglia initially contribute to neuronal protection and tissue regeneration, excessive or prolonged activation of the cells by alarm signals from exogenous and endogenous sources can lead to chronic overactivation and loss of autoregulatory mechanisms which contribute to retinal inflammation and degeneration (see 3.2.) (Langmann et al., 2007).

Resting microglia are programmed for immunological tolerance and display an antiinflammatory phenotype characterized, for example, by low NO and superoxide anion production (Stevenson et al., 2010; Forrester et al., 2010). The maintenance of the resting state of microglial cells involves antiinflammatory cytokines such as TGF-β and IL-10 produced, for example, by the retinal pigment epithelium (Zamiri et al., 2005). TGF-β induces the production of IL-10 in microglial cells which in turn downregulates antigen-presenting molecules including MHC class II and costimulatory CD80 and CD86 (D'Orazio and Niederkorn, 1998; Paglinawan et al., 2003). IL-10 also inhibits microglial migration and phagocytic activity (Broderick et al., 2000; Carter and Dick,

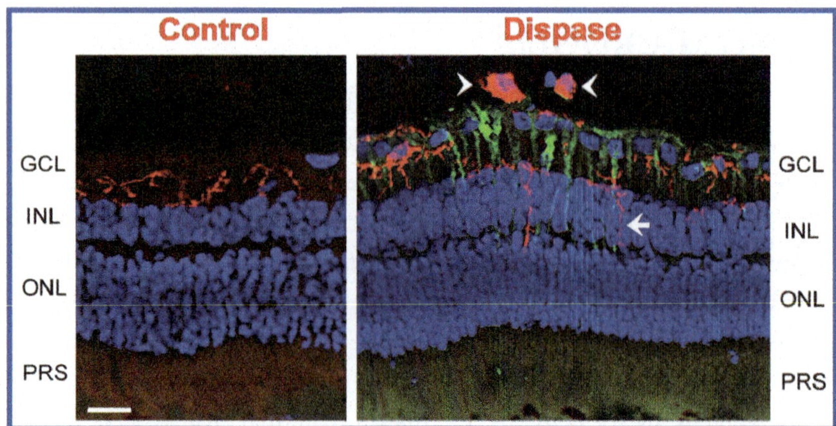

FIGURE 24: Interaction of blood-derived monocytes/macrophages and retinal glial cells in a rabbit model of early PVR induced by intravitreal injection of the protease dispase (Cantó Soler et al., 2002b). Retinal slices were stained against immune cells (*red*), GFAP (*green*; a marker of activated Müller glial cells), and cell nuclei (*blue*). Under control conditions, microglial cells (*red*) are restricted to the innermost retinal layers, and Müller cells do not express GFAP. The retinas from dispase-treated eyes display "hot spots" of glial cell reactivity characterized by an upregulation of GFAP in Müller cells (*green*) and activated microglia that begin to migrate towards the outer retina (*arrow*). Blood-borne monocytes/macrophages adhere to the vitreal surface of such hot spots (*arrowheads*), suggesting a relationship between the attachment of macrophages and glial cell activation. GCL, ganglion cell layer; INL, inner nuclear layer; ONL, outer nuclear layer; PRS, photoreceptor segments. Bar, 20 μm. Modified from Francke et al. (2003).

2003). The activation of latent TGF-β produced by the retinal pigment epithelium to its biologically active form is mediated primarily by thrombospondin-1 (Zamiri et al., 2005). Expression of thrombospondin-1, which is also produced by microglia, macrophages, and Müller cells (see 5.11.8.) is essential for maintaining the immune privilege of the retina. Deletion of thrombospondin-1 results in an proinflammatory retinal microenvironment and supports enhanced migration and activation of retinal microglia in response to injury (Ng et al., 2009). Retinal microglia constitutively secrete the antiinflammatory cytokine IL-27; photoreceptors constitutively express the IL-27 receptor and respond to IL-27 signaling by producing the antiinflammatory molecules IL-10 and suppressor of cytokine signalling 1 (Lee et al., 2011a). Direct cell-cell contacts mediated by membrane-bound molecules contribute to microglia quiescence. The immunoglobulin superfamily domain-containing molecule CD200 is a transmembrane glycoprotein expressed on neurons and vascular endothelial cells (Clark et al., 1985; McCaughan et al., 1987). The CD200 receptor is expressed on microglial cells; CD200 binding via cellular contact triggers signaling events that maintain the basal, deactivated state with mainly homeostatic functions of microglia cells (Hoek et al., 2000; Wright et al., 2000). Retinal microglia in CD200 knockout mice display normal morphology but are present in increased numbers and express inducible NO synthase, an activation marker (Broderick et al., 2002; Dick et al., 2003). Activation of the CD200 receptor also triggers secretion of IL-10 and is involved in mediating cellular migration after activation of the cells (Carter and Dick, 2004). The chemokine fractalkine (CX3CL1) also exists as a membrane-bound molecule on neurons and can restrain microglia activation (Bazan et al., 1997).

The process motility of resting microglia is not cell-autonomously regulated but modulated by endogenous neuro- and gliotransmission (Fontainhas et al., 2011). Under normal conditions, Müller glial cells are a source of extracellular ATP (see 5.6.3.1.). ATP regulates the activity-dependent microglial dynamic process motility (Damani et al., 2011; Wang and Wong, 2014). Retinal microglia express metabotropic (P2Y) and ionotropic purinergic (P2X) receptors (Morigiwa et al., 2000a,b; Fries et al., 2004a; Uckermann et al., 2005d; Pereira et al., 2010; Preissler et al., 2014). Activation of $P2Y_{12}$ receptors (that detect extracellular ATP and adenosine 5'-diphosphate

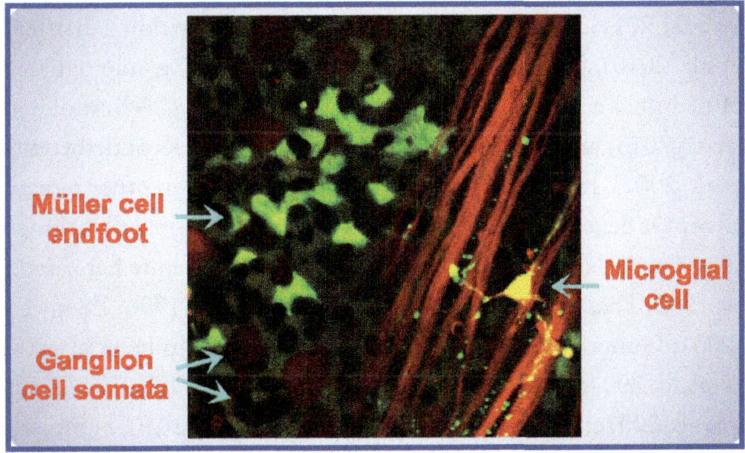

FIGURE 25: View onto the vitreal (inner) surface of a rabbit retina which was experimentally detached for 48 h. A freshly isolated retinal wholemount was stained with *Griffonia simplicifolia* agglutinin as a microglia/immune cell marker (*red*) and with Fura-Red (*green*). The calcium imaging record was obtained during administration of ATP (200 µM). ATP induced an increase of the cytosolic free calcium level in a subpopulation of Müller cell endfeet. Ganglion cell somata are *red-black*. The elongated structures are nerve fibers which are *red*-stained due to light reflection. Modified from Uhlmann et al. (2003).

[ADP]) induce membrane ruffling and filopodia extension while it has no effect on the distribution and ramified morphology of the cells (Haynes et al., 2006). Activation of $P2Y_{12}$ receptors is also required for the early microglia activation induced by ATP and ADP released from damaged neurons (Haynes et al., 2006). GPR34, a G protein-coupled receptor of the $P2Y_{12}$-like group, is involved in the regulation of microglia morphology and phagocytosis (Preissler et al., 2014). The microglial process motility is also increased by ionotropic glutamatergic neurotransmission and decreased by ionotropic GABA neurotransmission (Fontainhas et al., 2011). However, the neurotransmitter influences on retinal microglia are not directly mediated because microglial cells apparently do not express functional ionotropic glutamate receptors (iGluRs) and ionotropic GABA receptors (Fontainhas et al., 2011). Instead, these influences are mediated indirectly via extracellular ATP, released in response to glutamatergic neurotransmission (Fontainhas et al., 2011). Fractalkine signaling potentiates the rate of retinal microglial process motility and cellular migration (Liang et al., 2009).

3.3   MICROGLIA ACTIVATION

Microglial cells become early activated under pathological conditions (Figs. 10A-C, 12, D, E, 24) (Schuetz and Thanos, 2004). Microgliosis is associated with and may precede retinal degeneration (Zeiss and Johnson, 2004; Zeng et al., 2005; Gaucher et al., 2007; Kercher et al., 2007; Gehrig et al., 2007; Bosco et al., 2011). Microglial cells begin to migrate within 1 h after focal retinal laser damage (Paques et al., 2010). In experimental diabetic retinopathy, microglial cells are activated before the onset of neuronal cell death (Zeng et al., 2000b; Rungger-Brändle et al., 2000; Krady et al., 2005; Kezic et al., 2013) and proliferate already after three weeks of diabetes (Rungger-Brändle et al., 2000; Silva et al., 2007). In the further course of diabetes, like in other retinal pathologies such as inherited photoreceptor degeneration, retinal light injury, and retinal detachment (Figs. 10C, 24, 26A, B, D), migrating microglial cells invade the outer retina proliferate here, and phagocytize dead cell debris (Thanos, 1992; Thanos and Richter, 1993; Roque et al., 1996; Zeng et al., 2000b, 2008a; Ng and Streilein, 2001; Gupta et al., 2003; Francke et al., 2003; Koike et al., 2003; Hughes et al., 2003; Zeiss and Johnson, 2004; Chen et al., 2005; Zhang et al., 2005a; Lewis et al., 2005; Iandiev et al., 2006b; Yang et al., 2007c; Klebanov et al., 2009; Lewis et al., 2010; Santos et al., 2010; Collier et al., 2011; Sharma et al., 2012; Cebulla et al., 2012; Zhu et al., 2013; Kim et al., 2014). In the human retina of diabetic patients, activated microglia cluster around the retinal vasculature, especially the dilated veins, microaneurysms, hemorrhages, and cotton-wool spots (Zeng et al., 2008a). In proliferative diabetic retinopathy (PDR), microglial cells accumulate around the sites of neovascularization (Zeng et al., 2008a). Acute injury of the avian retina induces proliferation and migration of resident microglia and retinal immigration of exogenous microglia from the pecten (Jeon et al., 2004). Several months after injury, microglia regain their resting morphology, and the number of

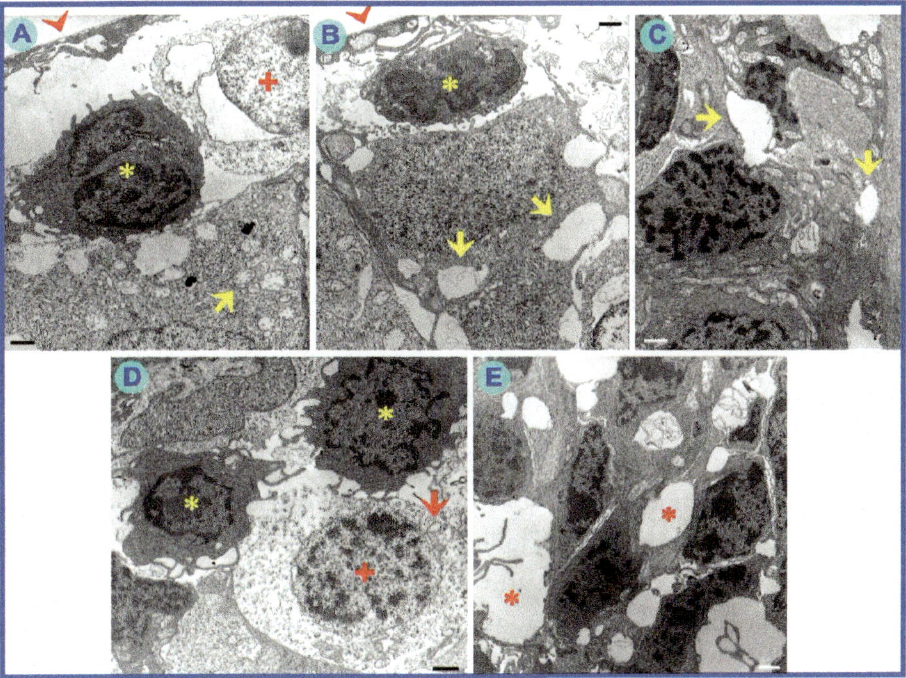

FIGURE 26: Early intra- and extracellular edema in the detached porcine retina. Electron microscopic images were taken from retinal areas that were experimentally detached for 24 h. **A.** A cell body in the ganglion cell layer displays intracellular edema (+), while another cell body contains swollen mitochondria (*arrow*). *Asterisk*, putative microglial cell. *Arrowhead*, inner limiting membrane. **B.** The ganglion cell layer contains edematous cystoid spaces (*arrows*) and a putative microglial cell (*). **C, D.** The inner nuclear layer contains cystoid spaces (*yellow arrows*), microglial cells (*), and several degenerating cells displaying intracellular edema (+) associated with an enlargement of the peri-nucleus space (*red arrow*). **E.** Cystoid spaces (*) in the outer nuclear layer of a detached retina. Bars, 1 μm. Modified from Hollborn et al. (2008).

microglial cells returns to control levels; the decrease in microglial cell number occurs at least in part by apoptosis of the cells (Jeon et al., 2004). Retinal detachment is associated with an early activation of a tripartite process involving inflammation, immune responses, and coagulation/fibrinolysis, which is probably triggered by the deconstruction of photoreceptors (because photoreceptor proteins are potent immunogens; Rahi and Addison, 1983; Adamus et al., 1994) and mediated by activation of immune cells (microglial cells in the retinal parenchyma, blood-derived macrophages in the subretinal space, and leukostasis in the blood vessels) (Hollborn et al., 2008).

Microglia activation is associated with a morphological transition from a stellate, ramified morphology to an amoeboid cell shape characteristic for the differentiation towards migratory phagocytes capable of clearing cell debris; activated microglial cells display an enlargement of their somata, shortening and thickening of their processes, and vacuolation (Fig. 10A) (Medana et al., 1997; Salvador-Silva et al., 2000; Jeon et al., 2004; Krady et al., 2005; Zhang et al., 2005b; Lee et al., 2008; Santos et al., 2010; Liu et al., 2012c; Ulbricht et al., 2013). Strongly activated, amoeboid microglial cells do not bear cell processes (Fig. 10A). Activation of purinergic $P2Y_1$ receptors accelerates the process retraction of activated microglia (Fig. 10A) (Uckermann et al., 2005d).

3.3.1   TRIGGER OF MICROGLIA ACTIVATION

Virtually all retinal injuries and diseases are associated with activation of inflammatory and immune processes, e.g., retinal detachment and diabetic retinopathy ("diabetic retinitis") (Gordon, 1967; Kern, 2007; Adamis and Berman, 2008; Hollborn et al., 2008; Tang and Kern, 2011). The local low-level inflammation in diabetic retinopathy is indicated by various molecular and cellular abnormalities such as adhesion of leukocytes to the vessel walls, increased expression of inflammatory factors like IL-1β and ICAM-1, vascular permeability, infiltration of blood-derived immune cells, complement deposition, activation of the redox-sensitive proinflammatory transcription factor NF-κB, and microglia activation (McLeod et al., 1995; Mizutani et al., 1998; Miyamoto et al., 1999; Barouch et al., 2000; Rungger-Brändle et al., 2000; Chakrabarti et al., 2000; Joussen et al., 2001; Zhang et al., 2002; Romeo et al., 2002; Kowluru et al., 2003; Ishida et al., 2003; Joussen et al., 2004; Dagher et al., 2004; Kowluru and Odenbach, 2004; Krady et al., 2005; Gerhardinger et al., 2005; Kaji et al., 2007; Gaucher et al., 2007; Silva et al., 2007; Pelikánová, 2007; Zeng et al., 2008a; Yang et al., 2009; Soufi et al., 2012; Liu et al., 2012a). Many of these features are seen also in high-fat diet-induced obesity resulting from insulin resistance (Marçal et al., 2013).

Microgliosis is triggered by various different molecules including lipopolysaccharide, IFN-γ, complement components, thrombin, aggregated, insoluble peptides, inflammatory cytokines, and chemokines such as IL-1β, IL-6, TNFα, IGF-1, VEGF, and fractalkine, as well as blood-derived advanced glycation end products (AGEs) and glycated albumin (Gregerson and Yang, 2003; Schuetz and Thanos, 2004; Krady et al., 2005; Ransohoff et al., 2007; Wang et al., 2007a,b, 2014a; Balasubramaniam et al., 2009; Ibrahim et al., 2010; 2011; Liu et al., 2011; Zelinka et al., 2012; Zhang et al., 2012; Xu et al., 2012; Couturier et al., 2014; Fischer et al., 2014; Zhao et al., 2014a). Among these molecules, lipopolysaccharide is the strongest inducer of microglia activation (Langmann, 2007). Lipopolysaccharide induces tissue plasminogen activator in microglial cells that contributes to the secretion of inflammatory factors like IL-1β and TNFα from the cells (Wang et al., 2009b).

Lipopolysaccharide also induces an immediate NADPH oxidase-dependent production of reactive oxygen species, NO production, and a NADPH oxidase-dependent increase in the activity of arginase-1 which contributes to retinal inflammation (El-Remessy et al., 2008; Zhang et al., 2009a). Experimental glaucoma induced by ocular hypertension results in a rapid upregulation of TNFα, followed sequentially by microglial activation, loss of optic nerve oligodendrocytes, and delayed loss of retinal ganglion cells (Nakazawa et al., 2006a).

There are further conditions that activate microglial cells. Hypoxia induces microglia proliferation (Morigiwa et al., 2000a), and a breakdown of the blood-retinal barrier elicits a thickening of microglial processes and a redistribution of microglia toward the vasculature (Medana et al., 2000). Gangliosides, hyaluronic acid, heparan sulfate, and extracellular heat shock proteins carry damage-associated molecular patterns and activate TLR in microglial cells (Mollen et al., 2006; Block et al., 2007; Luo et al., 2010). Early alarm signals released from degenerating neurons trigger TLR-dependent microglia activation which may also lead to attacks against healthy neurons by the release of cytotoxic cytokines and the initiation of immune responses against retinal antigens (Gehrig et al., 2007; Langmann, 2007). TLR4-mediated microglial activation, e.g., by lipopolysaccharide or endogenous photoreceptor proteins, aggravates retinal cell death, which is at least in part mediated by TNFα (Kilic et al., 2008; Ko et al., 2011; Kohno et al., 2013). Stimulation of TLR4 by damage-associated molecular patterns, which activates NLRP3 inflammasomes and induces the secretion of inflammatory factors like IL-1β and IL-18, is implicated in inducing tissue degeneration after retinal ischemia-reperfusion (Qi et al., 2014). TLR3-mediated microglia activation, in part mediated by NF-κB, contributes to retinal ganglion cell death after optic nerve transection (Lin et al., 2012). In diabetic retinopathy, hyperglycemic activation of the polyol pathway contributes to microglia activation (Chang et al., 2014). In experimental autoimmune uveitis, the oxidative stress-induced nitration of photoreceptor mitochondrial proteins and peroxidation of membrane lipids led to activation and migration of microglia toward the photoreceptors (Saraswathy and Rao, 2008).

M-CSF is a key factor for the initiation and maintenance of microglia activation, proliferation, and the phagocytic activity, independent of the initial trigger (Roque and Caldwell, 1993; Imai and Kohsaka, 2002; Langmann, 2007). In early experimental diabetic retinopathy, retinal astrocytes produce M-CSF that acts on its receptor (CSF-1R) expressed by microglial cells (Liu et al., 2009). M-CSF induces an inflammatory response in microglial cells characterized by an increased expression of TNFα, IL-1β, IL-6, macrophage inflammatory protein-1α (MIP-1α; Ccl3), M-CSF, and the inducible NO synthase (Mitrasinovic et al., 2001; Liu et al., 2011). The C-C chemokine MCP-1 is the most potent microglia chemoattractant (Fuentes et al., 1995; Kennedy et al., 1998; Fife et al., 2000; Izikson et al., 2000; Huang et al., 2001; Jiang et al., 2012b) and induces the accumulation of the cells at sites of pathology (Takata et al., 2007; Nakazawa et al., 2007a; Wang et al.,

2010a). Fractalkine is required for the accumulation of monocytes and microglia recruited by MCP-1 (Tacke et al., 2007). AGEs induces the expression of MCP-1 in retinal neurons which activates microglial cells (Dong et al., 2012). Retinal detachment induces MCP-1 in Müller cells (Nakazawa et al., 2007a; Hollborn et al., 2008). Intravitreal inflammatory factors like IL-1β induce MCP-1 in perivascular microglia, astrocytes, endothelial cells, and infiltrating macrophages (Cuff et al., 2000). MCP-1 also recruits bone marrow-derived monocytic precursor cells into the retina that replace resident microglial cells (Chen et al., 2012). Microglia migration is also under the control of the chemokine receptor-5 (Marella et al., 2004) which has various ligands including MIP-1α (Ccl3), MIP-1β (Ccl4), RANTES (Ccl5), and MCP-2 (Ccl8).

Activated microglia may also exacerbate retinal pathologies after systemic infections. In mice, systemic infection with the cytomegalovirus elicited an increase in the number of microglia in the subretinal space and an accumulation of iris macrophages; accumulation of microglia in the subretinal space does not occur by recruitment of circulating monocytes but by IFN-γ-dependent migration of resident retinal microglia (Zinkernagel et al., 2013). Activation of TLR3 (which recognizes viral double-stranded RNA) in microglial and retinal pigment epithelial cells induces microglia activation, suggesting that viral infections in the retinal pigment epithelium may have a proinflammatory influence on retinal microglia (Klettner et al., 2014). Furthermore, systemic fungal infection causes activation of retinal microglia (Maneu et al., 2014). Gram-positive bacteria, e.g., staphylococci which are a leading cause of endophthalmitis (Kumar et al., 2013a), increases the expression of TLR2 in retinal microglia; activation of TLR2 by bacterial cell wall components results in secretion of proinflammatory mediators like TNFα and MIP-2 (Kochan et al., 2012). Pretreatment of microglial cells with an TLR2 ligand reduces the production of proinflammatory factors but stimulates the phagocytosis of bacteria (Kumar et al., 2010; Kochan et al., 2012). Bacterial and viral infections of the cornea result in upregulation of TLR9 (which recognizes unmethylated CpG-DNA released by proliferating and dying microbes) in the retina, activate retinal microglia, and induce retinal infiltration of neutrophils and macrophages (Chinnery et al., 2012a).

3.3.2 CHARACTERISTICS OF ACTIVATED MICROGLIA

Microglia activation is characterized by the generation of reactive oxygen species, activation of tyrosine kinases, extracellular signal-regulated kinases 1 and 2 (ERK1/2), p38 mitogen-activated protein kinase (MAPK), and c-Jun N-terminal kinase (JNK), increased NF-κB expression and nuclear translocation of NF-κB, and endoplasmic reticulum stress (Krady et al., 2005; Sappington and Calkins, 2006, 2008; Shimazawa et al., 2007; Yang et al., 2007a,b; Wang et al., 2007a,b; El-Remessy et al., 2008; Zeng et al., 2008b; Ibrahim et al., 2010, 2011a; Ahmad et al., 2013; Zhao et al., 2014a). The translocation of NF-κB induced by elevated intraocular pressure is in part mediated by a calcium influx from the extracellular space through mechanosensitive transient receptor potential vanilloid-1 receptor (TRPV1) cation channels (Sappington and Calkins, 2008). Activation of microglial cells is also associated with an upregulation of intracellular calcium responses triggered by purinergic P2 receptor activation; increased calcium responses may account for the increase in the release of neurotransmitters and inflammatory mediators found in diabetic retinas, for example (Pereira et al., 2010). Activated microglia express both metabotropic P2Y and calcium-permeable $P2X_7$ receptors; activation of P2Y receptors induces microglia proliferation while activation of $P2X_7$ receptors suppresses microglia proliferation but increases the release of $TNF\alpha$ and IL-1β (Morigiwa et al., 2000a,b). High glucose increases the calcium responses of microglial cells mediated by both P2Y and calcium-permeable P2X receptors (Pereira et al., 2010).

Activated microglia upregulate the expression of chemokines (e.g., eotaxin and Ccl5), secrete proinflammatory cytokines like M-CSF, IL-1β, IL-6, IL-10, $TNF\alpha$, and MCP-1, release superoxide anions, produce neurotoxic MMPs and glutamate, increase the expression of the inducible NO synthase and cyclooxygenase-2 which produces NO and prostaglandins, respectively, and express Fas and Fas-ligand (Koeberle and Ball, 1999; Klöcker et al., 1999; Nakamura, 2002; Carter and Dick, 2003; Zeng et al., 2005; Krady et al., 2005; Wang et al., 2005a, 2007a,b; Ju et al., 2006; Sappington and Calkins, 2006, 2008; Zhang et al., 2007c; Yang et al., 2007a,b; El-Remessy et al., 2008; Balasubramaniam et al., 2009; Wu et al., 2009; Ibrahim et al., 2010, 2011a; Husain et al., 2011; Liu et al., 2011; Xu et al., 2012; Ahmad et al., 2013; Jiang et al., 2013; Wang et al., 2013a; Devarajan et al., 2014; Klettner et al., 2014; Zhao et al., 2014a). The majority of these microglia-secreted molecules can cause progressive neurodegeneration upon chronic exposure (Langmann, 2007). In diabetic retinopathy, glycated albumin induces the expression of adenosine deaminase-2 in microglial cells; the action of this adenosine-degrading enzyme results in a decreased level of the antiinflammatory mediator adenosine (see 3.6.) that is required for the microglial release of $TNF\alpha$ (Elsherbiny et al., 2013).

There are studies which described that microglial cells (as well as perivascular macrophages) constitutively express MHC class I and II molecules (Penfold et al., 1993; Liew et al., 1994; Provis et al., 1995; Diaz-Araya et al., 1995a; Cuff et al., 1996; Zhang et al., 1997; Yang et al., 2000; Chen et al., 2002; Gregerson and Yang, 2003; Huang et al., 2008). However, other studies showed no MHC class I- and II-positive cells in the normal retina (Dick et al., 1995; Yang et al., 1996a; Akaishi et al., 1998; Villarroya et al., 2001; Zhang et al., 2005b). Microglial expression of MHC class I and II molecules increases under pathological conditions, for example, in response to hypoxia, IFN-γ, amyloid-β peptide, oxidative stress, elevated intraocular pressure, and the exposure to extracellular heat shock proteins that induce TLR signaling (Akaishi et al., 1998; Matsubara et al., 1999;

Broderick et al., 2000; Walsh et al., 2005; Kaur et al., 2006; Luo et al., 2010; Gallego et al., 2012; Ebneter et al., 2010). IL-1 induces a migration of perivascular macrophages away from the blood vessels and upregulation of MHC class II in the cells (Cuff et al., 1996). Hematopoietically derived retinal perivascular microglia that express MHC class II molecules, IL-1β, and TNFα initiate uveo-retinitis in experimental autoimmune uveitis (Gullapalli et al., 2000).

3.4   MIGRATION OF MICROGLIA

Activation of microglia is associated with an increased expression of adhesion proteins which allows the cells to adhere to Müller cells; activated microglia translocate intraretinally in a radial direction using Müller cell processes as an adhesive scaffold (Sánchez-López et al., 2004; Wang et al., 2011). Microglia migrate towards the outer retina by the emission of a leading thin radial process that ramifies at the outer end before retraction of the rear of the cell (Sánchez-López et al., 2004). Through the inner nuclear layer to the outer plexiform layer, microglial cells migrate by another mechanism: they retract cell processes, become round, and squeeze through neuronal bodies (Sánchez-López et al., 2004). Tenascin plays a role in the stopping and ramification of radially migrating microglial cells (Sánchez-López et al., 2004). Levels where microglial cells stop and ramify are always between retinal strata with strong tenascin expression and strata with weak or no tenascin expression (Sánchez-López et al., 2004). When microglial cell radial migration ends, retinal tenascin expression is downregulated (Sánchez-López et al., 2004). The spread of retinal gliosis and retinal degeneration from the locally detached into the surrounding non-detached tissue might be mediated (in addition to the diffusion of growth and inflammatory factors) by migrating activated microglia (Figs. 10C; 12D, E; see 5.11.5.).

3.5   MICROGLIAL CONTRIBUTION TO NEURONAL DEGENERATION

Although inflammation normally protects from dangerous stimuli and restores normal tissue homeostasis, chronic, overstimulated, and dysregulated inflammation is a major cause of secondary tissue damage (Buschini et al., 2011). Activated microglia induces neuronal degeneration by the release of neurotoxins such as TNFα, IL-1β, reactive oxygen intermediates, NO, proteases, excitatory amino acids, and Fas-ligand (Banati et al., 1993; De Kozak et al., 1997; Krady et al., 2005; Ju et al., 2006; Wang et al., 2007b; Ibrahim et al., 2011; Sivakumar et al., 2011; Liu et al., 2012b; Roh et al., 2012; Kaur et al., 2013; Wang et al., 2013a; Zeng et al., 2014). Activated microglia induce death of photoreceptor cells and neurons *in vitro* (Roque et al., 1999; Srinivasan et al., 2004;

Krady et al., 2005; Nakazawa et al., 2007a; Yang et al., 2007a; Zhou et al., 2012; Jiang et al., 2013). Microglia-induced photoreceptor apoptosis *in vitro* is apparently independent on the expression of proinflammatory factors like IL-1β and TNFα (Jiang et al., 2013). Microglia-derived NGF or pro-NGF and activation of p75^{NTR} are required to induce apoptosis in the developing retina and in cultured photoreceptor cells (Frade and Barde, 1998; Roque et al., 1999; Srinivasan et al., 2004). In addition to NGF, TGF-β is required for the programmed cell death in the developing retina (Dünker et al., 2001). Microglia also initiate a cell death program in vascular cells of the developing retina by activation of the canonical wingless pathway (Lobov et al., 2005).

Inhibition of microglia activation slows hereditary and light-induced photoreceptor degeneration, the death of retinal ganglion cells after axotomy in rats, and has protective effects in the diabetic retina (Thanos et al., 1993, 1995; Krady et al., 2005; Ibrahim et al., 2011a,b; Zhang et al., 2012; Liu et al., 2012b; Zeng et al., 2014; Peng et al., 2014; Arroba et al., 2014). In hereditary photoreceptor degeneration, depletion of microglial cells reduces the level of photoreceptor cell death without affecting Müller gliosis (Arroba et al., 2014). Activated microglia may contribute to inherited retinal degeneration by phagocytosis of photoreceptor-derived lipids such as docosahexaenoic acid (Ebert et al., 2009). Phagocytotic monocytes/macrophages and microglial cells release oxygen and nitrogen free radicals and toxic cytokines that induce photoreceptor apoptosis (Cuthbertson et al., 1990; Nakazawa et al., 2006b, 2007a). In the light-injured retina, microglial cells produce MIP-1α that recruits polymorphonuclear leukocytes to the subretinal space; deficiency of MIP-1α attenuates the severity of hereditary and light-induced photoreceptor degeneration (Kohno et al., 2014).

Microglial cells may contribute to neuronal degeneration also indirectly, by the regulation of macroglial gliosis. There is a bidirectional cross-talk between activated microglia and macroglial cells in the normal and diseased retina (Wang and Wong, 2014; see 5.11.4.). Macroglial cells regulate the activation status of microglial cells and their capacity for phagocytosis of cellular debris (Dick et al., 2003). Reactive Müller cells produce cytokines and chemokines such as MCP-1 that recruit monocytes/macrophages to the site of injury, e.g., to the subretinal space in cases of retinal detachment and retinal light injury (Fig. 21A, C), where they phagocytize the cellular debris of deconstructed photoreceptor segments (Hisatomi et al., 2003; Nakazawa et al., 2006b, 2007a; Hollborn et al., 2008; Rutar et al., 2011a, 2012b). Activated microglia produce endothelin-2 which induces astrogliosis, retinal ganglion cell death, and vasoconstriction; microglia-mediated vascular dysfunction is involved, for example, in the development of glaucoma (Howell et al., 2011; Tonari et al., 2012). After retinal light injury, activated microglia modify the survival of photoreceptor cells by controlling the production of neurotrophic factors in Müller cells (Harada et al., 2002a;

see 5.11.7.). In the light-degenerated retina, activated microglia invade the photoreceptor layer and increase the production of NGF; NGF decreases the production of bFGF in Müller cells through activation of p75^{NTR}, resulting in enhanced photoreceptor apoptosis (Harada and Harada, 2004). Microglia-derived IL-6 also inhibits the neurogenesis from retinal progenitor cells (see 5.11.12.) and their neuronal differentiation in the injured retina (Balasubramaniam et al., 2009; Dick, 2009).

3.6   MICROGLIAL CONTRIBUTION TO NEURONAL SURVIVAL

Microglia activation can also promote neuroprotection and regeneration. Resting and activated microglia produce neurotrophic factors such as BDNF, CNTF, glial cell line-derived neurotrophic factor (GDNF), neurotrophin-3, neurotrophin-4, and bFGF, as well as antiinflammatory cytokines that support neuronal and photoreceptor survival (Srinivasan et al., 2004; Langmann, 2007; Sharma et al., 2012; McCarthy et al., 2013). Activated microglia release GDNF and CNTF that stimulate CNTF and bFGF production in Müller cells which together enhance photoreceptor survival (Harada et al., 2002a; see 5.11.7.). Microglial cells secrete further factors, e.g., oncomodulin, that stimulate the survival and regeneration of retinal ganglion cells (Yin et al., 2003, 2006). Microglia-derived IL-6 protects retinal ganglion cells from death by countering microglial proapoptotic signals and the apoptotic cascade intrinsic to ganglion cells (Sappington et al., 2006; Fisher et al., 2001). Activated microglia also benefit surviving cells by removing toxic byproducts, pathogens, extravasated serum proteins, and cell debris (Miller and Oberdorfer, 1981; Claudio et al., 1994; Bodeutsch and Thanos, 2000; Maneu et al., 2011). IGF-1 protects photoreceptor cells from death by a mechanism that includes microglia activation (Arroba et al., 2011). Experimental retinitis pigmentosa is associated with a proliferation of resident microglial cells and an recruitment of bone marrow-derived microglial precursors to the subretinal space and outer nuclear layer (Sasahara et al., 2008; Wang et al., 2013a). Depletion of the bone marrow-derived microglial precursors accelerates the retinal degeneration while systemic mobilization of hematopoietic precursors has a rescue effect (Sasahara et al., 2008; Wang et al., 2013a). In contrast to the recruited bone marrow-derived microglial cells, the proliferating resident microglial cells contribute to photoreceptor degeneration (Wang et al., 2013a).

Under normal conditions, retinal microglia suppress T cell activation (Gregerson et al., 2004). In autoimmune disease, microglia have dual functions: initiating uveoretinitis, but also limiting subsequent inflammation (Chen et al., 2002). It was shown that retinal autoimmunity may have also neuroprotective effects, via locally activated T cells that induce a microglial phenotype which reduces neuronal loss caused by amyloid-β, for example (Avidan et al., 2004). Activated microglia stimulate T cell proliferation; however, microglia direct the responding T cells toward the Th2 pathway, and release the immunosuppressive cytokine TGF-β (Ma and Streilein, 1999).

3.7   SUPPRESSION OF MICROGLIA ACTIVATION

At present, it is unclear why microglia are sometimes damaging and other times protective. In the injured mouse spinal cord, two distinct microglial populations with either neurotoxic or regenerative effects have been identified (Kigerl et al., 2009). Immunosuppressive cytokines such as thrombospondin-1 and TGF-β direct activated microglia cells to an antiinflammatory phenotype by blocking inflammatory gene expression (Paglinawan et al., 2003). The exacerbated expression of microglia-associated inflammatory genes in the thrombospondin-1-deficient retina correlates with a poor recovery from retinal injury (Ng et al., 2009). Microglia possess autoregulatory mechanisms that induce apoptosis of overactivated microglial cells; these mechanisms include the expression of the macrophage deactivation gene DAP12 and caspase 11 (Lee et al., 2001; Nakamura, 2002). Microglia overactivation might be also prevented by activation of TLR4 that triggers microglia apoptosis (Jung et al., 2005). Reprogramming of TLR4 by lipopolysacharide prevents the microglia activation induced by retinal ischemia; this is associated with a reduction of the neuronal degeneration upon a following ischemia (Halder et al., 2013). Stimulation with IFN-γ plus lipopolysacharide induces an IL-10-mediated downregulation of MHC class II molecules and a loss of migratory and phagocytic activity of microglia (Broderick et al., 2000). Multiple TLR ligands and IFN-γ induce the expression of the activated microglia/macrophage whey acidic domain protein (AMWAP) (Karlstetter et al., 2010b). AMWAP is a counter-regulator of microglia activation and reduces the microglial production of the proinflammatory cytokines IL-6 and IL-1β (Karlstetter et al., 2010b). The chemokine receptor CX3CR1 was also shown to negatively regulate microglia activation and retinal inflammation and degeneration after ischemia (Chen et al., 2013a). In addition, activation of adenosine A_{2A} receptors possess antiinflammatory properties, attenuates microglia activation, and inhibits the hypoxia- and lipopolysaccharide-induced release of TNFα from microglial cells (Ahmad et al., 2013). Prolonged activation of ionotropic $P2X_7$ receptors in retinal microglia by high concentrations of ATP induces the formation of large pores in the plasma membrane (Innocenti et al., 2004). Activation of $P2X_7$ receptors inhibits microglial proliferation and induces apoptosis of microglia (Morigiwa et al., 2000a,b).

In retinal inflammation and injury, astrocytes and Müller cells upregulate the expression of acyl coenzyme A-binding protein (ACBP; also known as "diazepam binding inhibitor"); ACBP-derived ligands activate the mitochondrial translocator protein (TSPO) which is increasingly expressed in activated microglial cells (Wang et al., 2014b; Karlstetter et al., 2014). Activation of TSPO negatively regulates features of microglial activation, including reactive oxygen species production, expression of TNF-α, MCP-1, IL-6, and inducible NO synthase, and microglia proliferation and migration (Wang et al., 2014b; Karlstetter et al., 2014). Activation of TSPO also promotes the formation of filopodia and increases the phagocytic capacity of activated microglial cells (Karlstetter et al., 2014). The increased macroglial expression of ACBP suggests that astrocytes and Müller cells limit the magnitude of inflammatory responses by facilitating the quiescence of microglial cells (Wang et al., 2014b).

Recent studies provide novel treatment options for the inhibition of overactivated microglia and the preservation of the trophic and homeostatic functions of the cells. Early inhibition of microglia activation, e.g., by peptides derived from the pigment epithelium-derived growth factor (PEDF) (Liu et al., 2012b), has protective effects in the diabetic retina. Antiinflammatory ω-3- and ω-6-polyunsaturated fatty acids such as docosahexaenoic acid inhibit the microglial production of TNFα and convert proinflammatory microglia to a neuroprotective phenotype that delays inherited retinal degeneration (Connor et al., 2007; Ebert et al., 2009; Mirza et al., 2013). A similar change to an antiinflammatory and neuroprotective phenotype was found after treatment with vegetable polyphenols like curcumin and luteolin (Dirscherl et al., 2010; Mirza et al., 2013). Luteolin downregulates the proinflammatory and proapoptotic gene expression (e.g., of proinflammatory cytokines and NO synthases) and upregulates the expression of genes related to antioxidant metabolism, phagocytic uptake, ramification, and chemotaxis (Dirscherl et al., 2010). Intravitral injection of the neuroprotectant pituitary adenylyl cyclase activating polypeptide (PACAP) alters the microglia status into an acquired deactivation subtype that favors their neuroprotective effects; this effect is associated with an increased microglial expression of antiinflammatory cytokines such as TGF-β1 and IL-10 and a decreased level of N-methyl-D-aspartate (NMDA)-induced cell loss in the retinal ganglion cell layer (Wada et al., 2013). Further molecules that inhibit microglia activation are, for example, the antioxidant agent N-acetylcysteine, carbon dioxide, IL-13, the tyrosine kinase inhibitor genistein, inhibitors of serotonin 5-HT$_{1A}$ receptors, Rho-kinase inhibitors, α-crystallin, IGFBP-3, cannabidiol, baicalein, blockers of voltage-gated potassium channels, the alkaloids sinomenine and sulforaphane, a chondroitin sulfate-derived disaccharide, clodronate, agonists of σ1 receptors, and the tetracycline derivative minocycline (Marie et al., 1999; Lemaitre et al., 2001; Hughes et al., 2004; Zhang et al., 2004a; Krady et al., 2005; Baptiste et al., 2005; Wang et al., 2005a, 2007b; Rolls et al., 2006; Bakalash et al., 2007; El-Remessy et al., 2008; Bosco et al., 2008; Tura et al., 2009; Yang et al., 2007b,c, 2009; Wu et al., 2009; Ibrahim et al., 2010; Koeberle and Schlichter, 2010; Kielczewski et al., 2011; Collier et al., 2011; Schallner et al., 2012; Yoshida et al., 2013; Peng et al., 2014 ; Zhao et al., 2014a; Wu et al., 2014). The effect of cannabidiol is mediated by inhibition of the adenosine uptake and subsequent activation of adenosine A_{2A} receptors in microglial cells (Liou et al., 2008). In addition, morphine inhibits the hypoxic and lipopolysaccharide-induced microglial production of TNFα; retinal microglia express δ-, κ-, and μ-opioid receptor subtypes (Husain et al., 2011). However, naloxone, an opioid receptor antagonist, was also shown to inhibit microglia activation and the microglial production of proinflammatory factors (Ni et al., 2008; Shen et al., 2011a; Xu et al., 2012). Furthermore, retinal microglia activation, as well as degeneration of retinal ganglion and photoreceptor cells, is inhibited by antiinflammatory steroids such as dexamethasone and fluocinolone acetonide (Glybina et al., 2009; Ryu et al., 2011). In another study, the antiinflammatory glucocorticoid triamcinolone acetonide suppressed microglia activation but not the death of retinal ganglion cells (Singhal et al., 2010; Huang et al., 2011c). However, it has been also described that acetylsalicylate and prednisolone may aggravate microglia activation (Sarra et al., 2005).

3.8   MICROGLIA IN THE AGING RETINA

With advancing age, microglia undergo changes in gene expression patterns that give rise to pathogenic phenotypes and to a dysregulation of the immune response (Ma et al., 2013a). In retinas of old animals, microglia, Müller glial cells, and astrocytes display increased signs of gliosis compared to retinas of young animals (Kim et al., 2004). Aged resting microglia have smaller and less branched dendritic arbors, and slower process motilities, which probably compromise their ability to survey and interact with their environment (Damani et al., 2011). While young microglia respond to extracellular ATP by increasing their motility and becoming more ramified, aged microglia exhibit a contrary response, becoming less dynamic and ramified (Damani et al., 2011). Upon retinal injury, aged microglia show slower acute responses with lower rates of process motility and cellular migration while the long term response is more sustained compared with young microglia (Damani et al., 2011). During aging, amyloid precursor protein (expressed by Müller cells; Chen et al., 1997a, 1998, 1999a) is upregulated in the retina; amyloid-β peptides represent one of the triggers of complement activation and microglia activation during the normal aging process (Seth et al., 2008).

In the healthy young adult retina, the outer nuclear layer and the subretinal space are devoid of microglia (Figs. 10C, 24) (Combadière et al., 2007; Xu et al., 2009). In the aging retina, oxidized photoreceptor lipoproteins and free radicals are major causes of tissue stress and serve as local triggers for microglia activation and other signs of inflammation such as complement activation and upregulation of inflammatory cytokines and chemokines (Saraswathy et al., 2006; Xu et al., 2009; Buschini et al., 2011). The subretinal accumulation of microglia is likely triggered by the inefficient clearance of oxidized lipids normally carried out by the retinal pigment epithelium (Favret et al.,

2013). Microglia migrate from the inner retina into the subretinal space to support the retinal pigment epithelium in the clearance of oxidized photoreceptor discs (Kunert et al., 1999; Kezic et al., 2008; Xu et al., 2009; Karlstetter et al., 2010a; Lei et al., 2012; Chinnery et al., 2012b). The subretinal and perivascular microglia contain autofluorescent lipofuscin granules (Combadière et al., 2007; Xu et al., 2008; Chinnery et al., 2012b) which is a "waste" material in the aging human retina and implicated in the formation of drusen, atrophy of the retinal pigment epithelium, and development of AMD (Anderson et al., 2002). In AMD, microglial cells and blood-borne macrophages are activated (Van der Schaft et al., 1993; Penfold et al., 1997) and accumulate in the subretinal space (Gupta et al., 2003; Combadière et al., 2007). Subretinal microglia/macrophages induce MCP-1 in the retinal pigment epithelium (Ma et al., 2009). Intracellular lipofuscin constituents induce microglial activation and decreases the microglial protection of photoreceptors (Ma et al., 2013b). Intracellular lipofuscin also suppresses microglial chemotaxis and may thus potentiate the subretinal microglia accumulation (Ma et al., 2013b). The subretinal microglia was suggested to form "crystallization" points for cellular deposits and complement-containing immune complexes, and activates retinal pigment epithelial cells (Xu et al., 2009). Amyloid-β, which increases with age in the outer retina (Begum et al., 2013), and proinflammatory factors secreted from activated retinal pigment epithelial cells further stimulate microglia migration and activation. Activated microglia in the subretinal space recruit microglial precursors from the bloodstream (Combadière et al., 2007) which may reach the subretinal space through pores in retinal pigment epithelial cells (Omri et al., 2011).

The chemokine MCP-1 and the chemokine receptor CX3CR1 are suggested to be critically involved in the subretinal microglia recruitment and the appearance of AMD-like characteristics in the aged mouse retina (Combadière et al., 2007; Chen et al., 2007a; Raoul et al., 2008; Ross et al., 2008; Luhmann et al., 2009). The production of MCP-1 in the retinal pigment epithelium is stimulated by amyloid-β, a major component of drusen (Wang et al., 2009c). Amyloid-β also increases the production of IL-1β and TNFα in microglia and macrophages (Wang et al., 2009c). Infiltrating macrophages and resident microglia are also a major source of the complement factor C3, a complement activator associated with retinal light damage and the pathogenesis of AMD (Nozaki et al., 2006; Yates et al., 2007; Tuo et al., 2007; Francis et al., 2009; Chi et al., 2010; Collier et al., 2011; Rutar et al., 2011b, 2012a). The microglial expression of the complement genes C3 and CFB, the main activator of the alternative complement pathway, increases with aging (Ma et al., 2013a). Hypoxia stimulates the expression of the complement 3 receptor in microglia (Kaur et al., 2006). In the presence of amyloid-β, microglia induce the expression of CFB in retinal pigment epithelium cells (Wang et al., 2009c). TNFα increases the expression of C3 and decreases the expression of CFH in retinal microglia (Luo et al., 2011). Intracellular lipofuscin induces the expression of CFB and decreases the expression of CFH in microglial cells, favoring increased complement activation and deposition in the outer retina (Ma et al., 2013b). Activated complement factors C3a and C5a participate in neutrophil and macrophage recruitment to the subretinal space in choroidal neovascularization (Nozaki et al., 2006), the key pathological event of wet AMD (see 5.11.8.). Deletion of the complement receptor 3 prevents microglia activation and the pathophysiological effects of ocular hypertension, suggesting that activated microglial cells play a crucial role in the loss of retinal ganglion cells under this condition (Nakazawa et al., 2006a).

Activated microglia containing phagocytosed photoreceptor debris may actively exit the subretinal space via retinal and choroidal vessels, and may reach the spleen, where they act as antigen-presenting cells and elicit systemic immune responses against retinal antigens (Raoul et al., 2008). Elevated levels of antiretinal antibodies have been found in the serum of patients with AMD (Penfold et al., 1990; Gu et al., 2003; Patel et al., 2005). Immunization of mice with protein-coupled carboxyethylpyrrole, an oxidation product of retinal fatty acids, triggers a systemic immune response with autoantibodies and a secondary infiltration of microglia into the subretinal space (Hollyfield et al., 2010). Microglia containing engulfed photoreceptor debris which leave the retina through optic nerve head capillaries into the circulation was also found in experimental light-induced retinal degeneration (Joly et al., 2009). Antibodies against retinal and optic nerve antigens are implicated in the retinal ganglion cell death and microglia activation in glaucoma (Joachim et al., 2012; Gramlich et al., 2013; Rieck, 2013). Autoimmunity against retinal antigens, e.g., photoreceptor and glial proteins and proteins of the retinal pigment epithelium, may also contribute to the pathogenesis of various other retinal diseases including retinitis pigmentosa, retinal detachment, retinal vasculitis, and diabetic retinopathy, and may be induced by argon laser photocoagulation, for example (Rahi and Addison, 1983; Adamus et al., 1994; Teplinskaia et al., 2006). Furthermore, antibodies to retinal antigens are also found in patients with systemic lupus erythematosus and other systemic immune disorders without ocular involvement (Rahi and Addison, 1983).

Activated microglia also contribute to the progression of AMD to a neovascular stage (wet AMD) (Combadière et al., 2007; Raoul et al., 2010). Microglia accumulate at sites of choroidal neovascularization by a process dependent on VEGF receptor-1 (Combadière et al., 2007; Huang et al., 2013b; Caicedo et al., 2005a). Transplantation of activated microglia into the subretinal space of mice triggers the development of choroidal neovascularization (Ma et al., 2009), and accumulation of microglia in the subretinal space of CX3CR1-deficient mice is associated with an exacerbation of experimental choroidal neovascularization (Combadière et al., 2007). Activated microglia produce angiogenic factors such as TNFα that stimulates the expression of angiogenic molecules like MCP-1, IL-8, and bFGF in macroglial cells (Yoshida et al., 2004a). In experimental choroidal neovascularization, infiltrating macrophages and resident microglia express VEGF, the major angiogenic factor implicated in wet AMD (see 5.11.8.), prior to the increased VEGF expression in the retinal pigment epithelium (Ishibashi et al., 1997; Liu et al., 2013a; Krause et al., 2014). The uptake of damaged retinal pigment epithelial cells induces the expression of VEGF in macrophages and microglia (Liu et al., 2013a). In animal models of choroidal neovascularization, activation of the pattern recognition receptor RAGE induces chemotactic migration of microglial cells (Chen et al., 2014). RAGE is a member of the Ig superfamily that has several ligands including AGEs, S100B, high-mobility group box-1 protein, amyloid-β, Mac-1, and phosphatidylserine (Hofmann et al., 1999; Taniguchi et al., 2003; Chavakis et al., 2003). High-mobility group box-1 is released from necrotic cells and by active secretion from immune cells such as macrophages and dendritic cells, and induces retinal inflammation associated with neuronal degeneration (Dvoriantchikova et al., 2011). Choroidal neovascularization is oftenly associated with subretinal hemorrhage. Subretinal hemorrhage induce microglial infiltration into the outer retina concurrently with photoreceptor degeneration; inhibition of microglia activation attenuates photoreceptor degeneration (Zhao et al., 2011). In addition, activated microglia are involved in the induction of retinal neovascularization (see 5.11.8.)

Breakdown of the blood-retinal barrier, MHC class II expression, microglia activation, and trafficking of activated T cells are associated with physiological aging (Chan-Ling et al., 2007). Activated microglia also contribute to the breakdown of the blood-retinal barrier resulting in vasogenic edema, a characteristic of wet AMD (see 5.11.9.1.). Microglia release several factors including VEGF, NO, and MMPs which dissolve the blood-retinal barrier and thus facilitate the retinal infiltration of leukocytes (Figs. 21C, 24). Invading monocytes/macrophages and neutrophils release cytotoxic cytokines and reactive oxygen species which normally kill microorganisms, but are also harmful to photoreceptors and neurons. However, whether activated microglia contribute, directly and indirectly, to the neuronal degeneration and the propagation of vascular damage (Feng et al., 2011), e.g., in the diabetic retina, remains to be further elucidated. In human subjects with diabetic macular edema, assumed to be primarily caused by vascular leakage (see 5.11.9.1.), oral administration of minocycline improves visual function, macular edema, and vascular leakage (Cukras et al., 2012).

C H A P T E R   4

Retinal Oligodendroglia

In most vertebrates, retinal ganglion cell axons are myelinated in the extraocular part of the optic nerve, but remain nonmyelinated in the retinal nerve fiber layer and the intraocular portion of the optic nerve (optic nerve head). Myelination of the optic nerve axons ceases abruptly in the region of the lamina cribrosa (Perides et al., 1990). Oligodendrocytes are present in the myelinated nerve fiber bundles in the retinas of some fish, of amphibians and birds, as well as of rabbits (Fig. 6C), hares, and dogs (Wolburg, 1980; Kalinina, 1983; Easter et al., 1984; Schnitzer, 1985; Reichenbach et al., 1988c; Perides et al., 1990; Nakazawa et al., 1993; Won et al., 2000). Due to an increase of light scattering (see 5.4.1.), myelination of axons in the nerve fiber layer must cause a decrease in the quality of image perception by the underlying photoreceptor cells (Leys et al., 1996; Hunter et al., 1997; Straatsma et al., 1979, 1981; Ali et al., 1994). Apparently this can be tolerated in some retinas such as that of rabbits and hares where a special course of the myelinated fibers (Fig. 6C) circumvents retinal areas that are crucial for vision (i.e., the 'visual streak').

In the adult avian retina, oligodendrocytes are distributed in the nerve fiber/ganglion cell layers throughout the retina, with a central-to-peripheral gradient; in addition, immature oligodendrocytes are present in the immediate vicinity of the optic head (Cho et al., 1997, 1999; Seo et al., 2001). Here, oligodendrocytes are closely associated with the soma and axons of ganglion cells (Cho et al., 1999; Seo et al., 2001). In the avian retina, myelin is produced only in the central retina, but not by oligodendrocytes in the retinal periphery, suggesting that oligodendrocytes also play a trophic role for retinal ganglion cells (Cho et al., 1999; Seo et al., 2001). Ganglion cell axons in the chicken retina are ensheathed by loose myelin in the retinal nerve fiber layer and by compact myelin in the intra- and extraocular optic nerve (Fujita et al., 2001).

In non-myelinated retinas, ganglion cell axons possess node-like specializations (Fig. 16A) which mediate a saltatory propagation of action potentials similar as, but slower than, in myelin ated axons of the same diameter (Chao et al., 1994b, and references therein). These node-like specializations are surrounded by finger-like processes extending from astrocytes and Müller cells (Fig. 16A, B) (Holländer et al.. 1991; Chao et al., 1994b). In myelinated retinas, oligodendrocytes secrete factors which induce the clustering of sodium channels in the nodes of retinal ganglion cell axons (Kaplan et al., 1997); myelination increases the conduction velocity of retinal ganglion cell axons (Tolhurst and Lewis, 1992). The blood vessels in the myelinated medullary rays of the rabbit retina (Fig. 6C) are surrounded by astrocytes and oligodendrocytes (Morcos et al., 1999), suggesting that both cell types contribute to the barrier properties of the vessels. Abnormal myelination of the retinal nerve fiber layer in humans was found to be associated with vascular anomalies (Rosen et al., 1999).

In vertebrate species with myelinated retinas, both oligodendrocytes and Müller glial cells form the loose myelin that enwraps the large ganglion cell axons (Yamada, 1989; Quesada et al., 2011). Müller cells of species with myelinated, but not of species with unmyelinated retinas (but see Stefansson et al., 1984), express (in addition to other myelin molecules) myelin oligodendrocyte-specific protein (Quesada et al., 2011). Müller cells of the embryonic chicken retina begin to express this protein just before myelination starts (Quesada et al., 2011).

4.1 DEVELOPMENT OF OPTIC NERVE AND RETINAL MYELINATION

Oligodendrocyte progenitor cells are generated in the preoptic area (localized in the ventral diencephalon) from where they colonize the developing optic nerve toward the retina (Small et al., 1987; Fulton et al., 1992; Pringle et al., 1992). In species with unmyelinated retinas, the progenitor cells stop their migration in the region of the lamina cribrosa, and differentiate into myelinating oligodendrocytes (Berliner, 1931; Black et al., 1985; Sefton and Lam, 1984; Hildebrand et al., 1985; Ffrench-Constant et al., 1988; Perry and Lund, 1990; Bartsch et al., 1994; Garcion et al., 2001). In the rat, myelination of retinal ganglion cell axons in the optic nerve starts at postnatal day 5 and proceeds at least the next three weeks (Black et al., 1982). In humans, the myelination of the optic nerve occurs by as early as 32 weeks of gestation and continues for several years into early childhood.

In humans, retinal ganglion cell axons remain nonmyelinated proximal to the lamina cribrosa. Various other mammals including marmoset, flying fox, cat, and sheep lack intraretinal myelination and possess a lamina cribrosa, while further mammals with nonmyelinated retinas such as rat and mouse lack a well-developed lamina cribrosa; here, fibrous astrocytes (which form a dense network proximal to the myelinated part of the optic nerve) act as barrier for migrating oligodendrocyte progenitors (Ffrench-Constant et al., 1988; Bartsch et al., 1994; Morcos and Chan-Ling, 2000; Ding et al., 2002). A dense network of fibrous astrocytes at the retinal-optic nerve junction of human fetuses is apparent at 13 weeks of gestation, prior to the myelination of the optic nerve; in contrast, the lamina cribrosa is not fully developed even at birth (Morcos and Chan-Ling, 2000). Astrocytes in the proximal region of the optic nerve express the extracellular matrix glycoprotein tenascin-C at elevated levels before the arrival of the first oligodendrocyte progenitor cells; tenascin-C was suggested to inhibit the adhesion and migration of oligodendrocyte progenitors (Bartsch et al., 1992, 1994; Kiernan et al., 1996; but see Kiernan et al., 1999). BMPs, expressed in the developing retina and at the retina-optic nerve junction, have also been implicated in preventing the intraretinal myelination (Gao et al., 2006). Further extracellular matrix proteins like anosmin-1 also impair the migration of oligodendrocyte progenitors (Bribián et al., 2008). The differentiation of oligodendrocytes is inhibited by activation of Notch1 receptors by Jagged1 derived from retinal ganglion cells; the expression of Jagged1 in retinal ganglion cell axons decreases with a time course that parallels the myelination in the optic nerve (Wang et al., 1998). Species with myelinated retinas lack a well-developed lamina cribrosa and a dense astrocytic network at the retinal-optic nerve junction (Ffrench-Constant et al., 1988; Morcos and Chan-Ling, 2000). In the rabbit retina, the outer limit of the migration of oligodendrocyte precursor cells is restricted by the outer limit of astrocyte spread (Morcos and Chan-Ling, 2000). Here, oligodendrocytes are coupled together and with astrocytes by gap junctions (Hampson and Robinson, 1995).

In species with myelinated retinas, retinal astrocytes, oligodendroglia, and diacytes (see Ch. 1) share a common progenitor (Rompani and Cepko, 2010). The proliferation of oligodendrocyte precursor cells depends on the electrical activity of retinal ganglion cell axons (Barres and Raff, 1993). Oligodendrocyte progenitor cells proliferate in response to different mitogens including PDGF-A, bFGF, VEGF-C, and neuregulin (Wolswijk et al., 1991; McKinnon et al., 1993; Canoll et al., 1996; Le Bras et al., 2006; Bribian et al., 2006). The migration of oligodendrocyte precursors is controlled by the interaction with molecules they find along their migratory routes (De Castro and Bribian, 2005). These molecules include secreted factors like semaphorins 3A and 3F, netrin-1, Shh, and CXCL1 (Sugimoto et al., 2001; Spassky et al., 2002; Tsai et al., 2002, 2003; Jarjour et al., 2003; Merchan et al., 2007), and growth factors such as PDGF-A, bFGF, and hepatocyte growth factor (HGF) (Pringle and Richardson, 1993; Milner et al., 1997; Yan and Rivkees, 2002; Bribian et al., 2006). Extracellular matrix proteins such as tenascin-C, laminin, fibronectin, and vitronectin and contact molecules like integrins, polysialylated-neuron cell adhesion molecule, ephrins, anosmin-1, and N-cadherin also influence the migration of oligodendrocyte precursors (Garcion et al., 2001; Prestoz et al., 2004; Bribian et al., 2006, 2008). Shh stimulates the migration of oligodendrocyte precursors likely via enhanced secretion of growth factors by astrocytes (Dakubo et al., 2008). The above-mentioned molecules also influence the migration of oligodendrocyte precursors in demyelinating diseases such as Devic's neuromyelitis and multiple sclerosis where optic neuritis is the most frequent initial symptom (Victor and Ropper, 2001; Frohman et al., 2005).

Shh and neuregulin derived from retinal ganglion cell axons induce the differentiation of oligodendrocytes from progenitor cells and the myelinating competence of the cells (Gao and Miller,

2006; Gibney and McDermott, 2009). Futher soluble factors like BDNF also induce the expression of myelin proteins in oligodendrocytes (Cellerino et al., 1997). In contrast, soluble factors released from Müller cells inhibit the differentiation of oligodendrocytes (Scherer et al., 1995). Phospholipids (and possibly myelin proteins) synthesized in the retinal ganglion cells are transported along their axons and transferred into the newly formed myelin (Prensky et al., 1975; Alberghina et al., 1982). Astrocytes control the onset of myelination by promoting the adhesion of oligodendrocyte processes to axons (Meyer-Franke et al., 1999) and contribute to the rate of myelin wrapping by oligodendrocytes (Watkins et al., 2008). In addition, thyroid hormone inhibits the proliferation of oligodendrocyte progenitors and triggers the terminal differentiation of oligodendrocytes (Baas et al., 2002).

Abnormal myelination of the retinal nerve fiber layer by ectopic oligodendrocytes or Schwann cells (the myelin-forming cells of the peripheral nervous system) was found in various mammalian species which normally lack intraretinal myelin including the mouse, rat, guinea pig, cat, and rhesus monkey (Jung et al., 1978; Büssow, 1978; Bellhorn et al., 1979; Wyse, 1980; Wyse and Spira, 1981; Berry et al., 1992; May, 2009). Abnormal myelination of the retinal nerve fiber layer also occurs in about 1% of humans (Duke-Elder, 1964; Straatsma et al., 1981; Aaby and Kushner, 1985; Williams, 1986; Kodama et al., 1990; Ali et al., 1994; Leys et al., 1996; Hunter et al., 1997; FitzGibbon and Nestorovski, 1997; Rosen et al., 1999). Intraretinal myelination in humans is associated with an increase in the diameter of the retinal ganglion cell axons (FitzGibbon and Nestorovski, 2013) and with visual problems, e.g., amblyopia (Leys et al., 1996; Hunter et al., 1997; Straatsma et al., 1979, 1981). In rats, myelination of the nerve fiber layer by Schwann cells can be also induced by lesioning the retina via the sclera and choroid (Perry and Hayes, 1985). Intraocular transplantation of myelinogenic cells such as oligodendrocyte lineage cells, Schwann cells, and neural progenitor cells, in developing or adult mammals with non-myelinated retinas results in myelination of the retinal nerve fiber layer (Huang et al., 1991; Laeng et al., 1996; Ader et al., 2000; Setzu et al., 2004, 2006; Woodhoo et al., 2007; Li et al., 2007b; Gibney and McDermott, 2009; Yang et al., 2013a). This suggests that normally non-myelinated retinal ganglion cell axons are receptive to myelination, once myelinating cells have access to the retinal nerve fiber layer.

4.2   OLIGODENDROGLIA IN OPTIC NERVE INJURY

Neuronal axons are capable to regenerate after transection in the adult CNS of lower vertebrates (fish, amphibia, reptiles) but not in the adult CNS of higher vertebrates (birds, mammals) (Wolburg, 1978, 1981). (In contrast, the peripheral nervous system is, to a varying degree, capable of regeneration also in adult higher vertebrates.) The failure of higher vertebrate CNS axons to regenerate is attributed to a programmed loss of the capability of neurons to elongate their axons (Cohen et al., 1986; Chen et al., 1995; Cai et al., 2001) and the presence of growth-inhibitory CNS myelin proteins like tenascin-R and other glial factors and molecules such as chondroitin sulfate proteoglycans (Schwab and Caroni, 1988; Cadelli et al., 1992; Kapfhammer et al., 1992; Bähr and Przyrembel, 1995; Bandtlow and Löschinger, 1997; Phokeo et al., 2002; Wang et al., 2002a; Leibinger et al., 2012; see 5.11.2.7.).

In the fish retina, oligodendrocytes with distinct cell adhesion proteins on their surface promote the growth of retinal ganglion cell axons after lesion of the optic nerve (Bastmeyer et al., Glia 1993; Ankerhold et al., 1998). However, the fish optic nerve is normally not permissive to the growth of adult retinal axons (because of the presence of myelin-associated growth-inhibitory molecules similar to the growth inhibitors present in the mammalian CNS myelin) but becomes growth permissive after injury (Sivron et al., 1994), likely by downregulation of the neurite growth inhibitors (Rachailovich and Schwartz, 1984; Stuermer et al., 1992; Wanner et al., 1995; Becker et al., 2000). Moreover, upon retinal injury, fish retinal ganglion cells reexpress a set of growth-associated cell surface molecules, suggesting that the cells reactivate the cellular machinery required for axonal regrowth and pathfinding (Stuermer et al., 1992). In reptiles, retinal ganglion cell axons are less sensitive to the growth-inhibitory myelin proteins and therefore are capable to regenerate after optic nerve injury (Lang et al., 1998).

In adult higher vertebrates, oligodendrocyte-derived CNS myelin proteins (but not Schwann cell-derived myelin of the peripheral nervous system) inhibit the aberrant sprouting and growth of retinal ganglion cell axons (Schwab and Caroni, 1988; Colello and Schwab, 1994; Cai et al., 2001; Becker et al., 2000; Phokeo et al., 2002; Wang et al., 2002a); the capacity for axon regeneration declines sharply with the appearance of mature oligodendrocytes and myelin. In addition to CNS myelin, mature astrocytes and Müller cells are nonpermissive for the growth of retinal ganglion cell axons. While embryonic neurons are capable of extending axons which is unaffected by myelin (because they are less sensitiv to the myelin-associated neurite growth inhibitors), developing neurons acquire the complete sensitivity for the growth-inhibitory myelin proteins around the time of myelination (Ard et al., 1991; Bandtlow and Löschinger, 1997). Soluble factors like bFGF stimulate the growth of embryonic unmyelinated axons, but not the growth of myelinated axons (Colello and Schwab, 1994). Myelin-associated glycoprotein promotes axon growth in the developing tissue, and inhibit axon growth in the mature tissue, via inducing different alterations in the neuronal cyclic adenosine 5'-monophosphate (cAMP) level (Cai et al., 2001). After optic nerve injury, oligodendrocytes and their precursor cells, as well as reactive astrocytes and Müller cells, inhibit the regeneration of retinal ganglion cell axons by repulsive axon guidance molecules, including ephrins, semaphorins, and repulsive guidance molecule A, and extracellular matrix constituents like tenascin-R (Becker et al., 2000; Goldberg et al., 2004; Schnichels et al., 2012; Joly et al., 2014a). On the other hand, the regeneration of transected retinal ganglion cell axons is permitted in the optic nerve of the adult Browman-Wyse mutant rat in which oligodendrocytes and CNS myelin are absent and Schwann cells are present; the axon growth is likely stimulated by trophic molecules from Schwann cells (Berry et al., 1989, 1992). In experimental glaucoma, the loss of optic nerve oligodendrocytes precedes the delayed loss of retinal ganglion cells, likely in response to activated microglia and the release of inflammatory factors such as TNFα (Nakazawa et al., 2006a). Oligodendrocytes and astrocytes are the primary infection sites after intravitreal virus administration which causes a demyelination of the retinal nerve fibers (Kristensson and Wiśniewski, 1978).

C H A P T E R   5

Müller Cells

5.1 MORPHOLOGY OF MÜLLER CELLS

Müller cells are specialized radial glial cells. In addition to biochemical and physiological specializations, Müller cells display a more complex morphology than embryonic radial glial cells (Fig. 27C). Radial glial cells have a bipolar morphology (Fig. 27C) and are present in the whole embryonic brain including the developing spinal cord (Fig. 27B) and retina (Fig. 27C). Their cell bodies pass through the whole neural tissue from the ventricles (and canalis centralis, respectively) to the pial surface of the tissue (Fig. 27B). Radial glial cells in the embryonic retina (Fig. 27C) and Müller cells in the mature retina (Fig. 27A) span their cell bodies from the subretinal space (which is a relict of the optic ventricle) to the vitreal surface of the neuroretina.

In comparison to other types of glial cells such as astrocytes and oligodendrocytes, Müller cells are relatively unspecialized cells; they have most of the possible types of glial cell processes (Reichenbach, 1989), for example, a process that has contact to a (ventricular, subretinal) fluid space, processes with contact to a mesenchymal borderline (basal laminas on the inner surface of the retina and around the vessels), and to neuronal compartments (Fig. 28). The cell processes are locally adapted to the neuronal microenvironment with which they are in contact (Reichenbach, 1989; Reichenbach et al., 1989). The side processes of Müller cells, which arise from the stem processes (Fig. 2A, E), insulate neuronal compartments and express suitable membrane properties for the glio-neuronal communication. These processes are present as fine perisynaptic side branches in the plexiform layers, as thin cytoplasmic "bubbles" ensheathing the neuronal somata in the nuclear layers, and as smooth processes that wrap ganglion cell axons in the thick (myelinated) nerve fibre layer of the central retina. The process that contacts the subretinal fluid has microvilli, tight junctions, and displays a high sodium-potassium-ATPase activity. Processes that are covered by a basement membrane contain gliofilaments and have a high potassium conductivity mediated by Kir channels (see 5.5.3.3.).

There is a great species-dependent diversity in the morphology of Müller cells, in particular of the structure of the inner stem process (Fig. 29). In many species such as lungfish, chameleon, lizard (Fig. 29), chicken (Fig. 27C), and dog (Fig. 27A), the inner process displays few or many

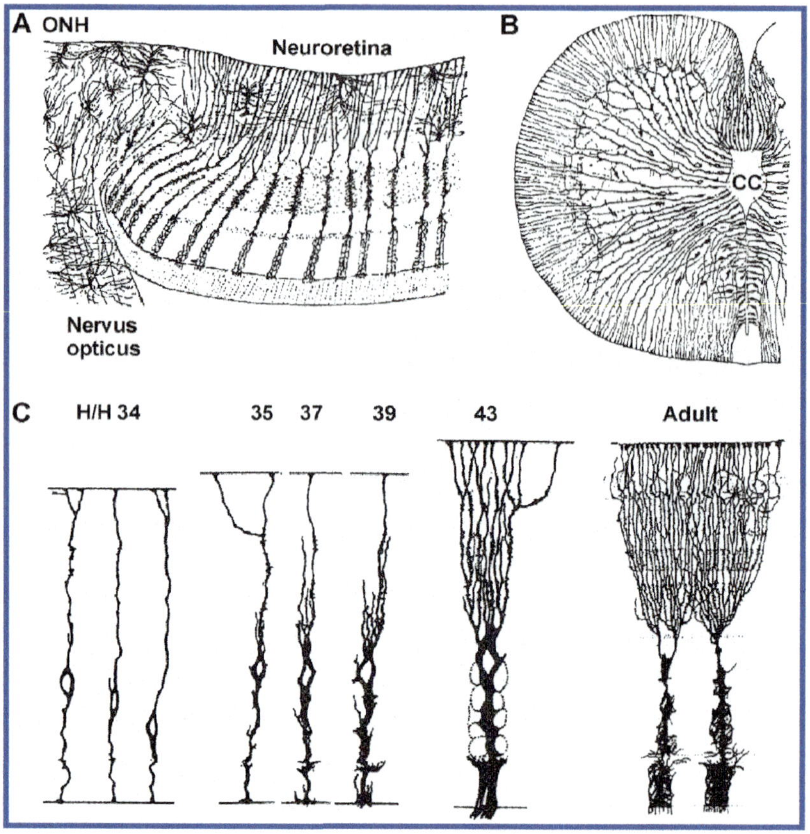

FIGURE 27: Müller cells are specialized radial glial cells. **A.** The slice through the neuroretina and optic nerve head (ONH) of an adult dog was stained with the Golgi technique. Müller cells pass through the whole retinal tissue from the vitreous-abutting surface to the subretinal space. **B.** Fetal radial glial cells pass through the whole lumbal spinal cord of a human embryo, from the canalis centralis (cc) to the pial surface. **C.** Morphological development of Müller cells in the chick (stages 34–43 after Hamberger and Hamilton, H/H). In the course of the development, the morphology of the cells becomes more complex. Modified from Ramón y Cajal (1952) and Prada et al. (1989).

branches at the level of the inner plexiform or ganglion cell layer; each branch ends with an extended endfoot at the inner limiting membrane. Müller cells of other species such as lamprey, salamander, rabbit, rat, and man, have only one inner stem process and one endfoot (Fig. 29). The tree shrew (*Tupaia*) is one of the few mammalian species whose retinas are strongly cone dominated, which is usually the case in reptilian and avian retinas. Unlike Müller cells in other mammalian species, but

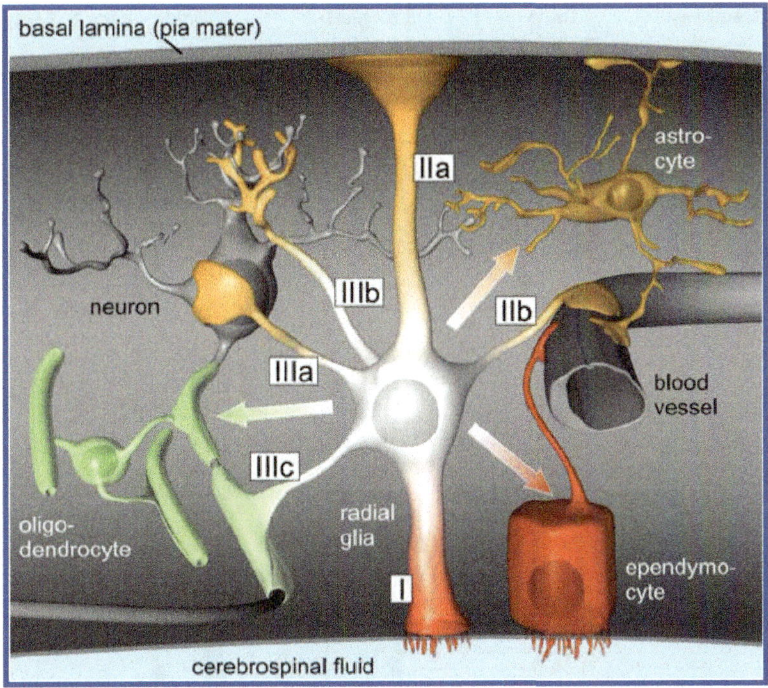

FIGURE 28: Hypothetical macroglial cell displaying all possible types of cell processes (and microenvironmental contacts, respectively), and its real derivatives. The presence *vs.* absence of the three basic types of cell processes defines the four basic macroglial cell types, *viz* radial glial cells (all three), ependymocytes (only two), astrocytes (only two), and oligodendrocytes (only one). *I*, ventricle-contacting process; *II*, pia- (*IIa*) or blood vessel- (*IIb*) contacting processes; *III*, neuroncontacting processes (*IIIa*, to neuronal somata; *IIIb*, to "neuropile" incl. synapses; *IIIc* to axons). Modified from Reichenbach (1989).

similar to reptilian and avian Müller cells, Müller cells of tree shrews commonly have two or more inner processes rather than one main trunk (Fig. 29) (Reichenbach et al., 1995a). The morphology of the inner stem process may also vary in dependence on the retinal topography. Cells in avascular areas of the rabbit retina have one process that is enlarged at the end to one endfoot while cells in the central retina beneath the vascularized visual streak send thin vitreal processes through the thick nerve fiber layer which are subdivided into several fine branches ending with multiple small endfeet (Fig. 30B) (Reichenbach, 1987). Similarly, the complexity of the endfeet tree of avian Müller cells (Fig. 27C) depends on the retinal topography (Anezary et al., 2001). It has been suggested that the splitting of Müller cell stem trunks into numerous filamentous processes terminating in small vitreal endfeet (Fig. 27C) represents a morphological adaptation for the effective spatial buffering

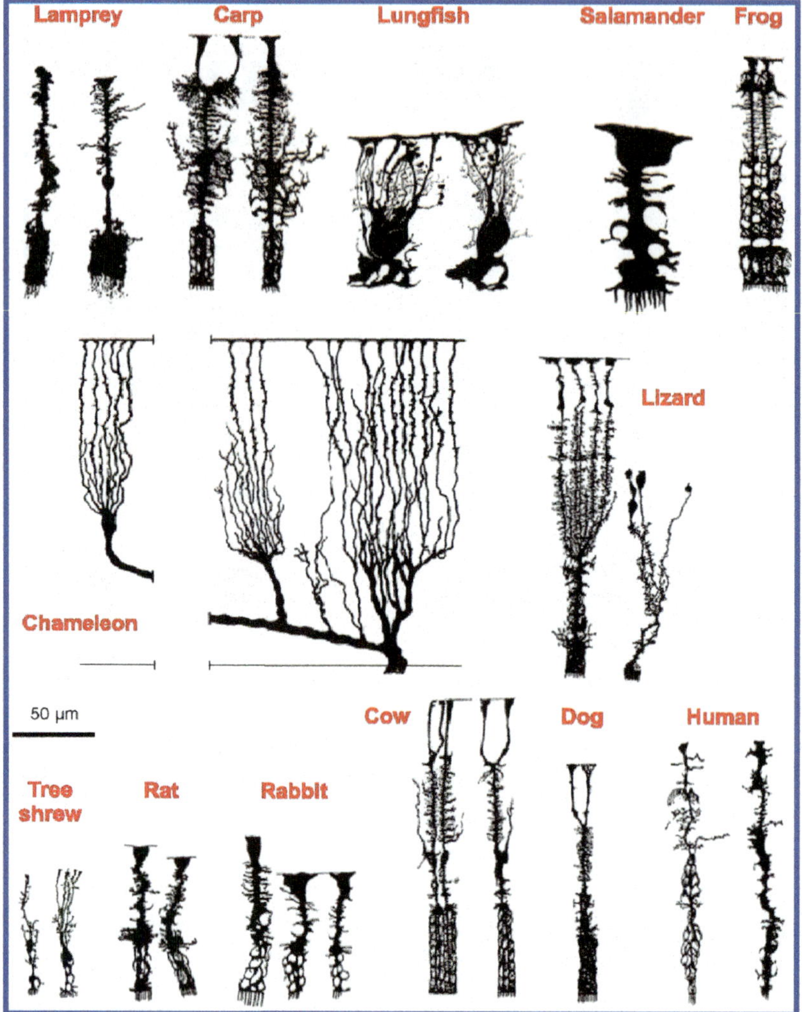

FIGURE 29: Adaptations of Müller cell morphology in various vertebrates. Most cells were drawn from Golgi-stained preparations, some are camera-lucida drawings of dye-filled cells. As far as possible, all cells are shown at the same magnification. Modified from Reichenbach and Wolburg (2005).

of potassium ions (see 5.5.3.) in the non-vascularized avian retina, and for the effective absorption and distribution of nutrients leaking from the pecten, the vitreally located supplemental nutritive organ of the avian eye (Dreher et al., 1994).

Müller cells are uniformly distributed within the retina (Figs. 2D, 3B,C, 4C), with a mean density of 8,000–13,000 cells per mm^2 (Dreher et al., 1992). The morphology of Müller cells var-

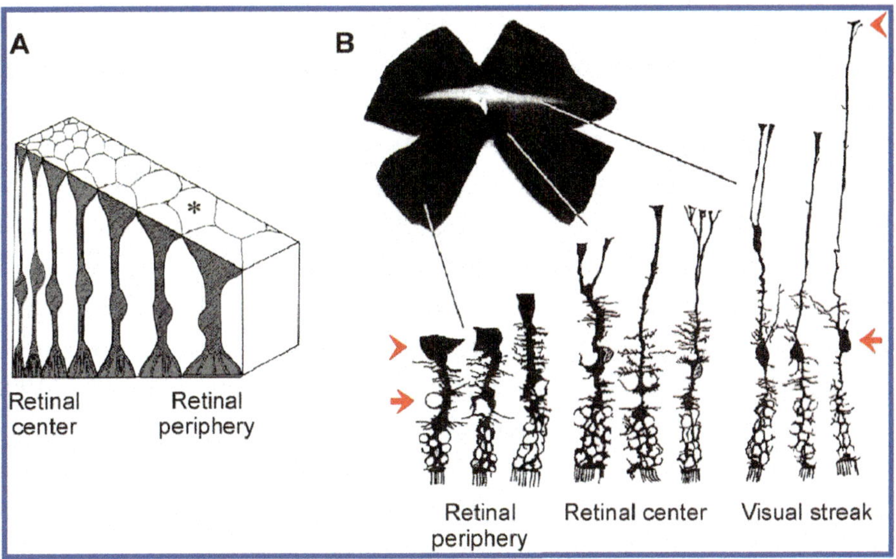

FIGURE 30: The morphology of rabbit Müller cells varies with the retinal topography. **A.** Schematic drawing of the rabbit retina containing single Müller cells. The Müller cell density is higher in the retinal center compared to the retinal periphery. In comparison to Müller cells of the retinal center, cells of the retinal periphery are shorter and thicker, and have larger vitreal endfoot membranes (*). The inner (vitreal) surface of the neuroretina consists of closely adjoined Müller cell endfeet. **B.** Topographical specialization of rabbit Müller cells. Single Müller cells from the retinal periphery, retinal center, and the myelinated visual streak are shown. *Arrows*, cell somata; *arrowheads*, cell endfeet. Modified from Reichenbach et al. (1989).

ies in relation to their retinal topography (Reichenbach, 1987). The central retina is thicker than the peripheral retina (Fig. 30A) and contains much higher densities of neuronal and Müller cells (Reichenbach et al., 1988a; Robinson and Dreher, 1990; Skatchkov et al., 1999). Müller cell density varies between 6000 cells/mm^2 in the far peripheral and peak densities of >30,000 cells/mm^2 in the parafoveal monkey retina (Distler and Dreher; 1996). Müller cells of central retinal regions are longer and thinner, and have smaller volumes but higher surface-to-volume ratios, than those of the periphery (Fig. 30B) (Pei and Smelser, 1968; Uga, 1974; Reichenbach and Wohlrab, 1986; Reichenbach et al., 1987, 1988a, 1989, 1995c; Prada et al., 1989; Distler and Dreher; 1996). In addition to Müller cells, also neurons of the retinal periphery are thicker than those of the center. When Müller cells become shorter and thicker, the area of the vitreal endfoot membrane (Fig. 30A) and the volume of the cells increase strongly (Reichenbach and Wohlrab, 1986; Reichenbach, 1987;

Prada et al., 1989). However, the contribution of Müller cell volume to the total volume of the retina (~7% in the rabbit), and the glia-neuron ratio (~1:15 in the rabbit) are constant, independent of the retinal topography (Reichenbach and Wohlrab, 1983; Reichenbach, 1987). The greater vitreal endfoot membranes of Müller cells in the peripheral retina contains lower densities of distinct membrane constituents, e.g., of orthogonal arrays of intramembranous particles (Richter et al., 1990).

Müller cells in vascular and avascular retinas differ in several morphological aspects. Paurangiotic retinas (that contain blood vessels only near the optic disc) and avascular retinas (e.g., of guinea pigs, rabbits, echidnas, horses, and zebras) are thinner than vascularized retinas (e.g., of mice, rats, cats, dogs, ungulates, and humans), mainly due to the smaller density of photoreceptors and thus the reduced thickness of the outer nuclear layer (Dreher et al., 1992; Chao et al., 1997). Therefore, Müller cells in vascularized retinas are longer and thinner, and have smaller volumes but higher surface-to-volume ratios, than their counterparts in avascular and paurangiotic retinas (Dreher et al., 1992; Chao et al., 1997). Due to the smaller density of photoreceptors in avascular retinas, there are fewer neurons per Müller cell (Dreher et al., 1992).

5.2   ULTRASTRUCTURE OF MÜLLER CELLS

Müller cells are strictly polarized cells; this includes the subcellular distribution of organelles (Fig. 31) (Reichenbach, 1989). The inner process endfoot of rabbit Müller cells are densely packed with smooth endoplasmic reticulum, the intermediate filament vimentin (Figs. 11A, 22C,D, 32, 33A), and glycogen granula, while the outer process mainly contains the Golgi apparatus, multivesicular bodies, and microtubules. Groups of polyribosomes are localized to the sites of the origin of the fine lateral processes within the plexiform (synaptic) layers and of the microvilli which extend into the subretinal space, suggesting that neuronal activity may stimulate the local synthesis of structural proteins and, thus, the growth of the perisynaptic processes and microvilli (Reichenbach et al., 1988a). The local protein synthesis required for the formation of glial sheaths with active potassium uptake capacity (as well as the expression of the sodium-potassium ATPase) is stimulated by extracellular potassium accumulation due to neuronal activity (Reichenbach et al., 1985, 1989). The release of other molecules by active synapses, such as neurotransmitters and metabolic waste products, may contribute to the local shaping of glial sheaths.

Multivesicular bodies, which are involved in active secretory processes (Akmayev and Popov, 1977), are located in Müller cells near the Golgi apparatus in the outer stem process, suggesting that Müller cells have a secretory function (Reichenbach et al., 1988a). The secretory function of Müller cells is also suggested by the expression of chromogranin B (Lorenz et al., 2011). Müller

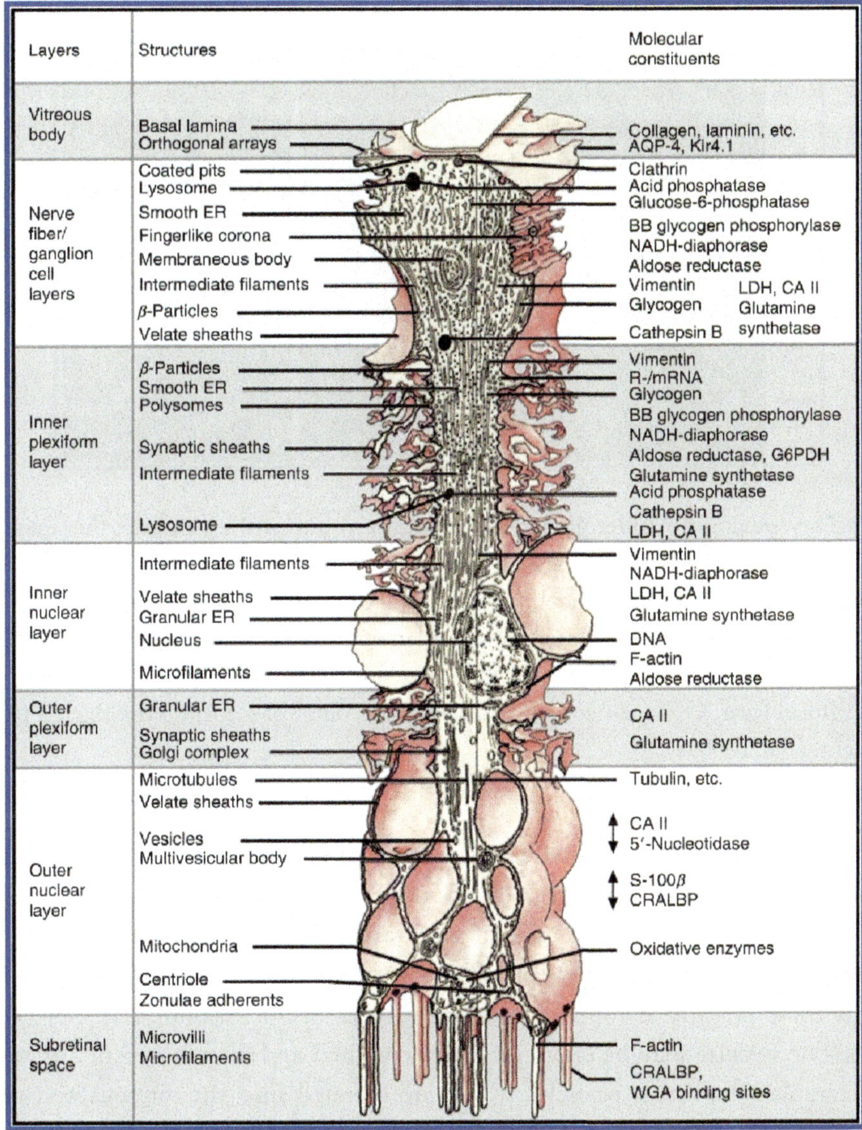

FIGURE 31: Cytotopographic specializations of a rabbit Müller cell (semi-schematic drawing). AQP-4, aquaporin-4 water channels; BB, brain-specific isozyme; CA II, carbonic anhydrase II; CRALBP, cellular retinoic acid binding protein; ER, endoplasmic reticulum; G6PDH, glucose-6-phosphate dehydrogenase; Kir4.1, inwardly rectifying potassium channels; LDH, lactate dehydrogenase; NADH, nicotinamide adenine dinucleotide (reduced form); S-100b, calcium-binding protein; WGA, wheat germ agglutinin. Modified from Reichenbach (1989).

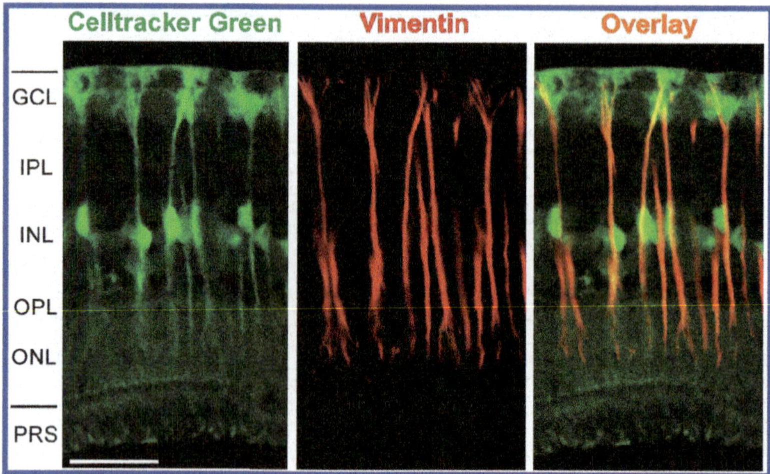

FIGURE 32: The somata of Müller glial cells are localized out of the cell axis; this may support the light-guiding function of the cells. In a freshly isolated slice of the guinea-pig retina, Müller cells and photoreceptor segments (PRS) were loaded with the vital dye Celltracker Green; after fixation, the slice was immunostained against the glial intermediate filament vimentin which marks the axis of Müller cells. Müller cell somata lie in the middle of the inner nuclear layer (INL). GCL, ganglion cell layer; IPL, inner plexiform layer; ONL, outer nuclear layer; OPL, outer plexiform layer. Bar, 25 µm. Modified from Uckermann et al. (2004a).

cells may exocytotically release glutamate (see 5.6.1.2.) and other neuroactive molecules such as growth factors, chemokines, and lipoproteins (Berka et al., 1995; Roesch et al., 2008), secrete lipoprotein particles (see 5.5.7.4.), and mediate the transcytosis of retinoschisin (Reid and Farber, 2005). The endfoot membrane of Müller cells show coated pits of approximately 150 nm basal diameter; near these pits, the cytoplasm contains vesicles of 90–100 nm diameter (Reichenbach et al., 1988a). The vesicles may be endocytotically engulfed and may represent structures of exocytosis, for example lipoprotein particles which are secreted into the vitreous and subsequently taken up by retinal ganglion cells (see 5.5.7.4.) as well as vesicles which contain material for the synthesis of the vitreal basement membrane.

The localization of the mitochondria in Müller cells (and in photoreceptor and pigment epithelial cells) depends on the retinal oxygen supply. Paurangiotic and avascular retinas (e.g., of salamanders, rabbits, and guinea pigs) display extremely low oxygen partial pressures proximal to the outer limiting membrane (Yu and Cringle, 2001). In Müller cells of these species, only a few

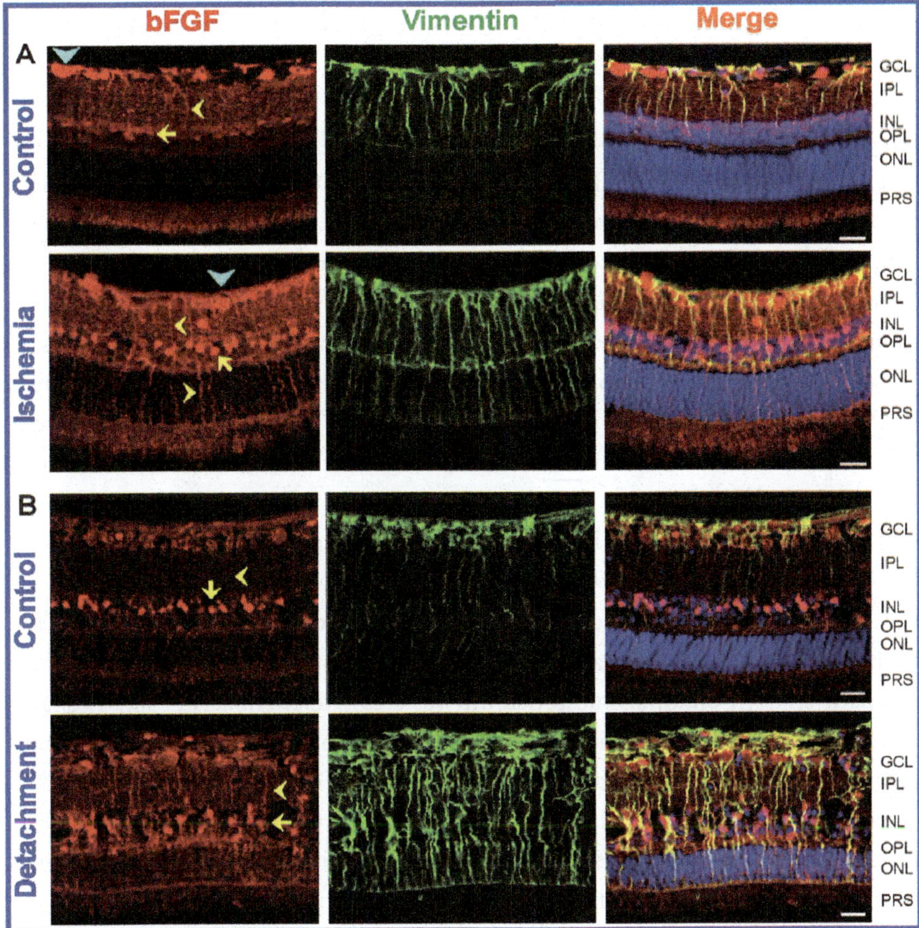

FIGURE 33: Increase of glial bFGF in the retina under pathological conditions. Retinal slices were labeled with antibodies against bFGF (*red*) and vimentin (*green*). Co-labeling yielded a *yellow* merge signal. Cell nuclei are *blue* stained. **A.** Experimental ischemia-reperfusion causes an increase of glial bFGF in the rat retina. Retinal slices were derived from a control eye (*above*) and an eye 3 days after a 1-h transient retinal ischemia (*below*). **B.** Experimental detachment of the porcine retina causes an increase of glial bFGF. The slices were derived from a control retina (*above*) and from a detached retina 3 days after surgery (*below*). *Blue arrowheads*, ganglion cell somata. *Arrows*, Müller cell somata. *Yellow arrowheads*, Müller cell processes. GCL, ganglion cell layer; INL, inner nuclear layer; IPL, inner plexiform layer; ONL, outer nuclear layer; OPL, outer plexiform layer; PRS, photoreceptor segments. Bars, 20 µm. Modified from Yafai et al. (2013) and I. Iandiev, Leipzig (unpublished results).

mitochondria are located at the outer end of the cells, i.e., close to the choroidal blood supply, while the other parts of the cells are devoid of mitochondria (Figs. 31, 34J,L) (Sjöstrand and Nilsson, 1964; Magalhães and Coimbra, 1972; Uga and Smelser, 1973; Reichenbach, 1988a, 1989a; Germer et al., 1998a,b; Poitry et al., 2000; Biedermann et al., 2002; Stone et al., 2008). In vascularized retinas, mitochondria are evenly distributed throughout the entire length of Müller cells (Fig. 35B) (Germer et al., 1998a). When the avascular retina of guinea pigs is kept in organotypic cultures where high pO2 levels are provided at the inner surface of the retina, the mitochondria migrate and rearrange to an even distribution within Müller cells (Germer et al., 1998b). The retinas of various species such as frogs and carps are overlaid by supraretinal (intravitreal) blood vessels; this corresponds to an accumulation of mitochondria in the Müller cell endfeet (in addition to the accumulation at the outer limiting membrane) (Uga and Smelser, 1973). In Müller cells of avascular retinas (e.g., of rabbits), aerob and anaerob metabolism occur in different cell compartments. While the mitochondria are located at the outer margin of the cells, the enzymes for the glycogen synthesis, glycogenolysis, and anaerobic glycolysis, as well as glycogen particles, are localized to the inner part of the cells (Kuwabara and Cogan, 1961; Lessell and Kuwabara, 1964; Cameron and Cole, 1964; Matschinsky, 1970; Magalhães and Coimbra, 1970, 1972; Reichenbach et al., 1988a). The endfoot of rabbit Müller cells contains a huge apparatus for the production of glucose from glycogen, in the form of abundant smooth endoplasmic reticulum vesicles (Reichenbach et al., 1988a) which are the site of glucose-6-phosphatase activity (Magalhães and Coimbra, 1972). In these cells, glucose is mainly taken up by the scleral microvilli (a certain amount of glucose may be also derived from the vitreal fluid), and is then either oxidatively metabolized by the mitochondria where it enters the cell, or transported into the inner (vitreal) part for glycogen storage and anaerobic metabolism. In contrast to Müller cells of avascular retinas, glycogen stores are uniformly distributed in Müller cells of vascularized retinas (Rungger-Brändle et al., 1996).

Müller cells have a continuous subplasmalemmal layer of filamentous actin (Vaughan and Fisher, 1987). At the level of the outer limiting membrane, Müller cells contain rings of filamentous actin that surround the photoreceptors; the actin rings are associated with the adherens junctions between Müller and photoreceptor cells and form a structural meshwork in which photoreceptor cells are embedded (Del Priore et al., 1987). The cytoplasmic plaques of the adherens junctions between Müller and photoreceptor cells contain actin, myosin, α-actinin, and vinculin (Drenckhahn and Wagner, 1985; Williams et al., 1990). In addition, Müller cells and photoreceptor cells are coupled by tight junctions at the level of the outer limiting membrane; this suggests that the outer limiting membrane represents a retinal barrier for fluid influx (Omri et al., 2010). Müller cells express myosin VI (Breckler et al., 2000) which may play a role in the retinomotor movements in response to changes in the light conditions.

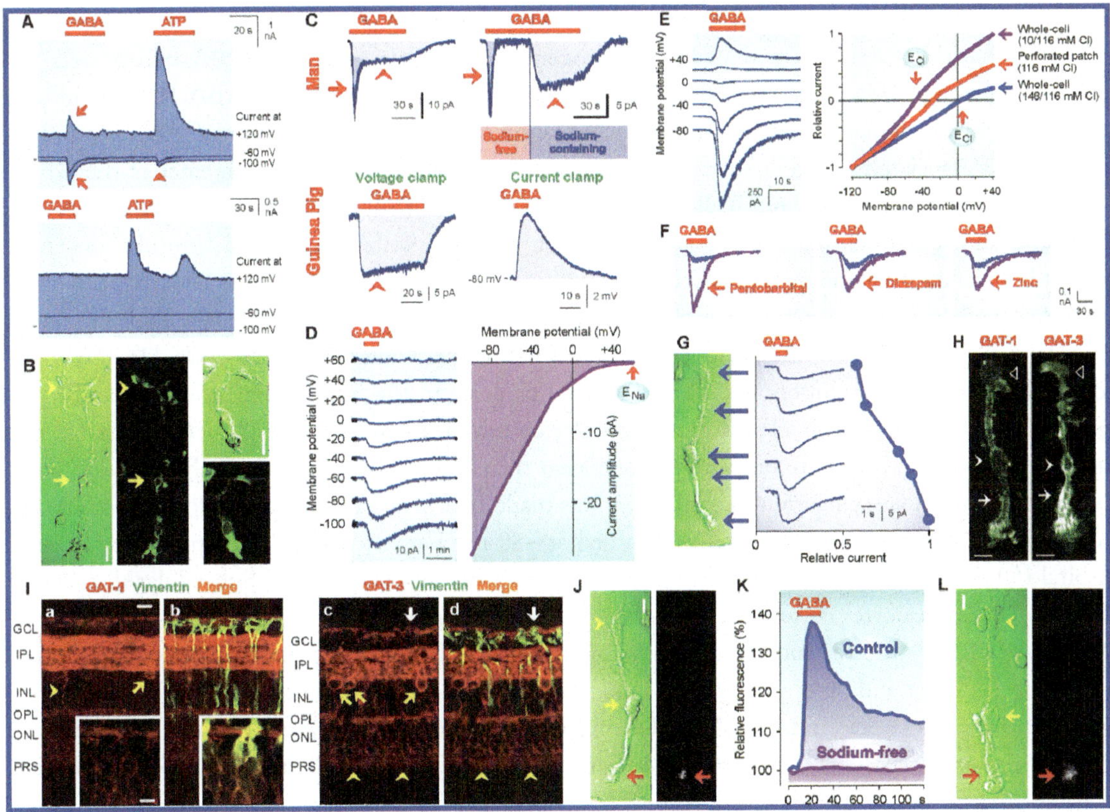

FIGURE 34: GABA$_A$ receptor currents and electrogenic GABA transport in Müller cells. The GABA-induced membrane currents were recorded in freshly isolated Müller cells from man (**A, C, E, F**) and guinea pigs (**C, D, G**). **A.** A subpopulation of human Müller cells express GABA$_A$ receptors. Extracellular administration of GABA (500 µM) induced a transient increase in the inward and outward membrane currents (*arrows*) in the record of one of the two cells shown. Administration of ATP (500 µM) evoked a transient increase in the BK channel-mediated outward potassium currents (at +120 mV) in nearly all Müller cells investigated. In the record shown *above*, ATP induced also a transient cation current (*arrowhead*). **B.** GABA receptors on acutely isolated Müller (*left*) and photoreceptor cells (*right*) of the human retina identified by staining with the fluorescent benzodiazepine derivative BODIPY FL Ro-1986 (*green*). *Arrow*, Müller cell soma. *Arrowhead*, Müller cell endfoot. **C.** Under potassium-free recording conditions, extracellular administration of GABA (100 µM) induces two kinds of inward currents in human Müller cells (*above left*): a transient, rapidly inactivating chloride current mediated by GABA$_A$ receptors (*arrow*) and a sustained current mediated by electrogenic GABA transporters

continued on next page

(*arrowhead*). The sustained current is depressed under extracellular sodium-free conditions (*above right*), indicating that this current is mediated by electrogenic (sodium-dependent) GABA transporters. *Below:* In guinea pig Müller cells (which lack GABA$_A$ receptors), extracellular GABA (1 mM) induces only a transporter-mediated inward current (*left*). The holding potential was −80 mV. Activation of the transporter is associated with a depolarization of the cells (*right*). **D.** Voltage dependency of the GABA transporter currents in guinea-pig Müller cells. The amplitude of the transporter currents is zero near the equilibrium potential of sodium ions (E$_{Na}$) when recorded with symmetrical chloride concentrations at both sides of the membrane. GABA was administered at a concentration of 100 µM. **E.** Voltage dependency of the GABA$_A$ receptor currents in human Müller cells. For the current-voltage relation of the receptor currents (*right*), the currents were recorded in the whole-cell mode (with 116 mM chloride in the extracellular solution and 10 or 146 mM chloride in the intracellular solution), and in the perforated-patch mode (with 116 mM extracellular chloride). In the whole-cell records, the receptor currents reverse from inward to outward currents near the equilibrium potentials of chloride ions (E$_{Cl}$). The example of whole-cell current records (*left*) was made with 146/116 mM chloride. **F.** The GABA$_A$ receptor currents in human Müller cells (recorded at −80 mV) are increased in the presence of pentobarbital (50 µM), diazepam (20 µM), and zinc ions (10 µM), respectively. **G.** Subcellular distribution of the GABA transporter currents. The distribution of the currents was determined by focal ejections of GABA (1 mM) onto the following membrane domains of Müller cells: endfoot (*above*), inner stem process, soma, inner and outer parts of the outer stem process. **H.** Distribution of GAT-1 and GAT-3 immunoreactivities (*white*) in isolated Müller cells of the guinea pig. *Filled arrows*, outer stem process. *Filled arrowheads*, cell soma. *Unfilled arrowheads*, cell endfoot. **I.** GAT-1 (**a, b**) and GAT-3 proteins (**c, d**) in slices of the guinea-pig retina. **a.** In the inner nuclear layer (INL), a labeled interplexiform cell (*arrowhead*) and an amacrine cell soma (*arrow*) express GAT-1 protein. A strong expression of GAT-1 protein is present in three sublayers of the inner plexiform layer (IPL). **b.** Double staining of GAT-1 protein (*red*) and vimentin (*green*). The *insets* show the outer nuclear layer (ONL) at higher magnification to visualize the double-labeled honeycomb meshwork of the outer Müller cell stem processes. **c.** GAT-3 protein is distributed across all retinal layers. *Arrows*, GAT-3 expressing amacrine cell somata. **d.** Double staining of GAT-3 protein (*red*) and vimentin (*green*). Both proteins are partially co-localized (*yellow*). Photoreceptor segments shows autofluorescence (*arrowheads*). Some vimentin-expressing Müller cell endfeet are outlined by GAT-3 protein (*white arrows*). **J.** Extracellular application of GABA (1 mM) causes an increase of the NAD(P)H fluorescence in the end of the outer process of an isolated guinea-pig Müller cell. *Red arrow*, outer process. *Yellow arrow*, soma. *Arrowhead*, endfoot. Because the guinea-pig retina is avascular, the mitochondria in guinea-pig Müller cells are localized in the outer end of the cells near the oxygen supply from the choriocapillaris *in situ*. **K.** Time dependence of the GABA-induced increase of the NAD(P)H fluorescence in the endfoot of the Müller cell. The fluorescence was recorded in control extracellular solution and in sodium-free extracellular solution. **L.** Immunostaining of the GABA transaminase in a single guinea-pig Müller cell. GCL, ganglion cell layer; OPL, outer plexiform layer; PRS, photoreceptor segments. Scale bars, 10 and 5 µm (*insets*). Modified from Bringmann et al. (2002a) and Biedermann et al. (2002, 2004).

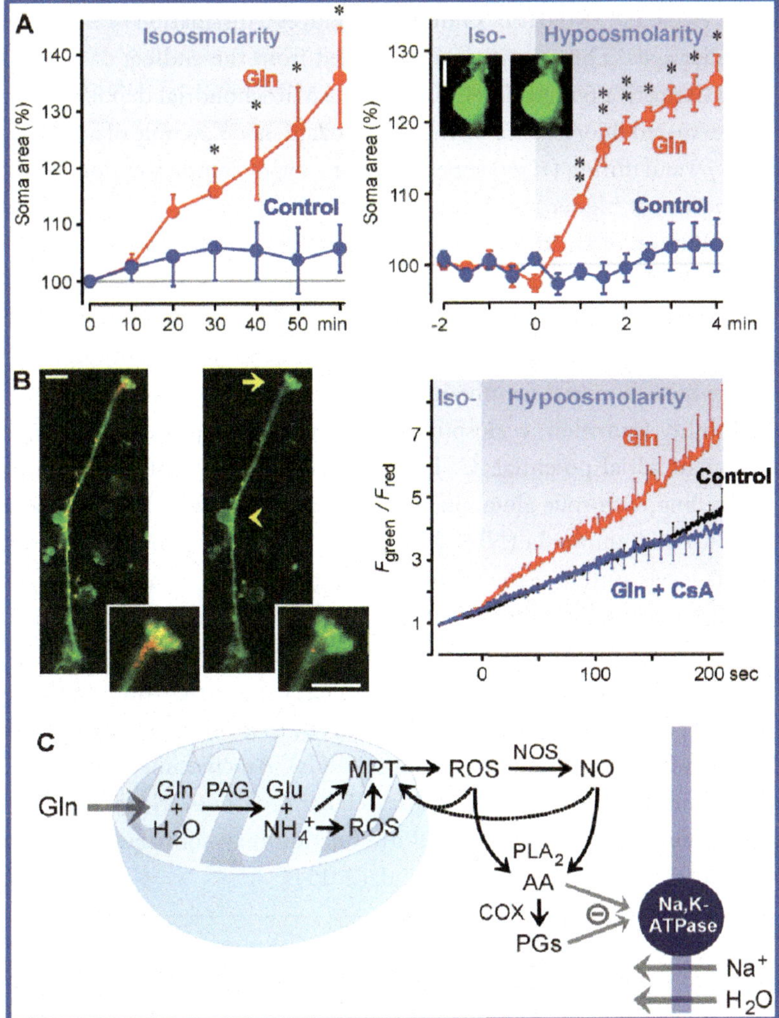

FIGURE 35: Glutamine (Gln) induces mitochondrial dysfunction and Müller cell swelling. Experiments were carried out in retinal slices (**A**) and isolated Müller cells (**B**) of the rat. **A.** Glutamine (5 mM) in isoosmotic extracellular solution induced a delayed swelling of Müller cells after 10 min of exposure (*left*) whereas glutamine (5 mM) in hypoosmotic solution (60% of control osmolarity) induced a rapid (within 1 min) swelling of Müller cells (*right*). The cross-sectional area of Müller cell somata was recorded and is expressed in percent of the value obtained before superfusion of the slices with the solutions (100%). The *images* display original records of a Müller cell soma obtained before (*left*) and during (*right*) superfusion with the glutamine-containing hypoosmotic solution. Scale bar, 5 μm. Significant

continued on next page

difference *vs.* control: *$P<0.05$; **$P<0.01$. **B.** Glutamine induces a dissipation of the mitochondrial membrane potential in Müller cells. The potential was recorded from the endfeet of freshly isolated cells by using the mitochondria-selective potentiometric dye JC-1. Mitochondrial depolarization is indicated by an increase in the green-to-red fluorescence intensity ratio. *Left side:* Example of a JC-1-loaded cell which was recorded before (*left*) and during (*right*) superfusion of a hypoosmotic solution containing glutamine (5 mM). *Insets,* cell endfoot at higher magnification. Note the decrease of the red fluorescence and the relatively uniform distribution of the mitochondria (*yellow*) in the cell. *Arrow,* cell endfoot. *Arrowhead,* cell soma. Bars, 10 μm. *Right:* Time-dependent change in the ratio of the green-to-red fluorescence of the JC-1 dye. The fluorescence was recorded in the absence and presence of glutamine (5 mM), before and during the transition of an isoosmotic to a hypoosmotic extracellular solution. Glutamine induced a faster dissipation of the mitochondrial membrane potential as compared to control. The inhibitor of the mitochondrial permeability transition, cyclosporin A (CsA; 1 μM), prevented the glutamine-induced dissipation of the mitochondrial potential. **C.** Hypothetical scheme of the mechanism of glutamine-induced Müller cell swelling. Cytosolic glutamine is transported into the mitochondria and is hydrolyzed there to glutamate (Glu) and ammonia (NH_4^+) by the action of the phosphate-activated glutaminase (PAG). High ammonia levels stimulate the mitochondrial production of reactive oxygen species (ROS) and induce mitochondrial permeability transition (MPT) that leads to mitochondrial dysfunction, energy failure, and enhanced free radical production. Mitochondria-derived free radicals activate cytosolic enzymes that generate reactive oxygen and nitrogen species, e.g., nitric oxide synthases (NOS). These radicals stimulate the activity of phospholipases A_2 (PLA_2), that produce arachidonic acid (AA), and cyclooxygenases (COX) which generate prostaglandins (PGs). Arachidonic acid and prostaglandins inhibit the sodium-potassium-ATPase resulting in intracellular sodium overload, water influx, and cellular swelling. The energy failure due to mitochondrial dysfunction may contribute to the inhibition of the sodium-potassium-ATPase. Modified from Karl et al. (2011).

5.3   MÜLLER CELLS AS CORES OF RETINAL COLUMNS

Müller cells are regularly arranged in the retina (Figs. 2B,D, 4C). Each Müller cell constitutes the core of a column of retinal neurons that represents the smallest functional unit of "forward information processing" (Fig. 5) (Reichenbach et al., 1994; Reichenbach and Robinson, 1995). This means that the Müller cell is responsible for all functional and metabolic interactions with this particular set of ("its") neurons. Such a column contains one cone per Müller cell (Fig. 13E,F) and (in dependence on the species) varying numbers of rods and inner retinal neurons. In the rabbit retina, for instance, a virtually perfect "constant set" of about 15 neurons (including 1 cone, 10 rods, 2 bipolar cells, and 1 amacrine cell) was observed throughout the retina, independent on local variations of absolute cell densities (Reichenbach et al., 1994). In the human retina, a column contains up to 10

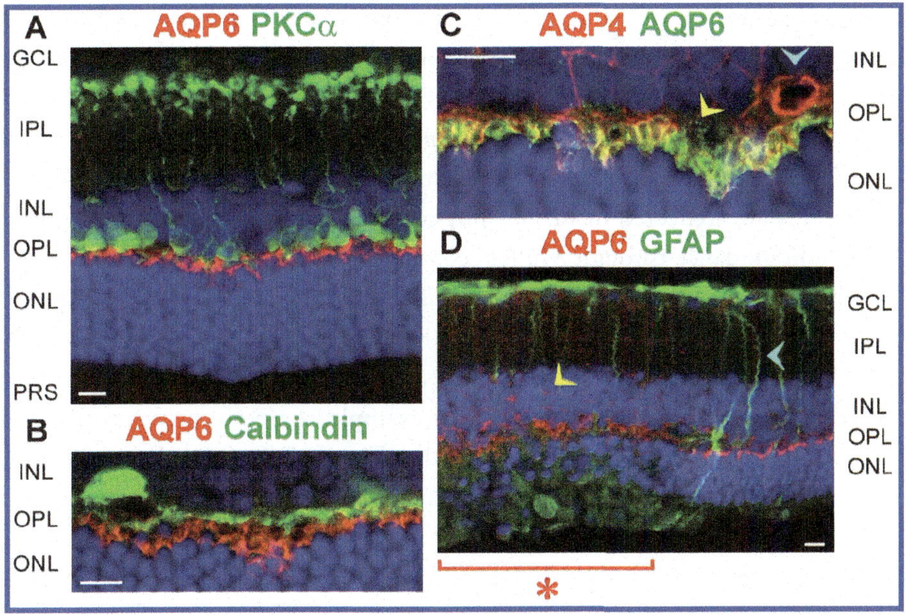

FIGURE 36: Localization of AQP6 in glial membranes that surround the ribbon synapses in the outer plexiform layer (OPL) of the rat retina. **A.** Immunolabeling of a retinal slice against AQP6 and protein kinase Cα (PKCα), the marker of rod bipolar cells and a subpopulation of amacrine cells. There is no colocalization of both proteins. **B.** There is also no co-localization of AQP6 and calbindin, a marker of horizontal cells. **C.** Immunolabeling of a slice against AQP4 and AQP6. AQP6 is selectively localized to the OPL and colocalized in part with AQP4 in glial membranes around ribbon synapses (*yellow*). In addition, AQP6 is present as punctate labeling in the OPL (*yellow arrowhead*). *Blue arrowhead*, perivascular staining of AQP4. **D.** Blue light injury of the retina causes redistribution of AQP6. The slice was immunolabeled against AQP6 and glial fibrillary acidic protein (GFAP) 3 days after light exposure for 30 min. In the light-injured retinal area (*), AQP6 staining around ribbon synapses in the OPL disappeared, whereas the punctate AQP6 labeling within the OPL remained and redistributed into the inner nuclear layer (INL; *yellow arrowhead*). *Blue arrowhead*, GFAP-labeled Müller cell fibers. Cell nuclei are *blue* labeled. GCL, ganglion cell layer; IPL, inner plexiform layer; ONL, outer nuclear layer. Bars, 10 µm. Modified from Iandiev et al. (2011).

rods, 4 (periphery) to 6 (fovea) inner nuclear layer neurons, and 0.3 (periphery) to 2.5 (fovea) ganglion cell layer neurons.

The cellular composition of the columnar units differs considerably among the diverse vertebrates, even among mammalian species; this depends mainly on the diurnal *vs.* nocturnal lifestyle, i.e., the photopic *vs.* scotopic specialization of the retina, which results in a wide variability of the number of rods in one retinal columnar unit. While the number of cones per Müller cell (~1) is similar in diurnal (tree shrew) and nocturnal animals (mouse), the number of rods per Müller cell is very low in the tree shrew retina (<0.1) and very high in the murine retina (27.27) (Reichenbach et al., 1995a; Jeon et al., 1998). This variability of the number of rods in one retinal columnar unit is also observed within the primate retina which contains only cones in the fovea and predominantly rods in the periphery. The distinct relationship between the Müller cell and the cone cell of one column is also reflected in various physiological and pathophysiological functions and events, e.g., the light guidance through Müller cells (see 5.4.), the recycling of photopigments (see 5.5.8.1.), the phagocytosis of cone outer-segment discs by Müller cells (see 5.5.8.), and the growth of subretinal Müller cell processes in association with cone photoreceptors after retinal detachment (see 5.11.2.6.). In addition to these columnar units, which represent cellular domains (Fig. 4B), subcellular Müller cell domains can be defined. For example, the periaxonal coronae of finger-like processes (Figs. 4A, 16A,B), the perisynaptic sheaths (Fig. 36A-C), and the perisomatic "honey-combs" (e.g., of the outer stem process; Fig. 2E), constitute sites of rather autonomous interactions between one Müller cell compartment and a distinct neuronal element. The macaque fovea contains one Müller cell per cone; however, the Müller cells that coat one cone terminal also partially coat the surrounding (approximately six) cone terminals, creating a common environment for the cones supplying the center/surround receptive field of foveal midget bipolar and ganglion cells (Burris et al., 2002). The entire Müller cell population of a retina forms a large macrodomain, as it interacts with virtually all retinal neurons (Fig. 4C).

5.4   LIGHT GUIDANCE THROUGH MÜLLER CELLS

5.4.1   LIGHT SCATTERING IN THE RETINAL TISSUE

The vertebrate retina is inverted; this allows an efficient metabolic and structural support of the outer photoreceptor segments by the retinal pigment epithelium and a short diffusion distance of oxygen and nutrients from the choriocapillaris to the mitochondria-containing inner photoreceptor segments (Fig. 1B). This is an important benefit because the photoreceptor cells are probably the cells of the body with the highest rate of oxidative metabolism (see 5.5.8.2.). However, in the inverted retina, light must pass the entire depth of the neuroretina before it arrives the photoreceptors. Retinal cells and their processes and organelles are phase objects, i.e., they scatter light (Zernike, 1955). In particular, the synapses in the plexiform layers have dimensions close to 500 nm, i.e., within the wavelength range of visible light (380–770 nm), which make them light-scattering structures (Fig. 37D,E) (Tuchin, 2000). The back-scattering of light by the retinal tissue is clinically used in the optical coherence tomography that delivers images of retinal layers in the

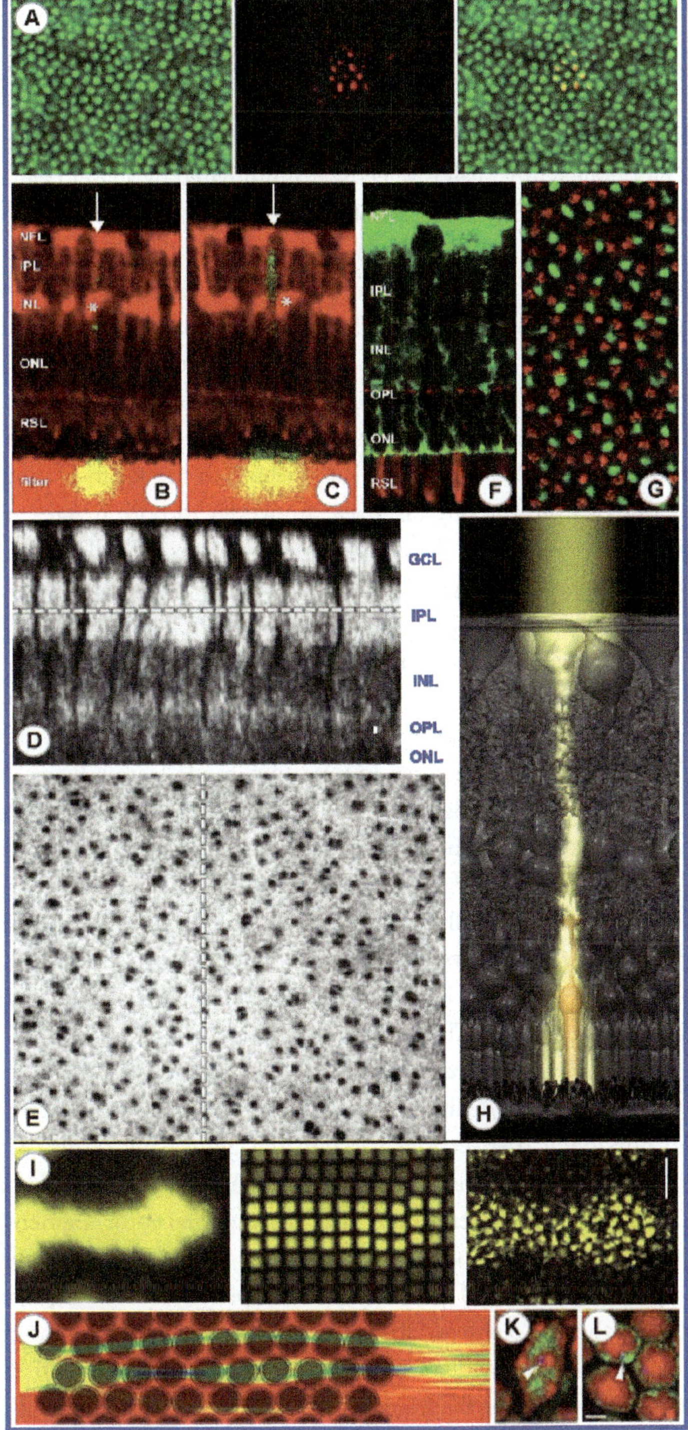

FIGURE 37: Müller cells are "optical fibers" guiding the light from the vitread retinal surface to the photoreceptor cells. Images shown in **A–I** were obtained in the guinea-pig retina. Images shown in **K** and **L**

continued on next page

were obtained in the murine retina. **A.** Müller cells illuminate the photoreceptor cells of their columnar units. When the endfoot of one Müller cell is selectively illuminated by a laser beam, light is transported to a distinct group of photoreceptor outer segments at the opposite surface of the retina. The number of photoreceptor cells is always 9–13, i.e., close to the average of 11.6 photoreceptor cells per Müller cell in the guinea-pig retina. **B, C.** Transretinal path of a thin laser light beam (*arrow*). A retinal slice is placed (together with the filter on which it was cut) in a movable chamber on the stage of a confocal microscope such that the retina and the filter are visible "from the cut side", and the retina can be moved perpendicular to its vitread surface. An optic fiber is placed close to this vitread surface, and illuminates small spots of it (diameter about 5 μm). Müller cells, photoreceptor cells, and the filter are filled with the vital dye, Mitotracker Orange, and thus display *red* fluorescence in the confocal mode. Laser light which is scattered from the tissue or from the filter, is *green*; an overlay of both images appears *yellow* if light is scattered by the dye-filled elements. **B.** When the laser beam hits a Müller cell endfoot, light scatter within the retinal tissue is almost absent, and at the level of the filter (i.e., behind the photoreceptor outer segments) a narrow, bright light beam arrives. **C.** When the sclice is moved by a few micrometers and the laser beam cannot longer enter endfoot/inner process of this Müller cell (*asterisk*), considerable light scatter occurs within the retinal layers, and the arriving spot at the level of the filter is large and blurred, due to beam divergence within the tissue. **D, E.** Light back-scattering occurs in the retinal neuropil but not in Müller cells. Confocal images were taken in reflection-mode from a living unstained guinea-pig retina oriented with the vitread side up. Back-scattering (reflection) of light from various retinal layers is indicated by the *white* structures. At the *black* structures, the light is not reflected. **D.** Orthogonal z-axis-reconstruction ("side view") of the confocal image stacks. The light is scattered (*bright* areas) predominantly by cells in the ganglion cell layer (GCL) and the synapses in the inner (IPL) and outer plexiform layers (OPL). Müller cell fibers spanning the whole retinal thickness are *dark*, indicating that Müller cells do not scatter light; the light can pass the Müller cells from the inner surface of the retina to the outer nuclear layer (ONL). The *dotted* line indicates the level at which image **E** was taken. **E.** View onto the inner plexiform layer. A regular pattern of non-reflecting (*black*) tubes is apparent which represent Müller cell stem processes. The light is back-scattered by the synaptic structures (*bright* areas). **F, G.** Vertical (**F**) and horizontal (**G**) sections through the guinea-pig retina. Müller cells were immunolabeled for cellular retinaldehyde-binding protein (CRALBP; *green*), and cones were labeled by peanut agglutinin (*red*). **F.** The cone inner segments in the photoreceptor segment layer (RSL) appear as "continuous" with the outer processes of Müller cells which envelop the cone perikarya in the ONL. **G.** The focus of the image is on the OPL. The number of cone pedicles (*red*) roughly equals that of Müller cell processes (*green*); often the two elements appear as pairs. Thus, each cone can receive its part of the image of the outside world by its "individual" light-guiding Müller cell. **H.** Artist's view of the optical path through the retina. Light arrives at the inner retinal surface where it hits Müller cell endfeet. Then it propagates trough the Müller cell stem processes (thus bypassing the light-scattering retinal structures, particularly in the two plexiform layers) until it arrives at the photoreceptor cells. Every Müller cell illuminates a distinct group of photoreceptors, about 10 rods and one cone in the human retina. **I.** By light guidance, Müller cells transport an image (*left*) like a fiberoptic plate (*middle*) with minimal loss of light intensity from the inner retinal surface to the photoreceptors; this image is resolved in "pixels" corresponding to individual Müller cells (*right*). **J–L.** The linear rows of rod nuclei in the ONL act as chains of lenses, allowing the light beam to pass the ONL. **J.** Mathematical simulation of light transport through the nuclei of adult mouse rod photoreceptors. **K, L.** Postnatal re-modeling of the chromatin structure and the shape of rod nuclei in the mouse retina. **K.** At early postnatal stages, the nuclei are elongated and display a conventional chromatin pattern. **L.** In the adult retina, the rod nuclei are spherical and show an inverted pattern of hetero- (*red*) and euchromatin (*green*). The nucleoli (*blue, arrowheads*) moved towards the nuclear surface. This inversion of the nuclear architecture (which is unique and occurs only in rods of nocturnal mammals) may be required to optimize the optical properties of these nuclei in the long "lens chains" of the thick outer nuclear layer in these species. NFL, nerve fiber layer; INL, inner nuclear layer. Modified from Franze et al. (2007), Solovei et al. (2009), and Agte et al. (2011).

living eye (Drexler and Fujimoto, 2008). The light scattering is expected to reduce the retinal light transmission resulting in decreased visual sensitivity in darkness and decreased visual acuity under daylight conditions. In order to minimize the retinal light scattering, primate retinas contain a fovea in which the inner retinal layers of the central area are shifted laterally and the light directly hits the photoreceptor cells (Reichenbach and Bringmann, 2010), while in non-foveal regions, Müller cells deliver the light through their cell bodies, bypassing the scattering elements of the inner retina and illuminating the photoreceptor cells.

5.4.2   LIGHT-GUIDING PROPERTIES OF MÜLLER CELLS

Müller cells act as living optical fibers that guide the light through the inner retinal layers towards the photoreceptors with minimal distortion and loss (Fig. 37H), similar to glass fiber optics (Fig. 37I) (Franze et al., 2007). When the endfoot of an enzymatically isolated individual Müller cell is illuminated by visible light, much more light arrived at the opposite side than when the outer stem process is illuminated, or when no Müller cell is placed into the optical path (Franze et al., 2007). This suggests that the funnel-shaped endfoot of Müller cells acts as light collector at the vitread surface of the retina, and that the stem processes are light-guiding fibers (Fig. 37H) (Franze et al., 2007). A thin laser light beam is transported through all retinal layers without much scattering and divergence if it hits a Müller cell endfoot (Fig. 37B) but causes intraretinal light scatter, and diverges considerably, if it hits the area between two adjacent Müller cells (Fig. 37C) (Agte et al., 2011). When confocal images are recorded from acutely isolated retinal wholemounts in the reflection mode, Müller cells remain dark whereas neuronal and vascular elements can be seen as bright structures (Fig. 37D, E) (Franze et al., 2007). This means that the light is passed through Müller cells but back-scattered by neuronal and vascular structures. The refractory index of Müller cell stem processes is slightly lower (1.38) than that of photoreceptor outer segments (1.4; which are also light-guiding fibers; Enoch and Tobey, 1981, and references therein) but higher than that of the surrounding retinal tissue (1.35–1.36) (Franze et al., 2007). On the other hand, the refractory index of Müller cell endfeet is rather low (1.35–1.36), about halfway between that of Müller cell stem processes and that of the vitreous body (1.335) (Franze et al., 2007). This allows a "soft coupling" of the light path between the vitreous and the retina, and reduces the light reflection at the inner retinal surface (Franze et al., 2007). The nuclei of Müller cells are usually localized out of the cell axis (Fig. 32) (Uckermann et al., 2004a); this is consistent with the light-guiding function of the stem processes.

Although Müller cell processes occupy <10% of the retinal cross-sectional area and tissue volume (Reichenbach et al., 1988a), Müller cells channel virtually all light from one side of the neuroretina to the other; this makes it possible that just few photons are detected by the photoreceptors of most vertebrates. By this way, they conserve the diameter of a beam that hits a single Müller cell endfoot (Labin and Ribak, 2010; Agte et al., 2011). The molecular basis of the light-guiding capacity of Müller cells is unknown and remains to be determined. Bundles of intermediate filaments are arranged along the light path (Fig. 32). In tissue edema (a characteristic of ischemic and inflammatory retinal diseases), the neuroretina loses its transparency (Iandiev et al., 2011a), and Müller cells upregulate the expression of intermediate filaments (see 5.11.3.). The milky opacity of the edematous tissue may suggest that the light guidance through Müller cells is deteriorated, resulting in increased light scattering in the neuroretinal tissue. In addition, crystallins were suggested to prevent the diffusion of light in cells (Reva et al., 2013).

By light guidance, Müller cells transport an image (like a fiberoptic plate) with minimal loss of light intensity from the inner retinal surface to the photoreceptors; this image is resolved in "pixels" corresponding to individual Müller cells (Fig. 37I) (Franze et al., 2007; Agte et al., 2011). Because the local densities of cones and Müller cells are roughly equal (Fig. 37F,G) (Agte et al., 2011), every cone has its "private" Müller cell which delivers its part of the image, while several rods (up to 10 in the human retina) are illuminated by one Müller cell (Fig. 37A,H). Müller cells are wavelength-dependent light guides; they concentrate the green-red part of the visible spectrum onto cones and allowing the blue-purple part to leak onto nearby rods (Labin et al., 2014). The array of light-guiding Müller cells will increase the number of photons arriving in the photoreceptor cell outer segment and, thus, contribute to a high sensitivity of the rods during night vision, will improve the contrast sensitivity of vision by enhancing the signal-noise ratio in the cone arrays, and will facilitate the detection of fast-moving objects (Franze et al., 2007; Labin and Ribak, 2010; Agte et al., 2011). Maximum possible resolution is achieved because, for each cone, there exists an individual light-guiding Müller cell. The retinas of reptiles and birds contain Müller cells with many thin branches (Fig. 29) which appear not to be suitable for light guidance. It may be speculated that this is (one of) the reason(s) for the presence of up to three foveas in the same retina of some birds.

The outer stem process of Müller cells in the outer nuclear layer is irregularly shaped (Fig. 2B,E), and intermediate filaments are absent in the (outer part of) this layer (Figs. 31, 32). Thus, this part is not suitable as an optic fiber. Instead, light is guided through this layer by rod nuclei which are arranged in linear vertical rows providing a chain of lenses which collect and transport the light to the photoreceptor segments (Fig. 37J) (Solovei et al., 2009; Kreysing et al., 2010). In nocturnal animals, which have a thick outer nuclear layer, this function of rod nuclei might be supported by the spherical shape of the nuclei and the inverted arrangement of chromatin, i.e., heterochromatin localizes to the nuclear center and euchromatin lines the nuclear border, rather than *vice versa* as in "normal" nuclei (Fig. 37K,L) (Solovei et al., 2009). At the border between the outer plexiform and outer nuclear layers, the light is transferred from Müller cells to photoreceptor nuclei. Here, the outer stem process of Müller cells taper and split into thin branches. A similar tapering can be observed on cone outer segments in many species; it has been speculated that these tapered cylinders are light radiators which transfer the light (that has been guided but not absorbed in the cone outer segments) to the adjacent rod outer segments (Miller and Snyder, 1973). As an analogy, the tapered outer process of Müller cells may act as light radiators which illuminate a chain of rod nuclei.

5.5   HOMEOSTATIC AND METABOLIC SUPPORT OF RETINAL NEURONS

5.5.1   MECHANICAL TISSUE HOMEOSTASIS

5.5.1.1 Mechanical Forces in the Retinal Tissue

Neuronal activity is associated with rapid ion shifts between intra- and extracellular spaces. Sodium, calcium, and chloride ions flow into activated neurons while potassium ions are released from neurons. Because ion fluxes are associated with water fluxes, neuronal activity causes also rapid alterations in the size of neuronal synapses and cell bodies, in particular in the plexiform layers which contain many ionotropic receptors and sodium-dependent transporters. Glutamate induces a swelling of inner retinal neurons (Figs. 3B,E, 38B, 39A,B, 40A,B) (Uckermann et al.,

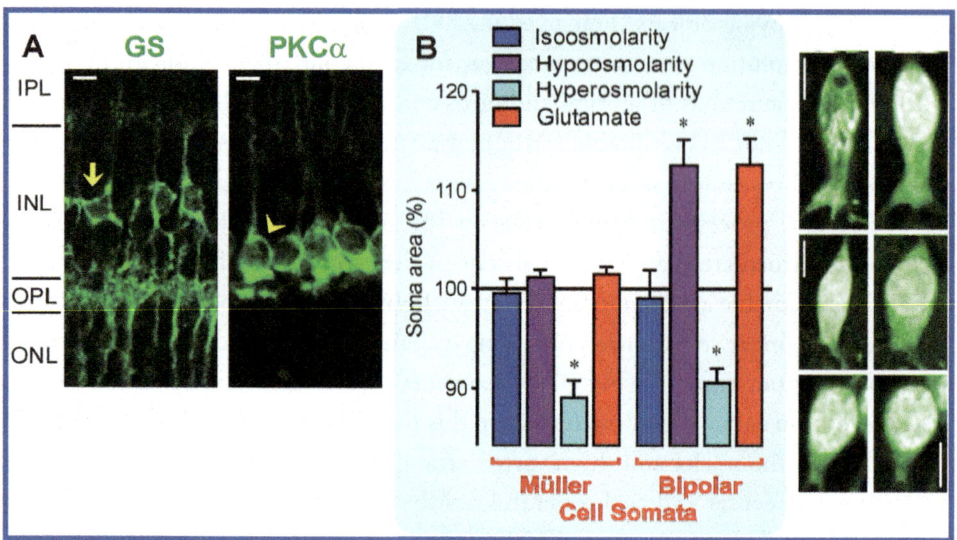

FIGURE 38: Glutamate and hypoosmolarity of the extracellular fluid induce a swelling of bipolar cells but not Müller cells in slices of the rat retina. **A.** Retinal slices stained for the glial marker glutamine synthetase (GS) and the rod bipolar cell marker protein kinase Cα (PKCα). The focus is at the inner nuclear layer (INL). *Arrow*, Müller cell soma. *Arrowhead*, bipolar cell soma. Note that Müller cell somata are localized in the central part of the INL while bipolar cell somata are localized near the outer border of the INL. IPL, inner plexiform layer; ONL, outer nuclear layer; OPL, outer plexiform layer. Bars, 5 μm. **B.** The slices were superfused with an isoosmotic, a hypoosmotic (60% of control osmolarity), and a hyperosmotic solution (which was made up by addition of 100 mM sucrose to the extracellular solution), respectively, and the cross-sectional area of cell somata was recorded after 4 min of superfusion. Glutamate (1 mM) was applied for 15 min in isoosmotic solution. Müller cell somata did not increase their size in hypoosmotic solution and in the presence of glutamate, respectively, whereas bipolar cell somata swelled under both conditions. The hyperosmotic solution caused a shrinking of both Müller and bipolar cells. The *images* display examples of bipolar cell somata recorded before (*left*) and after hypoosmotic swelling (*right*). Bars, 5 μm. *$P<0.05$. Modified from Vogler et al. (2013a) and Garcia et al. (2014).

2004b; Wurm et al., 2008a; Vogler et al., 2013a). In retinal ganglion cells, activation of AMPA/KA receptors by glutamate causes a net uptake of sodium chloride which is associated with a water influx, resulting in a swelling of the cell bodies and synapses (Figs. 3B,D, 39A,B) (Uckermann et al., 2004b). Glutamate induces a swelling of bipolar cells via a sodium influx due to activation of NMDA and AMPA/KA receptors, sodium-dependent glutamate transporters, and voltage-gated sodium channels (Vogler et al., 2013a). Neuronal activity is also associated with a decrease of the

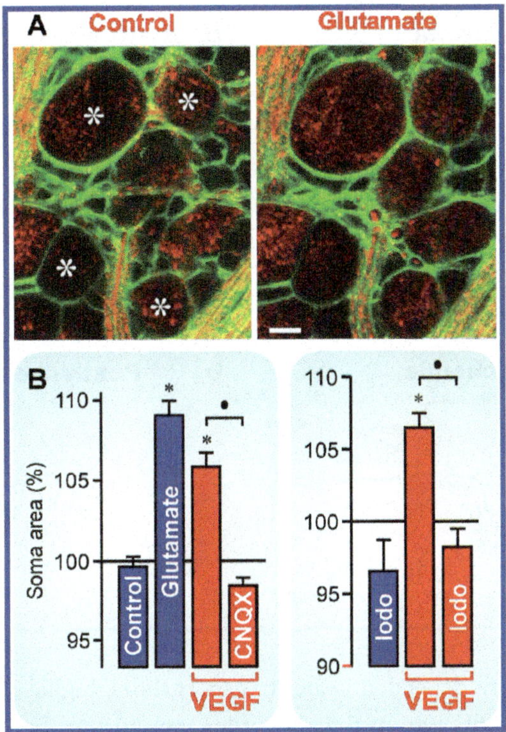

FIGURE 39: Müller cell-derived glutamate may induce swelling of neuronal cell somata in the ganglion cell layer of the rat retina. The plasma membranes in retinal wholemounts were stained with a FM dye. **A.** The size of neuronal cell bodies (*) in the ganglion cell layer of retinal wholemounts increases upon administration of glutamate (1 mM, 15 min). Bar, 5 μm. **B.** The cross-sectional area of neuronal somata shows an increase upon administration of glutamate and VEGF (10 ng/ml, 15 min), respectively. The effect of VEGF is prevented by the competitive inhibitor of AMPA/kainate receptors, cyanonitroquinoxalinedione (CNQX; 50 μM), suggesting that VEGF evokes a release of endogenous glutamate that subsequently activates ionotropic glutamate receptors expressed by retinal neurons. **C.** The VEGF-evoked swelling of retinal neurons is prevented in the presence of the gliotoxin iodoacetate (iodo; 1 mM), suggesting that Müller cell-derived glutamate contributes to neuronal cell swelling. *$P<0.001$. Bar, 5 μm. Modified from Wurm et al. (2008a).

osmolarity of the extracellular fluid because the activity-dependent decrease of the sodium chloride concentration in the extracellular fluid exceeds the increase of the potassium concentration by a factor of two (Dmitriev et al., 1999). The reduction of the extracellular osmolarity leads to an osmotic gradient that favors water flux from extracellular to intracellular spaces. Hypoosmolarity of the extracellular fluid causes a swelling of bipolar cells (Fig. 38B) that is induced by a release of

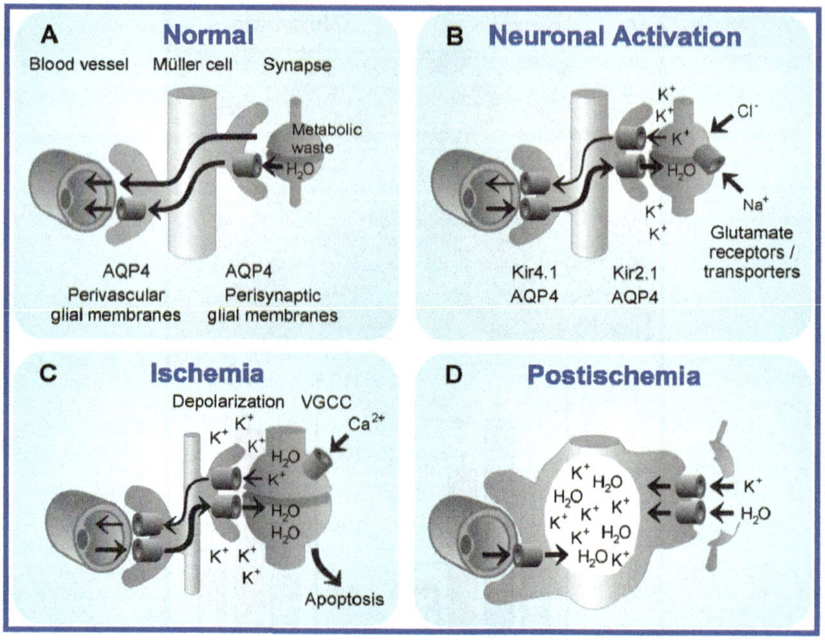

FIGURE 40: Model of activity-dependent water transport through glial AQP4 in the plexiform layers of the retina and possible contribution of the glial water transport to the ischemic injury of the retina. **A.** Under resting conditions, Müller cells mediate the constitutive dehydration of the inner retina. The water transport from the retinal interstitium through the Müller cell bodies into the blood vessels is facilitated by AQP4 water channels expressed at high amount in the perivascular and perisynaptic membrane domains of Müller cells. The transport of metabolic water may be coupled to the transglial transport of metabolic waste. **B.** Intense neuronal activity results in a sodium flux into the synapses mediated by ionotropic and metabotropic glutamate receptors, glutamate transporters, and voltage-gated sodium channels. The sodium influx is associated with a chloride and water flux. The water flux results in synapse swelling. Because the plexiform layers are high-resistance barriers of extracellular water movement (Antcliff et al., 2001), the water which flows into activated synapses is delivered from the Müller cell interior through AQP4 localized in their perisynaptic membranes; this is followed by a water flux from the vessels into Müller cells. Activated neurons release potassium ions which flow through Kir channels into Müller cells; simultaneously, an equal amount of potassium ions are released by Müller cells into the blood mediated by Kir4.1 channels. Note the different direction of the water transport in dependence on the level of neuronal activity. **C.** In the ischemic retina, over-excited neurons release a huge amount of potassium and glutamate. The strong activation of glutamate receptors and transporters, as well as the high extracellular potassium level, cause (in addition to synaptic swelling) a long-lasting depolarization of neurons resulting in activation of voltage-gated calcium channels (VGCCs). The intracellular calcium overload activates the apoptosis machinery of the cells. In this model, closure of AQP4 will inhibit the water flux from the blood into the Müller cells and subsequently into the synapses. Because ion currents

are necessarily associated with a water flux, inactivation of AQP4 will hinder the rapid flux of sodium and calcium ions into the synapses, resulting in a reduced extent of neuronal cell swelling and apoptosis. **D.** Within days after reperfusion, Müller cells downregulate the expression of Kir4.1 channels in the perivascular membranes while Kir channels in the perisynaptic sheets are largely unaltered. This results in an accumulation of potassium within the Müller cell bodies that causes an osmotical driving force for water movement from the blood into the cells, resulting in Müller cell swelling. Modified from Bringmann et al. (2005).

---

endogenous glutamate which induces a sodium influx resulting from activation of metabotropic glutamate receptors (mGluRs) and sodium-dependent transporters associated with a water flux (Vogler et al., 2013a). The swelling of neuronal cells results in a thickening of the inner retinal tissue (Fig. 3G) (Uckermann et al., 2004b). Müller cells adapt their morphology to the increased size of activated retinal neurons with an extension (Fig. 3G) and thinning of the inner stem process (Fig. 3B,D,H) (Uckermann et al., 2004b). Similar morphological alterations of Müller cells and a thickening of the inner retinal tissue are also observed during retinal ischemia and during administration of a high-potassium extracellular solution (Fig. 3C,D,F,I); both conditions induce a release of endogenous glutamate in the retinal tissue (Uckermann et al., 2004b). The glutamate-induced thickening of the inner retina may be a reason for the predominant distribution of the intermediate filament vimentin in the inner stem process of Müller cells (see 5.2.) which provides mechanical stability during the activity-dependent Müller cell elongation. Cellular swelling results in a shrinkage of the extracellular space (Fig. 3H) (Dmitriev et al., 1999; Uckermann et al., 2004b) which, if uncompensated, will cause neuronal hyperexcitation (Dudek et al., 1990; Chebabo et al., 1995). The morphological alterations of Müller cells limit the glutamate-induced decrease of the extracellular space volume, i.e., the decrease is smaller than expected when only the neuronal swelling is considered (Uckermann et al., 2004b). Thus, the compensatory reshaping of Müller cells is a homeostatic response to prevent deleterious decreases of the extracellular space volume.

In addition to morphological alterations due to glutamatergic neurotransmission, there are tractional forces onto Müller cells deriving from the retinomotor movements in response to changes of the light conditions as well as from the vitreous body. In the human retina, the vitreous body adheres to the retinal tissue at the peripheral retina, the major superficial retinal vessels, the optic disc, and the macula (Schubert et al., 1989). At sites of vitreo-retinal attachments, the basement membrane of the inner limiting membrane can become thinner, and vitreous fibers adhere directly to Müller cells (Schubert et al., 1989). Under normal conditions, many vitreous fibers distribute tractional forces evenly to numerous Müller cells. However, in cases of vitreous shrinkage and partial posterior vitreous detachments as occurring during aging, fewer vitreous fibers and Müller cells endure most of the traction; this may result in chronic irritation of Müller cells and local release of factors that, in turn, induce Müller cell gliosis and vascular leakage (Schubert et al., 1989; see 5.11.11.3.).

5.5.1.2 Viscoelastic Properties of Müller Cells

The reshaping of Müller cell processes during glutamatergic neurotransmission (Fig. 3B,D) or induced by tractional forces is supported by the viscoelastic properties of the cells. Müller cells are softer than neurons, e.g., about twice as soft as bipolar and amacrine cells (Lu et al., 2006). The inner and outer stem processes of Müller cells are even softer than the endfoot (Fig. 41A) and the soma (Lu et al., 2006, 2013). The difference of the viscoelastic properties between neuronal

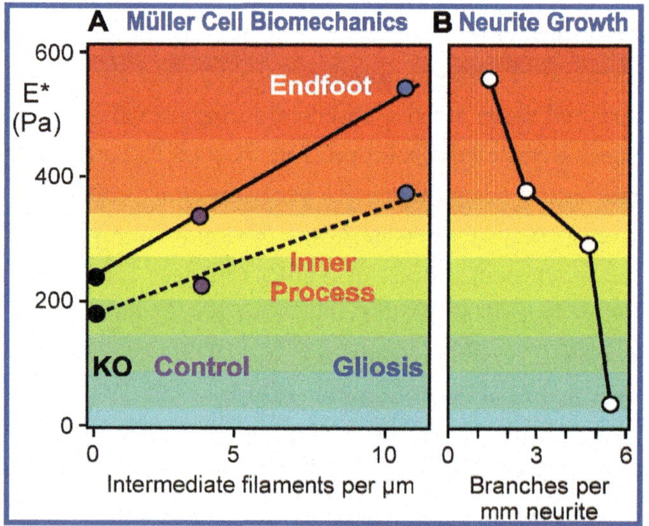

FIGURE 41: Stiffness of murine Müller cells (**A**) and dependence of neurite branching on the stiffness of the culture substrate (**B**). The stifness (elastic modulus, E^*) of Müller cells was measured at the inner stem process (localized in the inner plexiform layer *in situ*) and the endfoot of isolated cells derived from retinas of wildtype mice, from retinas of transgenic (KO) mice which lacked the intermediate filaments GFAP and vimentin, and in gliotic Müller cells from wildtype mice. Müller cell gliosis was induced by high-intraocular pressure-induced transient retinal ischemia for 1 h; the cells were isolated 6–8 days after ischemia. Gliosis is associated with an increased density of intermediate filaments (as counted in electron microscopical images of radial sections of Müller cells). There is a linear regression between the elastic modulus of the endfeet and inner processes and the density of intermediate filaments in the cells. Modified from Flanagan et al. (2002) and Lu et al. (2011).

and glial cells may generally occur in CNS cells because it was found that hippocampal pyramical neurons are stiffer than hippocampal astrocytes (Lu et al., 2006). Because Müller cells are softer than neurons, they may act as soft, compliant embedding for neurons (Lu et al., 2006). The relative softness of Müller cells is also apparent in the inner nuclear layer where glial somata are impressed by the surrounding neuronal somata (Fig. 3E) (Lu et al., 2006). Synaptic plasticity and glutamatergic synaptic swelling occurs primarily in the inner plexiform layer (Fig. 3B,D) (Uckermann et al., 2004b). This corresponds with the notable softness of the inner stem process (Fig. 41A) which is localized in this layer *in situ* (Lu et al., 2006, 2011, 2013). The softness of Müller cells enables them to flexibly alter their morphology in dependence on the activity-dependent swelling of neurons and synapses. Growing neurites prefer soft substrates (Fig. 41B) (Flanagan et al., 2002; Discher et al., 2005; Georges et al., 2006); neuronal growth cones are actively guided by soft substrates and avoid rigid substrates (Franze et al., 2009). Thus, Müller cells may act as deformable substrates for neurite outgrowth and branching implicated in both retinal development and adult synaptic plasticity (Lu et al., 2011). Synaptogenesis and synaptic plasticity might be particularly stimulated by the viscoelastic properties of the inner stem process lying in the inner plexiform layer *in situ* which is the softest region of Müller cells (Lu et al., 2013) and which display the greatest glutamate-induced morphological alterations due to the high density of synapses. In addition, Müller cells may protect neurons from mechanical stress which might be caused, for example, by traumatic craniocerebral injuries or, in the aged human eye, by the movements of the shrinked vitreous body.

When isolated entire Müller cells is subjected to a global deformation induced by an optical cell stretcher device, the cell stretching and subsequent relaxation behavior is analogous to the behavior of two Voigt elements in series (Lu et al., 2006). The Voigt element is a viscoelastic object composed of a restoring spring (elastic part) and a dissipative dashpot (viscous part), connected in parallel. The resulting overdamped viscoelastic behavior of the cells is comparable to that of shock absorbers (Lu et al., 2006). Because Müller cells behave as elastic, restoring but highly compliant soft solids, they cannot serve as structural support cells (because they are too soft) or as glue (because restoring forces are dominant) for neurons (Lu et al., 2006). The molecular basis of the subcellular inhomogeneities in the viscoelasticity of Müller cells is presently unknown but might be partly caused by the inhomogeneous distribution of cellular organelles, the actin cytoskeleton, and intermediate filaments (Fig. 31) (Reichenbach et al., 1988a,b, 1989).

5.5.1.3 Increased stiffness of reactive Müller cells

Intermediate filaments contribute to the biomechanical properties of Müller cells. Müller cells of mice lacking the intermediate filaments GFAP and vimentin display an enhanced fragility upon mechanical challenge compared to cells from wildtype mice (Lundkvist et al., 2004). Basically,

Müller cells of GFAP- and vimentin-knockout mice have similar biomechanical properties as cells from wildtype mice (Fig. 41A) (Lu et al., 2011). This may reflect the relative scarcity of intermediate filaments in normal wildtype Müller cells. Reactive gliosis, associated with an upregulation of intermediate filaments (Bringmann et al., 2009b; see 5.11.3.), alters the biomechanics of Müller cells. As shown in Figure 41A, the stiffness of the endfeet and inner stem processes of gliotic Müller cells is strongly increased when compared to that of control cells; the increased stiffness correlates with the increased density of intermediate filaments in the cells (Lu et al., 2011). In contrast, Müller cells of mice that lack intermediate filaments do not undergo any alterations of their biomechanics under pathological conditions (Lu et al., 2011). This suggests that the upregulation of intermediate filaments is one major factor which defines the viscoelastic properties of reactive Müller cells (Lu et al., 2011). Rigid glial scars will impair neurite growth and may contribute to the poor regenerative capabilities of the mammalian retina (Lu et al., 2011). Therapeutic suppression of the upregulation of intermediate filaments in reactive Müller cells may facilitate the regeneration of injured retinal tissue including neurite growth and plasticity (Wilhelmsson et al., 2004; Cho et al., 2005), migration and differentiation of endogenous or transplanted cells (Kinouchi et al., 2003; Widestrand et al., 2007), and the maturation of stem cell-derived neurons (Teixeira et al., 2009). The enhanced stiffness of reactive Müller cell endfeet and inner processes may be also (at least in part) responsible for the fact that, in retinal ischemia, new blood vessels grow towards the vitreous rather than within the retinal tissue (Lundkvist et al., 2004). In GFAP- and vimentin-knockout mice, intraretinal vessel growth rather than an intravitreal neovascularization was observed under pathological conditions, suggesting that reactive Müller cells normally provide a physical barrier to the growth of new blood vessels (Lundkvist et al., 2004). However, upregulation of GFAP *per se* does not inhibit the growth of new neurites from retinal ganglion cells (Toops et al., 2012b), likely by inducing a permissive glial environment for retinal remodeling (see 5.11.2.8. and 5.11.3.3.).

5.5.1.4 Sensing Mechanical Tissue Deformations

Müller cells sense mechanical deformations of the retinal tissue by calcium-dependent mechanisms. Stretching of the retinal tissue induces calcium responses, activation of ERK1/2, and upregulation of the transcription factor c-Fos and of bFGF in Müller cells (Fig. 42A–F) (Lindqvist et al., 2010). Thus, mechanical stress triggers molecular responses in Müller cells that could prevent retinal damage, e.g., activation of MAPKs and the release of neuroprotective factors such as bFGF (Fischer et al., 2009a; Bringmann et al., 2009b). This might have implications also for the postnatal eye growth. Because bFGF counteracts the development of form deprivation-induced axial myopia (Rohrer and Stell, 1994), Müller cell-derived bFGF may prevent retinal over-stretching and the

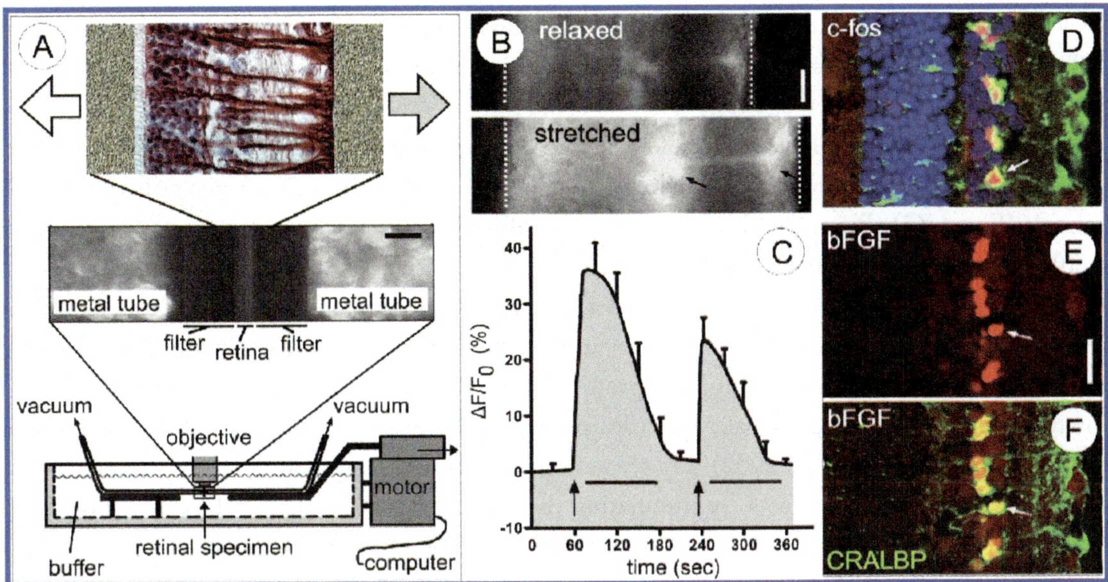

FIGURE 42: Müller cells sense and respond to mechanical stretch. **A.** Experimental setup to stretch retinal pieces (orthogonally to their surfaces) under microscopic control. **B.** Müller cells in adult guinea pig retinae were stained with the fluorescent and calcium-sensitive dye X-Rhod-1; two images of the same section of a retina where the image on *top* shows the unstretched, relaxed retina with weakly fluorescent Müller cells. The retina was stretched to a 20% increase in retinal thickness using a speed of 2 µm per s, and an immediate increase of fluorescence intensity in Müller cells could be observed as shown in the image *below*. **C.** The change in the cytosolic free calcium level over time was calculated relative to the fluorescence at time point 0 ($\Delta F/F_0$). The *arrows* indicate the start of the stretch, the *horizontal bars* indicate the time period during which the retina was kept in a stretched position; note that the fluorescence decreased during this time. **D.** After 60 min in stretched retinae, immunoreactivity for c-Fos (*red*) was significantly increased in Müller cell bodies (*arrow*), as revealed by counter-staining with the Müller cell-selective marker, cellular retinaldehyde-binding protein (CRALBP; *green*). Hoechst 33258 was used to identify cellular nuclei (*blue*). **E, F.** 180 min after stretch, the staining for basic fibroblast growth factor (bFGF) was increased in somata in the inner nuclear layer (*arrow*). **F.** Double-staining for bFGF and CRALBP was used to identify Müller cells as bFGF-expressing cells. Scale bars, 25 µm. Note that in this figure the retina is turned by 90° to the right in comparison with the other figures. Modified from Lindqvist et al. (2010).

development of myopia during ocular growth (Lindqvist et al., 2010). Mechanical stretching of Müller cells induces extensive changes in the expression of genes implicated in cell proliferation, tissue remodeling, and vasculogenesis (Namba et al., 2001; Wang et al., 2013c).

Human Müller cells have stretch-activated calcium-permeable cation channels (Puro, 1991a). Calcium influx results in increased activity of calcium-activated, big-conductance potassium (BK) channels (Fig. 43G) (Puro, 1991b). The potassium efflux through BK channels is associated with an efflux of cell water and results in a decrease of the Müller cell volume (Puro, 1991b). Tractional forces onto Müller cells (e.g., after partial detachment of the vitreous from the retina as occurring during aging) will increase the calcium influx into the cells and will activate BK channels; both events are involved in mediating the proliferation of Müller cells induced by high-potassium, growth factors or ATP (Puro et al., 1989; Puro and Mano, 1991; Kodal et al., 2000; Bringmann et al., 2000a, 2001; Moll et al., 2002). Thus, tractional forces may trigger neuroprotective effects but may also have detrimental effects, by stimulating the development of Müller cell gliosis and proliferation (see 5.11.11.3.). Murine Müller cells express the TRPV4 cation channel known to mediate osmotransduction and mechanotransduction (Ryskamp et al., 2011).

5.5.2   NEUROTRANSMITTER RECYCLING

Glial cells enhance the synaptic efficacy of retinal neurons (Pfrieger and Barres, 1997). In the retina, both chemical and electrical synapses transmit visual signals from the photoreceptors to the ganglion cells. Müller cells are involved in the synaptic signaling of the retina by the rapid uptake of neurotransmitter molecules and providing the precursor of neuronal transmitter synthesis. The precise shaping of the synaptic activity depends upon the kinetics of both the presynaptic release of neurotransmitter and the cellular reuptake of the transmitter molecules. In the retina, photoreceptor cells, neurons, and macroglial cells express high-affinity transporters for neurotransmitters. Müller cells express uptake and exchange systems for various neurotransmitters including glutamate, GABA, glycine, and adenosine. The uptake and metabolization of glutamate and GABA by Müller cells are key steps of the glutamate-glutamine cycle (see 5.5.2.1.9.), and link neuronal excitation with the release of lactate and other molecules that nourish retinal neurons (see 5.5.7.2.), the defense against oxidative stress (see 5.5.2.1.15.), the shaping and termination of the synaptic glutamate action in the inner retina (see 5.5.2.1.1.), the release of gliotransmitters (see 5.6.1.), and the detoxification of excess ammonia (see 5.5.2.1.14.). Alterations in the Müller cell's transmitter recycling contribute to the neuroprotective and detrimental effects of retinal gliosis. A malfunction (see 5.5.2.1.6.) and even a reversal of glial glutamate transporters (see 5.6.1.1.) is a common phenomenon in retinopathies associated with increased extracellular glutamate. However, the pathogenic mechanisms resulting in a decreased glial glutamate clearance capacity are incompletely understood.

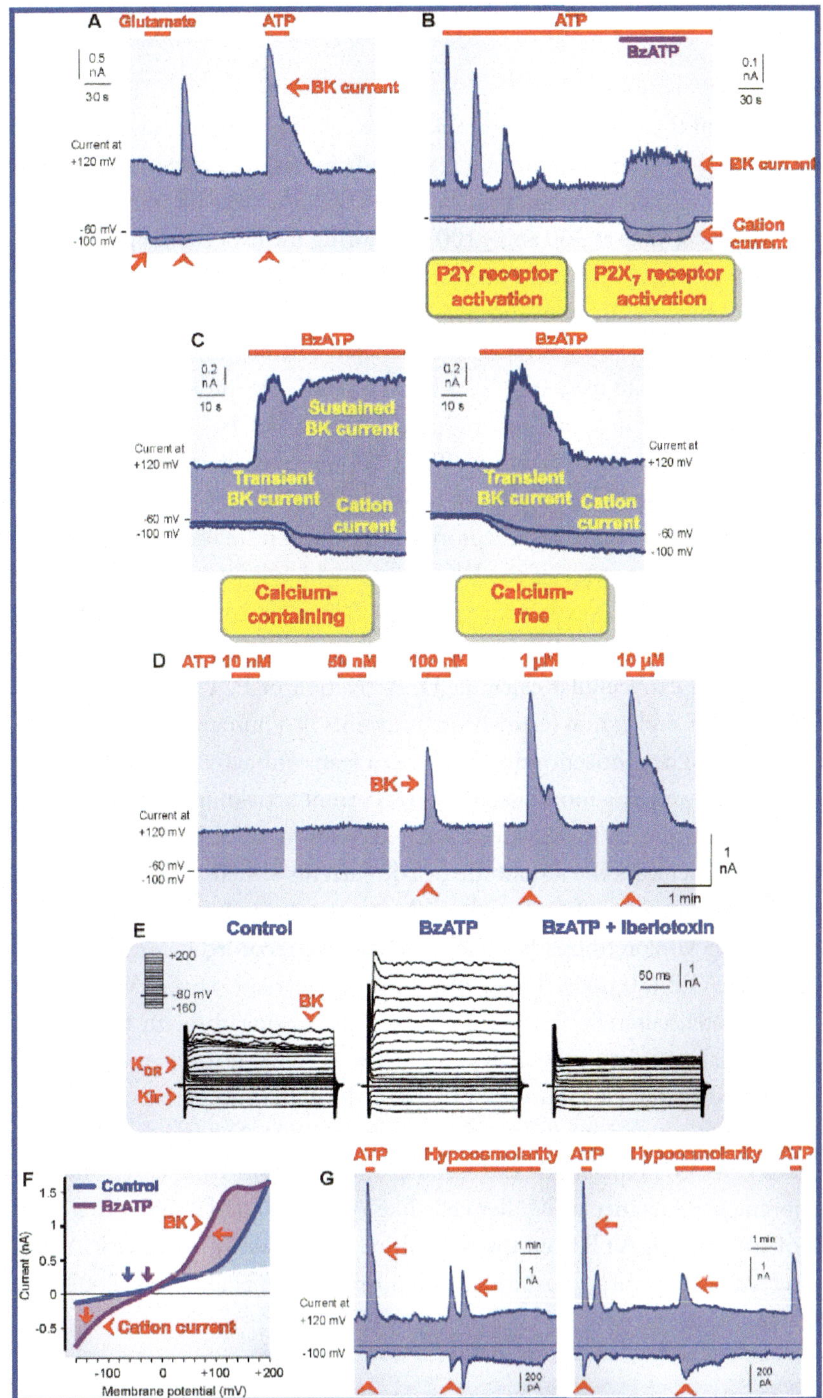

FIGURE 43: Activation of metabotropic glutamate receptors, glutamate transporters, P2Y and P2X$_7$ receptors, as well as hypoosmotic stress alter the membrane conductance of human Müller cells. **A, B.**

continued on next page

Time-dependent record of the whole-cell currents in one cell. The currents at +120 mV are mainly mediated by BK channels. **A.** The BK currents are transiently inreased in response to P2Y receptor activation by ATP (500 μM). Extracellular glutamate (500 μM) evoks a delayed transient increase in BK currents. The increase in the currents at −60 and −100 mV during the exposure of glutamate (*arrow*) reflects the activation of electrogenic glutamate transporters. The *arrowheads* indicate transient activation of calcium-induced cation channels. **B.** Activation of P2Y and P2X$_7$ receptors in another cell. Activation of P2Y receptors by ATP (100 μM) evokes repetitive transient calcium-induced activation of BK currents (recorded at the potential of +120 mV; *left*). Activation of P2X$_7$ receptors by the P2X$_7$ receptor agonist BzATP (50 μM) evokes a sustained calcium-induced activation of BK currents, as well as cation currents through P2X$_7$ receptor channels (*right*). **C.** The P2X$_7$ receptor channels are permeable for calcium ions. *Left:* Administration of BzATP (50 μM) to a human Müller cell evokes a transient increase of the BK currents (through stimulation of P2Y receptors and subsequent release of calcium from intracellular stores) followed by a sustained increase of the BK currents which is caused by an influx of calcium from the extracellular space through P2X$_7$ receptor channels. *Right:* Under extracellular calcium-free conditions, the sustained component of the BK current response is absent, whereas the transient BK current increase is independent on extracellular calcium. **D.** Activation of P2Y receptors with increasing ATP concentrations activates BK and cation (arrowheads) currents in a human Müller cell from a patient with PVR. Note that ATP at higher concentrations induces a transient activation of BK and cation currents (*arrowheads*) which is followed by a more sustained BK current activation that results from a calcium influx from the extracellular space. **E.** In an acutely isolated cell from a donor eye, activation of P2X$_7$ receptors by BzATP (50 μM) increases the amplitude of BK currents which is inhibited by coadministration of the BK channel blocker iberiotoxin (100 nM). **F.** Mean current-voltage relations of Müller cells from patients with proliferative vitreoretinopathy. The currents were recorded before and during activation of P2X$_7$ receptors with BzATP (50 μM). The BzATP-evoked increase of the currents at hyperpolarized (negative) membrane potentials reflects the cation currents flowing through the P2X$_7$ receptor channels. At positive potentials, a shift in the activation of BK currents towards more negative potentials is apparent which is caused by the calcium influx through the P2X$_7$ receptor channels. Activation of the cation conductance results in a positive shift of the zero-current (0 pA) potential (*arrows*) that reflects the depolarization of the cells. **G.** Hyposmotic extracellular solution (60% osmolarity) induces similar alterations of the membrane conductance of Müller cells like ATP (100 μM), suggesting that osmotic stress induces a release of endogenous ATP from the cells which subsequently activates P2Y receptors. *Arrows,* BK current. *Arrowheads,* cation current. Modified from Bringmann et al. (2001, 2002a) and unpublished results (A. Bringmann, Leipzig).

Generally, the driving force of the uni- or bidirectional substrate transport across membranes is the transmembrane gradient of the substrate itself and of ions which are cotransported with the substrate. The bulk of the neurotransmitter uptake by Müller cells is sodium-dependent (Biedermann et al., 2002; Sarthy et al., 2005) and allows uphill transport of substrates into the cells against a concentration gradient. The driving force for these transporters is the electrochemical gradient of sodium ions over the plasma membrane that is generated by the energy-consumptive activity of the sodium-potassium-ATPase. In the case of electrogenic sodium-dependent transporters, there is a net influx of positive charges into the cells, while in electroneutral transporters, the inward shift of positive charges is balanced by the cotransport of other ions.

5.5.2.1 Glutamate Uptake and Metabolism

The principal amino acid neurotransmitters in the retina are L-glutamate, GABA, and L-glycine. Glutamate is the main excitatory neurotransmitter in the retina (Thoreson and Witkovsky, 1999) and is used in the retinal forward transmission of visual signals by photoreceptors, bipolar, and ganglion cells (Massey and Miller, 1987, 1990; Islam and Atoji, 2009; Reichenbach and Bringmann, 2012). In addition, a subpopulation of amacrine cells may release glutamate (Du et al., 2008). In the outer retina, glutamate is released continuously from photoreceptor terminals in the dark; this release is inhibited by light (Reichenbach and Bringmann, 2012). In the inner plexiform layer, ON-bipolar cells release glutamate in the light, and OFF-bipolar cells release glutamate in the dark. Photoreceptor and bipolar cells do not generate action potentials but respond to light with graded potentials that modulate the continuous release of glutamate. Ganglion cells and a subpopulation of amacrine cells are the only retinal neurons that generate action potentials.

5.5.2.1.1 Functional Role of the Glial Glutamate Uptake   In the CNS, glial glutamate transporters are responsible for the bulk of the glutamate uptake, while neuronal glutamate transporters have more specialized roles in shaping the time course of synaptic responses and the termination of the presynaptic glutamate release (Wersinger et al., 2006; Beart and O'Shea, 2007). In the neural retina, photoreceptors, neurons, and macroglial cells express high-affinity glutamate transporters (Derouiche, 1996; Rauen and Wiessner, 2000). Müller cells remove the bulk of extracellular glutamate in the inner retina (White and Neal, 1976; Ladanyi and Beaudet, 1986; Harada et al., 1998; Rauen et al., 1998; Rauen, 2000; Pow et al., 2000; Holcombe et al., 2008). Under pathological conditions (when the transport into Müller cells is reduced; see 5.5.2.1.6.), a higher amount of glutamate is also transported into retinal neurons (Barnett et al., 2001; Holcombe et al., 2008). It has been suggested that the bulk of glutamate released from photoreceptor terminals is removed by presynaptic transporters of photoreceptor cells (Hasegawa et al., 2006) and by postsynaptic transporters localized to horizontal and bipolar cells (Rauen et al., 1996). However, a study done in the rabbit retina showed that inhibition of the main glutamate uptake carrier of Müller cells (GLAST; see 5.5.2.1.2.) is highly effective in blocking the synaptic transmission in the outer plexiform layer and in inducing a permanent electroretinogram deficit, whereas inhibition of GLT1 (see 5.5.2.1.2.)

caused no permanent electroretinogram deficit (Levinger et al., 2012). Whether the opposing data reflect species differences remains to be clarified.

The role of glial transporters in shaping the time course of excitatory transmission may vary in dependence on the type of synapses investigated. The glutamate uptake by Müller cells in the inner retina contributes to the rapid termination of the postsynaptic action of glutamate in non-spiking retinal neurons and ganglion cells (Matsui et al., 1999; Higgs and Lukasiewicz, 2002). Here, Müller cell's glutamate uptake is an active part in synaptic transmission. When the retinal glutamate transport is blocked with a competitive inhibitor, the amplitude and duration of ganglion cell's excitatory postsynaptic currents increase dramatically; when only the neuronal transport is blocked, little change in synaptic current is observed (Higgs and Lukasiewicz, 2002). In the outer plexiform layer which contains the photoreceptor terminals (Fig. 2A), Müller cells take up glutamate which is diffused out of the synaptic clefts; this prevents a lateral spread of the transmitter, separates individual synapses from each other, and thus ensures visual resolution (Rauen et al., 1996). The diffusion of glutamate out of the synaptic cleft of photoreceptor terminals proceeds with a time constant of less than 1 ms (Vandenbranden et al., 1996) which is 10–100 times faster than the time constants of the light-induced responses in second-order neurons (Copenhagen et al., 1983). Müller cell processes are 1–3 µm away from the sites of glutamate release (Sarantis and Mobbs, 1992), and thus are located within diffusion times of a few milliseconds from the synaptic cleft. However, the finding of a significant glutamate spillover between cone photoreceptors (Szmajda and Devries, 2011) makes it likely that the diffusion barrier constituted by Müller cells is at least temporarily switched off.

There are further indications for the assumption that the glutamate uptake and metabolism of Müller cells is more directly involved in the regulation of the activity of inner retinal neurons than of photoreceptors. These include, for example, the cellular distribution of glutamate-metabolizing enzymes: aspartate aminotransferase is predominantly localized to photoreceptors and some horizontal cells (Gebhardt, 1991), glutamate dehydrogenase is localized to photoreceptor inner segments and Müller cells (Gebhardt, 1992), and glutamine synthetase to Müller cells (Riepe and Norenburg, 1977). The precursor of the glutamate synthesis in bipolar and ganglion cells (glutamine) is derived almost exclusively from Müller cells whereas photoreceptor cells synthesize only a part of their glutamate from Müller cell-derived glutamine (Pow and Robinson, 1994). In addition, a significant amount of GABA in amacrine cells is synthesized from glutamate after uptake of Müller cell-derived glutamine (Pow and Robinson, 1994).

The clearance of the synaptic glutamate by Müller cells is required for the prevention of neurotoxicity; malfunction of the glutamate transport into Müller cells results in an increased extracellular glutamate level that can be toxic to neurons through overstimulation of iGluRs (Choi, 1988). After experimental inhibition of the glial glutamate uptake, even low concentrations of extracellular glutamate become neurotoxic (Kashii et al., 1996; Izumi et al., 1999, 2002). Alterations in the activity of glial glutamate transporters induced by alterations of the membrane potential might be also involved in the regulation of the glial support of the neuronal signal transfer from photoreceptors to retinal ganglion cells (glial forward signaling; see 5.7.).

5.5.2.1.2 Glial Glutamate Transporters Müller cells regulate the extracellular glutamate level via sodium-dependent and -independent uptake systems (Sarthy et al., 2005). The sodium-dependent removal of glutamate from extracellular sites in the retina involves at least five EAATs (EAAT1-5) (Kanai and Hediger, 2004). EAATs mediate the transport of L-glutamate and L- and D-aspartate (but not D-glutamate) (Kanai and Hediger, 2004). The major glutamate transporter of Müller cells is the electrogenic, sodium-dependent, high-affinity glutamate-aspartate transporter (GLAST or EAAT1) (Otori et al., 1994; Derouiche and Rauen, 1995; Rauen et al., 1996, 1998; Lehre et al., 1997; Rauen, 2000). In Müller cells of the mouse, approximately 50% of extracellular glutamate is taken up via GLAST, another 40% through electroneutral, sodium-dependent (presently undefined) glutamate transporters, and 10% via sodium-independent transporters or exchangers (Sarthy et al., 2005). One of the sodium-independent glutamate uptake systems of Müller cells is the cystine-glutamate antiporter (Mysona et al., 2009; Oliveira et al., 2010; see 5.5.2.1.15.). Rat Müller cells express, in addition to normally spliced GLAST, the splice variants GLAST1a and 1b which lack exon 3 and 9, respectively (Macnab et al., 2006; Macnab and Pow, 2007). While GLAST is localized throughout the Müller cell bodies, GLAST1a is localized preferentially to the endfeet and inner stem processes of the cells, suggesting a selective regulation of GLAST function in different membrane domains (Macnab et al., 2006). In addition, the splice variant GLAST1c, where exons 5 and 6 are skipped, may be expressed (Lee et al., 2012b). Normally, GLAST1c exhibits an intracellular peri-nuclear distribution; this protein rapidly redistributes to the cell surface upon activation of protein kinase C (PKC) (Lee et al., 2012b).

In addition to GLAST, the presence of other EAATs in Müller cells of various species has been described: glutamate transporter-1 (GLT1 or EAAT2; goldfish, rat, man), excitatory amino acid carrier 1 (EAAC1 or EAAT3; carp, bullfrog, rat, man), EAAT4 (rat, cat), and EAAT5 (rat) (Vandenbranden et al., 2000a; Rauen, 2000; Zhao and Yang, 2001; Kugler and Beyer, 2003; Fyk-Kolodziej et al., 2004; Ward et al., 2005). Müller cells of the salamander express at least four distinct EAAT subtypes (Eliasof et al., 1998). Similar to Müller cells, retinal astrocytes express multiple EAAT subtypes (GLAST, EAAC1, EAAT4) (Rauen et al., 1996; Lehre et al., 1997; Pow and Barnett, 1999; Rauen, 2000; Kang et al., 2000; Kugler and Beyer, 2003; Ward et al., 2004).

Knockout or antisense knockdown of GLAST results in a marked suppression of the electroretinogram b-wave (reflecting the depolarization of glutamatergic ON-bipolar cells in response to activation by photoreceptor cells; Stockton and Slaughter, 1989) and oscillatory potentials (originating in the inner plexiform layer; Karwoski and Kawasaki, 1991), whereas GLT1 knockout mice exhibit a minimal compromise of the retinal function (Harada et al., 1998; Barnett and Pow, 2000). This suggests that GLAST is essential for the maintenance of the normal synaptic transmission in the retina. In GLAST knockout mice, the total retinal levels of glutamate and GABA (which is produced from glutamate; Fig. 44) is increased about twofold compared to that in the wild type (Sarthy et al., 2004). While the retinas of GLAST and GLT1 knockout mice show a benign phenotype, retinal damage after ischemia is exacerbated, suggesting that both transporters play a neuroprotective role in the ischemic retina (Harada et al., 1998).

In addition to astrocytes and Müller cells, photoreceptors and retinal neurons take up glutamate and express multiple EAAT subtypes (reviewed in Bringmann et al., 2013). A direct recycling of glutamate by photoreceptor terminals (Winkler et al., 1999; Hasegawa et al., 2006) is in agreement with the observation that only a part of glutamate used by photoreceptor cells is derived from the glutamate-glutamine cycle (Pow and Robinson, 1994). Apparently, a direct recycling of glutamate is energetically more efficient than the use of glutamine-derived glutamate. In addition to the uptake of glutamate, neuronal glutamate transporters have also other functional roles in the regulation of synaptic events. Presynaptic transporters, in particular such with a high chloride conductance (EAAT4/5), act as glutamate receptors that mediate a fast inhibitory feedback regulation on the glutamate release (Wersinger et al., 2006; Gameiro et al., 2011).

5.5.2.1.3 Ion Dependency of the Glial Electrogenic Glutamate Transport   Close to the resting membrane potential of Müller cells (approximately −80 mV; Figs. 8H, 45E, 46A,B,D), the glutamate concentration that half-maximally activates the electrogenic transporters is 10-20 µM in amphibian Müller cells, and 2 µM in rat Müller cells (Barbour et al., 1991; Rauen et al., 1998; Matsui et al., 1999). The transport of glutamate by EAATs involves the cotransport of 3 sodium ions (Fig. 47B) and 1 proton, and the counter-transport of 1 potassium ion, with each glutamate anion (Barbour et al., 1988; Amato et al., 1994; Pannicke et al., 1994; Kanai and Hediger, 2004; Owe et al., 2006; Beart and O'Shea, 2007). The coupling of the glutamate transport with the ion transport allows an uphill transport of glutamate into the cells against a concentration gradient. The transport of an excess of (positively charged) sodium ions into the cell generates an inward current (Fig. 47A–D) (Brew and Attwell, 1987; Barbour et al., 1988, 1991; Schwartz and Tachibana, 1990; Pannicke et al., 1994; Sarthy et al., 2005). By the electrogenic glutamate transport, the intracellular concentration of glutamate in Müller cells can rise at a rate of ~0.5 mM per second if no metabolization of glutamate occurs (Barbour et al., 1993). The influx of both glutamate and sodium ions may result in a swelling of Müller cells after prolonged (1 h) incubation of retinal slices with high glutamate (Casper et al., 1982; Izumi et al., 1996, 1999).

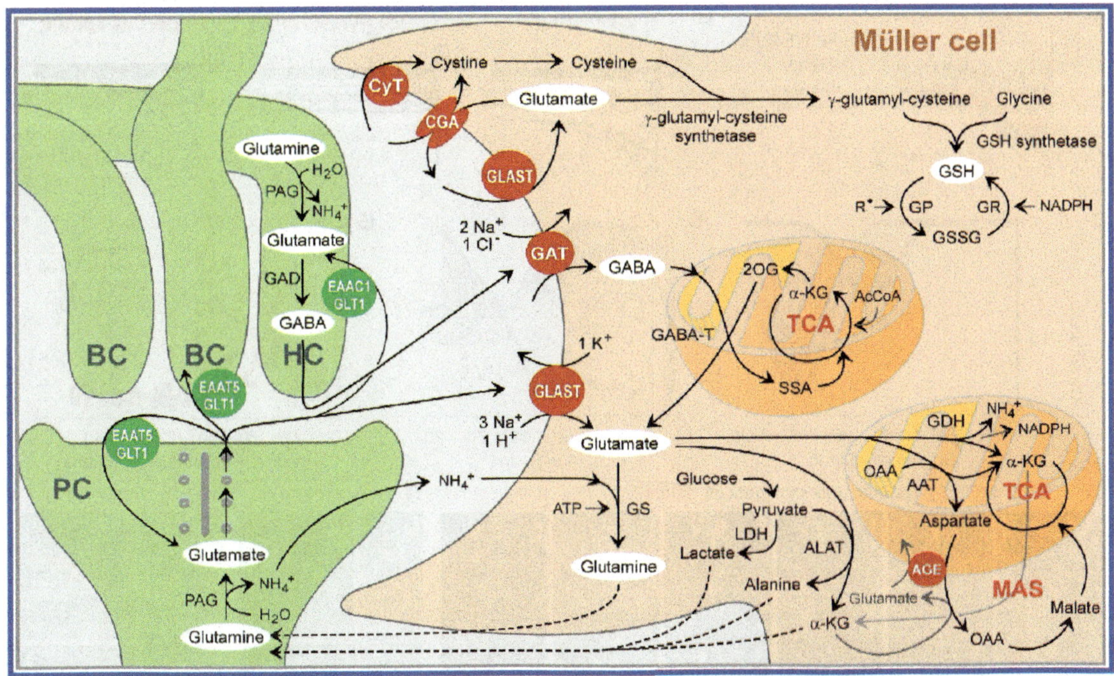

FIGURE 44: Recycling of amino acid neurotransmitters in the outer plexiform (synaptic) layer. The ribbon synapse of a photoreceptor cell (PC) synthesizes glutamate which is continuously released in the dark. The postsynaptic elements are dendrites of bipolar (BC) and horizontal cells (HC). Horizontal cells release GABA which is formed from glutamate. The synaptic complexes are surrounded by Müller cell sheets. The *right side* shows neurotransmitter uptake systems and some metabolic pathways of Müller cells. Glutamate, GABA and ammonia (NH_4^+) are transported into Müller cells and transformed to glutamine, alanine, and α-ketoglutarate (α-KG). Glutamine is released from Müller cells and serves as precursor for the transmitter synthesis in neurons (glutamate-glutamine cycle). Lactate, alanine, pyruvate, α-ketoglutarate, and glutamine are utilized by neurons as substrates for their energy metabolism. The mitochondrial enzyme GABA transaminase (GABA-T) catalyzes the formation of glutamate from 2-oxoglutarate (2OG), coupled to a conversion of GABA to succinate semialdehyde (SSA). Glutamate is also used for the production of reduced glutathione (GSH) which is an antioxidant, released from Müller cells and taken up by neurons under oxidative stress conditions. AcCoA, acetyl coenzyme A; ALAT, alanine aminotransferase; AAT, aspartate aminotransferase; CGA, cystine-glutamate antiporter; CyT, cystine transporter; EAAC1, excitatory amino acid carrier 1; EAAT5, excitatory amino acid transporter 5; GAD, glutamic acid decarboxylase; AGC, aspartate-glutamate carrier; GAT, GABA transporter; GDH, glutamate dehydrogenase; GLAST, glutamate-aspartate transporter; GLT-1, glutamate transporter-1; GlyT, glycine transporter; GP, glutathione peroxidase; GR, glutathione reductase; GS, glutamine synthetase; GSSG, glutathione disulfide; LDH, lactate dehydrogenase; MAS, malate-aspartate shuttle; OAA, oxaloacetate; PAG, phosphate-activated glutaminase; R•, free radicals; TCA, tricarboxylic acid cycle. Modified from Bringmann et al. (2009a).

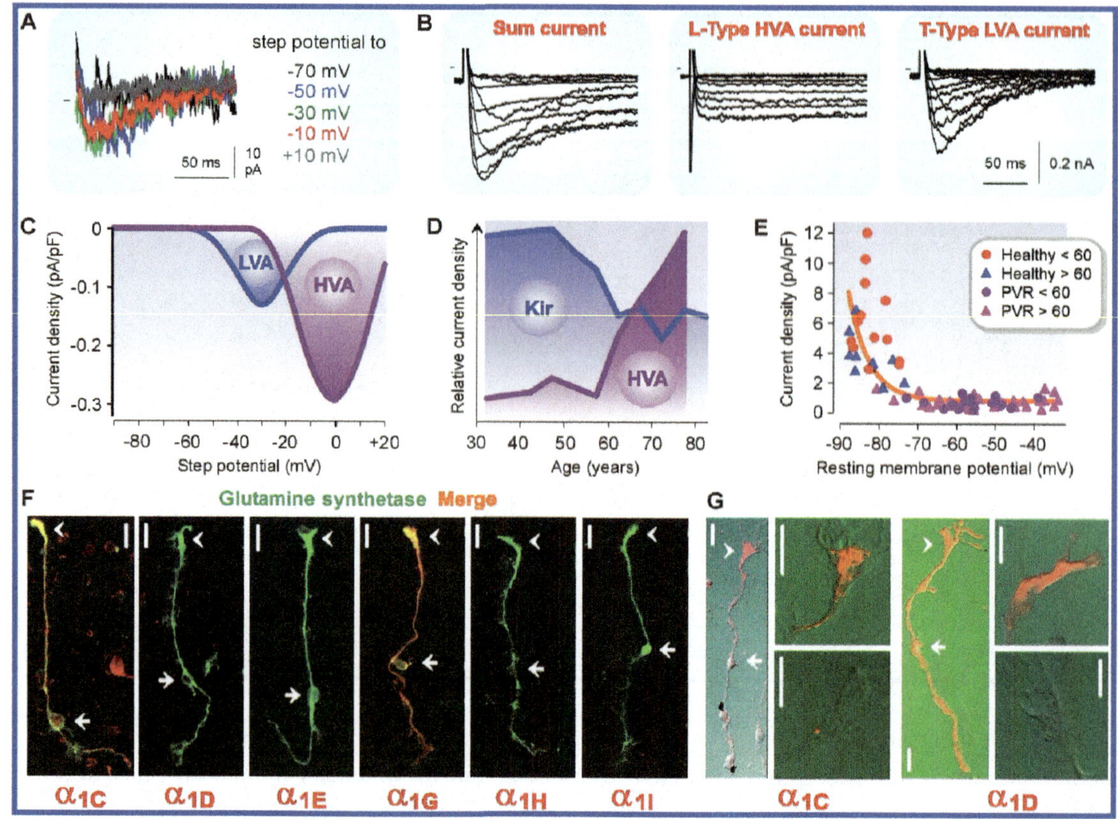

FIGURE 45: Voltage-gated calcium channels of Müller cells and age-dependent and gliotic alterations of the Kir conductance of human Müller cells. **A.** Sodium currents through low voltage-activated calcium channels of a Müller cell from an adult rat. **B, C.** Acutely isolated human Müller cells display transient (T-type) calcium currents through low voltage-activated (LVA) channels and long-lasting (L-type) calcium currents through high voltage-activated (HVA) channels. **B.** Example of sodium currents through voltage-gated calcium channels in one cell. The sum currents were evoked by depolarizing voltage steps (increment, 10 mV) from pre-pulses to −120 mV. The non-inactivating HVA currents were evoked by depolarizing voltage steps from pre-pulses to −70 mV. The difference between both records revealed the presence of transient LVA currents. Sodium ions were used as charge carrier in order to increase the amplitude of the currents through the calcium channels. **C.** Mean peak current density-voltage relationships of calcium currents through LVA and HVA channels. LVA channels activate at potentials positive to −60 mV, while HVA channels activate at voltages positive to −40 mV. **D.** Age-dependent alterations in the densities of Kir and HVA calcium currents in human Müller cells. Whereas the Kir currents display an age-dependent decrease, the currents through HVA channels increase in the course af aging. **E.** Relation between the Kir current density and the resting membrane potential of Müller cells from human donors of different age. The cells were derived from donors without apparent

retinal disease (Healthy) and from patients with PVR. **F.** Immunolabeling of isolated rat Müller cells for the α_{1C}, α_{1D}, α_{1E}, α_{1G}, α_{1H}, and α_{1I} subunits of voltage-gated calcium channels (*red*). The cells were counterstained against the glial cell marker glutamine synthetase (*green*). Co-localization yielded a *yellow* merge signal. Müller cells were stained for α_{1C} and α_{1G} subunits and not for α_{1D}, α_{1E}, α_{1H}, and α_{1I} subunits. *Arrows*, cell soma. *Arrowheads*, cell endfoot. **G.** Immunolabeling of isolated human Müller cells for the α_{1C} and α_{1D} subunits of voltage-gated calcium channels (*yellow-red*). *Small images:* Müller cell endfeet at higher magnification. The *small images above* display specific immunostaining; the *small images below* are negative controls obtained after omission of the first antibody. Scale bars, 20 µm. Modified from Bringmann et al. (2000b,c, 2003c) and Linnertz et al. (2011), and unpublished results (S. Schopf, Leipzig).

The amplitude of the electrogenic glutamate transporter currents in Müller cells is strongly voltage-dependent (Fig. 47C,D); a very negative membrane potential is essential for the efficient uptake of glutamate (Brew and Attwell, 1987; Sarantis and Attwell, 1990; Barbour et al., 1991; Pannicke et al., 1994). Cell depolarization, for example by an increase in extracellular potassium or by activation of glial ionotropic receptors (Fig. 47E), decreases the uptake rate substantially (Pannicke et al., 2000a). A decrease in the intracellular glutamate level stimulates the uptake of glutamate by Müller cells (Ola et al., 2011b).

EAATs subserve at least dual functions both as glutamate transporter and chloride channel (Ryan et al., 2004). The glutamate-elicited chloride conductance is recognizable in electrophysiological recordings as an outward current at positive membrane potentials (Fig. 47A) (Eliasof and Jahr, 1996; Billups et al., 1996; Sarthy et al., 2005). The glutamate transport and the chloride conductance are independent from each other (Billups et al., 1996; Grewer and Rauen, 2005). The chloride conductance of GLAST is relatively low when compared to EAAT4/5 (Grewer and Rauen, 2005). The glutamate-induced chloride conductance observed in Müller cells from GLAST knockout mice (Fig. 47A) might be mediated by EAAT5 (Sarthy et al., 2005).

5.5.2.1.4 Regulation of GLAST   The expression and activity of GLAST in Müller cells is regulated by the availability of extracellular glutamate. Short-term hypoxia, known to be associated with elevated extracellular glutamate and oxidative stress, stimulates the glutamate transport by a mobilization of transporters to the cell membrane and due to the depletion in cell glutathione (Payet et al., 2004). Extracellular glutamate increases the expression of GLAST in cultured Müller cells (Taylor et al., 2003; Imasawa et al., 2005; Xia et al., 2008) while extended exposure to high concentrations of glutamate induces a time-dependent internalization of the transporter proteins (Gadea et al., 2004). Glutamate receptor activation in cultured Müller cells results in an increase in

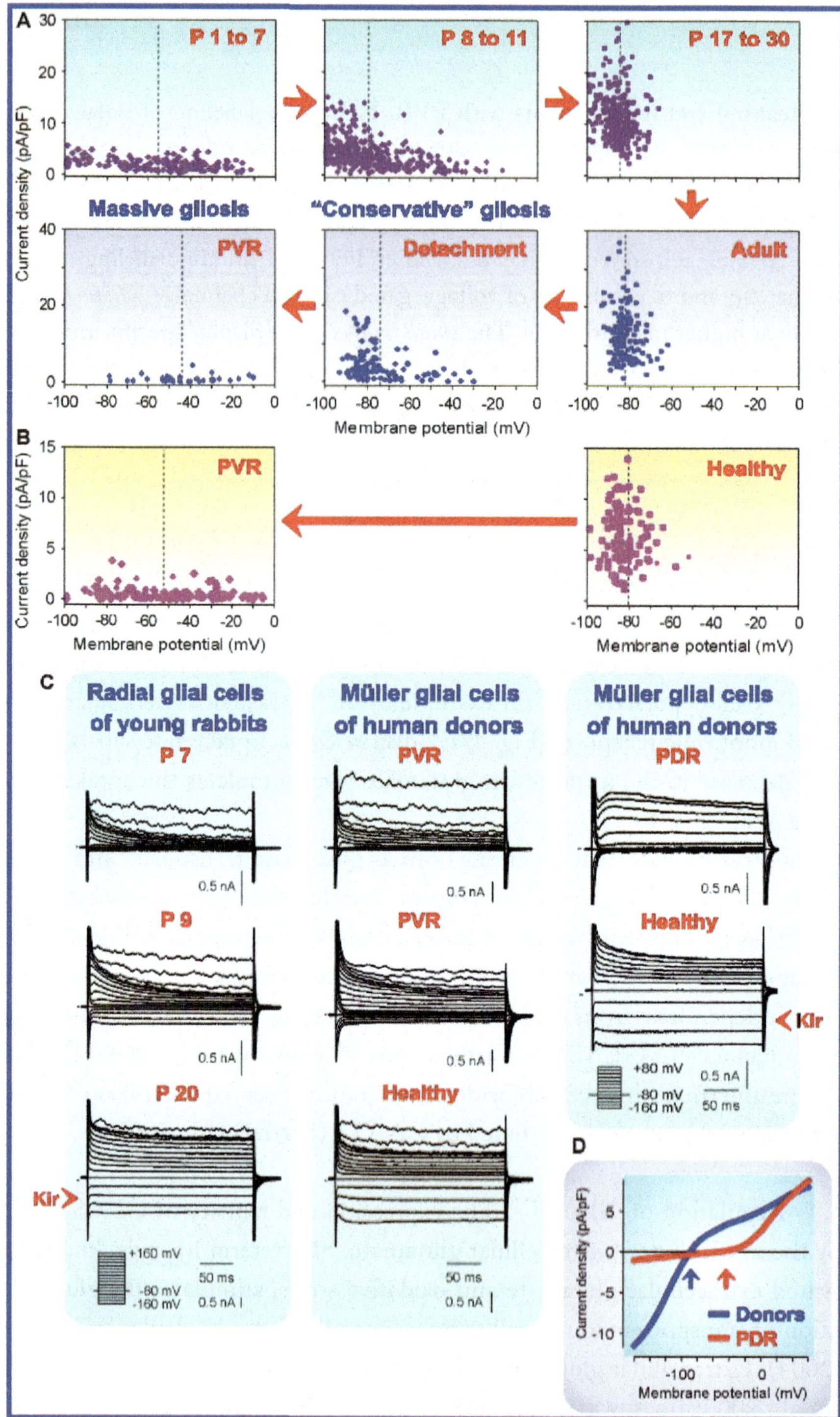

FIGURE 46: Relation between the Kir conductance and the resting membrane potential of rabbit (A) and human Müller cells (B). A. The Kir conductance and the membrane potential of rabbit Müller

cells display alterations during "conservative" and massive gliosis (*below*) which recapitulate the properties of maturing Müller cells (*above*; postnatal days 8–11) and late progenitor/stem cells (*above*; postnatal days 1–7) during the ontogenetic development of the retina. The *diagrams* display scatter plots of the Kir current density *vs.* the membrane potential for radial glial/Müller cells derived from young (*above*) and adult rabbits (*below*). In the case of adult animals, data from control retinas and from animal models of retinal detachment and proliferative vitreoretinopathy (PVR) are shown. *Dotted lines* indicate the mean resting membrane potential of the cells. **B.** The data were obtained from Müller cells of adult human donors without apparent retinal disease (Healthy) and of patients with PVR. **C.** Representative traces of the whole-cell potassium currents obtained in radial glial/Müller cells of young postnatal rabbits (*left*) and of adult human donors. Human cells were obtained from donors without eye diseases (Healthy) and from patients with proliferative vitreoretinopathy (PVR) and proliferative diabetic retinopathy (PDR), respectively. Note that the Kir currents are almost fully absent in the patient's cells. **D.** Current density-voltage relations of the whole-cell potassium currents of human cells from healthy donors and PDR. The *arrows* mark the zero-current (0 pA) potential of the currents which is close to the resting membrane potential of the cells. The zero-current potential is ~–80 mV in donor cells and ~–40 mV in patient's cells; this shift towards more positive potentials reflects the depolarization of Müller cells without functional Kir channels. Modified from Bringmann et al. (1999a,b, 2000a, 2002b) and Francke et al. (2001a).

---

the cytosolic free calcium and activation of PKC (Lopez-Colome et al., 1993; Lopez et al., 1998). Phosphorylation by PKC increases the activity of GLAST (but not of neuronal glutamate transporters) (Bull and Barnett, 2002; Gonzalez et al., 1999). The glutamate uptake by GLAST represents a receptor-independent mode of glutamate signaling in cultured Müller cells that stimulates the protein synthesis (Lopez-Colome et al., 2012). The intracellular signaling induced by GLAST activation involves calcium influx and activation of PI3K, Akt, mTOR, and p70S6K, as well as activator protein 1 (AP-1) binding to the DNA (Lopez-Colome et al., 2012). However, it is unclear whether these mechanisms observed in cultured Müller cells are also functional *in situ*. In tissue preparations of rabbit, guinea pig (Fig. 17B), and rat retinas, exogenous glutamate does not induce calcium responses in Müller cells (Newman and Zahs, 1997; Uckermann et al., 2003, 2004b, 2006; Newman, 2005; Rillich et al., 2009). In subpopulations of human Muller cells, small glutamate-induced calcium responses were observed; Fig. 48B; Bringmann et al., 2002a. Other factors that increase the GLAST expression in Müller cells are cAMP (Sakai et al., 2006), neurotrophic factors such as GDNF, BDNF, neurturin, and PEDF, as well as taurine (Naskar et al., 2000; Delyfer et al., 2005a; Koeberle and Bähr, 2008; Zeng et al., 2010b; Shen et al., 2012; Dai et al., 2012; Xie et al., 2012). Adenosine acting at A_{2A} receptors was described to downregulate GLAST in cultured Müller cells (Yu et al., 2012).

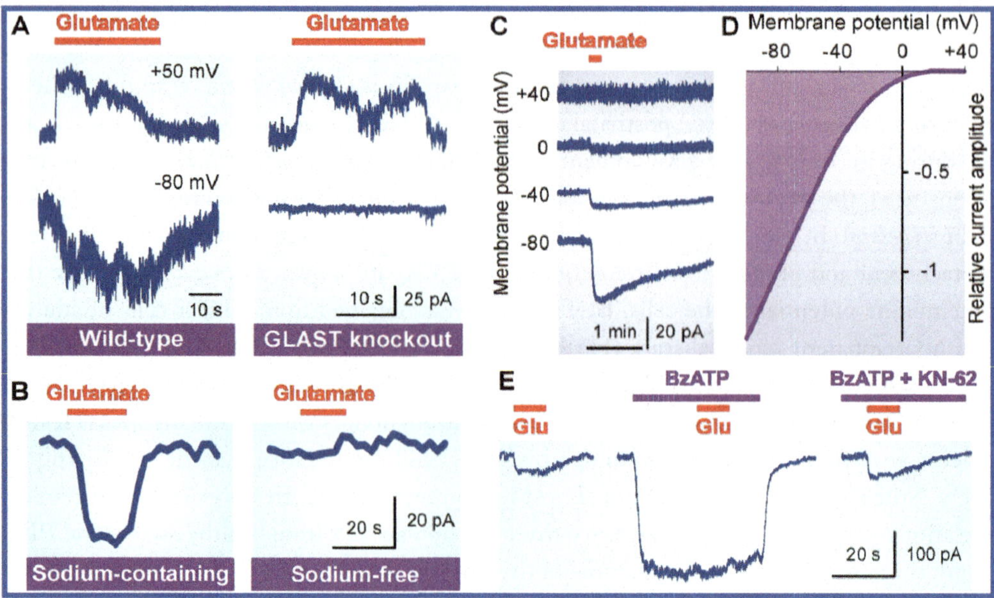

FIGURE 47: Electrogenic glutamate transport in Müller cells. Whole-cell records of membrane currents were made in freshly isolated cells. **A.** Administration of glutamate (1 mM) to a Müller cell of a wild-type mouse evoked inward currents at −80 mV, and outward currents at +50 mV. The inward currents were mediated by the sodium-dependent glutamate uptake, while the outward currents were mediated by the anionic (chloride) conductance of the glutamate transporter. (The amplitude of the anionic conductance was increased by replacing extracellular chloride with thiocyanate.) In a cell of a GLAST knockout mouse, glutamate did not evoke inward currents, whereas outward currents remained. The absence of inward currents may suggest that at the resting membrane potential of murine Müller cells the electrogenic glutamate uptake is mediated by GLAST. The presence of the chloride conductance may suggest that EAAT5 (which has a large chloride conductance and minimal glutamate transport capability) is also expressed in the cells. **B.** The electrogenic glutamate transport in Müller cells is dependent on extracellular sodium ions. Omission of sodium from the extracellular solution results in abolishment of the glutamate (100 µM)-induced inward currents. The traces were recorded in a rat Müller cell at a potential of −80 mV. **C.** Administration of glutamate (1 mM) to a rabbit Müller cell evokes inward currents at negative membrane potentials. The increase in current noise at 0 and +40 mV is caused by activation of voltage-dependent potassium channels. **D.** Current-voltage relation of the glutamate transporter currents in Müller cells of the guinea pig. (The anionic outward conductance is minimal because extracellular chloride instead of thiocyanate was used to record the currents.) **E.** Activation of ionotropic P2X$_7$ receptors (which mediate cation currents and thus a depolarization of the cells) decreases the electrogenic uptake of glutamate in human Müller cells. The uptake currents evoked by glutamate (Glu; 100 µM) were diminished in the presence of the P2X$_7$ receptor agonist 2′-/3′-O-(4-benzoylbenzoyl)-ATP (BzATP; 10 µM). Inhibition of P2X$_7$ activation by KN-62 (1 µM) suppressed the BzATP-evoked current (and cell depolarization), resulting in glutamate uptake currents similar in amplitude as under control conditions. Modified from Pannicke et al. (2000a, 2005a) and Sarthy et al. (2005).

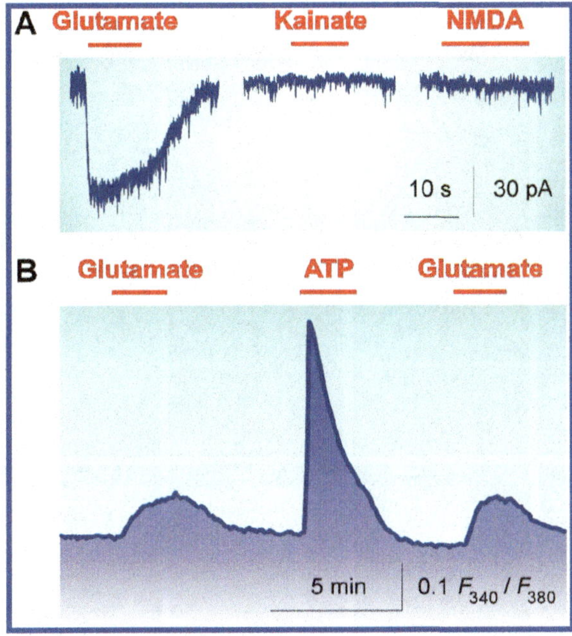

FIGURE 48: Freshly isolated Müller cells express metabotropic but not functional ionotropic glutamate receptors. **A.** In rat Müller cells, glutamate (100 μM) induces inward currents through electrogenic glutamate transporters while the glutamate receptor agonists kainate (500 μM) and NMDA (100 μM, in the presence of 10 μM glycine and the absence of magnesium) do not induce membrane currents. The current traces were recorded at a membrane potential of −80 mV. **B.** Administration of glutamate (100 μM) and ATP (500 μM) to a human Müller cell induces intracellular calcium responses, suggesting the presence of metabotropic glutamate receptors. The calcium imaging record was done in a cell from a patient with PVR. Modified from Bringmann et al. (2002a) and Pannicke et al. (2005a).

5.5.2.1.5 Glutamate Uptake in Retinal Development

In the human fetal retina, Müller cells express GLAST after cessation of the proliferation of late progenitor cells, shortly before synaptogenesis commences at 10 weeks gestation (Walcott and Provis, 2003; Diaz et al., 2007). In the rat retina, GLAST and GLT-1 are present in glia-like cells and in neuronal elements early in the development (embryonic day 12), before the onset of synaptogenesis (Williams et al., 2006). Weak immunoreactivity for GLAST in presumptive Müller cells is seen in rat retinas at postnatal day 0, and a rapid increase occurs between postnatal days 7 and 10 (Pow and Barnett, 1999) in correlation with a rise in the expression of the glutamine synthetase (Fig. 49) (Wurm et al., 2006b). In the course of the development of the rat retina, there is a gradual reduction in the numbers of cells that take up glutamate; the uptake is initially associated with a wide variety of cells including

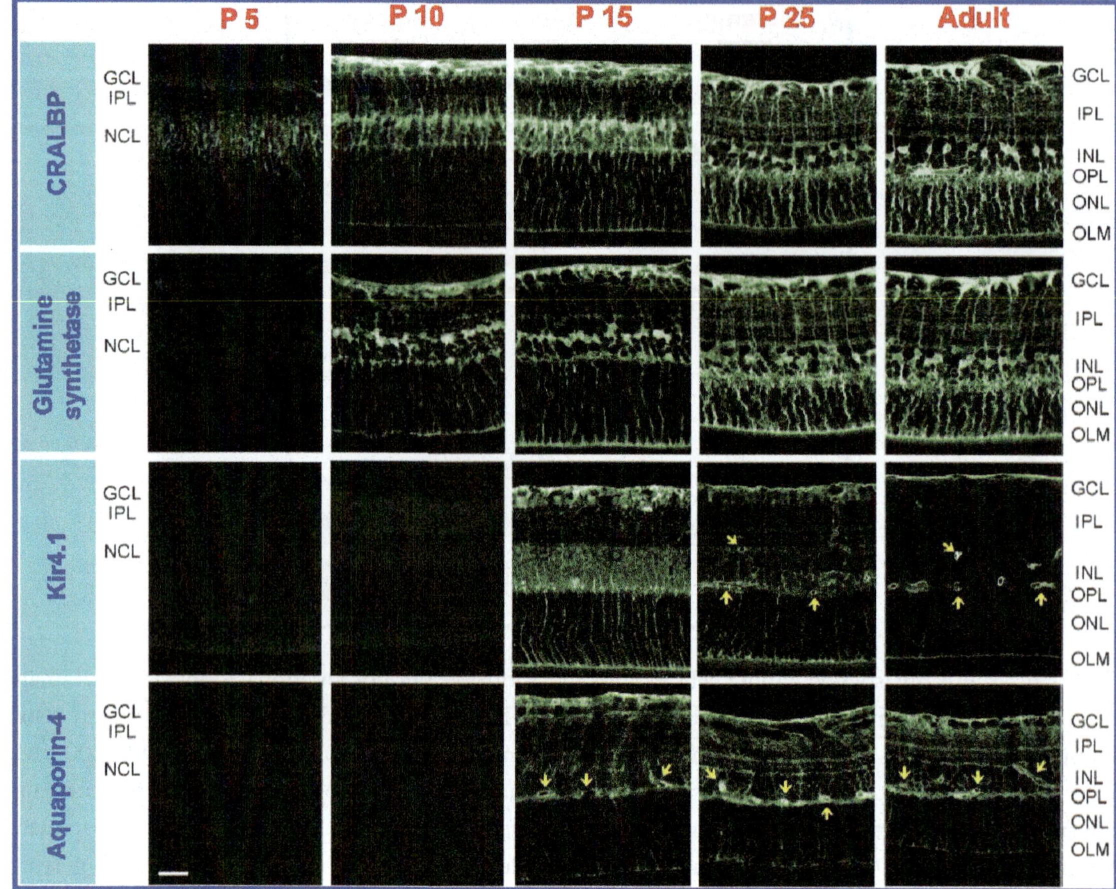

FIGURE 49: Expression of Müller cell proteins in the developing rat retina. Retinal slices from animals of different postnatal days (P), and of adult animals, were immunostained against CRALBP, glutamine synthetase, Kir4.1, and aquaporin-4 proteins. The Kir4.1 protein displays a relatively uniform distribution across the whole length of Müller cell fibers at P 15, and redistributes towards a prominent localization around the retinal vessels (*arrows*) and at the limiting membranes of the retina in the further course of development. On the other hand, aquaporin-4 protein displays a distribution similar to adult tissues from the very beginning of developmental expression. GCL, ganglion cell layer; INL, inner nuclear layer; IPL, inner plexiform layer; NCL, neuroblastic cell layer; OLM, outer limiting membrane; ONL, outer nuclear layer; OPL, outer plexiform layer. Bar, 20 μm. Modified from Wurm et al. (2006b).

neuroblasts, presumptive Müller cells, and astrocytes while in adult tissues, the uptake is predominantly mediated by Müller cells and astrocytes (Pow and Barnett, 1999).

5.5.2.1.6 Glutamate Uptake Under Pathological Conditions

Elevated levels of extracellular glutamate and the resulting glutamate toxicity have been implicated in the excitotoxic degeneration of retinal neurons in many ophthalmic disorders including glaucoma, ischemia-hypoxia, diabetic retinopathy, inherited photoreceptor degeneration, and autoimmune optic neuritis (Lucas and Newhouse, 1957; Louzada-Junior et al., 1992; Osborne and Larsen, 1996; Kitano et al., 1996; Ambati et al., 1997; Brooks et al., 1997; Lieth et al., 1998; Dkhissi et al., 1999; Kowluru and Kennedy, 2001; Martin et al., 2002; Osborne et al., 2004; Delyfer et al., 2005b; Villarroel et al., 2010; Ola et al., 2013; Hernández et al., 2013; Sühs et al., 2014). Relatively low concentrations of extracellular glutamate (10 µM–1 mM) decrease the survival rate of retinal neurons via activation of NMDA and non-NMDA receptors (Lucas and Newhouse, 1957; Kashii et al., 1996; Izumi et al., 1999, 2002; Baptiste et al., 2002; Lebrun-Julien et al., 2009a; Anccasi et al., 2013). Müller cells protect photoreceptors and retinal neurons from the excitotoxic action of high glutamate by the uptake of glutamate from the extracellular space (Izumi et al., 1999; Kawasaki et al., 2000; Koeberle and Bähr, 2008; Furuya et al., 2012) and by the secretion of antioxidative and neurotrophic factors (see 5.5.2.1.15. and 5.11.7.). A malfunction of the glial glutamate transport contributes to the increase in the extracellular glutamate to excitotoxic levels. Conditional ablation of Müller cells in a transgenic mouse model was shown to result in photoreceptor apoptosis which could be prevented by exogenous CNTF and the antiinflammatory corticosteroid triamcinolone acetonide, respectively (Shen et al., 2012, 2014a). CNTF causes also a shift of retinal glial cells toward a more neuroprotective phenotype which is characterized by, among others, a more efficient buffering of excess glutamate (Van Adel et al., 2005).

Various studies showed that transient retinal ischemia and diabetes do not significantly alter the plasma membrane expression and localization of GLAST but reduce the efficiency of the glutamate transport into Müller cells (Barnett et al., 2001; Li and Puro, 2002; Ward et al., 2005; Pannicke et al., 2005a, 2006). Under these conditions, a high amount of glutamate is transported into photoreceptor, bipolar, and ganglion cells (Barnett et al., 2001). Other studies showed a downregulation of GLAST in the diabetic retina (Saïdi et al., 2011; Silva et al., 2013; Hernández et al., 2013). A decrease in the GLAST-induced membrane currents in Müller cells was observed already at 2–4 weeks of experimental diabetes (Li and Puro, 2002). Because a reducing agent restored the activity of the glutamate transporter, it was suggested that the dysfunction of the glutamate transport in the diabetic retina is caused by oxidative stress (Li and Puro, 2002). Hypoxia elevates the mitochondrial peroxide production; the resulting lipid peroxidation was suggested to disrupt the glutamate transport into Müller cells (Muller et al., 1998). In addition, oxygen radicals, hydrogen peroxide, and peroxynitrite (which is formed by combination of superoxide and NO) directly inhibit the GLAST-mediated glutamate transport (Trotti et al., 1996). Dietary taurine ameliorates diabetic retinopathy at least in part via an increase in GLAST expression resulting from its antioxidant activity (Yu et al., 2008; Zeng et al., 2009, 2010b). Topical administration of somatostatin prevents the downregulation of GLAST induced by diabetes mellitus (Hernández et al., 2013).

Functional disorders of the glutamate uptake in Müller cells might be one of the etiologies of the secondary ganglion cell death in glaucoma (see 2.4.), in particular in patients with satisfactory control of intraocular pressure (Dreyer et al., 1996; Kawasaki et al., 2000; Harada et al., 2007). Conflicting data were published regarding the regulation of GLAST expression in glaucomatous eyes. Human retinas of patients with glaucoma were described to display a downregulation of GLAST, but not GLT1 (Naskar et al., 2000) while no alteration in GLAST expression, but an upregulation of GLT1, was found in experimental glaucoma (Park et al., 2009). Other studies described an increase in GLAST protein, especially in Müller cell processes which encompass the ganglion cells (Taylor et al., 2003; Woldemussie et al., 2004). In cultured Müller cells, elevated hydrostatic pressure was described to increase GLAST expression (Yu et al., 2012). Experimental glaucoma causes a decrease of the GLAST activity that results in a decreased accumulation of glutamate in Müller cells and a significant glutamate uptake by retinal ganglion cells; the failure of GLAST activity coincides with the excitotoxic damage of the retina (Holcombe et al., 2008). The decreased efficiency of the glial glutamate uptake results (at least in part) from the decrease of the glutamine synthetase expression and activity (Harada et al., 2007; Chen et al., 2008; Ishikawa et al., 2011; see 5.5.2.1.12.). Deletion of GLAST in mice results in spontaneous degeneration of retinal ganglion cells and optic nerve without elevated intraocular pressure, similar to normal tension glaucoma in human patients (Harada et al., 2007). An increase of the intraocular pressure causes retinal hypoxia (by the compression of blood vessels) that results in stimulation of the free radical formation in the mitochondria and lipid peroxidation which disrupts the glutamate transport in Müller cells. Hypoxia and high glucose, which both result in oxidative stress, were shown to induce a downregulation of GLAST in cultured Müller cells (Chen et al., 2010; Zeng et al., 2010b; Xie et al., 2012; but see Otori et al., 1994). A similar mechanism (malfunction of the glutamate transport into Müller cells caused by free radicals formed in the mitochondria) may explain the retinal ganglion cell death in Leber hereditary optic neuropathy (Beretta et al., 2006).

The amplitude of the GLAST-mediated glutamate uptake by Müller cells is strongly voltage-dependent (Fig. 47C,D; see 5.5.2.1.3.). A major condition that decreases the efficiency of the electrogenic glial glutamate transporters is depolarization of Müller cells (Napper et al., 1999; see 5.5.2.1.3.). The depolarization of Müller cells may be strong enough to reverse the operation mode of glutamate transporters resulting in an efflux of accumulated glutamate from the cells (see 5.6.1.1.).

Depolarization of Müller cells can be induced by various mechanisms. The limiting factor of the glutamate uptake is the activity of the sodium-potassium-ATPase which decreases very rapidly under diabetic conditions, for example (MacGregor and Matschinsky, 1986; Greene et al., 1987; Ottlecz et al., 1993; Kowluru et al., 1996). Inflammatory lipid mediators such as arachidonic acid and prostaglandins are produced under oxidative stress and hyperglycemic conditions, and after activation of NMDA receptors, by the sequential activation of PKC and cytosolic phospholipases A_2 (PLA_2) (Asano et al., 1987; Birkle and Bazan, 1989; Xia et al., 1995; Davidge et al., 1995; Landino et al., 1996; Du et al., 2004; Offer et al., 2005; Lambert et al., 2006; Balboa and Balsinde, 2006). Arachidonic acid and prostaglandins are potent inhibitors of the sodium-potassium-ATPase; the inhibition results in intracellular sodium overload and cellular depolarization (Lees, 1991; Staub et al., 1994; Owada et al., 1999). Arachidonic acid inhibits also directly the electrogenic glutamate transporters (Barbour et al., 1989). The decrease of the efficiency of the electrogenic glutamate uptake by Müller cells under pathological conditions might be counterregulated by an increased membrane insertion of sodium-potassium-ATPase molecules. IL-1 activates the p38 MAPK/caspase 11 pathway in Müller cells; activation of this pathway destabilizes the actin cytoskeleton and allows an accelerated membrane redistribution of sodium-potassium-ATPase molecules (Namekata et al., 2008). The IL-1-induced membrane redistribution of the sodium-potassium-ATPase increases the glutamate uptake by suppressing the intracellular sodium accumulation (Namekata et al., 2009). Thus, IL-1 may act as a neuroprotective factor via stimulation of the glutamate uptake by Müller cells, in addition to its detrimental effects (see 5.11.1.2.).

There are further conditions that may contribute to the depolarization-induced reduction of the glutamate transport into Müller cells under pathological conditions. The very negative membrane potential of Müller cells (around -80 mV; Figs. 8H, 45E, 46A,B,D) is constituted by the ample expression of Kir channels, in particular Kir4.1 (see 5.5.3.1.). The potassium efflux through Kir4.1 channels also counterbalances the increase of the intracellular osmolarity induced by the uptake of sodium-glutamate which will otherwise result in intracellular edema of Müller cells (see 5.11.9.2.2.). Under various pathological conditions, Müller cells are depolarized as a consequence of a functional inactivation and downregulation of Kir channels (Figs. 45E, 46A,B,D; see 5.5.3.5.). An age-dependent decrease in Kir currents found in human Müller cells (Fig. 45D) (Bringmann et al., 2003c) will lower the threshold for membrane depolarization in cells of the elderly. Chick and human Müller cells express ionotropic $P2X_7$ receptors which are ATP-gated cation channels (see 5.10.2.2.). Activation of the receptors induces a membrane depolarization which decreases the rate of the glial glutamate uptake (Fig. 47E) (Pannicke et al., 2000a). The resulting elevated extracellular glutamate level induces an excitotoxic death of retinal neurons (Anccasi et al., 2013). High-glucose conditions were shown to induce a downregulation of GLAST and Kir4.1 in cultured Müller cells (Zeng et al., 2010b; Xie et al., 2012; Mysona et al., 2009). Treatment with PEDF or taurine inhibits the effects of high glucose (Zeng et al., 2010b; Xie et al., 2012). Dietary taurine supplementation ameliorates experimental diabetic retinopathy in part via an increase in retinal GLAST expression (Yu et al., 2008; Zeng et al., 2009). Further factors which reduce the glutamate transport into Müller cells are a reduction of the extracellular pH, as occurring in ischemia, zinc ions (Billups and Attwell, 1996; Spiridon et al., 1998; Vandenberg et al., 1998) which are released from photoreceptors (Wu et al., 1993; Qian et al., 1994; Redenti et al., 2007), internalization of the transporter proteins in response to long-term exposure to glutamate (Billups and Attwell, 1996; Gadea et al., 2004; Gowda et al., 2011), and an increase in the intracellular glutamate level as observed after retinal detachment and in experimental diabetic retinopathy (Marc et al., 1998b; Gowda et al., 2011); high levels of intracellular glutamate impair the glutamate uptake by the decrease of the driving force.

Ischemic and inflammatory retinal diseases are associated with a breakdown of the blood-retinal barrier and a leakage of serum into the retina. Blood serum decrease the glutamate uptake by Müller cells (López-Colomé and Romo-de-Vivar, 1996). Glutamate is a normal constituent of the blood plasma at concentrations between 100 and 300 µM (Castillo et al., 1997). Administration of plasma or glutamate activates electrogenic glutamate transporters in bovine and human Müller cells but also inhibits Kir channels and induces cellular depolarization (Kusaka et al., 1999). A decrease in Kir currents and a depolarization of Müller cells is also induced by other blood-derived molecules like thrombin (Puro and Stuenkel, 1995). A reduced efficiency of the glutamate transport into Müller cells may explain in part the clinical observation that the presence of hemorrhages at sites of vascular leakage is associated with a greater reduction in the retinal function (Gass, 1997).

On the other hand, human Müller cells from patients with various retinopathies such as retinal detachment, PVR, and glaucoma were found to display an increase in the density of the glutamate transporter currents compared to cells from donors without eye disease (Reichelt et al., 1997a). An increase in GLAST expression was also observed in experimental retinal detachment and following transient retinal ischemia (Otori et al., 1994; Sakai et al., 2001). One may assume that the increased expression of electrogenic glutamate transporters is a counterregulation in response to the cellular depolarization, in order to protect the Müller cells from the toxic effects of glutamate.

5.5.2.1.7 Uptake of Ammonia   Ammonia is generated in glutamatergic and GABAergic neurons during the generation of glutamate from glutamine (Fig. 44). It is released from neurons and taken up by glial cells (Coles et al., 1996; Tsacopoulos et al., 1997a, b). Ammonia ions induce an alkalinization of the Müller cell interior; the cytosolic alkalinization stimulates the glutamate uptake through GLAST, via an increase in the driving force for the transporter-mediated uptake of protons. In addition, ammonia speeds the glutamate uptake by Müller cells by a separate, likely direct effect on the glutamate transporter molecule (Mort et al., 2001).

The mechanisms of the ammonia uptake by Müller cells are unclear. At the physiologic pH of 7.4, the majority of ammonia is charged (NH_4^+) and only a small fraction (less than 2%) is uncharged (NH_3) and can passively penetrate the plasma membrane. Ammonia is not transported by electrogenic glutamate transporters (Mort et al., 2001). The water channel AQP8 was identified in the inner mitochondrial membrane of various tissues and was shown to mediate the mitochondrial ammonia transport (Calamita et al., 2005; Soria et al., 2010; Molinas et al., 2012). AQP8 gene transcripts are present in the neuroretina and cultured Müller cells (Tenckhoff et al., 2005; Hollborn et al., 2011a, 2012a; see 5.5.4.2.). However, the plasma membrane, but not the mitochondrial membrane, of Müller cells is permeable for ammonia (see 5.5.2.1.14.). Other possibilities of facilitated ammonia transport are the transport through aquaporins 3 and 9, glycoproteins of the Rh family, and potassium channels (see discussion in Lichter-Konecki et al., 2008). However, results of own unpublished investigations make it rather unlikely that potassium channels of mammalian Müller cells are permable for ammonium ions (T. Pannicke, Leipzig, personal communication). The presence of ammonia-transporting systems in the plasma membrane of Müller cells remains to be established. Retinal glial cells of the bee take up ammonia via a chloride cotransporter selective for ammonia over potassium (Marcaggi and Coles, 2001; Marcaggi et al., 2004).

5.5.2.1.8   Removal of N-acetylaspartylglutamate

The neuropeptide N-acetylaspartylglutamate (NAAG) is expressed by retinal ganglion and amacrine cells (Tieman and Tieman, 1996). NAAG is an agonist at mGluRs and an antagonist at NMDA receptors (Coyle, 1997). Müller cells hydrolize extracellularly NAAG by the membrane-bound glutamate carboxypeptidase II which results in liberation of glutamate (Berger et al., 1999). In addition, Müller cells may take up NAAG via the peptide transporter PEPT2 (Berger and Hediger, 1999). The liberation of glutamate by the glutamate carboxypeptidase II might be implicated in excitotoxicity under pathological conditions such as ischemia (Harada et al., 2000).

5.5.2.1.9   Production of Glutamine

After being taken up by Müller cells, glutamate is rapidly amidated to glutamine by the enzyme glutamine synthetase (Fig. 44). Glutamate can be also transaminated to α-ketoglutarate which is released and taken up by neurons as a substrate for their oxidative metabolism, utilized for the production of glutathione, or loaded into secretory vesicles. In the neural retina, glutamine synthetase is localized in astrocytes and Müller cells (Riepe and Norenburg, 1977; Linser and Moscona, 1979; Derouiche and Rauen, 1995; Prada et al., 1998). Glutamine synthetase is distributed throughout the cytosol of Müller cells (Figs. 2G, 21A, 45F, 49, 50E) (Derouiche and Rauen, 1995). Glutamine is released from Müller cells and taken up by neurons as a precursor for the synthesis of glutamate and GABA (Fig. 44) (Pow and Crook, 1996);

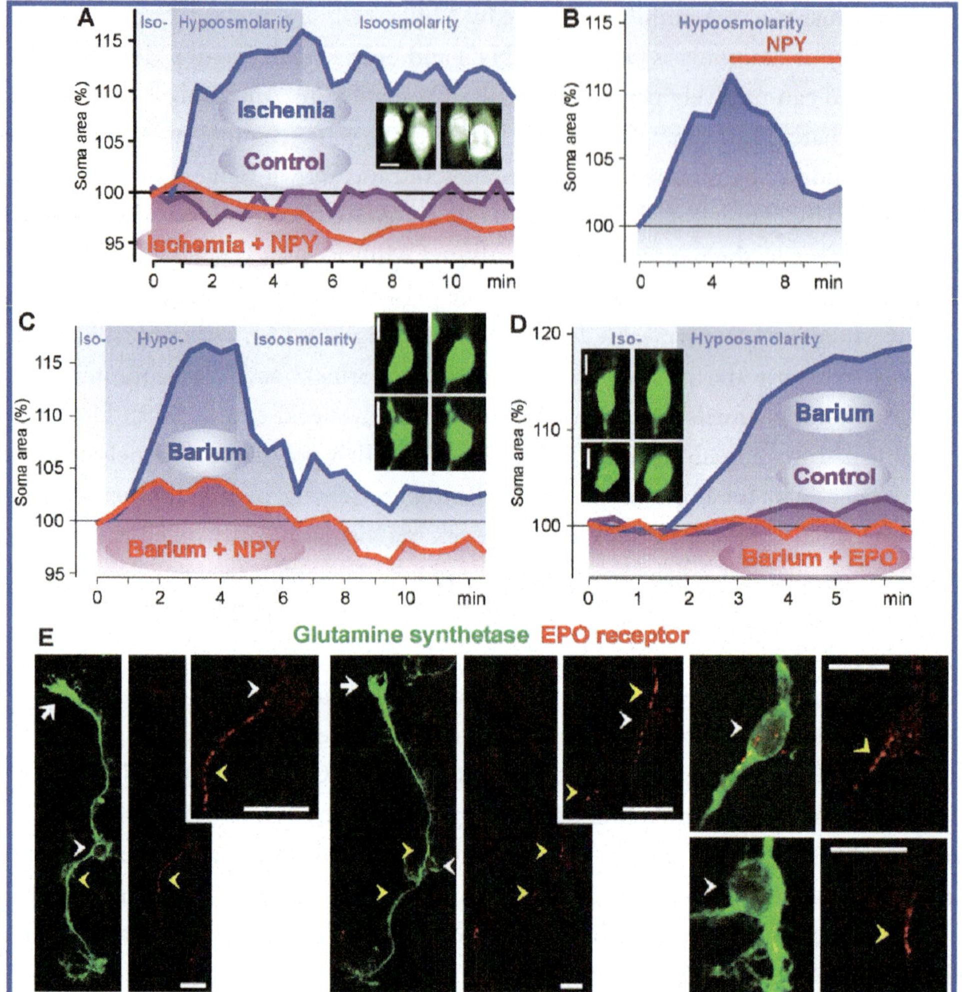

FIGURE 50: Neuropeptide Y (NPY; **A–C**) and erythropoietin (EPO; **D**) inhibit the osmotic swelling of rat Müller cells. **A.** NPY (20 nM) inhibits the osmotic swelling of Müller cell somata induced by superfusion of a hypoosmotic extracellular solution onto retinal slices isolated 3 days after a 1-h transient retinal ischemia. *Control*, healthy control retina. The *insets* show Müller cell somata in the postischemic retina before (*left*) and during (*right*) hypoosmotic exposure. **B.** Addition of NPY (20 nM) to swollen Müller cells in 3 days-postischemic retinas caused a volume reduction of their somata. **C.** Müller cells in healthy control retinas reversibly increased the volume of their somata in the presence of barium ions (1 mM). The soma swelling was largely inhibited by NPY (10 nM) simultaneously applied with the hypoosmotic solution. **D.** EPO (20 nM) prevents the swelling of Müller cells in control retinas induced by a hypoosmotic extracellular solution in the presence of barium ions. *Control*, hypoosmotic stimulation

in the absence of barium. The *insets* show Müller cell somata before (*left*) and during (*right*) hypo-osmotic exposure in the presence of barium. **E.** Immunolabeling of EPO receptor protein (*red*) in isolated Müller cells. The cells were co-stained against glutamine synthetase (*green*). The *small images* show the peri-somatic region of the cells at higher magnification. *Yellow arrowheads*, EPO receptor labeling. *White arrowheads*, cell somata. *Arrows*, cell endfeet. Scale bars, 10 and 5 µm (*small images*). Modified from Uckermann et al. (2006) and Krügel et al. (2010).

---

glutamate and GABA are then sequestered in synaptic vesicles, and exocytotically released into the extracellular space upon neuronal activation (or, as in the case of GABA, released via a reversal of its transporters; Duarte et al., 1998; Andrade da Costa et al., 2000; Calaza et al., 2006). Alternatively, glutamine in Müller cells can be transported into the mitochondria where it is hydrolyzed to glutamate and ammonia by the phosphate-activated glutaminase (Takatsuna et al., 1994; see 5.5.2.1.14.). The shuttle of glutamate and glutamine, respectively, between neurons and Müller cells is known as glutamate-glutamine cycle.

The activity of the glutamine synthetase enhances the rate of the glutamate uptake by Müller cells (Rauen et al., 1998; Shaked et al., 2002). The rapid metabolization of glutamate to glutamine causes a stronger driving force for the glutamate uptake in Müller cells than in neurons which have intracellular free glutamate concentrations two orders of magnitude higher than Müller cells (Marc et al., 1995). Due to the efficiency of the glutamine synthetase, free glutamate in Müller cells can be immunohistochemically demonstrated only when the glutamine synthetase activity is inhibited pharmacologically or under pathological conditions (Pow and Robinson, 1994; Marc et al., 1998b; Rauen, 2000; Takeo-Goto et al., 2002). Semi-quantification of immunohistochemically stained retinal slices revealed a free glutamate concentration in Müller cells of ~50 µM or less, and a glutamine concentration of 1–3 mM (Marc et al., 1990, 1998b; Pow and Robinson, 1994). The amino acid signature of Müller cells of most vertebrate classes investigated so far is dominated by glutamine and taurine (Kalloniatis et al., 1994, 1996; Marc et al., 1995, 1998a; Marc and Cameron, 2001).

When the glutamine synthetase in Müller cells is pharmacologically blocked, bipolar and ganglion cells lose their free glutamate content, and the animals become rapidly (within 2 min) functionally blind (Pow and Robinson, 1994; Barnett et al., 2000). This is associated with a considerable reduction of the electroretinogram b-wave (Barnett et al., 2000). The lack of immunohistochemically detectable free glutamate in bipolar and ganglion cells after inhibition of the glutamine synthetase suggests that these neurons do not synthesize significant amounts of glutamate from other substrates than glutamine (Pow and Robinson, 1994). On the other hand, inhibition of the glutamine synthesis decreases (but not abolishes) the level of detectable free glutamate in photoreceptor cells (Pow and Robinson, 1994). This suggests that photoreceptor cells take up significant amounts of glutamate from the synaptic cleft (Hasegawa et al., 2006) and are capable to synthesize glutamate by transamination of α-ketoglutarate (Pow and Robinson, 1994; Bui et al., 2009).

Müller cells possess enzymes that are involved in the *de novo* synthesis of glutamate from pyruvate, e.g., pyruvate carboxylase, that catalyzes the carboxylation of pyruvate to oxaloacetate as substrate of the Krebs cycle, and glutamate dehydrogenase, that converts α-ketoglutarate to glutamate; both enzymes are preferentially localized to glial cells (Gebhard, 1992; Hertz et al., 1992; Lieth et al., 2001; Ola et al., 2011a). Glutamate dehydrogenase, a mitochondrial enzyme (Fig. 44), is capable to metabolize glutamate at a relatively low pH (Zaganas et al., 2012) that prevails in glial cells following glutamate uptake (Bouvier et al., 1992). The activity of the malate-aspartate shuttle in Müller cells (Fig. 44) is low (LaNoue et al., 2001) due to the low expression of the aspartate aminotransferase (Gebhard, 1991) and of glutamate-aspartate exchangers (Xu et al., 2007b). Thus, the bulk of glutamate is converted to glutamine, and only a small fraction of glutamate is transported into the mitochondria (Poitry et al., 2000). The low activity of the malate-aspartate shuttle is also the reason why Müller cells are not capable to oxidize completely glucose or lactate within the mitochondria; instead, they display a high rate of aerobic glycolysis resulting in the production of lactate and pyruvate that is released into the extracellular space and taken up by photoreceptors (LaNoue et al., 2001; Xu et al., 2007b; see 5.5.7.2.). However, the expression level of the glutamate-aspartate exchanger is dependent on the differentiation degree of the cells and is increased under pathological or culture conditions when the cells dedifferentiate and proliferate, and the expression of the glutamine synthetase is decreased (see 5.5.2.1.12.). Glucocorticoids inhibit the glutamate-induced increase of mitochondrial NADH (Psarra et al., 2003); hydrocortisone increases the expression of the glutamine synthetase in Müller cells (see 5.5.2.1.11.) and decreases the level of the glutamate-aspartate exchanger (Ola et al., 2005, 2011a). When the expression of the glutamine synthetase is decreased under pathological conditions (see 5.5.2.1.12.), more glutamate enters mitochondria. The loss of the glucocorticoid-mediated inhibition of the expression of the glutamate-aspartate exchanger (Ola et al., 2011a) under these conditions may increase the importance of the oxidative glutamate metabolism. The functional relevance of the recently discovered biotin-coupled bifunctional enzyme p42, which displays glutamine synthetase and glutamate decarboxylase activities (Arunchaipong et al., 2009), remains to be determined.

5.5.2.1.10 Glutamine Transport A bidirectional transport of glutamine across plasma membranes can be mediated by various neutral amino acid carriers known as systems A and L, and the sodium-dependent amino acid exchanger ASCT2 (Varoqui et al., 2000; Kanai and Hediger, 2004; Sáenz et al., 2004). The principal glutamine transporters in rodent Müller cells are amino acid transporters of the system N, consisting of SN1/SNAT3 (system N1/sodium-coupled neutral amino acid transporter 3) and SN2/SNAT5 (system N2/sodium-coupled neutral amino acid transporter 5); these transporters are responsible for ~70% of the glutamine transport across Müller cell membranes (Umapathy et al., 2005). The sodium-dependent system A (ATA1/SNAT1, ATA2/SNAT2) and the sodium-independent system L (LAT1, LAT2) contribute to a lesser extent to the glutamine transport of rodent Müller cells (Umapathy et al., 2005). The presence of SN1 in Müller cells in the intact retina was shown by immunohistochemical techniques (Boulland et al., 2002). Melatonin increases the retinal glutamine transport (Sáenz et al., 2004).

5.5.2.1.11 Regulation of Glutamine Synthetase Expression in Retinal Development   The expression of the glutamine synthetase is a key event in the differentiation of Müller cells from retinal progenitors (Figs. 49, 51) and is induced by Müller cell-photoreceptor interaction (Germer et al., 1997b; Prada et al., 1998; Wurm et al., 2006b). The gene transcription of both GLAST and glutamine synthetase is stimulated by glucocorticoids (Juurlink et al., 1981; Moscona and Degenstein, 1981a; Vardimon et al., 1988, 1993; Gorovits et al., 1996; Prada et al., 1998; Rauen and Wiessner, 2000; Ola et al., 2005). The glucocorticoid receptor NR3C1 has been localized in the retina predominately to Müller cells (Gorovits et al., 1994; Grossman et al., 1994; see 5.10.11.). The upstream region of the glutamine synthetase gene contains a glucocorticoid response element that binds the glucocorticoid receptor protein (Zhang and Young, 1991). There is an inverse relation between the expression of glutamine synthetase and Müller cell proliferation in the developing retina, under pathological conditions in the mature retina, and under culture conditions (Linser and Moscona, 1983; Vardimon et al., 1993; Gorovits et al., 1996; Kruchkova et al., 2001). At early developmental stages, the c-Jun protein (a component of the AP-1 complex of transcription factors that regulates cellular proliferation) is abundant in proliferating retinal cells. This protein renders the glucocorticoid receptor molecules transcriptionally inactive, and glucocorticoids cannot induce the expression of glutamine synthetase (Ben-Dror et al., 1993; Berko-Flint et al., 1994). Concomitant with the decreases in cell proliferation and c-Jun expression, the developing retina acquires the cabability to express glutamine synthetase in response to glucocorticoids (Vardimon et al., 1993). This capability can be suppressed by introduction of the oncogene v-src which stimulates retinal cell proliferation (Vardimon et al., 1991) or by dissociation of the retinal tissue into separated cells (Linser and Moscona, 1979; Vardimon et al., 1988; Reisfeld and Vardimon, 1994). Cell dissociation results in a rapid increase in c-Jun expression, stimulation of glial cell proliferation, and inactivation of the glucocorticoid receptor. Under these conditions, glutamine synthetase expression cannot be induced (Linser et al., 1982; Linser and Moscona, 1983). Cell contacts to neurons reestablish the hormonal induction of the glutamine synthetase, in part via an increased glucocorticoid receptor expression (Linser et al., 1982; Linser and Moscona, 1983). The expression of the glutamine

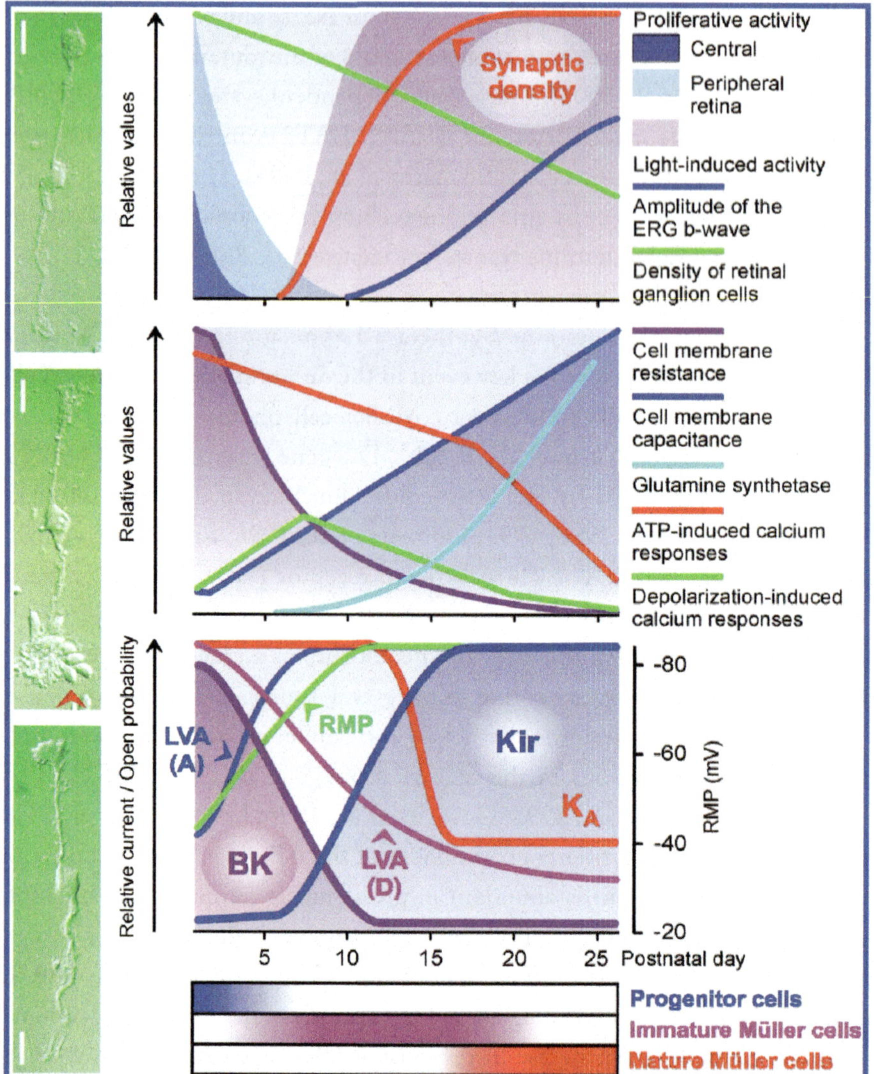

FIGURE 51: Developmental alterations of the plasma membrane characteristics of rabbit Müller cells. *Above:* Markers of the retinal development: proliferative activity in the retina (Schnitzer, 1990; Reichenbach et al., 1991a; Sharma and Ehinger, 1997), incidence of light-responsive ganglion cells (Masland, 1977), density of ribbon synapses (McArdle et al., 1977), and the amplitude of the electroretinogram b-wave (Noell, 1958). The density of the ganglion cell somata decreases during the postnatal development (Uckermann et al., 2002) while the size of the ganglion cell somata increases (not shown). *Middle:* Markers of Müller cell maturation: cell membrane resistance, cell membrane capacitance, glutamine synthetase content of Müller cells (Germer et al., 1997b), and incidence of radial glial/Müller cells that

display ATP- and depolarization (50 mM potassium)-induced calcium responses, respectively (Uckermann et al., 2002). The alteration of the cell membrane resistance reflects the decrease of the resistance against (Kir channel-mediated) potassium fluxes over the plasma membranes of radial glial/Müller cells. The increase of the cell membrane capacitance reflects the increase of the plasma membrane area. The depolarization-induced calcium responses are in part mediated by activation of an autocrine/paracrine ATP signaling. *Below:* Mean alterations of the open probability of BK channels at the resting membrane potential (RMP), of the amplitudes of Kir and K_A currents, of the amplitude (LVA-A) and the density (LVA-D) of currents through low voltage-activated calcium channels, and of the RMP in dependence on the postnatal age. Note that a RMP of around −80 mV is achieved when the Kir currents are greater than ~40% of the maximal amplitude. The *schedule below* shows stages of Müller cell development from mitotically active late progenitor cells. The *images* show Müller cells isolated from retinas of postnatal day 6 (*above*), 9 (*middle*), and 14 rabbits (*below*). Photoreceptor cells are attached to the outer stem process of the postnatal day 9 cell (*arrowhead*). Scale bars, 15 μm. Modified from Bringmann et al. (1999a, 2000d).

---

synthetase in Müller cells increases directly with an increase of the extracellular glutamate concentration (Germer et al., 1997a). In the developing rat retina, Müller cells express glutamine synthetase when the glutamatergic synapses mature; the first expression of glutamine synthetase occurs around postnatal day 6 (Fig. 49) (Fletcher and Kalloniatis, 1997), before the expression of other glia-specific proteins such as Kir4.1 and AQP4 (Wurm et al., 2006b).

5.5.2.1.12 Regulation of the Glutamine Synthetase Under Pathological Conditions   The expression of the glutamine synthetase is regulated by glutamate (Shen et al., 2004). When the major glutamate-releasing neuronal population, the photoreceptors, degenerate (for example, in inherited photoreceptor degeneration and after retinal light injury [Figs. 14B, 18A–C, 21A, 36D, 52] or detachment [Figs. 10C, 53A, B, 54A], but not in rodent models of slowly developing inherited photoreceptor degeneration [Fig. 14D,E]), the expression of the glutamine synthetase in Müller cells is reduced (Lewis et al., 1989; Härtig et al., 1995; Grosche et al., 1995; Germer et al., 1997a; Marc et al., 1998b; Reichenbach et al., 1999; Iandiev et al., 2006e; Vogler et al., 2013b). Decreases in the glutamine synthetase expression and activity were also observed under ischemic, inflammatory, and traumatic conditions, in the glaucomatous retina, in the presence of xenobiotics which inhibit the neuronal activity like diazepam and cadmium, and after separation of the neuroretina from the retinal pigment epithelium (Reinhardt and Schein, 1995; Nishiyama et al., 2000; Jablonski and Iannaccone, 2001; Kruchkova et al., 2001; Moreno et al., 2005; Hauck et al., 2007; Chen et al., 2008; Fernandez et al., 2009; Dorfman et al., 2013; but see Carter-Dawson et al., 1998). In addition,

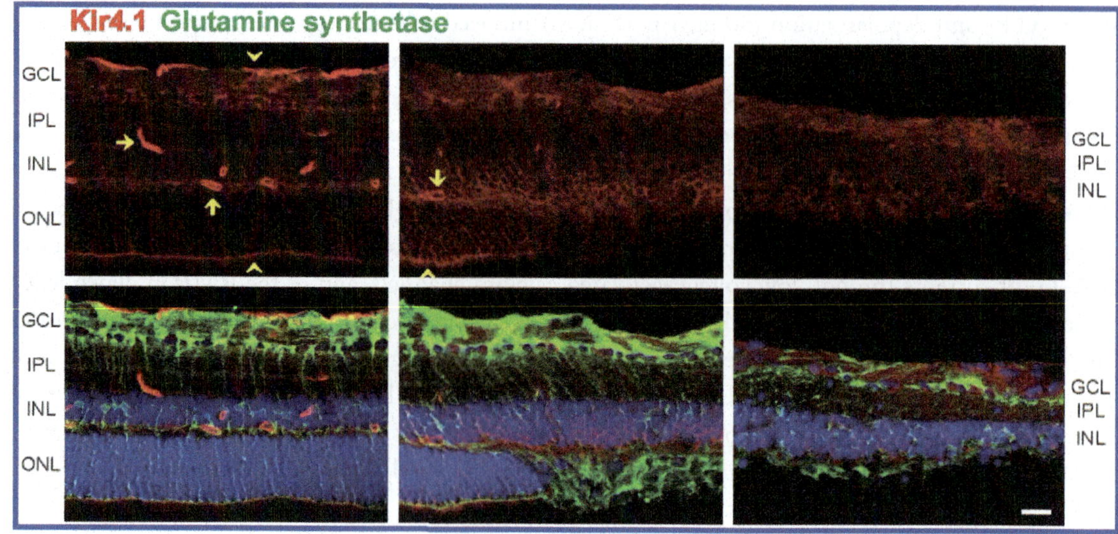

FIGURE 52: Local irradiation of the rat retina with excessive blue light causes degeneration of the photoreceptor cells and gliotic alterations of Müller cells, as indicated by the alteration in the immunolocalization of the potassium channel Kir4.1. Retinal slices were stained against Kir4.1 (*red*) and glutamine synthetase (*green*) three days after light exposure. Cell nuclei were labeled with Hoechst 33258 (*blue*). Injured retinal areas are shown *right*, uninjured areas are shown *left*, and transition zones are shown in the *middle*. The *arrows* point to perivascular labeling of Kir4.1, and the *arrowheads* indicate the inner (ILM) and outer limiting membranes (OLM). GCL, ganglion cell layer; INL, inner nuclear layer; IPL, inner plexiform layer; ONL, outer nuclear layer. Bar, 20 μm. Modified from Iandiev et al. (2008a).

cell separation or depolymerization of the actin or microtubule network represses glutamine synthetase induction by a mechanism that involves induction of c-Jun and inhibition of the glucocorticoid receptor transcriptional activity (Oren et al., 1999). While glutamate does not induce an increase in the glutamine synthetase activity in Müller cells in the absence of neurons, the activity is stimulated by glutamate when neurons are present (Heidinger et al., 1999).

The downregulation of the glutamine synthetase under conditions of high hydrostatic pressure and in glaucomatous eyes, which is associated with a swelling of ganglion cells axons, was suggested to be a result of the decreased GLAST activity and a depletion of neuronal glutamate (Gionfriddo et al., 2009; Ishikawa et al., 2011). It has been shown that decreases of the glutamate uptake and glutamine synthetase activity precede the functional and histological alterations induced by ocular hypertension, suggesting that alterations in the glutamate-glutamine cycle carried out by Müller cells contribute to the death of retinal ganglion cells in glaucoma (Moreno et al., 2005). In

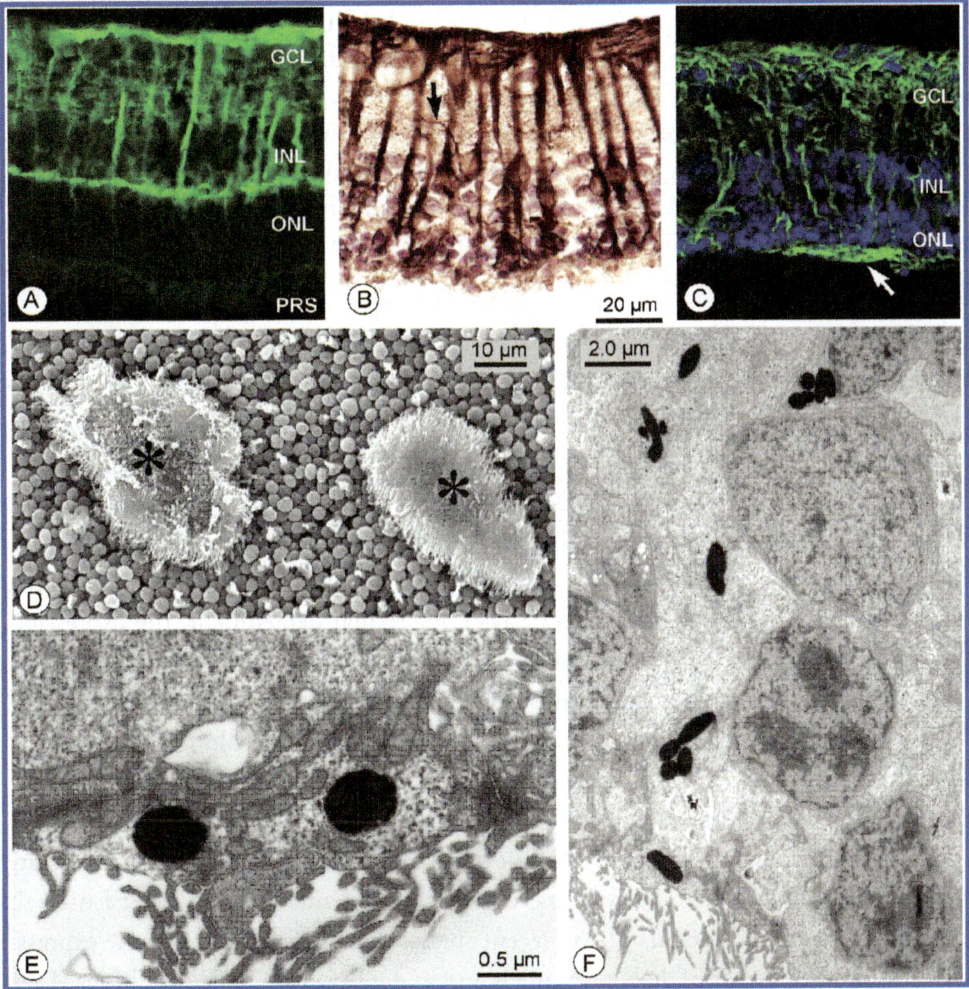

FIGURE 53: Reactive gliosis after experimental retinal detachment and in proliferative vitreoretinopathy (PVR). GFAP immunoreactivity (*green* fluorescence in **A** and **C**; *brown* DAB-nickel reaction product in **B**) after 2 days (**A**) and 1 week (**B**) of detachment. **C.** PVR. Cell nuclei are *blue* stained. **A.** Two days after detachment, no morphological indications of neurodegeneration are obvious. The Müller cells are immunopositive for GFAP within their inner processes (up to the inner nuclear layer, INL). **B.** After 1 week, many photoreceptor cells are already degenerated as indicated by the thin outer nuclear layer (ONL). Müller cells display GFAP immunoreactivity throughout their length, and some cells extend additional side branches (*arrow*). **C.** When a PVR develops, some Müller cells grow out of the retina into

continued on next page

the subretinal space (*arrow*). The *scale bar* in **B** is valid for **A-C. D.** Raster electron micrograph of the rabbit retina obtained immediately after experimental detachment. The view is onto the photoreceptor segments. Some pigment epithelial cells are adhering (*asterisks*). **E.** Transmission electron micrograph of the sclerad retinal surface after 3 weeks of detachment. The Müller cell cytoplasm contains many mitochondria and two typical melanin granules. **F.** Outer retina after 6 weeks of detachment. A Müller cell contains melanin granules scattered throughout the sclerad stem process up to the level of the INL (*top*). GCL, ganglion cell layer; PRS, photoreceptor segments. Modified from Francke et al. (2001a,b).

Müller cells of Royal College of Surgeons (RCS) rats with inherited photoreceptor degeneration (due to a genetic defect within the retinal pigment epithelium), the degradation of glutamate is prolonged; this dysfunction of Müller cells is obvious before apparent histological and functional changes of the retina (Fletcher and Kalloniatis, 1996; Fletcher, 2000). After experimental retinal detachment, retinal neurons display a depletion of glutamate beginning within 5 min of detachment, which is followed by an increase in the glutamine content of Müller cells, suggesting that an acute efflux of neuronal glutamate contributes to the excitotoxicity in the detached retina (Sherry and Townes-Anderson, 2000). Within three days after retinal detachment, the expression of the glutamine synthetase in Müller cells declines resulting in glutamine depletion and an increase in Müller cell's glutamate content to supramillimolar levels (Lewis et al., 1989; Marc et al., 1998b). The failure of Müller cell's capacity to metabolize glutamate persists as long as the retina remains detached (Marc et al., 1998b).

Conflicting data were published regarding the regulation of the glutamine synthetase expression in experimental diabetic retinopathy. While most previous studies showed no alteration or a slight enhancement of the glutamine synthetase expression (Mizutani et al., 1998; Lo et al., 2001; Gerhardinger et al., 2005; Silva et al., 2013), recent studies described decreases of the expression and enzyme activity in Müller cells of diabetic animals and under hyperglycemic conditions (Lieth et al., 2000; Yu et al., 2009; El-Remessy et al., 2010; Shen et al., 2010b, 2011b; Saïdi et al., 2011; Fernandez et al., 2012). A malfunction of the glutamine synthetase might be caused by tyrosine nitration of the enzyme (Görg et al., 2007; El-Remessy et al., 2010) which results from the oxidative-nitrosative stress present in the diabetic retina (Madsen-Bouterse and Kowluru, 2008; Zheng and Kern, 2009; Silva et al., 2009; Pazdro and Burgess, 2010). Cannabidiol preserves the glutamine synthetase activity by blocking the tyrosine nitration of the enzyme (El-Remessy et al., 2010). When diabetic retinopathy develops to a proliferative state, the glutamine synthetase of Müller cells will be increasingly downregulated. Müller cells in diabetic epiretinal membranes display a progressive loss of glutamine synthetase (Guidry et al., 2009; see 5.11.11.2.). An increase of the glutamine synthetase expression in Müller cells was observed under conditions of increased ammonia levels; here, elevated glutamine synthetase is required to detoxify excess ammonia (see 5.5.2.1.14.).

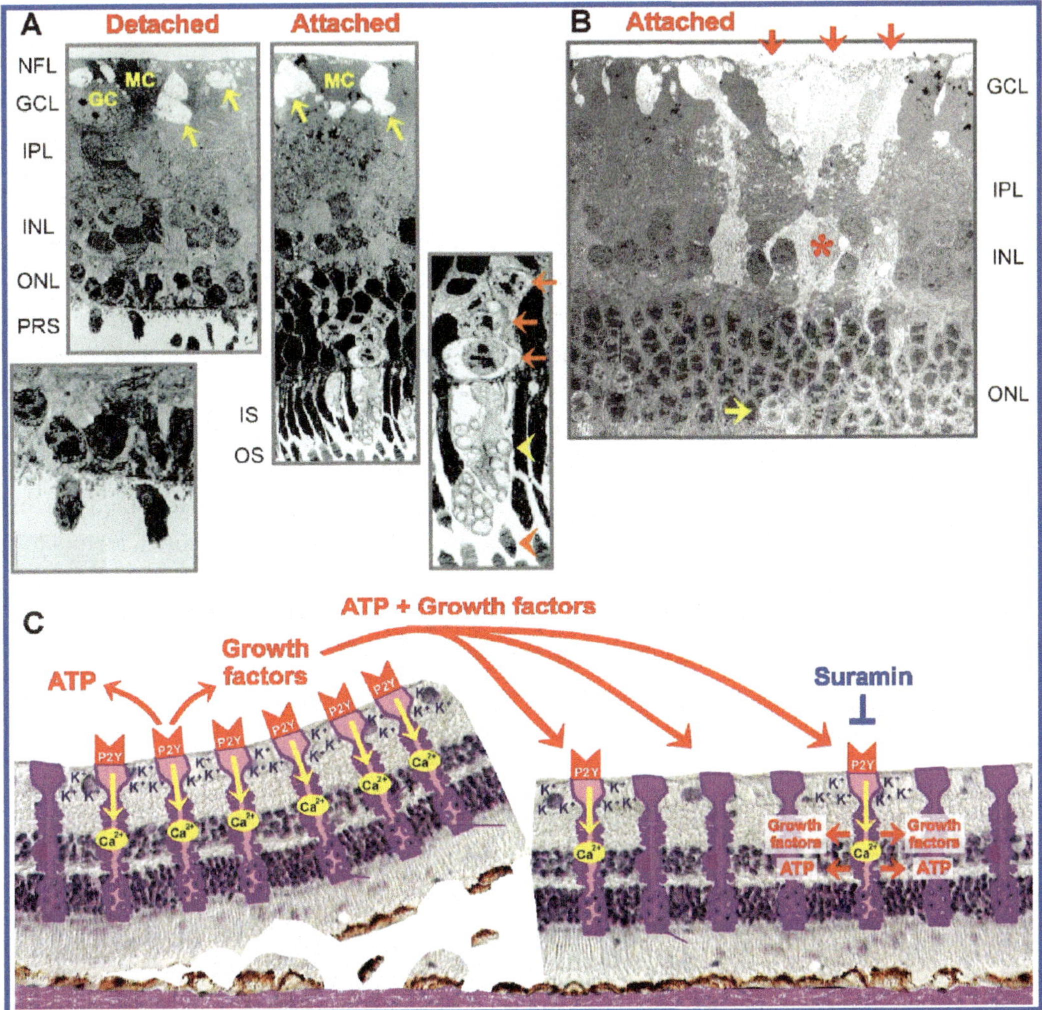

FIGURE 54: In the locally detached rabbit retina, retinal degeneration is not restricted to the detached retina but is observed also in the surrounding non-detached tissue. **A.** Ultrastructure of slices through a detached (*left*) and a non-detached retinal area (*right*) of a rabbit retina which was focally detached for 6 weeks. In the detached tissue, photoreceptor segments degenerate that is followed by the death of photoreceptor cells. The outer nuclear layer (ONL) is severely reduced in its thickness; however, two rows of photoreceptor cell nuclei are preserved. The remaining photoreceptor cells are devoid of outer segments and, in many cases, of inner segments (IS). In addition to ganglion cell (GC) bodies and Müller cell (MC) endfeet, the innermost retina contains edematous cysts (*yellow arrows*). In the non-detached area (*right*), the ONL and the photoreceptor segments (PRS) are much better preserved compared to the

continued on next page

detached area; however, several groups of adjacent photoreceptor cells are in the process of degeneration. These cells show swollen cell bodies with altered chromatin morphology (*red arrows*) and swollen inner segments (*yellow arrowhead*) while the outer segments (OS; *red arrowhead*) are relatively well preserved. Such groups of degenerating photoreceptor cells were rarely found after 1 week but regularly after 3 weeks, and abundantly after 6 weeks of detachment. **B.** Edematous degeneration of a group of Müller cells in the attached portion of a focally detached rabbit retina. The cells and their nuclei (*) and mitochondria swell, the cytoplasm is vacuolized, and the cells die after disruption of the plasma membranes. The cell death is associated with a disruption of the inner limiting membrane (*red arrows*) and with degeneration of photoreceptor cell bodies (*yellow arrow*). **C.** Hypothetical scheme of the gliosis-induced spread of retinal degeneration in the locally detached rabbit retina. Soluble factors such as extracellular nucleotides and growth factors may diffuse from the detached area into the surrounding non-detached tissue, and may activate P2Y and growth factor receptors expressed by Müller cells. Gliotic alterations of activated Müller cells, e.g., the decrease of the potassium conductance, may disrupt the ion and water homeostasis within the non-detached tissue, resulting in photoreceptor cell degeneration and the formation of edematous cysts. Suramin (which inhibits the binding of nucleotides and growth factors to their respective receptors) may inhibit the spread of gliosis into formerly non-affected retinal areas (Uhlmann et al., 2003). GCL, ganglion cell layer; INL, inner nuclear layer; IPL, inner plexiform layer; NFL, nerve fiber layer. Modified from Faude et al. (2001) and Francke et al. (2005).

Experimental downregulation of the glutamine synthetase in the rat retina by using siRNA or the glia-selective toxin DL-α-aminoadipic acid (Pedersen and Karlsen, 1979; Wakakura and Ishikawa, 1982; Karlsen et al., 1982; Ishikawa and Mine, 1983; Pow, 2001a) induces glial dysfunction and gliosis which results in a breakdown of the inner blood-retinal barrier associated with a reduced expression of the tight junction protein claudin-5 (Shen et al., 2010a). This suggests that an impairment of Müller cell's glutamate metabolism results in a dysfunction of the cells which disturbs the integrity of the blood-retinal barrier. An increase in the glutamine synthetase expression in retinal glial cells (via induction of the endogenous gene or supply of purified protein) may represent a therapeutical approach that protects against neuronal degeneration in the injured retinal tissue (Gorovits et al., 1997).

5.5.2.1.13 Regulation of Glutamine Synthetase by Soluble Factors   The decline of the glutamine synthetase expression in Müller cells under various pathological conditions is mediated (at least in part) by soluble factors such as bFGF, EGF, TGF-α, IL-1β, insulin, and adenosine (Kruchkova et al., 2001; Shen and Xu, 2009; Shen et al., 2010b, 2011b; Ola et al., 2011a; Yu et al., 2012). bFGF and IL-1ß increase the level of c-Jun and inhibits the glucocorticoid-induced expression of the glutamine synthetase (Kruchkova et al., 2001; Shen and Xu, 2009). Retinal IL-1β is upregulated in the diabetic retina, and high glucose induces increased IL-1β expression in vascular endothelial cells (Liu et al., 2012a). bFGF is rapidly released in the retina after detachment (Geller et al., 2001) and increasingly expressed (e.g., in Müller cells; Fig. 33A,B) under ischemic conditions, after light injury and retinal detachment, and in response to inherited photoreceptor degeneration and mechanical injury (Miyashiro et al., 1988; Gao and Hollyfield, 1995a,b, 1996; Matsushima et al., 1997; Cao et al., 1997a; Kruchkova et al., 2001; Yafai et al., 2013). Although bFGF is one of the major neuroprotective factors which supports the neuronal survival in the retina (Faktorovich et al., 1990, 1992; see 5.11.7.7.), the bFGF-induced downregulation of the glutamine synthetase might rather aggravate the process of neuronal degeneration. The decrease of the glutamine synthetase expression after retinal detachment is likely also a result of the separation of Müller cells from the pigment epithelium and the subsequent interruption in the supply with PEDF (Jablonski et al., 2001; Jablonski and Iannaccone, 2001). PEDF also prevents the IL-1ß-induced decrease of the glutamine synthetase expression in diabetic retinopathy and under high glucose conditions (Shen et al., 2010b, 2011b). In addition to PEDF, hydrocortisone (see 5.5.2.1.11.), taurine, lactose, and BDNF increase the expression of the glutamine synthetase in Müller cells (Jablonski and Iannaccone, 2001; Ola et al., 2005, 2011a, b; Zeng et al., 2010b; Chen et al., 2010; Toops et al., 2012a; Dai et al., 2012; but see Chen and Weber, 2002). Cannabidiol preserves the glutamine synthetase activity by blocking tyrosine nitration which inhibits the glutamine synthetase, e.g., in retinas of diabetic rats (El-Remessy et al., 2010). Melatonin increases the glutamine synthetase activity and decreases the glutaminase activity (Sáenz et al., 2004).

5.5.2.1.14 Ammonia-Dependent Regulation of the Glutamine Synthetase—Hepatic Retinopathy   The expression of the glutamine synthetase is also regulated by the availability of ammonia. Exposure to elevated levels of ammonia causes an upregulation of the glutamine synthetase expression in Müller cells (Reichenbach et al., 1995b,d; Germer et al., 1997a; Albrecht et al., 1998; Bringmann et al., 1998a). As the glutamine synthethase of Müller cells is the most important enzyme available for ammonia detoxification in the retina (in addition to the mitochondrial enzyme glutamate dehydrogenase; Fig. 44), this is an important additional function of neurotransmitter recycling.

The glutamine synthetase protein is located evenly in the cytosol (Figs. 2G, 21A, 45F, 49, 50E) while mitochondria are unevenly distributed in Müller cells from avascular retinas such as of guinea pigs (Fig. 34J, L; see 5.2.). Thus a major part of ATP used by the glutamine synthetase is suggested to be produced through the cytosolic glycolytic pathway. Glutamate and ammonia cause a large increase in lactate (and glutamine) production and release from Müller cells; in addition, ADP and P_i produced by the glutamine synthetase reaction stimulate mitochondrial respiration (Poitry et al., 2000). Lactate and pyruvate are preferentially utilized by photoreceptors and neurons as fuel for their oxidative metabolism (Fig. 44; see 5.5.7.2.).

The availability of ammonia is a major factor that determines the metabolic fate of glutamate. When enough ammonia is available, the bulk of glutamate in Müller cells is metabolized to glutamine (Poitry et al., 2000), as indicated by the observation that blockade of the glutamine synthetase results in a dramatic increase in the glutamate level of Müller cells (Pow and Robinson, 1994). When the concentration of ammonia decreases, more glutamate enters into mitochondria (Poitry et al., 2000). Inhibition of the glutamine synthetase suppresses the stimulatory effect of both agents on the glycolysis and induces a massive entry of glutamate into the mitochondria (Poitry et al., 2000). The rate of glutamine production also determines the amount of pyruvate transaminated by glutamate to alanine and α-ketoglutarate.

The major complication of fulminant hepatic failure, responsible for the death of a large percentage of patients with liver disease (Blei, 2007), is the development of brain edema characterized by a swelling of astrocytes (Willard-Mack et al., 1996; Häussinger et al., 2000). In the neural retina, pathological alterations are likewise found primarily in Müller cells and astrocytes; glial alterations include cellular swelling (Fig. 35A), mitochondrial dysfunction (Fig. 35B), vacuolization, and necrosis (Reichenbach et al., 1995b,d; Albrecht et al., 1998; Karl et al., 2011). An increased level of blood ammonia, which is associated with an increase in the cerebral concentration of ammonia to values up to 5 mM (Swain et al., 1992; Tofteng et al., 2006), is a key pathogenic factor of hepatic encephalo- and retinopathy (Reichenbach et al., 1995b; Albrecht and Norenberg, 2006). The ammonia-induced swelling of brain astrocytes and Müller cells depends on glutamine synthesis rather than ammonia *per se* (Willard-Mack et al., 1996; Jayakumar et al., 2006; Karl et al., 2011). The swelling-inducing effect of glutamine in Müller cells (Fig. 35A) is maximally at a concentration of ~0.5 mM (Karl et al., 2011). The glutamine-induced swelling of Müller cells is accelerated under hypoosmotic conditions (Fig. 35A) (Karl et al., 2011). Such conditions occur *in situ*; osmotic gradients across the glio-vascular interface are a result of ionic disbalances in the blood caused by, for example, hyponatremia and hypoalbuminemia in cases of renal and hepatic failures. Hyponatremia acts synergistically with hyperammonemia in the development of hepatic encephalopathy (Córdoba et al., 2010), and low serum sodium predicts the mortality in end-stage liver disease (Heuman et al., 2004; Ruf et al., 2005).

In the retina, the detoxification of excess ammonia occurs in astrocytes and Müller cells by the glutamate dehydrogenase reaction and in particular by the formation of glutamine from ammonia and glutamate (Fig. 44). Excess cytosolic glutamine is transported into the mitochondria where it is hydrolyzed to glutamate and ammonia by the mitochondrial enzyme phosphate-activated glutaminase (Fig. 35C). In the rodent retina, both neurons and glial cells express this enzyme (Takatsuna et al.,

1994). Retinal ischemia-reperfusion induces an irreversible decrease of the phosphate-activated glutaminase activity which results in increased retinal ammonia levels (Tomita et al., 1999).

The generation of high levels of ammonia in the mitochondria results in mitochondrial permeability transition (Fig. 35B,C) (Ziemińska et al., 2000; Rama Rao et al., 2003; Albrecht and Norenberg, 2006; Karl et al., 2011). The consequences of mitochondrial permeability transition are mitochondrial dysfunction, energy failure, and generation of free oxygen radicals. Mitochondria-derived free radicals activate cytosolic enzymes that generate oxygen and nitrogen radicals, e.g., NO synthases (Fig. 35C) (Karl et al., 2011). These radicals stimulate the activity of enzymes that produce inflammatory lipid mediators, i.e., PLA_2 and cyclooxygenases (Fig. 35C) (Landino et al., 1996; Du et al., 2004; Offer et al., 2005; Balboa and Balsinde, 2006). Arachidonic acid and prostaglandins are potent inhibitors of the sodium-potassium-ATPase; inhibition of the ATPase results in intracellular sodium overload, water influx, and cellular swelling (Fig. 35C) (Lees, 1991; Staub et al., 1994; Owada et al., 1999). The energy failure due to mitochondrial dysfunction and the high energy consumption of the glutamine synthetase reaction (Meister, 1974) contributes to the inhibition of the sodium-potassium-ATPase. The necessity to detoxify the retina from excess ammonia results in an enhanced consumption of glutamate for glutamine synthesis; the competition with the glutathione formation (Fig. 44) causes a decline of the cellular glutathione level which accelerates the pathogenic mechanisms involving free radicals (Reichenbach et al., 1999). High ammonia may also induce a downregulation of Kir channels and a depolarization of Müller cells (Bringmann et al., 1998a).

The glutamine-induced swelling of Müller cells is inhibited by ATP and adenosine (acting at adenosine A_1 receptors) (Karl et al., 2011). However, adenosine does not prevent the glutamine-induced dissipation of the mitochondrial membrane potential, suggesting that adenosine acts by promoting a potassium and chloride efflux across the plasma membrane (Karl et al., 2011; see 5.5.5.3.). The use of A_1 receptor agonists may aid in the treatment of brain and retinal edema in acute liver failure (Karl et al., 2011).

5.5.2.1.15 Production of Glutathione   The uptake of GABA and glutamate by Müller cells links neuronal excitation with the defense against oxidative stress. The retina has a high need of antioxidant protection. This results from the light exposure together with the high oxygen consumption (see 5.5.8.2.) and the presence of high levels of polyunsaturated fatty acids in the photoreceptors; these factors lead to peroxidation of photoreceptor lipids and proteins which represents a major pathogenic factor of AMD (Kopitz et al., 2004; Hollyfield et al., 2008). In addition, the outer retina underlies circadian periods of severe hypoxia (in the dark) and hyperoxia (in the light) (Alder et al., 1990; Linsenmeier, 1986; Linsenmeier et al., 1998; see 5.5.8.2.); both cause oxidative stress. Oxidative stress is a major factor which contributes to the retinal degeneration under various pathological conditions, e.g., ischemia-hypoxia, diabetic retinopathy, and retinal light injury (Remé et al., 1998; Wenzel et al., 2005).

Müller cells provide photoreceptors and neurons with an antioxidative environment by the upregulation and release, respectively, of pyruvate, α-ketoglutarate, metallothionein, lysozyme, the ferroxidase ceruloplasmin, heme oxygenase, and reduced ascorbate (Woodford et al., 1983; Klomp et al., 1996; Ulyanova et al., 2001; Miyahara et al., 2003; Chen et al., 2003a; Arai-Gaun et al., 2004; Frenzel et al., 2005; Hollborn et al., 2008; Wunderlich et al., 2010). The major glia-derived antioxidant is reduced glutathione which is a tripeptide produced from glutamate, cysteine, and glycine (Fig. 44) (Pow and Crook, 1995). Glutathione protects against oxidative and nitrosative stress by scavenging free radicals. The glial release of antioxidants like glutathione, and of further neuroprotective factors like adenosine and bFGF (see 5.5.2.1.15. and 5.11.7.7.), is implicated in the protection of the photoreceptors from the harmful effects of the circadian light exposure (see 5.5.8.2.). Various glial antioxidants, e.g., glutathione and ascorbate, may also function as neuromodulators. Via its γ-glutamyl moiety, glutathione at micromolar concentrations binds to iGluRs, and via its free cysteinyl thiol group, glutathione at millimolar concentrations modulates the redox site of NMDA receptors, resulting in increased receptor channel currents (Janaky et al., 1999). Ascorbic acid enhances $GABA_A$ and $GABA_C$ receptor currents and, thus, may act as an endogenous agent capable of potentiating GABAergic neurotransmission in the retina (Calero et al., 2011).

Under normal conditions, retinal glutathione is concentrated in glial and horizontal cells (Pow and Crook, 1995; Schütte and Werner, 1998; Huster et al., 1998; Marc and Cameron, 2001). It has been estimated that the intracellular glutathione concentration in Müller cells is 3–5 mM and that glutathione represents approximately 2% of the total Müller cell protein (Paasche et al., 1998). Under conditions associated with oxidative and nitrosative stress, e.g., during retinal ischemia, glutathione is rapidly released from Müller cells, and provided to neurons (Schütte and Werner, 1998). Here, glutathione acts as cofactor of various enzymes which remove toxic peroxides, control the redox state of the cells, and regulate the protein function through thiolation and dethiolation, e.g., glutathione peroxidase, reductase, transferase, and glutaredoxin. Glutathione peroxidase reduces peroxides to water or alcohol. During this process, glutathione peroxidase is oxidized and must subsequently be regenerated by oxidizing two molecules of glutathione to glutathione disulfide (GSSG). GSSG is recycled by glutathione reductase, which utilizes NADPH as reducing agent (Fig. 44). Müller cells have sodium-dependent and -independent transport systems for glutathione (Kannan et al., 1999). Whether the sodium-independent cystine-glutamate antiporter mediates a release of glutathione, as recently suggested (Oliveira et al., 2010), remains to be confirmed by further investigations. Glutamate and aspartate induce a GLAST-mediated release of glutathione from cultured Müller cells; this mechanism may be involved in the cellular defense against glutamate toxicity (Garcia et al., 2011).

The production of glutathione in Müller cells is critically dependent on the availability of extracellular glutamate and cystine (Fig. 44) (Reichelt et al., 1997b). Pharmacological blockade of glutamate transporters or knockout of GLAST result in a decreasd glutathione level in Müller cells (Reichelt et al., 1997b; Harada et al., 2007). Cysteine is formed by reduction of cystine that is taken up from the extracellular space via the cystine-glutamate antiporter (Fig. 44); inhibition of the antiporter results in a large decrease in the retinal glutathione level (Kato et al., 1993). Inhibition of the antiporter can also result from an increase in the extracellular glutamate concentration (see 5.6.1.1.). The expression of the γ-glutamyl-cysteine synthetase, which is implicated in the glutathione synthesis (Fig. 44), is increased upon oxidative stress and decreased during prolonged hyperglycemia; the latter results in reduced glutathione levels (Lu et al., 1999).

Pathological conditions associated with oxidative-nitrosative stress cause a reduction of the retinal gluthatione level. During hypoxia and hypoglycemia, the glutathione levels in Müller cells decrease dramatically (Huster et al., 2000), and under nitrosative stress conditions, the glutathione content of Müller cells drops to 50% within 2 h (Frenzel et al., 2005). In diabetes, hyperglycemia leads to a decrease of cellular gluthatione because the glucose metabolization through the polyol pathway entails reduced NADPH (Feldman et al., 1997). In the retina, the concentration of glutathione normally exceeds that of GSSG by a factor of 7 to 9 (Kern et al., 1994). In experimental diabetes, the retinal content of glutathione decreases while the GSSG level increases (Kern et al., 1994; Pinto et al., 2007; Gupta et al., 2011; Soufi et al., 2012; Kumar et al., 2013b, 2014). Because the synthesis of glutathione is dependent on the availability of extracellular glutamate and cystine (Reichelt et al., 1997b; Harada et al., 2007), the decreased glutamate uptake by Müller cells in the diabetic retina (see 5.5.2.1.6.) reduces the glutathione synthesis and results in an upregulation of glutaredoxin which induces nuclear translocation of NF-κB and expression of proinflammatory factors like ICAM-1 (Shelton et al., 2007, 2009). The downregulation of the glutamine synthetase occurring under various pathological conditions such as glaucoma (see 5.5.2.1.12.) leads to a depletion of neuronal glutamate resulting in a decrease of retinal glutathione (Gionfriddo et al., 2009).

Müller cells of aged animals contain reduced levels of glutathione compared to cells of young animals (Paasche et al., 1998). The age-dependent glutathione deficiency is associated with mitochondrial damage, membrane depolarization, and reduced cell viability (Paasche et al., 2000), suggesting that aging Müller cell mitochondria are impaired by accumulating oxidative damage. The age-dependent decrease of the Müller cell-mediated defense against free radicals accelerates the pathogenesis of retinopathies in the elderly. Externally applied radical scavengers like *Ginkgo biloba* extract enhance the intrinsic glutathione content of aged Müller cells and protect the mitochondria from the damaging actions of free radicals (Paasche et al., 1998, 2000). The retinal glutathione content in diabetic rats is also increased by dietary flavonoids like curcumin, hesperetin, quercetin, and green tea polyphenols (Gupta et al., 2011; Kumar et al., 2013b, 2014; Silva et al., 2013). The increased glutathione content and the elevated activity of antioxidant enzymes like superoxide dismutase and catalase after flavonoid intake is associated with improvements in various degenerative and inflammatory signs of diabetic retinopathy including the retinal expression of caspase-3, NF-κB, GFAP, TNFα, and IL-1β, and the rate of ganglion cell apoptosis (Kumar et al., 2013b, 2014).

5.5.2.2 GABA Uptake and Metabolism

GABA is the main inhibitory neurotransmitter in the vertebrate retina. Subclasses of horizontal, amacrine, ganglion, bipolar, and interplexiform cells utilize GABA as transmitter. The termination of the synaptic action of GABA is achieved by the uptake into presynaptic neuronal terminals and surrounding glial cells. In addition to neurons such as amacrine and interplexiform cells (Moran et al., 1986; Pow et al., 1996; Johnson et al., 1996) and (in the fish retina) horizontal and bipolar cells (Malchow and Ripps, 1990; Nelson et al., 2008; Jiang et al., 2009b), Müller cells and (at least under pathological conditions) astrocytes and microglia take up GABA from the extracellular space (Neal et al., 1979; Sarthy, 1982; Redburn and Madtes, 1986; Osborne et al., 1995). It was suggested that in the retinas of most lower vertebrates and birds, the GABA removal is almost exclusively mediated by neuronal cells, whereas in the mammalian retina, neurons and Müller cells remove GABA from the extracellular space (Yazulla, 1986; 5.5.2.2.3.). In mammals, GABA is taken up predominantly by amacrine and Müller cells in the inner retina (Fig. 34I), and almost exclusively by Müller cells in the outer retina (Redburn and Madtes, 1986; Marc, 1992; 5.5.2.2.3.). During the postnatal maturation of the rabbit retina, GABA uptake is shifted from various types of neurons to Müller cells and a subpopulation of amacrine cells (Redburn and Madtes, 1986).

5.5.2.2.1 GABA Uptake   The uptake of GABA by Müller cells is mediated by sodium- (Fig. 34C) and chloride-dependent high-affinity GABA transporters (GATs). Per transport step, 2 sodium ions and 1 chloride ion are cotransported with 1 GABA molecule (Qian et al., 1993; Biedermann et al., 2002). Omission of sodium or chloride from the extracellular solution fully inhibits the transport of GABA (Fig. 34C) (Biedermann et al., 2002, 2004). Because GABA is electrically neutral at physiological pH, the transport process causes inwardly directed membrane currents (Fig. 34C) (Biedermann et al., 1994). The shift of one positive charge from the extra- to the intracellular side of the plasma membrane results in a depolarization of the cells (Fig. 34C). The electrogenic transport of GABA is concentration-dependent, with near-maximal currents at

100 µM GABA (Biedermann et al., 2002). At a membrane potential of −80 mV (which is close to the resting membrane potential of Müller cells; Figs. 8H, 45E, 46A, B, D), the GABA concentration that half-maximally activates the electrogenic transporters is 5.7 and 7.9 µM in Müller cells of guinea pigs and man, respectively (Biedermann et al., 2002). The GABA transporter currents are voltage-dependent. The amplitude of the currents increases (Fig. 34D) and the affinity of GABA to the transporter molecules decreases with hyperpolarization of the plasma membrane (Biedermann et al., 2002). The GABA transporter currents are unevenly distributed over the plasma membranes of guinea-pig Müller cells, with the largest currents at the end of the outer stem processes which envelop the terminals and somata of photoreceptor cells *in situ* (Fig. 34G) (Biedermann et al., 2002). The time dependence of the GABA clearance from the extracellular space surrounding one Müller cell was estimated; at a membrane potential of −80 mV, a pulse of 100 µM extracellular GABA is fully cleared after 70 ms (Biedermann et al., 2002). Due to the high efficiency of the GABA uptake, Müller cells are suggested to be involved in the rapid termination of the GABAergic transmission in the mammalian retina.

5.5.2.2.2 GABA Release Rat and primate Müller cells were suggested to release GABA, e.g, after activation with KA, high potassium, and GABA mimetics (Neal and Bowery, 1979; Sarthy, 1983; Andrade da Costa et al., 2000). Membrane depolarization and glutamate are known to induce a transporter-mediated GABA release from retinal neurons (Calaza et al., 2006; Guimarães-Souza et al., 2011). Such a transporter-mediated GABA release was not found in chick and rabbit Müller cells (Bauer and Ehinger, 1977; Bauer, 1978; De Sampaio Schitine et al., 2007). However, rabbit Müller cells release GABA after inhibition of the sodium-potassium-ATPase (Agardh and Bauer, 1984). Whether Müller cells are capable to release GABA via a reversal of GABA transporters, or via other mechanisms, remains to be determined in future experiments. The enzyme glutamic acid decarboxylase (GAD), which synthesizes GABA from glutamate in GABAergic neurons (Fig. 44), was found in cultured Müller cells (Kubrusly et al., 2005). However, it is unknown whether this enzyme is also present in Müller cells *in situ*. It was suggested that retinal glial cells may also produce GABA from 4-aminobutyraldehyde, independently of the GAD pathway (Matsushima et al., 1987).

5.5.2.2.3 Expression of GABA Transporters To date four GABA transporter subtypes have been described (GAT1-4) in addition to the vesicular transporter (VGAT), with GAT-3 being the predominant glial form (Schousboe, 2003). The expression of GAT subtypes in Müller cells varies among species. Müller cells of the guinea pig display immunoreactivities for GAT-1 and GAT-3 (Fig. 34H, I), but not GAT-2 (Biedermann et al., 2002). The transporter proteins, which are located in the whole plasma membrane of guinea-pig Müller cells, show an elevated expression level in the outer stem process (Fig. 34H) (Biedermann et al., 2002). Müller cells of the chick and rat also express GAT-1 and -3 (Brecha and Weigmann, 1994; Honda et al., 1995; Johnson et al., 1996; Kim et al., 2003; De Sampaio Schitine et al., 2007) while Müller cells of the rabbit express GAT-3 but not GAT-1 (Hu et al., 1999). On the other hand, Müller cells of the bullfrog retina express GAT-1 and GAT-2 but not GAT-3 (Zhao et al., 2000), and Müller cells of other lower vertebrate species such as tiger salamander and salmon apparently do not express GAT proteins (Yang et al., 1997; Ekström and Anzelius, 1998).

Following excitotoxic injury of the adult rat retina, Müller cells accumulate GABA (Andrés et al., 2003). Cultured avian Müller cells, but not avian Müller cells *in situ*, were shown to accumulate GABA (Marshall and Voaden, 1974; Pow et al., 1996; Calaza et al., 2001; De Sampaio Schitine et al., 2007). However, a failure in demonstrable GABA uptake in Müller cells of distinct lower vertebrates and birds should be used with caution. It cannot be ruled out that GABA is rapidly converted by the GABA transaminase in Müller cells but not in neurons, resulting in a failure of detectable GABA in Müller cells (see 5.5.2.2.4.). It has been shown, for example, that turtle Müller cells display a very little GABA transport activity but high levels of GABA transaminase (Sarthy and Lam, 1978). A failure in the immunohistochemical detection of GAT proteins in Müller cells of lower vertebrates may be due to poor cross reactivity of antibodies directed against rodent sequences.

Whether or not neuronal cells participate in the GABA clearance of the outer mammalian retina is unclear and apparently dependent on the species investigated. Horizontal cells of guinea pigs and mice do not express GATs (Guo et al., 2010; Deniz et al., 2011). In these cells, GABA is synthesized from glutamate or glutamine (Fig. 44), taken up into synaptic vesicles by VGAT, and released by a vesicular mechanism (Deniz et al., 2011). On the other hand, monkey rod bipolar and horizontal cells express GAT3 (Lassová et al., 2010). It has been suggested that monkey rod bipolar cells tonically release GABA from their dendrites using a reverse action of GAT3 (Lassová et al., 2010).

5.5.2.2.4   GABA Metabolism   When GABA enters the interior of Müller cells, it is readily converted to glutamate by the GABA transaminase via a NAD(P)-dependent process (Fig. 44). GABA transaminase, which catalyzes the formation of glutamate from 2-oxoglutarate (Fig. 44), coupled to a conversion of GABA to succinate semialdehyde, is localized in the mitochondria (Fig. 34J-L) (Schousboe et al., 1977). In the avascular retina of the guinea pig, the mitochondria (and thus the GABA transaminase; Fig. 34L) are solely located within the end of the outer stem processes, near to the choroidal blood supply *in situ* (see 5.2.). Extracellular administration of GABA induces a NAD(P)H fluorescence signal (caused by the reduction of NAD(P) to NAD(P)H) selectively in the mitochondria of Müller cells (Fig. 34J,K) (Biedermann et al., 2002). Due to the efficiency of the GABA transaminase reaction as the primary mechanism of GABA turnover, Müller cells display a very low level of intracellular GABA (<100 µM) which is hardly detectable with immunohistochemical methods (Davanger et al., 1991; Marc et al., 1998a). GABA immunoreactivity in Müller cells is only detectable under pathological conditions or after pharmacological inhibition of the GABA transaminase (Cubells et al., 1988; Neal et al., 1989; Barnett and Osborne, 1995; Perlman et al., 1996; Ishikawa et al., 1996a; Yazulla et al., 1997; Takeo-Goto et al., 2002).

In diabetic and ischemic retinas of the rat, GABA rapidly accumulates in Müller cells due to a decrease in the GABA transaminase activity (Barnett and Osborne, 1995; Ishikawa et al., 1996a, b; Kobayashi et al., 1999; Napper et al., 2001). During ischemia, Müller cell energy levels are sufficient to allow the active uptake of released GABA, but insufficient to metabolize it to glutamine (Barnett and Osborne, 1995). An intracellular GABA accumulation will impair the efficiency of the GABA uptake into Müller cells due to a decrease in the transmembrane driving force.

5.5.2.3 Uptake of Glycine and Arginine

In the vertebrate CNS, glycine acts both as an inhibitory neurotransmitter and as a coagonist at post-synaptic NMDA receptors. In the retina, populations of amacrine, bipolar, and interplexiform cells utilize glycine as transmitter (Davanger et al., 1991; Pow, 2001b). The termination of the synaptic action of glycine is achieved by reuptake. In retinas of a variety of mammalian and non-mammalian species, Müller cells apparently do not take up glycine, and the expression of glycine transporters is restricted to neurons (reviewed by Pow, 2001b). However, in amphibian retinas, both neurons and Müller cells express glycine transporters (GlyTs). GlyT1-like transporters are expressed in Müller cells while GlyT2-like transporters are present in neurons such as amacrine and horizontal cells (Du et al., 2002; Lee et al., 2005; Jiang et al., 2007). GlyTs are electrogenic, sodium-dependent transporters; thus, extracellular glycine induces inward currents in amphibian Müller cells (Du et al., 2002a). In human Müller cells which do not express glycine transporters, extracellular glycine does not induce alterations in the membrane conductance (Bringmann et al., 2002a). The species-dependent expression of glycine transporters suggests that Müller cells participate in the termination of the glycinergic neurotransmission in retinas of lower vertebrates, and do not play a significant role in the removal of extracellular glycine in retinas of higher vertebrates. On the other hand, Müller cells of the rat retina express the glycine cleavage system (Sato et al., 1991), suggesting that they are capable to degrade glycine. In retinas of lower vertebrates, the regulation of the glycine transport in Müller cells may contribute to the modulation of the NMDA receptor activity. Whereas Müller cells of higher vertebrates, e.g., chicken, rat, and man, do not express glycine transporters *in situ*

(Pow and Hendrickson, 1999; Bringmann et al., 2002a) they have the capacity to take up glycine and express GlyT1 when placed into culture (Beale and Osborne, 1983; Gadea et al., 1999, 2002; Reye et al., 2001). These data underline the assumptions that results obtained in cultured cells do not necessarily reflect the *in-situ* siuation, and that Müller cells in pathological tissues may exhibit different patterns of transporter expression than in normal tissues (Pow, 2001b).

Cultured chick Müller cells were shown to take up arginine by various transport systems (Cossenza and Paes de Carvalho, 2000). The availability of arginine is important for the synthesis of NO (see 5.6.5.).

5.5.2.4 Uptake of Dopamine and Anandamide

Dopamine is the predominant biogenic amine in the retina. It has been shown that cultured chicken Müller cells express dopamine D_1 receptors, tyrosine hydroxylase, L-DOPA decarboxylase (two of the enzymes that synthesize dopamine), but not the dopamine transporter DAT (Kubrusly et al., 2005). Although acutely isolated mammalian Müller cells may express functional D_2 receptors (see 5.10.7.), it remains to be determined whether Müller cells *in situ* also express these enzymes and transporters. In the rat retina, only catecholaminergic amacrine cells express tyrosine hydroxylase (Iandiev et al., 2006d). In the carp retina, Müller cells (in addition to retinal neurons) may take up serotonin (Negishi and Teranishi, 1990). In the mammalian retina, retinal ganglion and amacrine cells take up serotonin (Ehinger and Florén, 1980; Wässle et al., 1987; Osborne et al., 1995; Jo et al., 1998). In the retina, free tryptophan is mainly present in Müller cells and photoreceptors, suggesting that serotonergic neurons are dependent upon the transfer of tryptophan from Müller cells to produce serotonin (Pow and Cook, 1997). Müller cells are capable to take up histidine, the precursor of histamine synthesis (Morgan et al., 1999b).

Cannabinoid ligands have electrophysiological effects on cones and bipolar cells. Müller cells and cone inner segments in the goldfish retina express the fatty acid amide hydrolase (Glaser et al., 2005) which hydrolyzes the endocannabinoid anandamide. Goldfish Müller cells and cone photoreceptors take up anandamide; the bulk anandamide clearance occurs as a consequence of a concentration gradient created by the fatty acid amide hydrolase activity (Glaser et al., 2005). In contrast, in the monkey retina, fatty acid amide hydrolase is localized to photoreceptors and neurons, but not to Müller cells (Bouskila et al., 2012).

5.5.3   RETINAL POTASSIUM HOMEOSTASIS

Neuronal activity induced by the onset of light stimuli results in increases of the extracellular potassium concentration (by ~1 mM) in the plexiform (synaptic) layers, and a decrease of the potassium concentration (by 2–3 mM) in the subretinal space because photoreceptors hyperpolarize in response to light stimulation (Oakley and Green, 1976; Steinberg et al., 1980; Karwoski et al., 1985, 1989). Cessation of illumination causes an increase in the potassium level of the subretinal space fluid. If uncorrected, increases of extracellular potassium will cause neuronal depolarization and hyperexcitability. Homeostasis of the extracellular potassium concentration is a precondition of regular neuronal information processing. A major functional role of glial cells in the CNS including the sensory retina is to buffer the activity-dependent variations in the extracellular potassium level by permission of transcellular potassium currents, a process termed spatial potassium buffering or potassium siphoning (Orkand et al., 1966; Newman et al., 1984; Karwoski et al., 1989; Reichenbach et al., 1992; Newman and Reichenbach, 1996). Müller cells take up excess potassium from the extracellular space especially in the plexiform layers, and release equal amounts of potassium into fluid-filled spaces outside the neural retina where the potassium concentration is constant (blood, vitreal fluid) or decreased (subretinal space) during light stimulation (Fig. 55) (Newman et al., 1984; Karwoski et al., 1989; Reichenbach et al., 1992). The light-induced potassium efflux from Müller cells into the subretinal space in association with the potassium influx into the inner end of the cells establish a dipole with a positive field potential in the outer retina (underlying the slow PIII response of the electroretinogram) (Witkovsky et al., 1975; Newman and Odette, 1984; Yanagida and Tomita, 1984; Reichenbach and Wohlrab, 1985; Dmitriev et al., 1985; Xu and Karwoski, 1997; Kofuji et al., 2000). The spatial buffering potassium currents through Müller cells limit the lateral spread of excitation beyond the borders of the light-stimulated retinal columns and thus help to maintain visual acuity (Reichenbach et al., 1993a).

As a consequence of the high expression of potassium channels, the plasma membranes of Müller cells are highly permeable to potassium ions (Newman, 1984, 1985a). In Müller cells of the frog, the potassium-to-sodium membrane permeability ratio is approximately 490:1, while the chloride permeability is (under resting conditions) very low (Newman, 1985a). The high potassium permeability of the plasma membrane is the basis of the very negative resting membrane potential of the cells (around −80 mV; Figs. 8H, 45E, 46A,B,D) which is close to the equilibrium potential of potassium ions (−80 to −90 mV) (Witkovsky et al., 1985; Brand and Hanke, 1996; Kofuji et al., 2000). Recordings of the whole-cell currents of isolated Müller cells (Figs. 8F, 12L, 21D, 46C, 56A,B, 57A, 58A) reveal different kinds of potassium currents (Fig. 56C) (Newman, 1985b; Chao et al., 1994a). Around the resting membrane potential and upon membrane hyperpolarization, Kir channel-mediated inward potassium currents can be recorded (Fig. 56C). These channels are characterized by their capability to mediate greater inward potassium currents (into the cell) than outward currents (out of the cell). Depolarization of the plasma membrane of Müller cells may activate various kinds of voltage-gated outwardly rectifying potassium currents including fast transient

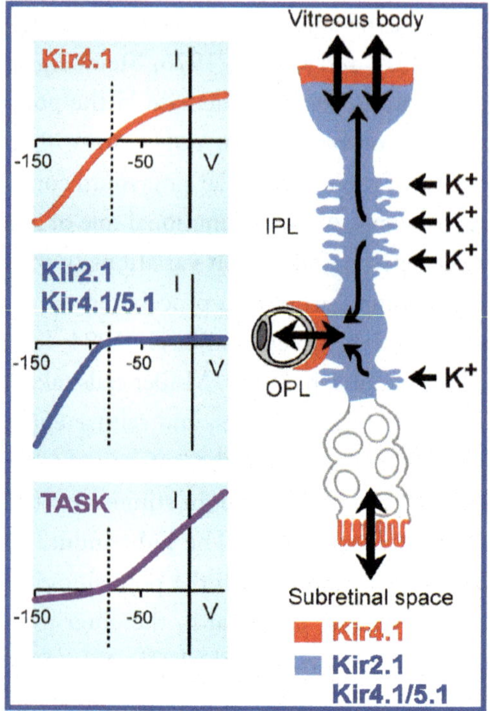

FIGURE 55: The subcellular distribution of different Kir channel subtypes determines the direction of the spatial buffering potassium currents through Müller cells. *Left:* Current-voltage (I-V) relations of various glial potassium channels. Kir4.1 channels mediate inward and outward currents with similar amplitudes at the resting membrane potential (*broken line*), whereas Kir2.1 and Kir4.1/5.1 channels mediate inward currents and two-pore domain (TASK) channels mediate outward potassium currents. *Right:* Scheme of the potassium buffering currents that flow through Müller cells during neuronal activation. Activated neurons release potassium ions predominantly into both plexiform (synaptic) layers. The ions are absorbed by Müller cells through Kir2.1 and Kir5.1/4.1 channels, and distributed into the blood vessels, the vitreous, and the subretinal space through Kir4.1 channels. Kir4.1 channels mediate in- and outward currents and, thus, contribute to the osmohomeostasis between the neuroretina and extra-retinal fluid-filled spaces. Modified from Kofuji et al. (2002).

(A-type) potassium (K_A) currents, delayed rectifying potassium (K_{DR}) currents, and currents through calcium-activated potassium channels of big conductance (BK currents) (Fig. 56C). Although the sodium-potassium-ATPase (which is concentrated in glial membranes in the plexiform layers and in the microvilli; Ueno et al., 1981; Stirling and Sarthy, 1985; Reichenbach et al., 1988b; and which is more active in response to external potassium accumulation; Reichenbach et al., 1985; Reichelt et al., 1989) and transporter molecules (e.g., the K/Na/2Cl cotransporter) contribute to the Müller

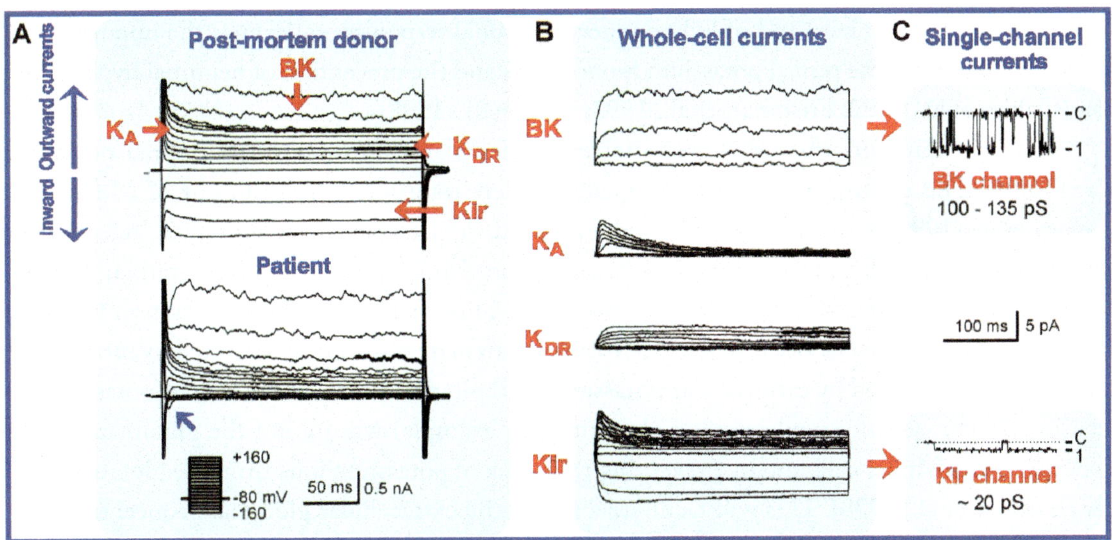

FIGURE 56: Four different types of potassium currents can be recorded in human Müller cells. **A.** Potassium currents of human Müller cells. The currents were recorded in the whole-cell mode of the patch-clamp technique in a cell from a post-mortem donor without apparent eye diseases (*above*) and a cell from a patient with proliferative vitreoretinopathy (*below*). Outward currents (*upwardly* depicted) were induced by step-wise depolarization up to +160 mV from a holding potential of −80 mV. Inward currents (*downwardly* depicted) were induced by hyperpolarizing voltage steps up to −160 mV. Note the complete absence of inward potassium currents in the trace of the patient's Müller cell. The *blue arrow* indicates transient inward currents induced by depolarizing voltage steps which are mediated by voltage-gated sodium channels. **C.** The whole-cell currents of Müller cells are composed of at least four different kinds of potassium currents: inwardly rectifying potassium (Kir) currents, and three kinds of outwardly rectifying currents: BK, currents through calcium-activated potassium channels of big conductance; K_A, transient (A-type) potassium currents; and K_{DR}, delayed rectifying potassium currents. **D.** The currents through single potassium channels recorded in cell-attached membrane patches display the different conductance of BK and Kir channels. C, closed state; 1, open state current levels. Modified from Bringmann et al. (1999b).

cell-mediated potassium homeostasis (Reichenbach et al., 1986, 1992; Arrindell et al., 1992), passive currents through Kir channels play the major role in the clearance of the retinal tissue from excess potassium. Kir channels are the only potassium channels that display a high open probability at the very negative resting membrane potential characteristic for Müller cells (Fig. 59A,C) (Brew et al., 1986; Newman, 1993; Bringmann et al., 1999a,b). The facts that a blockade of the Kir channels with barium ions is associated with strong increases of the light-induced alterations in the extracellular potassium level and of light-induced neuronal responses underlines the importance of glial Kir channels for the retinal potassium homeostasis and the prevention of neuronal hyperexcitation (Oakley et al., 1992; Frishman et al., 1992; Linn et al., 1998).

The ion transport through transporter molecules may contribute to the retinal potassium homeostasis. The electrogenic glutamate uptake carriers transport potassium out of Müller cells (Amato et al., 1994; see 5.5.2.1.3.). The light-induced suppression of the glutamate release from photoreceptor cells reduces the efflux of potassium from Müller cells in the outer retina; this may contribute to the light-induced decrease in the extracellular potassium concentration in the outer retina (Amato et al., 1994). Because the electrogenic glutamate transport is activated by intracellular potassium and inhibited by extracellular potassium, pathological rises in extracellular potassium (as occuring during ischemia, epilepsy, and glaucoma, for example) will inhibit the glutamate uptake by depolarizing Müller cells and by preventing the efflux of potassium ions from the glutamate carrier (Barbour et al., 1988). This will facilitate a rise in the extracellular glutamate concentration to neurotoxic levels.

The classical view of the mechanism how glial cells buffer imbalances in the extracellular potassium concentration suggests that a local increase in the extracellular potassium level causes the driving force for the passive potassium currents through the glial cells (Orkand et al., 1966). An increase in extracellular potassium shifts the equilibrium potential of potassium ions towards more positive voltages. When this increase is localized to a small area (around few synapses, for example), the equilibrium potential of potassium becomes more positive than the resting membrane potential of the cell (which is only slightly shifted towards more positive voltages because the surrounding non-affected membrane holds the potential at a high value). As a result, potassium moves down its electrochemical gradient and enters the glial cell interior. At sites distant from the local increase in extracellular potassium, the slight depolarization of the membrane enhances the electrogenic driving force for the efflux of potassium from the cells. Thus, potassium enters the Müller cell where the extracellular potassium concentration is elevated and exits where the extracellular potassium level is unchanged. Such a spatial buffering mechanism is estimated to clear excess potassium from the retina up to ~4 times faster than extracellular diffusion (Newman et al., 1984; Eberhardt and Reichenbach, 1987; Reichenbach et al., 1992). However, this classical view needs a supplement because it would imply that potassium can be also released from Müller cells at sites near the local increase in extracellular potassium, e.g., into spaces around non-activated synapses. To avoid affection of neuronal activity due to Müller cell-derived potassium, Müller cells release potassium solely through membrane domains which have contact to fluid-filled spaces outside the neuroretina. The direction of this potassium flux out of the neuroretina is determined by the subcellular localization of different Kir channel subtypes.

5.5.3.1 Kir Channels

Single Kir channels (Figs. 59A,D, 60B) of Müller cells from various vertebrate species have conductances between 17 and 28 pS (Fig. 59B), in dependence on the recording conditions (Newman, 1993; Ishii et al., 1997; Kusaka and Puro, 1997; Tada et al., 1998; Rojas and Orkand, 1999; Bringmann et al., 1999a, 2000e). The conductance of Kir channels increases when the extracellular potassium concentration raises (Newman, 1993). Kir channels have a high open probability (>0.8) over a wide voltage range around the resting membrane potential (Fig. 59C) (Kusaka and Puro, 1997; Bringmann et al., 1999a,b). This high open probability of Kir channels is a precondition for the mediation of prompt passive potassium currents across the plasma membrane when the local level of the extracellular potassium alters.

Among the various subtypes of Kir channels expressed by Müller cells (Raap et al., 2002), Kir4.1, Kir2.1, and Kir4.1/5.1 channels were suggested to be implicated in mediating the potassium buffering currents (Ishii et al., 1997; Tada et al., 1998; Kofuji et al., 2000, 2002). Homomeric Kir4.1 channels are weakly rectifying channels, i.e., they mediate inward and outward potassium currents with similar amplitudes (Fig. 55) (Takumi et al., 1995; Kubo et al., 1996; Shuck et al., 1997; Tada et al., 1998). Kir2.1 channels are strongly rectifying channels and mediate predominantly inward potassium currents and almost no outward currents (Fig. 55) (Kubo et al., 1993). Kir5.1 subunits are not functional by themselves, but are capable to coassemble with Kir4.1; the assembling alters the gating properties of Kir4.1, resulting in a steeper degree of inward rectification (Pessia et al., 1996).

Different Kir channel subtypes are expressed in a polarized fashion in the plasma membrane of Müller cells. Homomeric Kir4.1 channels are prominently localized in such membrane domains across which Müller cells extrude potassium into spaces outside of the neural retina, i.e., in perivascular membranes, in membranes of the endfeet which have contact to the vitreous chamber, and in the microvilli that extend into the subretinal space (Figs. 2G, 7G,H, 8C, D, 9A, 12A, 18C, 19, 23A, 49, 52, 55) (Nagelhus et al., 1999, 2004; Kofuji et al., 2000; Poopalasundaram et al., 2000; Ishii et al., 2003a). In addition, Kir4.1 is localized at a lower density in neuron-abutting membrane domains, e.g., in the plexiform layers (Fig. 9A). In avascular retinas such as of the guinea pig and rabbit, the Kir4.1 protein is localized prominently at the inner and outer limiting membranes, and as spots throughout the retinal tissue (Fig. 7G) (Francke et al., 2005). Kir2.1 protein is localized in membrane domains of Müller cells that face retinal neurons (Figs. 7I, 8C, 12B, 55) (Kofuji et al., 2002; Iandiev et al., 2006c; Ulbricht et al., 2008). Single spots of Kir5.1 immunoreactivity have been found to be distributed diffusely at the cell body and the outer portions of rat Müller cells (Ishii et al., 2003a). Thus, heterotetrameric Kir4.1/5.1 channels may be expressed in Müller cell membranes across which excess potassium is taken up from the interstitium (Ishii et al., 2003a). The polarized expression of different subtypes of Kir channels (together with the local transmembraneous potassium gradients) determines the direction of the transglial potassium currents: excess potassium is absorbed by Müller cells from the interstitial space around excited neurons, and is distributed into the blood, the vitreous fluid, and the subretinal space (Fig. 55) (Kofuji et al., 2002). It has been suggested that the predominant expression of strongly rectifying Kir channel subtypes at the glio-neuronal interface constitutes a mechanism that avoids affection of neuronal information processing by depolarization due to unwarranted efflux of potassium from Müller cells (Kofuji et al., 2002). However, the expression and subcellular distribution of different Kir channel subtypes in Müller cells of various species remains to be clarified. It was found that Kir5.1 is not expressed in Müller cells of frogs, mice, and guinea pigs (Skatchkov et al., 2001; Kofuji et al., 2002; Raap et al., 2002). Other studies described a neuronal, but not glial, expression of Kir2.1 in the rat retina (Tian et al., 2003; Raz-Prag et al., 2010).

Kir4.1 and Kir2.1 are ATP-dependent channels (Fakler et al., 1994; Takumi et al., 1995). The opening of the channels requires the generation of ATP by local glycolysis near the channel proteins and subsequent hydrolysis of ATP by an ATPase (Fakler et al., 1994; Kusaka and Puro, 1997). The activity of Kir2.1 channels is also regulated by protein kinases; phosphorylation of the channel protein by the protein kinase A (PKA) stimulates the opening of the channels whereas phosphorylation by PKC reduces the channel activity (Fakler et al., 1994).

5.5.3.2 Whole-Cell Kir Currents

The membrane conductance of whole Müller cells is dominated by large currents through Kir channels which are inwardly directed when the membrane is hyperpolarized, and outwardly directed at potentials positive to the resting membrane potential of approximately -80 mV (Figs. 7A, 8H, 21D, 23E, 46C, 56B,C, 57A,B, 61A, 62, 63B). The current-voltage relation of the whole-cell currents reveals weak inward rectification of the potassium currents around the resting membrane potential, suggesting that a large portion of the currents is mediated by weakly rectifying Kir4.1 channels. However, the rectification degree of the whole-cell currents differs in Müller cells from different species, e.g. from man (Figs. 46C, 56B) and rat (Figs. 8F, 21D, 23E, 57A,B, 58A, 61A), reflecting a species-dependent variation in the expression of distinct Kir channel subtypes. The rectification of the Kir currents may be in part regulated by intracellular polyamines such as spermine/spermidine (Lopatin et al., 1994; Biedermann et al., 1998; Skatchkov et al., 2000; Kucheryavykh et al., 2007). Kir currents are blocked by extracellular barium ions (Fig. 57A,B) (Newman, 1989; Reichelt and Pannicke, 1993; Chao et al., 1994a).

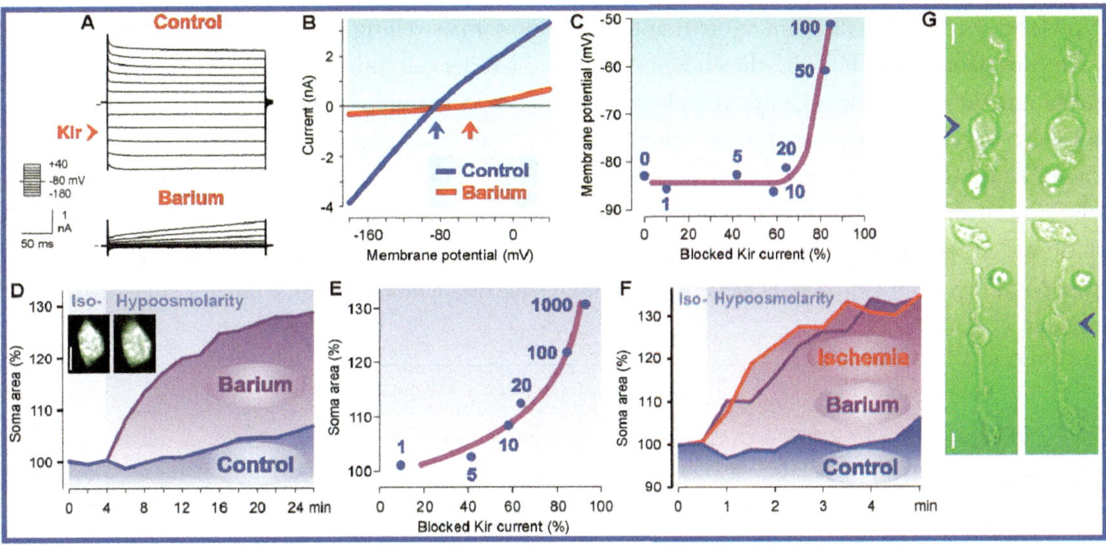

FIGURE 57: Inhibition of Kir channel-mediated potassium currents of rodent Müller cells by barium ions induces an osmotic swelling of the cells under hypoosmotic conditions. **A.** Examples of whole-cell potassium current records in an isolated rat Müller cell before (control) and during extracellular administration of barium chloride (100 μM). Note the absence of Kir currents in the presence of barium. **B.** Current-voltage relations of the whole-cell currents of rat Müller cells. Note the weak inward rectification of the currents under control conditions, and the positive shift of the zero-current (0 nA) potential (*arrows*) in the presence of barium chloride (100 μM) that reflects the depolarization of the cells. **C.** Relation between the resting membrane potential (RMP) of rat Müller cells and the amplitude of their Kir currents which were blocked by barium chloride. The barium concentrations (in μM) are given in the diagram. Note that the cells depolarize to potentials positive to -80 mV when the Kir currents are decreased to amplitudes lower than ~40% of control. **D.** Superfusion of freshly isolated slices of the murine retina with a hypoosmotic solution (60% of control osmolarity) results in a swelling of Müller cell somata in the presence, but not absence (control), of barium chloride (1 mM). The mean time-dependent alteration of the cross-sectional area of Müller cell somata during the change from the iso-osmotic to the hypoosmotic extracellular solution is shown. Note that Müller cells maintain their soma size for at least 10 min under hypoosmotic conditions (in the absence of barium). The *images* display original records of a dye-filled Müller cell soma obtained before (*left*) and during (*right*) superfusion of the hypoosmotic solution in the presence of barium. **E.** Relation between the amplitude of Kir currents, which was blocked by barium chloride, and the mean soma area of rat Müller cells measured in hypoosmotic solution in the presence of different concentrations of barium chloride. The barium concentrations

continued on next page

(in µM) are given in the diagram. Note that the osmotic soma swelling is positively related to the extent of Kir current blockade. **F.** Time-dependent swelling of Müller cell somata recorded in retinal slices from control rats (in the absence [Control] and presence of 1 mM barium chloride) and in slices which were obtained 3 days after a transient retinal ischemia of 1 h. Note that ischemia and barium induced a similar swelling of Müller cell somata under hypoosmotic conditions. **G.** Freshly isolated rat Müller cells display a swelling of their somata (*arrowheads*) after 4 min of exposure to a barium-containing hypoosmotic solution. The records were obtained before (*left*) and during (*right*) hypoosmotic exposure. Scale bars, 5 µm. Modified from Pannicke et al. (2004, 2005a), Uckermann et al. (2006), Linnertz et al. (2011), and Brückner et al. (2012).

Kir4.1 channels mediate ~90% of the potassium conductance of Müller cells at the resting membrane potential (Kofuji et al., 2000). Müller cells of Kir4.1 knockout mice display a depolarization of their membranes (Kofuji et al., 2000), suggesting that the Kir4.1 channel is the major determinant of the very negative membrane potential of approximately −80 mV. A full blockade of the Kir channels with barium ions results in a depolarization of the cells to values between −60 and −40 mV (Fig. 57B, C) which is the activation threshold of outwardly rectifying K_A and K_{DR} currents (Pannicke et al., 2000b). There is a nonlinear relation between the Kir current amplitude and the membrane potential of Müller cells, i.e., Müller cells depolarize when the Kir currents are decreased to values lower than ~40% of control (Figs. 8H, 57C) (Bringmann et al., 2000a; Pannicke et al., 2005a). This nonlinear relation is also reflected in the physiological properties of developing Müller cells where the resting membrane potential increases faster than the Kir currents (Fig. 51) (Bringmann et al., 1999a). Apparently, Müller cells express more Kir channels in their membranes than required to maintain a negative membrane potential; this provides a distinct safety against membrane depolarization when the expression of functional Kir channels decreases under pathological conditions (see 5.5.3.5.).

5.5.3.3 Subcellular Distribution of the Potassium Conductance

Müller cells display a non-uniform distribution of the potassium conductance across their plasma membrane. Cells of species with avascular retinas (fish, amphibians, rabbit, guinea pig) have the highest potassium conductance in the membranes of their endfeet that face the vitreous cavity, and at the outer (photoreceptor) end of the cells (Fig. 7C,D) (Newman, 1984, 1985a, 1986, 1987; Francke et al., 2005). In dogfish, amphibian, and rabbit Müller cells, 80–95% of the total membrane conductance is localized in the endfoot membrane (Newman, 1984, 1985a, 1988; Reichenbach and

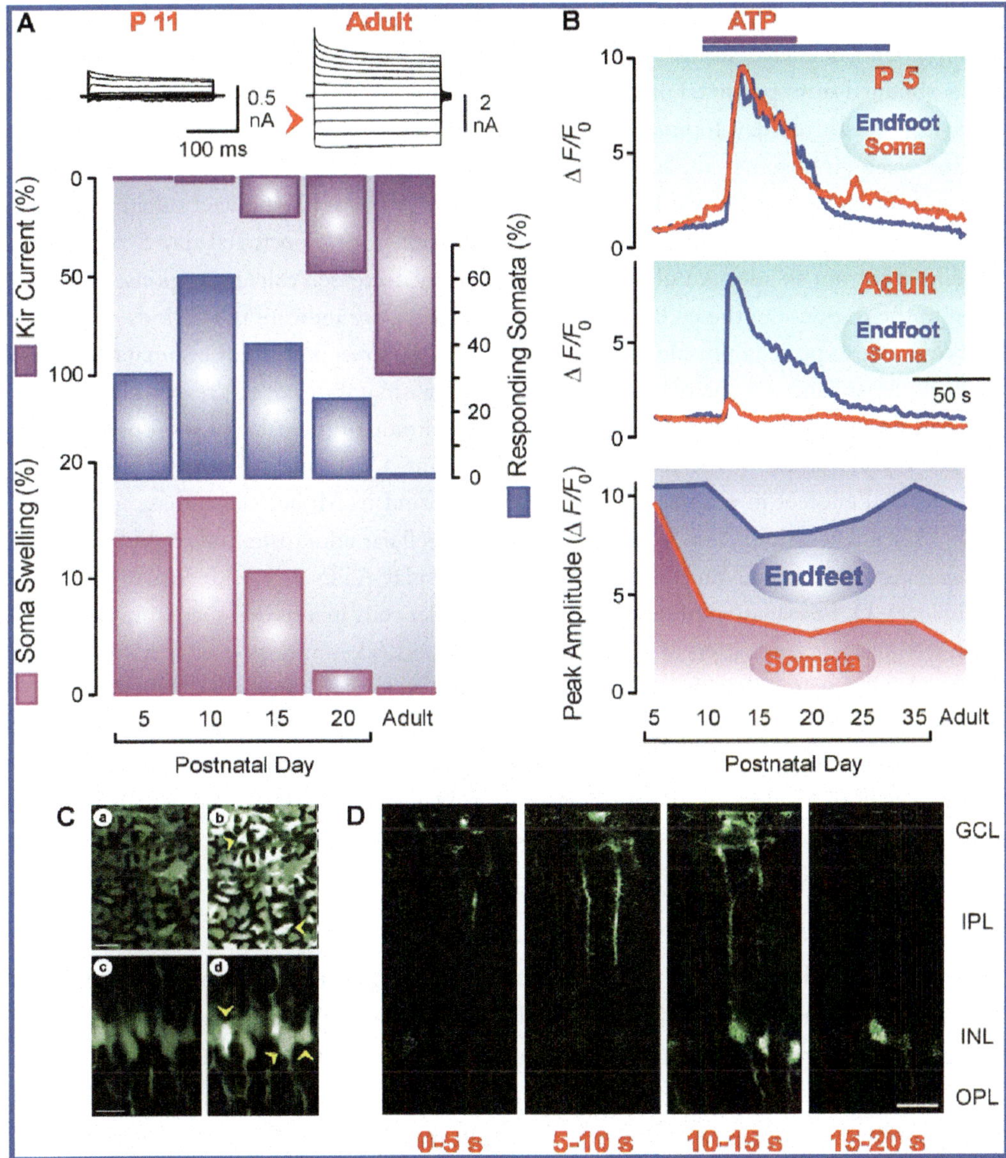

FIGURE 58: P2Y signaling in developing Müller cells of the postnatal rat retina. **A.** During the postnatal differentiation of immature Müller cells to mature Müller cells, the incidence of Müller cell somata that respond to exogenous ATP with intracellular calcium mobilization displays a peak at postnatal day 10 and declines thereafter (*middle*). The decline is related to the increase in the Kir currents of the cells

continued on next page

(*above*) and to the extent of the osmotic swelling of Müller cell somata recorded under hypoosmotic conditions (*below*). The *images* shown *above* display examples of potassium current records in individual Müller cells obtained from postnatal day (P) 11 and adult animals. The Kir currents are depicted *downwardly* (*arrowhead*). In the developing rat retina, synaptic activity is firstly detected at the end of the first postnatal week (Johnson et al., 2003) when the proliferation of late progenitors is ceased; the eye opening occurs around postnatal day 15. **B.** The amplitude of the ATP-induced calcium response was similar in the endfoot and soma of an immature Müller cell from a postnatal day-5 rat (*above*). The mature Müller cell from an adult rat displayed a dramatically decreased calcium response in the soma in comparison to the response in the endfoot (*middle*). The *bars above* indicate the periods of ATP administration. *Below*: Mean peak amplitude of ATP-induced calcium responses in the somata and endfeet of Müller cells in dependence on the developmental age. At postnatal day 5, the responses in the endfeet and somata display similar amplitudes. Thereafter, the amplitude of the calcium response in the somata declines while the amplitude of the endfeet response remains. **C.** Records of the cytosolic free calcium level in Müller cell endfeet in a retinal wholemount (**a, b**) and in Müller cell somata in a retinal slice (**c, d**) of a postnatal day 15 rat before (**a, c**) and during extracellular administration of ATP (50 µM; **b, d**). The *arrowheads* indicate some Müller cell structures that display ATP-induced increases in the cytosolic free calcium level. **D.** Propagation of calcium waves in Müller cells in a retinal slice from a postnatal day 15 rat. Extracellular administration of ATP (50 µM) induced calcium responses that were initiated in the endfeet of Müller cells within the ganglion cell layer (GCL; 0-5 s). Thereafter, the calcium responses propagated to the inner stem processes of Müller cells in the inner plexiform layer (IPL; 5-10 s). Then, the calcium responses appeared in the somata of Müller cells in the inner nuclear layer (INL) and in the outer stem processes of Müller cells in the outer plexiform layer (OPL; 10-15 s). Thereafter, the calcium responses disappeared but were still visible in the somata of the cells (15-20 s). Scale bars, 20 µm. Modified from Wurm et al. (2006b, 2009a).

Eberhardt, 1988; Skatchkov et al., 1995). The non-uniform distribution of the potassium conductance corresponds with the density of single Kir channels that is far higher in the endfoot membrane than in other cell regions (one salamander Müller cell possess ~54,000 Kir channels; ~90% of the channels are located in the endfoot membrane), and with the distribution of the Kir4.1 protein which is predominantly located in the endfoot membrane (Fig. 7G) (Brew et al., 1986; Newman, 1993; Rojas and Orkand, 1999; Francke et al., 2005). Müller cells of some species with vascularized retinas (man, *Macaca*, pig) also display the highest potassium conductance in their endfeet membranes (Fig. 7E) (Pannicke et al., 2005c; Iandiev et al., 2006b), while cells of other species with vascularized retinas (rat, mouse, *Aotus*) have the highest conductance in the middle portion of the cells, i.e., at the soma and the inner part of the outer stem process (Figs. 7B, 15D) (Newman, 1987; Connors and Kofuji, 2002; Pannicke et al., 2004). These cell portions are located in the inner nuclear layer *in situ* where retinal blood vessels form a sheath-like network, and where Kir4.1 channels are located in perivascular membranes of Müller cells (Figs. 7G,H, 15A,B). In Müller cells of the cat (vascularized retina), the highest potassium conductance is localized in the outer (photoreceptor) end of the cells that has contact to the subretinal space (Newman, 1987). The distribution of the potassium conductance (that reflects mainly the distribution of currents through Kir4.1 channels) suggests that Müller cells of avascular retinas extrude the greatest amount of excess potassium into the vitreous fluid (some release also occurs into the subretinal space) whereas Müller cells of various species with vascularized retinas dissipate excess potassium ions predominantly into retinal capillaries and (to a lower extend) into the vitreous fluid (Newman, 1987). In cats, excess potassium from the inner retina is predominantly redistributed towards the subretinal space (Frishman and Steinberg, 1989). Potassium released into the subretinal space may buffer the large light-induced decrease of the extracellular potassium produced by photoreceptors (Steinberg et al., 1980) and may be transferred across the retinal pigment epithelium by spatial buffering currents (Immel and Steinberg, 1986).

The efficiency of the potassium buffering depends on the morphology of Müller cells. In Müller cells of non-vascularized retinas, the resistance for the intracellular potassium currents running through the inner process of the cells depends on the distance between the sites of potassium influx (plexiform layers) and efflux (endfoot and subretinal microvilli), as well as on the diameter of the inner process (Reichenbach and Wohlrab, 1986). Müller cells of the retinal center are longer and thinner compared to cells from the retinal periphery (Fig. 30A,B) (Reichenbach et al., 1989) and thus have a higher resistance for intracellular potassium currents. In addition, the smaller area of the vitreal endfoot membrane (Fig. 30A) increases the output resistance of the cells (Reichenbach and Wohlrab, 1986). It has been calculated that rabbit Müller cells are unable to mediate spatial buffering potassium currents through the whole cell bodies when they are longer than ~150 μm (Reichenbach and Wohlrab, 1986; Eberhardt and Reichenbach, 1987). Thus, the potassium clearance function of Müller cells may represent one reason for the fact that Müller cells in avascular retinas are shorter than those in vascularized retinas (Dreher et al., 1992).

5.5.3.4 Increase of Kir Currents in Developing Müller Cells

A high expression level of Kir channels (in particular Kir4.1) is the precondition for a stable negative membrane potential (Kofuji et al., 2000) and is required for various fundamental functions of Müller cells such as the maintenance of the retinal potassium homeostasis, the effective clearance of neurotransmitters through electrogenic transporters (see 5.5.2.1.3. and 5.5.2.2.1.), and the cell volume homeostasis (see 5.5.5.1.). Therefore, a high expression level of functional Kir channels is a major characteristic of differentiated Müller cells (Bringmann et al., 2000a). In the course of the ontogenetic development of the retina, Müller cells differentiate from mitotically active late progenitor cells. In the rabbit retina, late progenitors proliferate up to postnatal days 4 (central retina) and 10 (peripheral retina) (Schnitzer, 1990; Reichenbach et al., 1991a; Sharma and Ehinger, 1997). In the course of the maturation of rabbit Müller cells from progenitor cells after the postnatal day 5, the profile of the membrane potassium conductance alters from a current pattern with prominent K_A currents and a high BK channel activity into a pattern with large Kir and K_{DR} currents (Fig. 51) (Bringmann et al., 1999a). The maturation of Müller cells is associated with an increase in the density of single Kir channels in membrane patches (Fig. 59D) (Bringmann et al., 1999a). The resting membrane potential is increased to values negative to -80 mV (around the postnatal day 12) when the amplitude of the Kir currents is increased to ~40% of the adult level (Fig. 51) (Bringmann et al., 1999a). The developmental increase of the Kir currents between postnatal days 6 and 20 occurs along with the light-induced ganglion cell activity and the increase of the density of retinal synapses (Fig. 51).

In developing rat Müller cells, the Kir currents increase after the postnatal day 11 (Fig. 61A) which is associated with the emergence of Kir4.1 protein in the retina (Fig. 49) (Wurm et al., 2006b). The developmental expession of the Kir4.1 protein occurs in two phases. Around the postnatal day 15, the Kir4.1 protein is distributed relatively uniformly along the Müller cell fibers; thereafter, the Kir4.1 protein is redistributed towards a prominent localization in Müller cell membranes that surround the blood vessels and at the limiting membranes of the retina (Fig. 49) (Wurm et al., 2006b). The redistribution of the Kir4.1 protein is reflected in the developmental alteration of the cellular distribution of the potassium conductance of Müller cells. The potassium conductance displays a relatively uniform distribution in Müller cells around the postnatal day 15, before the development of the prominent conductance in the middle portion of the cells (Fig. 7F) (Wurm et al., 2006b). The developmental increase of the Kir currents and the decrease of K_A currents are delayed by visual deprivation (Wurm et al., 2006b), suggesting that light-driven neuronal activity accelerates the maturation of Müller cells.

5.5.3.5 Kir Currents in Gliotic Müller Cells

Under various pathological conditions, there is a downregulation and/or mislocation of Kir4.1 channels which is associated with a decrease of the potassium conductance of Müller cells indicating a functional inactivation of the channels. Such a decrease of the Kir current amplitude and a redistribution of the Kir4.1 protein from the prominent expression sites around the vessels and at the limiting membranes of the retina (resulting in a more even distribution along the Müller cell fibers which traverse the retinal tissue) were observed in animal models of retinal ischemia-reperfusion,

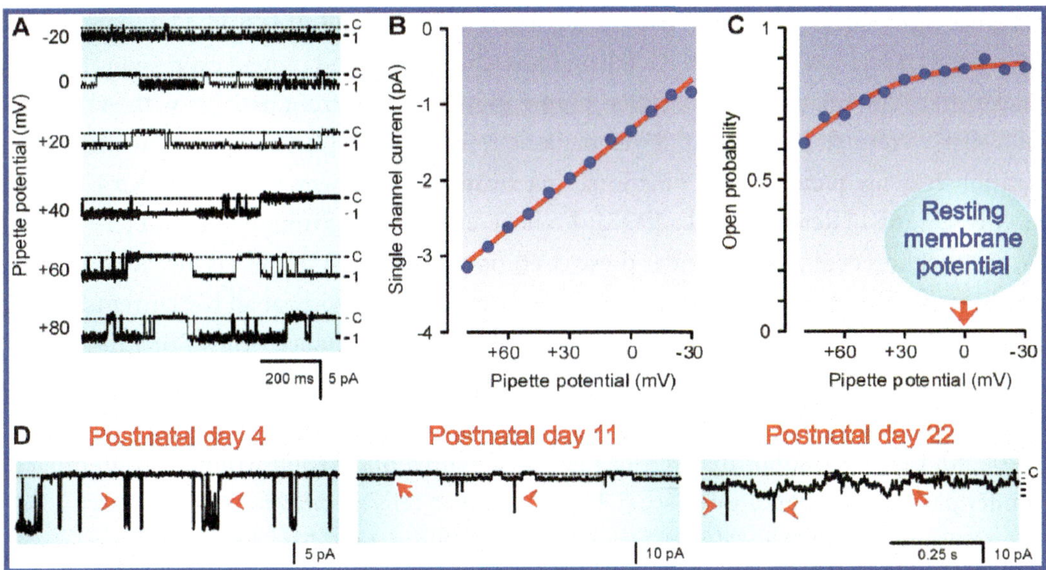

FIGURE 59: Single Kir channels of Müller cells. **A.** Activity of one Kir channel in a membrane patch which was recorded at the soma of a human cell. Downward deflections reflect channel openings. C, closed state; 1, open state current levels. **B.** Mean current-voltage relation of single Kir channels of human Müller cells, with a slope conductance of 21 pS. **C.** Mean open-state probability of Kir channels of human Müller cells in dependence on the pipette potential (which is inversely related to the membrane potential of the cells). A pipette potential of 0 mV means that the patch potential is near the resting membrane potential of the cells. **D.** The density of single Kir channels in membrane patches increases during the postnatal maturation of Müller cells. Examples of channel records in soma membrane patches of Müller cells from rabbits of various postnatal stages (pipette potential +80 mV). The patch of the cell from the postnatal day 4 cell contained no Kir channel but one BK channel (*arrowheads*). The patch of the postnatal day 11 cell contained one Kir channel (*arrow*) and a BK channel, while the patch of the postnatal day 22 cell contained at least 4 Kir channels together with a BK channel. The recordings were made in the cell-attached mode with 130 and 3 mM potassium in the pipette and bathing solution, respectively. Modified from Bringmann et al. (1999a,b).

retinal vein occlusion, ocular inflammation, diabetic retinopathy, retinal blue light injury, retinal detachment, dispase-induced retinopathy, and PVR (Figs. 7D,E, 8C,D,F, 11B, 12K,L, 15A-C, 19, 21D, 46A,C, 61A, 63B,E) (Francke et al., 2001a, 2002, 2003; Uhlmann et al., 2003; Pannicke et al., 2004, 2005a,b, 2006; Uckermann et al., 2005a,b; Wurm et al., 2006a; Iandiev et al., 2006b,c, 2008a; Bringmann et al., 2007; Kuhrt et al., 2008; Ulbricht et al., 2008; Sene et al., 2009; Rehak et al., 2009, 2011; Hirrlinger et al., 2010; Drechsler et al., 2012; Berner et al., 2012; Köferl et al., 2014). PVR is a frequent complication of retinal detachment and vitreoretinal surgery in human subjects that is associated with a massive proliferation of Müller cells (see 5.11.11.). After transient retinal ischemia, there is a decrease in Kir4.1 (but not Kir2.1) gene and protein expression (Fig. 8C,D) (Pannicke et al., 2004; Iandiev et al., 2006c). Human Müller cells from patients with various retinopathies such as retinal detachment, PVR, diabetic retinopathy, PDR, and glaucoma display a depolarization as consequence of the functional inactivation and downregulation of Kir4.1 channels (Figs. 46B–D, 56B) (Reichelt et al., 1997a; Francke et al., 1997; Bringmann et al., 1999b, 2001, 2002a, b; Tenckhoff et al., 2005). Under these conditions, the Kir4.1 protein is distributed relatively uniformly across the Müller cell membranes. The current pattern with small Kir currents, as well as the uniform distribution of the Kir4.1 protein and the Kir conductance (Figs. 7B, 15D) in Müller cells, resemble the characteristics of developing Müller cells in the postnatal period, before they differentiate into mature cells (Figs. 7F, 49) (Bringmann et al., 1999a; Pannicke et al., 2002; Wurm et al., 2006b); these alterations may reflect the dedifferentiation of adult Müller cells to progenitor cells under pathological conditions (see 5.11.12.). Müller cells of *taiep* rats (which carry a myelin mutation causing a progressive deterioration of the CNS due to a disturbance of the microtubule network of oligodendrocytes) display low-amplitude Kir currents compared to control as well as signs of gliosis such as upregulation of GFAP; this suggests that the progressive dysmyelination process of the optic nerve, accompanied by functional deficits of retinal ganglion cells, induces induces a malfunction and gliosis of Müller cells (Chávez et al., 2003, 2004).

However, Müller cell gliosis is not necessarily associated with a reduction of the Kir currents, i.e., Müller cells (of various species) respond in a different fashion to various pathological stimuli. Relatively severe pathological conditions may occur without any significant decrease in the Kir conductance of Müller cells, e.g., Borna disease virus-induced retinitis, inherited photoreceptor degeneration in *rds* mice, *rd/rd* mice, and RCS rats, inherited glaucoma, damage to the optic tract, or bright white light-induced retinal degeneration (Fig. 18C), whereas other signs of gliosis (e.g., increase in GFAP expression and cellular hypertrophy) are obvious (Pannicke et al., 2001; Felmy et al., 2001; Iandiev et al., 2006e, 2008b; Bolz et al., 2008; Chua et al., 2013; and T. Pannicke, Leipzig, unpublished results). In *rds* mice that display a slow degeneration of photoreceptor cells, only a slight transient decrease in the Kir current density (but no alteration in the Kir4.1 protein) was found which was ascribed to a transient hypertrophy of the cells (Iandiev et al., 2006e). On the other hand, in a transgenic rat model of slow primary photoreceptor degeneration due to a mutant polycystin-2 gene which is a cilia protein (Feng et al., 2009), the retinal Kir4.1 protein displays an age-dependent redistribution (with a more even distribution along Müller cell membranes and a downregulation of perivascular Kir4.1; Fig. 23A) while the Kir conductance of Müller cells displays only a slight decrease compared to control (Fig. 23D) (Vogler et al., 2013b).

A decrease of functional Kir4.1 channels is associated with a depolarization of the Müller cells when the Kir currents are decreased to values lower than ~40% of control (Figs. 8H, 12K, 63E,F) (Pannicke et al., 2005a). (Decreases of the Kir current amplitude lesser than ~60% are not associated with a cell membrane depolarization, e.g., in a transgenic rat model of slow photoreceptor degeneration; Fig. 23D; Vogler et al., 2013b.) Although other types of potassium channels such as K_{DR}, BK or two-pore domain (TASK) channels may maintain a less negative membrane potential between −60 and −40 mV (Pannicke et al., 2000b; Skatchkov et al., 2006), the potassium siphoning by Müller cells must be impaired because membrane hyperpolarization is a precondition for the passive transglial potassium currents, and because BK and likely TASK channels are not continuously open (like Kir channels) but active only after receptor stimulation. When the potassium flux through Kir channels is impaired, Müller cells are stimulated to remove excess potassium by an active uptake through the sodium-potassium-ATPase (Reichenbach et al., 1986, 1992). Elevations in extracellular potassium increase the activity of the sodium-potassium-ATPase in cultured Müller cells (Reichelt et al., 1989) which lack functional Kir channels (Kuhrt et al., 2008; Wurm et al., 2009b). This activation may finally cause a functional overload and metabolic exhaustion of the cells. The depolarization of Müller cells after functional inactivation of Kir channels will also result in an impairment of the electrogenic neurotransmitter uptake by the cells (Napper et al., 1999). Because the Kir conductance of Müller cells is is required for effective potassium homeostasis, neurotransmitter recycling (see 5.5.2.1.6. and 5.5.2.2.1.), retinal water homeostasis (see 5.5.4.1.), and the regulation of the Müller cell and extracellular space volumes (see 5.5.5.1.), the dysfunction of Müller cells caused by the downregulation of functional Kir4.1 channels represents one major factor that contributes to neuronal hyperexcitation (Ivens et al., 2007), glutamate toxicity, and the development of tissue edema under pathological conditions. Human Müller cells display an age-dependent decrease of the Kir current amplitude, in the mean by approximately the half between the ages of 40 and 80 years (Fig. 45D) (Bringmann et al., 2003c) which is near the threshold (~40% of control) for a decrease of the resting membrane potential of Müller cells (Fig. 8H) (Bringmann et al., 2000a; Pannicke et al., 2005a). The age-dependent decrease of the Kir conductance is associated with other gliotic signs such as upregulation of GFAP (Wu et al., 2003) and will increase the likelihood of Müller cell dysfunction when additional pathogenic factors such as oxidative stress and inflammation are present. This contributes to the increased vulnerability of the retinal tissue to pathogenic factors in the elderly. Glutamate, blood plasma (which contains glutamate), and thrombin decrease the Kir (and K_A) currents in Müller cells; the effect of glutamate is mediated by activation of PKA (Schwartz, 1993; Puro and Stuenkel, 1995; Kusaka et al., 1999). This suggests that a leakage of blood serum compromises the potassium homeostasis mediated by Müller cells (see 5.11.9.3.).

Selective inactivation of Kir4.1 in the rat retina decreases electroretinogram components (Raz-Prag et al., 2010). Patients with EAST syndrome, which carry mutations in the Kir4.1 gene, show delayed electroretinogram b-waves and a reduced retinal sensitivity (Thompson et al., 2011).

The mechanism of the decrease of the Kir currents under distinct pathological conditions is unclear. In experimental ocular inflammation, a transient downregulation of Kir4.1 was shown at the mRNA and protein level (Liu et al., 2007). A decrease in the retinal content of Kir4.1 mRNA and protein was also shown in experimental retinal ischemia and in tissues from patients with PVR (Pannicke et al., 2004; Tenckhoff et al., 2005; Iandiev et al., 2006c; Rehak et al., 2009), whereas in an animal model of PVR, a mislocation and functional inactivation of Kir4.1 was not associated with a decrease of the Kir4.1 mRNA and protein content of Müller cells (Ulbricht et al., 2008). Oxidative stress and chronic inflammation are conditions that are associated with a downregulation of functional Kir4.1 channels in Müller cells (Pannicke et al., 2004, 2005a,b; Iandiev et al., 2006c). It has been shown that astrocytes surrounding ischemic brain lesions display a reduction of their potassium currents, and that a similar reduction can be observed in cultured astrocytes in the presence of TNF (Köller et al., 2000). The redistribution of Kir4.1 from perivascular Müller cell processes in the diabetic retina is, at least in part, caused by AGEs/advanced lipoxidation end products (ALEs) which increase the oxidative stress level in the retina (Curtis et al., 2011; Berner et al., 2012). ALEs were shown to reduce the Kir4.1 protein level in Müller cells (Yong et al., 2010). In addition, extravasated serum albumin may induce a downregulation of Kir4.1, via activation of TGF-β receptors (see 5.11.9.3.). On the other hand, minocycline, intravitreal bevacizumab (a VEGF scavenger), and glucocorticoids were shown to increase the expression of Kir4.1 in the retina and to prevent the ischemic downregulation of Kir4.1 gene expression (Zhao et al., 2010; Iandiev et al., 2011b; Zhang et al., 2011b; Rehak et al., 2011). Upregulation of the purinergic calcium signaling observed in gliotic Müller cells (see 5.10.2.5.) seems to be involved in triggering the downregulation of Kir4.1 in cells of the ischemic retina. P2Y$_1$ receptor-deficient mice display a significant weaker decrease of the Kir currents upon transient retinal ischemia than wildtype mice (Pannicke et al., 2014).

Extracellular matrix components are involved in the distribution of the Kir4.1 protein. The membrane anchoring and clustered distribution of Kir4.1 channels, as well as the gene and protein expression of Kir4.1 and the amplitude of Kir currents, depend on the presence of the extracellular matrix molecules laminins β2 and γ3 (Ishii et al., 1997; Hirrlinger et al., 2011). The channel clustering enhances the activity of Kir4.1 (Horio et al., 1997). The clustering activity of laminin is translated into a subcellular localization signal for Kir4.1 in a PDZ-ligand domain-mediated fashion by α-dystroglycan, a central element of the dystrophin-associated protein complex (Noel et al., 2005) which links cytoskeletal actin to the basal lamina. In the retina, α-dystroglycan is concentrated in the inner limiting membrane, around blood vessels, and in the outer plexiform layer (Blake and

Kröger, 2000; Takahashi et al., 2011). At its core, the dystrophin glycoprotein complex includes α-syntrophin, the short dystrophin isoform Dp71, the transmembrane protein β-dystroglycan, and the extracellular matrix receptor α-dystroglycan (Claudepierre et al., 2000). In the retina, β-dystroglycan is localized to glial cell endfeet (Koulen et al., 1998). Laminin and dystrophin are localized at the inner limiting membrane and around the vessels (Fig. 8B) (Pannicke et al., 2004), suggesting that the prominent expression of Kir4.1 in the vitreous-abutting endfeet membranes and in the perivascular membranes (Fig. 8C,D) is regulated by these molecules (but see Rurak et al., 2007). After transient ischemia of the rat retina, which causes a dislocation of the Kir4.1 protein (Fig. 8C,D), the immunolabelings of laminin and type IV collagen remain unaltered (Fig. 8B) whereas dystrophin shows a redistribution similar to that of Kir4.1 protein (Fig. 8B), suggesting that the redistribution of Kir4.1 occurs secondary to a disruption of the dystrophin complex (Pannicke et al., 2004).

The spatial redistribution and the functional inactivation of Kir4.1 under pathological conditions are likely two different phenomenons. The slow photoreceptor degeneration in transgenic rats with a defective polycystin-2 is associated with an age-dependent redistribution of Kir4.1 (Fig. 23A) while the Kir conductance displays only a slight decrease compared to control (Fig. 23D) (Vogler et al., 2013b). A similar disrupted distribution of the Kir4.1 protein (but no decrease of the potassium currents) has been observed in retinas of mdx^{3Cv} mice that lacks the expression of dystrophin (Connors and Kofuji, 2002), and of mice with a genetic inactivation of Dp71 (Dalloz et al., 2003; Fort et al., 2008; Sene et al., 2009); Dp71 is expressed by Müller cells and perivascular astrocytes (Claudepierre et al., 1999) and involved in the clustering (but not membrane insertion) of Kir4.1 channels (Connors and Kofuji, 2002; Noel et al., 2005). The more diffuse distribution of Kir4.1 protein in Dp71-null mice is associated with an increased retinal vascular permeability (Sene et al., 2009) and an enhanced vulnerability of retinal ganglion cells to ischemia-reperfusion injury (Dalloz et al., 2003) which is known to be (at least in part) mediated by the toxicity of excess glutamate (Osborne et al., 2004). Because the gating of Kir4.1 channels depends on the presence of ATP (see 5.5.3.1.), a functional inactivation of the channels may disturb retinal potassium homeostasis in ischemic tissue areas even already before the dislocation of the channel protein is apparent.

5.5.3.6 BK Channels

In addition to Kir channels, BK channels may be involved in the activity-dependent buffering of extracellular potassium (Puro et al., 1996a; Ishii et al., 1997). This assumption is supported by the facts that extracellular nucleotides (Fig. 64A,B) and glutamate (Fig. 64D,E) stimulate the activity of single BK channels at the resting membrane potential of Müller cells (Bringmann and

Reichenbach, 1997; Bringmann et al., 2002a). This suggests that BK channels of Müller cells are a target of neuron-derived signaling molecules. BK channels are potassium channels of big conductance between 100 and 135 pS in cell-attached membrane patches with high (130 mM) potassium in the pipette solution (Bringmann et al., 1997, 1998b, 1999a,b; Schopf et al., 1999). These channels are frequently found (in addition to Kir channels) in membrane patches of Müller cells from various species (Figs. 59D, 60A,B, 64B,E, 65A) (Bringmann et al., 1998b, 1999a,b). Single Kir and BK channels are well discernible due to their different channel conductance, the different voltage dependence of channel opening, as well as the different gating properties with the presence (BK) and absence (Kir) of flickery closures during the opening of the channels (Figs. 56D, 59D, 60A,B, 65A).

BK channels are mainly activated by membrane depolarization (Fig. 65A) and an increase in the free calcium level at the intracellular side of the plasma membrane (Fig. 65B,C) (Bringmann et al., 1997, 1999a). The sigmoid activation curve of the channel (reflecting the increase in channel opening in response to membrane depolarization) shifts towards more negative (i.e., physiologically relevant) potentials when the intracellular calcium level increases (Fig. 65C) (Bringmann et al., 1997, 1999a). The calcium-dependent open probability of human BK channels indicates a Hill coefficient of 1.7 (Bringmann et al., 1997), suggesting that two calcium binding sites are involved in channel opening. BK channels in excised membrane patches of Müller cells from various mammalian species display a half-maximal activation between 0 and +10 mV when the cytosolic calcium concentration is 10 μM (Bringmann et al., 1997, 1998a, 1999a; Schopf et al., 1999). This low calcium sensitivity suggests that Müller cells express the pore-forming α-subunit but not the regulatory β-subunit of BK channels (Wallner et al., 1996). On the other hand, cultured human Müller cells express the β2-subunit of BK channels after treatment with 17β-estradiol; the β-subunit-induced shift of the channel gating towards more negative membrane potentials may be implicated in the apoptosis-preventing effect of this sex steroid (Li et al., 2006).

There are several coactivating factors of BK channels in Müller cells (Fig. 65I). Intracellular magnesium ions increase the activity of BK channels (shift of the activation curve of the channel towards more negative potentials) but inhibit the potassium currents through the channel pore (resulting in a decrease in the amplitude of the channel currents; Fig. 65H) (Bringmann et al., 1997). The channel activity is regulated by the cytosolic pH; an increase in the proton concentration decreases the channel opening (Fig. 65D) (Bringmann et al., 1997), likely via interaction of protons with the calcium binding sites of the channel protein. Arachidonic acid, which is produced under oxidative stress conditions (Asano et al., 1987; Birkle and Bazan, 1989; Offer et al., 2005; Lambert et al., 2006; Balboa and Balsinde, 2006), strongly activates the BK channel activity in Müller cells (Bringmann et al., 1998b). In addition to arachidonic acid, various other polyunsaturated fatty acids (such as docosahexaenoic acid) stimulate the activity of BK channels (Bringmann et al., 1998b).

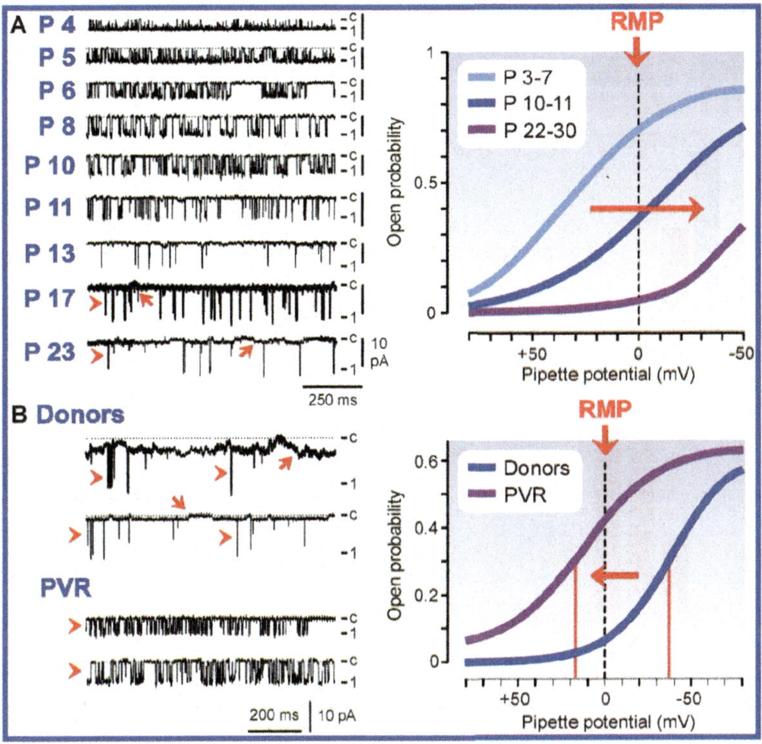

FIGURE 60: Alterations of the BK channel activity in radial glial/Müller cells of the young postnatal rabbit retina (**A**) and in Müller cells of adult human donors without apparent retinal disease and of patients with proliferative vitreoretinopathy (PVR), respectively (**B**). The channel current traces at *left* display activities of single BK (*arrowheads*) and Kir channels (*arrows*) recorded in cell-attached membrane patches near the resting membrane potential (RMP). The *right side* displays the mean relations between the open probability of BK channels and the pipette potential (which is inversely related to the membrane potential of the cells). **A.** In the course of the postnatal development, the activation curve of BK channels shifts towards more negative pipette potentials (i.e., towards more positive membrane potentials). **B.** Human Müller cells of patients with PVR display an increased open probability of BK channels at the RMP in comparison to cells from healthy donor eyes. The shift of the pipette potential that induced a half-maximal activation of BK channels (*red lines*) suggests a depolarization of Müller cells from patients with PVR by ~55 mV compared to the donor cells. P, postnatal day. C, closed state; 1, open state current level. Modified from Bringmann et al. (1999a,b).

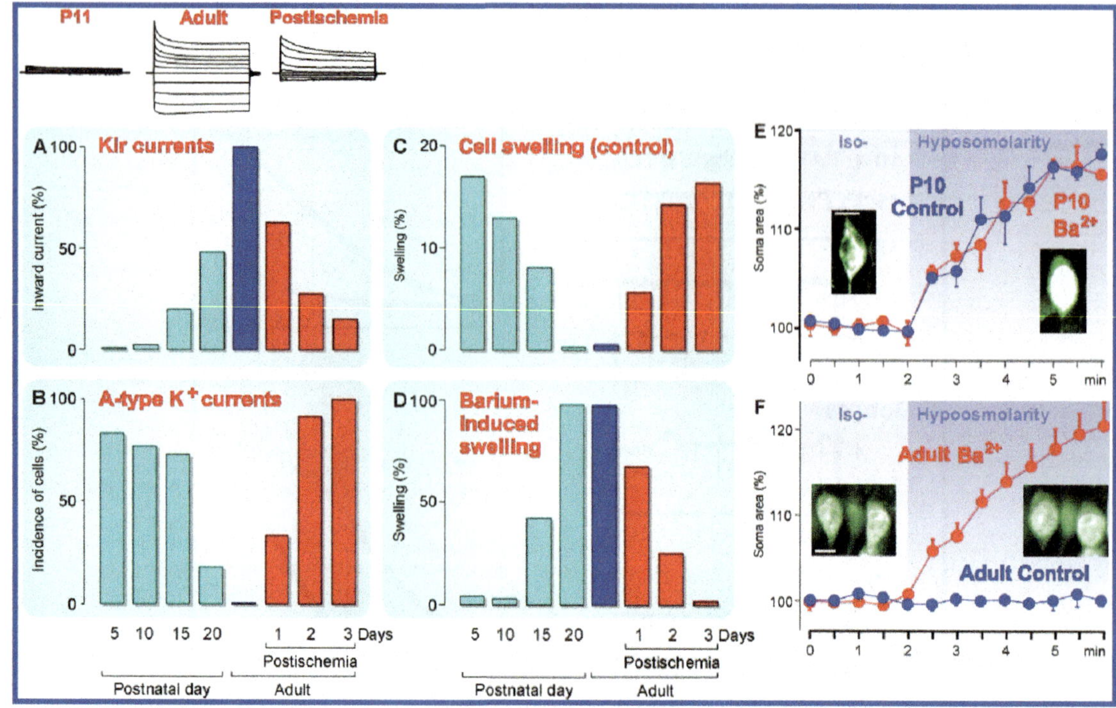

FIGURE 61: The extent of osmotic swelling in rat Müller cells is associated with alterations of the potassium conductance during postnatal development and after a 1-h transient ischemia of the adult retina. **A.** Alterations of the Kir current amplitude in dependence on the postnatal age and the time period after ischemia. **B.** Incidence of cells that display A-type K⁺ currents. **C.** Severity of Müller cell swelling during hypoosmotic stress. **D.** Severity of Müller cell swelling during hypoosmotic stress in the presence of Kir channel-blocking barium ions. Modified from Wurm et al. (2006b) and Pannicke et al. (2004, 2005a).

Membrane stretch increases the activity of BK channels (Fig. 65E), likely after opening of stretch-activated calcium-permeable cation channels (Puro, 1991a). The BK channel protein is also a target of protein kinases. While PKA-mediated phosphorylation of the channel protein increases the channel activity (Fig. 65F), PKC-mediated phosphorylation reduces the activity of the channels (Fig. 65G) (Bringmann et al., 1997; Schopf et al., 1999). The inhibitory action of PKC may limit the time period of channel activation when receptor agonists cause an increase in cytosolic calcium. The PKA-mediated activation of BK channels is a further indication for a lack of a regulatory β-subunit in BK channels of Müller cells (Dworetzky et al., 1996).

There are various inhibitors and activators of BK channels in Müller cells (Fig. 65I). The flavoid phloretin is a BK channel opener (Bringmann and Reichenbach, 1997) thought to act di-

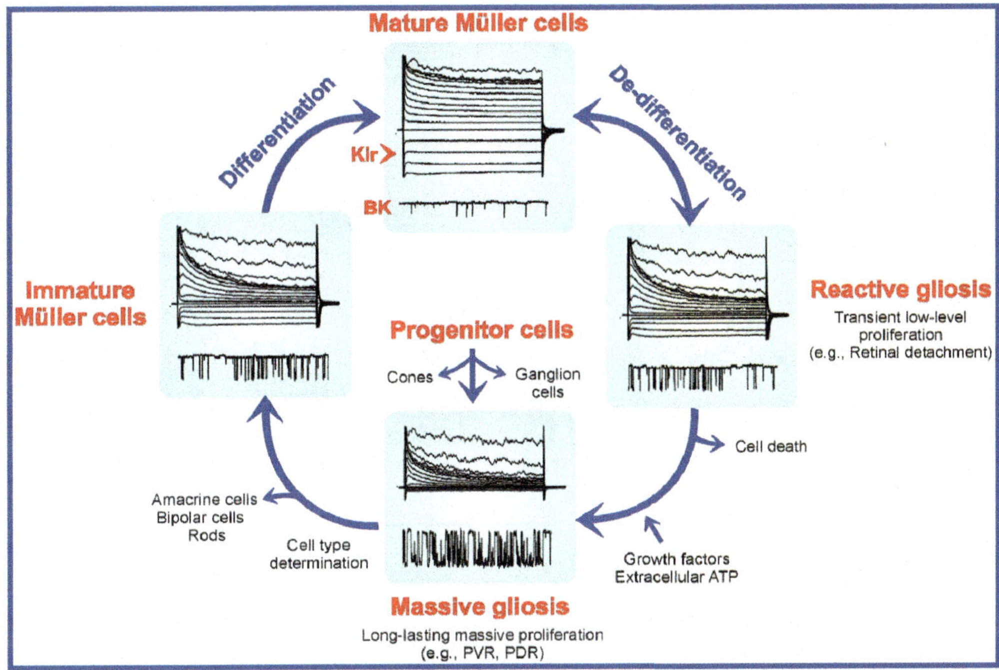

FIGURE 62: The amplitude of Kir currents and the activity of BK channels at the resting membrane potential alter inversely in dependence on the differentiation degree of Müller cells. During retinal development, progenitor cells do not display Kir currents; a high activity of BK channels supports the proliferation of the cells. In the course of the maturation of Müller cells from progenitor cells, the amplitude of the Kir currents increases and the activity of BK channels at the resting membrane potential decreases. Mature Müller cells display large-amplitude Kir currents and a small activity of BK channels. Gliosis under pathological conditions (e.g., after retinal detachment) is associated with a de-differentiation of Müller cells reflected by the decrease in the amplitude of Kir currents and the increase in the activity of BK channels. In proliferative vitreoretinopathy (PVR) and proliferative diabetic retinopathy (PDR), Müller cells do not display Kir currents and have a high activity of BK channels at the resting membrane potential. Modified from Bringmann et al. (2000a).

rectly at the fatty acid binding sites of the pore-forming α-subunits (Gribkoff et al., 1997). Tetraethylammonium at a concentration of 1 mM is a selective blocker of BK channels in Müller cells, exerting essentially no effects onto currents through Kir, K_A, or K_{DR} channels (Bringmann et al., 1997, 2007). Tetraethylammonium is an open channel blocker, and the binding site is localized at the outer (but not inner) side of the pore region of the channel. A further selective blocker of open BK channels is iberiotoxin (Latorre, 1994). Barium ions, when applied to the cytosolic (but not to the extracellular) side of membrane patches, inhibits the channel activity (Bringmann et al.,

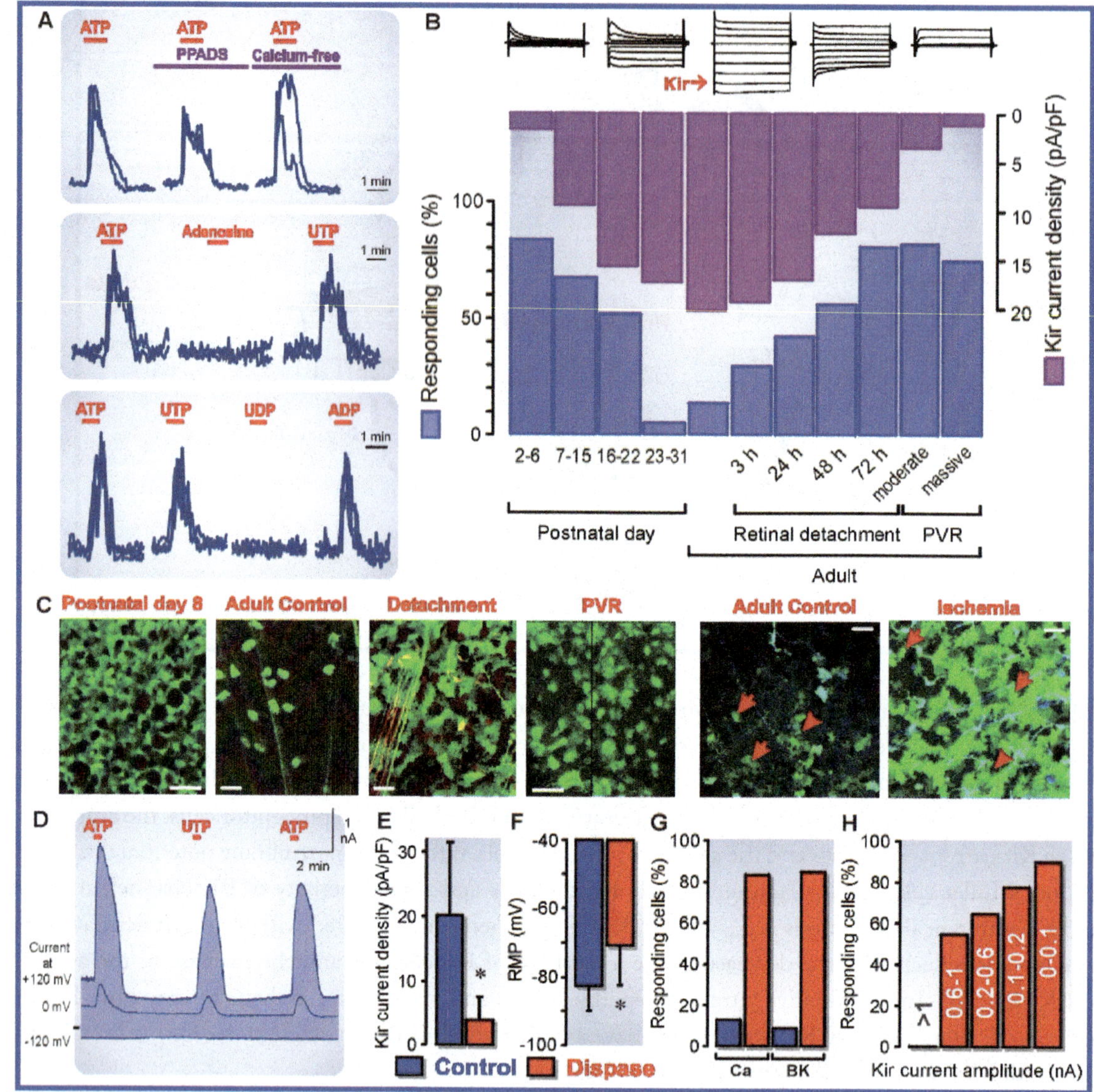

FIGURE 63: P2Y receptor-induced calcium and BK current responses in rabbit Müller cells. The responses were recorded in Müller cell endfeet of retinal wholemounts. **A.** *Above:* The ATP (200 μM)-induced calcium response is mainly mediated by activation of metabotropic P2Y receptors. The P2 receptor blocker PPADS (100 μM) decreased the ATP-evoked calcium response, and the response remained largely unaffected in extracellular calcium-free conditions. *Middle:* UTP (200 μM) induced a similar calcium response as ATP, while adenosine (200 μM) had no effect. *Below:* ADP and UTP induced

similar responses as ATP while UDP had no effect. The agents were applied at 10 μM. **B.** The incidence of Müller cells that respond to exogenous ATP (200 μM) with a rise in the cytosolic free calcium (*diagram, below*) is inversely related to the density of inwardly rectifying potassium (Kir) currents (*diagram, above*). This relation was observed during the postnatal development (*left side*) and during experimental retinal detachment and moderate and massive PVR (*right side*). The *traces above* represent examples of whole-cell potassium current records in single isolated Müller cells. **C.** *Left:* Examples of peak calcium responses (*green areas*) to ATP (200 μM) at the inner surface of the retinas. While nearly all Müller cell endfeet display a calcium response in the retina of the postnatal day-8 rabbit and of rabbits with retinal detachment and PVR, only some Müller cell endfeet responded in the retina of the adult control animal. In the rabbit retina, the proliferation of late progenitor cells ceases between the postnatal days 2 and 7 (Reichenbach et al., 1991). *Right:* ATP (200 μM)-induced peak calcium responses in Müller cell endfeet in a control retina and a retina isolated 8 days after a transient retinal ischemia of 1 h. The *arrows* indicate endfeet which show calcium responses while the *arrowheads* indicate non-responding endfeet. **D-H.** Increased responsiveness of Müller cells upon P2Y receptor stimulation in experimental dispase-induced retinopathy which causes a non-proliferative Müller cell gliosis and retinal degeneration. Intravitreal administration of the proteolytic enzyme dispase (0.1 U) was carried out 3 weeks before the recordings. **D.** Activation of P2Y receptors by ATP and UTP (both 100 μM) induces transient increases of the BK currents (recorded at the membrane potentials of +120 and 0 mV) of a Müller cell derived from a dispase-treated eye. **E.** The Kir currents of Müller cells from dispase-treated retinas decreased compared to control. **F.** This was associated with a decrease of the resting membrane potential (RMP). **G.** The number of Müller cells that showed ATP (100 μM)-induced cytosolic calcium responses (Ca) and ATP-induced transient increases of the BK currents increased compared to control. **H.** Relation between the percentage of ATP-responsive cells and the amplitude of the Kir currents of Müller cells from dispase-treated retinas. The Kir current amplitude (in nA) is given in the bars. Cell with large Kir currents (>1 nA) displayed no ATP-induced BK current responses. The percentage of responding cells increased with the extent of the decrease of the Kir currents. Scale bars, 25 μm. Modified from Bringmann et al. (1999a), Francke et al. (2001a, 2003), Uckermann et al. (2002, 2003, 2005a), and Uhlmann et al. (2003).

1997), likely via competition with calcium ions for the calcium binding sites of the channel protein. The various possibilities of regulation of the channel activity (Fig. 65I) together with the large conductance of the channel (resulting in a strong hyperpolarization of the membrane around open channels) suggest that BK channels provide an important link between various intracellular second messenger systems and the membrane conductance of Müller cells. Extracellular signaling molecules that induce an increase in cytosolic calcium or cAMP, a stimulation of the production of arachidonic acid, or a depolarization by activation of electrogenic uptake carriers, may cause an opening of BK channels. An increase in extracellular potassium concentration is associated with

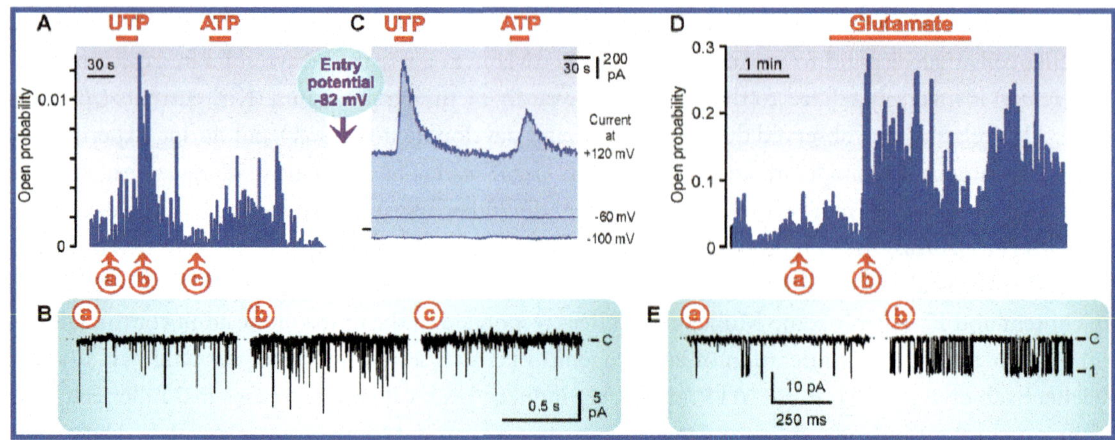

FIGURE 64: Agonists of P2Y (**A–C**) and metabotropic glutamate receptors (**D, E**) induce activation of single BK channels in human Müller cells. The channel currents were recorded in cell-attached membrane patches at the resting membrane potential. **A.** Time dependency of the open probability of single BK channels. Extracellular administration of UTP (100 μM) and ATP (100 μM) resulted in transient increases of the open probability of the channels. **B.** Examples of channel records at the three time points indicated in **A.** The downward deflections represent potassium currents through single BK channels. **C.** After the end of the cell-attached record, the whole-cell mode was established and the agonists were tested again to verify that they induce increases of the whole-cell BK currents. The whole-cell currents were recorded at three potentials. Shortly after the rupture of the cell membrane, the membrane potential of the cell was measured in the current clamp mode and was found at −82 mV. **D, E.** Extracellular glutamate (200 μM) increased the activity of a single BK channel. **D.** Time dependency of the open probability. **E.** Original records of the channel activity. C, closed state; 1, open state current levels. Modified from Bringmann and Reichenbach (1997) and Bringmann et al. (2002a).

intracellular alkalinization (Newman, 1996). Intracellular alkalinization stimulates the opening of BK channels (Fig. 65D); the resulting membrane hyperpolarization supports the uptake of excess extracellular potassium and the electrogenic uptake of neurotransmitter molecules.

5.5.3.7 Decrease of the BK Channel Activity in Developing Müller Cells

The ontogenetic development of Müller cells from mitotically active late progenitor cells is characterized by an increase in the expression of Kir channels (Figs. 46A,C, 51, 61A, 62, 63B) which causes a negative shift of the resting membrane potential from values around −40 mV to approximately −80 mV (Figs. 46A, 51). The developmental membrane hyperpolarization causes a strong

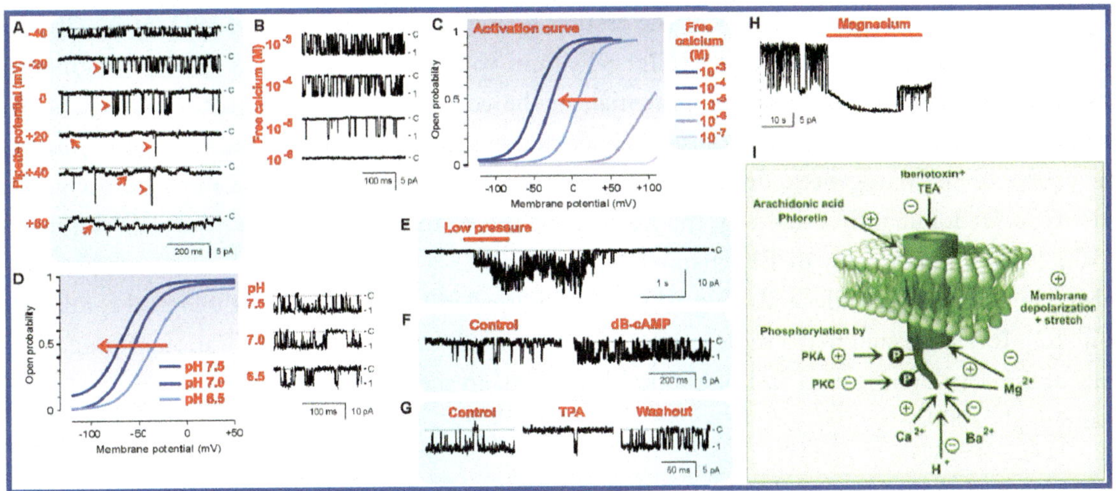

FIGURE 65: Regulation of the BK channel activity in Müller cells. **A.** Membrane depolarization activates BK channels. The currents were recorded in a cell-attached membrane patch of a human Müller cell. The images display the activity of one BK channel (*arrowheads*) and at least three Kir channels (*arrows*) at different pipette potentials (that is inversely related to the membrane potential of the cell). A pipette potential of 0 mV is near the resting membrane potential of the cell. Note that the activity of the BK channel increases with membrane depolarization (negative pipette potentials). C, closed state current level. **B.** Elevation of the calcium concentration at the cytosolic side of an excised membrane patch from a rabbit Müller cell increases the activity of a BK channel. **C.** The activation curve of BK channels (recorded in excised membrane patches of human Müller cells) is shifted towards more negative membrane potentials when the calcium concentration at the cytosolic side of the patches increases. **D.** The open probability of a BK channel in an excised membrane patch from a porcine Müller cell depends upon the cytosolic pH (*right*). Increasing cytosolic pH cause a shift of the activation curve of BK channels towards more negative membrane potentials (*left*). **E.** Membrane stretch induced by applying low pressure to the patch pipette interior activates BK channels in a cell-attached membrane patch of a human Müller cell. **F.** The activity of a BK channel in a cell-attached membrane patch of a rabbit Müller cell is increased during administration of dB-cAMP (100 μM), a cell-permeable activator of the protein kinase A. **G.** The activity of a BK channel in a cell-attached membrane patch of a rabbit Müller cell is decreased during administration of TPA (10 μM), a cell-permeable phorbol ester that activates the activity of the protein kinase C. **H.** Intracellular magnesium (10 mM) decreases the conductance of a single BK channel that was recorded in an excised inside-out membrane patch of a porcine Müller cell. Note the decrease of the channel current amplitude. **I.** Summary of factors and agents that increase (+) and decrease (−) the activity and conductance, respectively, of BK channels in Müller cells. Modified from Bringmann et al. (1997) and Schopf et al. (1999).

decrease in the BK channel activity at the resting membrane potential (Figs. 59D, 60A) (Bringmann et al., 1999a). BK channels in Müller cells from young postnatal rabbits display a high open probability at the resting membrane potential; in the course of development, the activity of the channels decreases (Fig. 60A). Because the calcium sensitivity of the channels does not alter in the course of the ontogenetic development, it is suggested that the decrease in the BK channel activity is predominantly caused by the increase of the resting membrane potential (Bringmann et al., 1999a). The activity of BK channels and the expression level of Kir channels are inversely related in developing Müller cells (Fig. 51) and in gliotic Müller cells under pathological conditions (Fig. 62). It is suggested that a high activity of BK channels support the proliferation of progenitor cells in the developing retina and of gliotic Müller cells in the adult retina (see 5.11.10.2.) (Bringmann et al., 2000a).

5.5.3.8 Whole-Cell BK Currents

In whole-cell records, BK currents are activated at positive membrane potentials (Figs. 43E,F, 56B,C) (Newman, 1985b; Bringmann et al., 2002a). Activation of whole-cell BK channels at positive membrane potentials is suggested to be a recording artifact because single channel activity is observed at the resting or slightly depolarized potentials in cell-attached membrane patches (Fig. 64A–C). The positive shift of the activation threshold is likely caused by the loss of essential cytoplasmic components that coactivate the channels (such as activators of PKA) when the cell interior is filled with the pipette solution.

There is a conspicuous species dependency in the expression of BK channels. While all Müller cells from toads, rabbits, and man investigated so far displayed BK currents in whole-cell currents records (Bringmann et al., 1998a,b, 1999a,b, 2000e), about half of porcine Müller cells investigated displayed such currents (Bringmann and Reichenbach, 1997), whereas no BK currents could be recorded in Müller cells from mice, rats, guinea pigs, sheeps, horses, and the cynomolgus monkey, *Macaca fascicularis* (Pannicke et al., 2005a,c). (However, guinea pig Müller cells in culture have BK channels [Kodal et al., 2000], suggesting that the expression level of the channels depends on the differentiation degree of the cells.) In porcine Müller cells, BK channels are localized in a clustered fashion especially in the membranes of the inner processes (Fig. 11A) (Bringmann et al., 2007), suggesting a role of these channels in the interaction between Müller cells and second- and third-order neurons of the retina. This interaction may be mediated by activation of the channels by neuron-derived transmitters such as glutamate (Figs. 43A, 64A,B) and nucleotides (Figs. 43B,D,G, 64A,B, 66). In gliotic Müller cells, the BK channel activity is required for the sustained calcium influx from the extracellular space mediated by cation and voltage-gated calcium channels (see 5.11.10.2.).

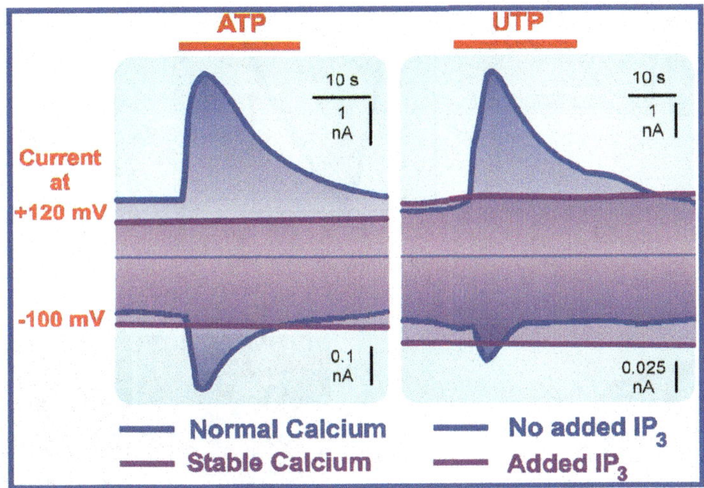

FIGURE 66: The P2Y receptor-induced activation of BK channels in human Müller cells is mediated by IP$_3$-induced intracellular calcium mobilization. The cells were derived from patients with proliferative vitreoretinopathy (PVR). The images display time-dependent records of the whole-cell currents at +120 mV (which are mainly mediated by BK channels) and at −100 mV. *Left:* ATP (100 μM) induced a transient increase of the BK currents (at +120 mV) and a cation current at −100 mV which is mediated by calcium-activated, calcium-permeable cation channels (Puro, 1991b). Clamping the intracellular free calcium concentration to a stable level of ~20 nM (by a high [10 mM]-EGTA pipette solution) abrogated the transient increase of the BK currents induced by ATP (100 μM). *Right:* The UTP (100 μM)-induced current activation is inhibited in the presence of IP$_3$ (50 μM) in the pipette solution. Due to the excess cytosolic IP$_3$, the IP$_3$-gated intracellular calcium stores become empty. UTP was applied 5 min after establishing the whole-cell configuration. Modified from Bringmann et al. (2002a).

5.5.3.9 K$_A$ Currents

As in the case of BK channels, there is a variation in the expression of fast transient K$_A$ currents (Fig. 8G) among Müller cells of various mammalian species. Approximately 75% of human Müller cells (Fig. 56C), 60% of monkey Müller cells, and 35% of rabbit Müller cells (Fig. 51) investigated so far express K$_A$ currents (Bringmann et al., 1999a,b; Pannicke et al., 2005a,c) whereas almost all Müller cells of the rat and mouse investigated do not normally express such currents (Figs. 8G,H, 23D,E, 61B, 67D) (Pannicke et al., 2002, 2005a; Vogler et al., 2013b). However, the expression of K$_A$ currents is dependent on the differentiation degree of Müller cells. The incidence of cells displaying K$_A$ currents (Figs. 61B, 67D) and the amplitude of these currents (Fig. 51) decrease in the course of the ontogenetic maturation of Müller cells (Bringmann et al., 1999a; Wurm et al., 2006b).

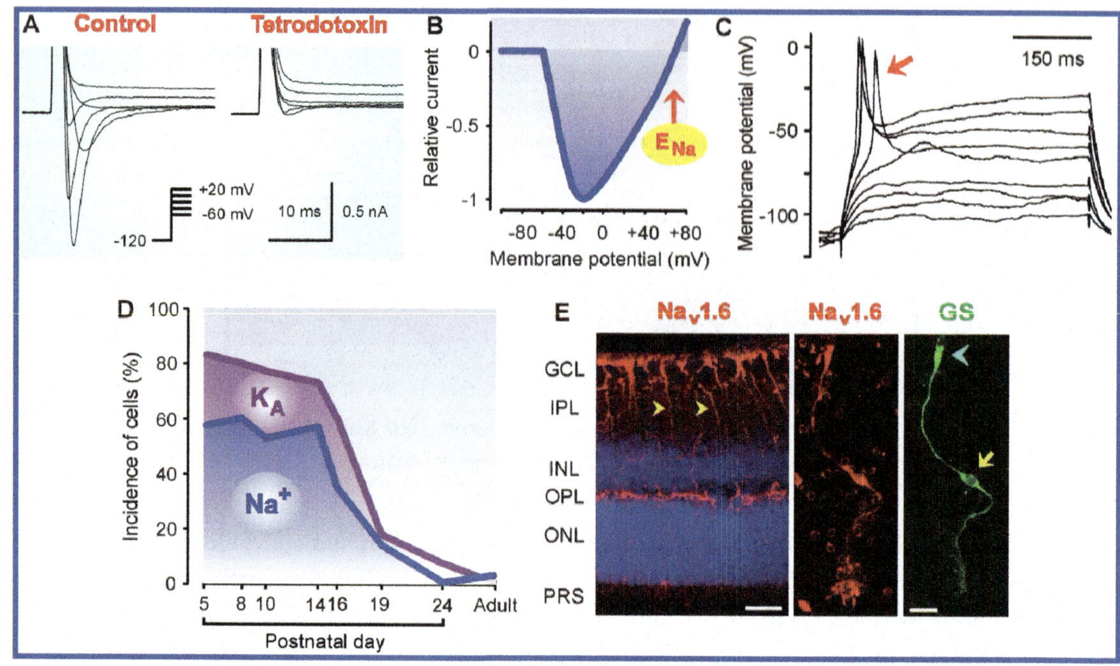

FIGURE 67: Voltage-gated sodium channels of Müller cells. **A.** The transient inward sodium currents of a human Müller cell derived from a patient with PDR are blocked by tetrodotoxin (1 μM). **B.** Current-voltage relation of the sodium currents of human Müller cells. The currents activate beyond −60 mV, peak at −20 mV and reverse the direction close to the reversal potential of sodium ions (E_{Na}). **C.** Single action potential-like discharges can be induced by large depolarizing current steps in a Müller cell of a patient with PVR. Depolarizing currents from 40–200 pA (increment, 20 pA) were applied after administration of a hyperpolarizing current of 250 pA (resulting in a membrane potential between −100 and −125 mV). **D.** Incidence of Müller cells isolated from the developing retina of the rat which display tetrodotoxin-sensitive, voltage-gated sodium (Na^+) and K_A potassium currents in whole-cell records. **E.** Müller cells of the adult rat retina display immunoreactivity for voltage-gated sodium channels. A retinal slice (*left*) and an acutely isolated Müller cell (*right*) were stained against the $Na_v1.6$ channel. *Yellow arrowheads*, Müller cell fibers that traverse the inner plexiform layer (IPL). *Blue arrowhead*, cell endfoot. *Arrow*, cell soma. Cell nuclei are *blue* stained. GCL, ganglion cell layer; INL, inner nuclear layer; NFL, nerve fiber layer; ONL, outer nuclear layer. PRS, photoreceptor segments. Bars, 10 μm. Modified from Francke et al. (1996), Bringmann et al. (2002b), Wurm et al. (2006b), and Linnertz et al. (2011).

Under various pathological conditions in the retina of adult rats, a decrease in the Kir channel-mediated potassium currents of Müller cells is associated with an emergence of K_A currents (Pannicke et al., 2005a,b, 2006). While Müller cells of the mature rat normally do not express such currents at a detectable level, the incidence of cells displaying K_A currents strongly increases after transient ischemia (Figs. 8G,H, 61B), in diabetic retinopathy, and during photoreceptor degeneration (Fig. 23D,E), for example (Pannicke et al., 2005a, 2006; Chavira-Suárez et al., 2012; Vogler et al., 2013b). In Müller cells of the rat, an increase in the incidence of cells which display K_A currents is an early sign of gliosis, even when the Kir channels are not downregulated (Fig. 23D) (Pannicke et al., 2001). In diabetic retinopathy and in resposne to high glucose, the potassium channel interacting protein 3 (KChIP3) is upregulated in Müller cells which may underlie the increase in K_A currents; KChIP3 is associated with voltage-gated potassium channels of the $K_V4.2$-4.3 subtype (Chavira-Suárez et al., 2011, 2012). The kinetics of the K_A currents is modulated by intracellular factors (Bringmann et al., 1998b, 2000g) and extracellular ions and protons (Bringmann et al., 1999c) which are altered in their concentration during neuronal activity.

The functional role of the increase in K_A currents under pathological conditions is unclear. K_A channels mediate (together with voltage-dependent sodium channels) rapid fluctuations of the membrane potential (Wurm et al., 2006b). Rapid fluctuations of the membrane potential are necessary for the activation of voltage-gated calcium and sodium channels, for example (see 5.9.1. and 5.9.2.). Currents through voltage-dependent calcium channels mediate the mitogen-induced calcium entry required for the proliferation of Müller cells (see 5.11.10.2.). It can be speculated that an increase in the activity of K_A channels support the proliferation of retinal progenitor cells and Müller cells of the diseased adult retina.

5.5.3.10 Other Types of Potassium Channels

Under distinct pathological conditions, when the Kir channels are downregulated or inactivated, other kinds of potassium channels (in addition to BK channels) may contribute to the potassium clearance by Müller cells. Müller cells of different amphibian and mammalian species express two pore-domain (TASK-like) channels (Eaton et al., 2004; Skatchkov et al., 2006). Currents through these outwardly rectifying potassium channels (Fig. 55) may contribute to the K_{DR} currents and may be implicated in the maintenance of the resting membrane potential when Kir channels are inactivated. These channels may have also functional importance in the neuron-abutting membrane domains of Müller cells which are poorly equipped with Kir4.1 channels but express strongly rectifying Kir2.1 channels (Figs. 7I, 8C, 12B, 55). Here, these channels may help to stabilize the negative membrane potential of Müller cells that is necessary to reach the opening threshold of Kir2.1

channels. TASK-like channels are also implicated in the agonist-mediated regulation of the Müller cell volume under osmotic stress conditions when the Kir4.1 channels are inactivated or downregulated (see 5.5.5.3.).

Another kind of potassium channels expressed by Müller cells are K_{ATP} channels which are inhibited in their activity by intracellular ATP. The pore-forming subunit of K_{ATP} channels (Kir6.1) is expressed in Müller cells of various vertebrate species (Skatchkov et al., 2001, 2002; Eaton et al., 2002). In frog Müller cells, the Kir6.1 protein is enriched in the endfeet membranes of the cells, and displays a colocalization with the Kir4.1 protein. Under conditions of ATP depletion, e.g., ischemia, spatial buffering potassium currents through K_{ATP} channels may help to protect the neurons from excitotoxic cell death. Activation of K_{ATP} channels inhibits the osmotic swelling of Müller cells in the diabetic retina (Krügel et al., 2011) which results (at least in part) from the downregulation of Kir4.1 channels (see 5.5.5.1. and 6.11.9.2.3.).

5.5.4   RETINAL WATER HOMEOSTASIS

5.5.4.1 Retinal Water Transport

Retinal glial cells maintain the retinal water homeostasis by allowing a rapid transcellular water transport. Under normal conditions, water accumulates in the retinal tissue due to at least three processes: endogenous production of water by the oxidative glucose metabolism, influx of water from the blood into the retina coupled to the uptake of metabolic substrates such as glucose, and a continuous forcing of water into the retina due to the intraocular pressure (Fig. 68) (Marmor, 1999). The accumulation of metabolic water is especially high in the macular tissue because of the high densities of cone photoreceptors and second- and third-order neurons, and the high metabolic activity of photoreceptor cells (see 5.5.8.2.). This generates the necessity of a substantial constitutive efflux of water out of the neural retina into the blood. In addition to the flux of metabolic water, there are rapid transmembrane ion and water shifts associated with neuronal activity (in particular with the glutamatergic signaling; see 5.5.1.1.) which should be buffered to avoid osmotic imbalances in the tissue. Furthermore, the transglial water transport is required to balance osmotic gradients which may occur between extra-retinal fluids (vitreous, blood) and the retinal parenchyma.

The redistribution of excess water from the retinal tissue into the blood is carried out by retinal glial and pigment epithelial cells. The pigment epithelium dehydrates the subretinal space and the outer part of the neural retina (Pederson, 1994) while Müller cells dehydrate the inner retinal tissue (from the inner limiting membrane up to the level of the outer plexiform layer; Fig. 68) (Bringmann et al., 2004). The water clearance from the retinal tissue is mediated by an osmotically

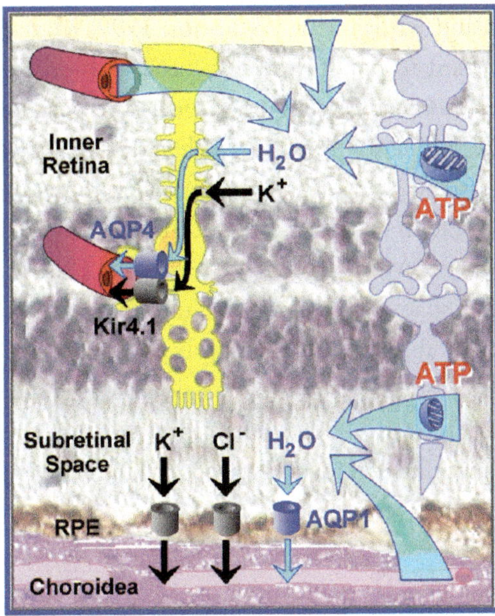

FIGURE 68: Water fluxes through the retina. Under normal conditions, water accumulates in the neural retina and subretinal space due to an influx from the blood (coupled to the uptake of nutrients such as glucose) and vitreous chamber (due to the intraocular pressure), and the oxidative synthesis of ATP in the mitochondria that generates carbon dioxide and water. The excess water is redistributed into the blood by a transcellular water transport through Müller cells and the retinal pigment epithelium (RPE). The water transport across cell membranes is facilitated by aquaporin (AQP) water channels. RPE cells express AQP1, while Müller cells express AQP4. The transcellular water transport is osmotically coupled to the transport of osmolytes, in particular of potassium and chloride ions. The ion flux across the cell membranes is facilitated by transporter molecules and ion channels. In Müller cells, the Kir4.1 potassium channel is co-localized with AQP4 in membranes that surround the vessels, and at both limiting membranes of the retina. Modified from Reichenbach et al. (2007).

driven transcellular water transport that is coupled to a transport of osmolytes, in particular potassium and chloride ions (Fig. 68) (Bialek and Miller, 1994; Pederson, 1994; Nagelhus et al., 1999; Bringmann et al., 2004). The water flux through the membranes of Müller and pigment epithelial cells is facilitated and directed by AQP water channels which increase the water permeability of membranes.

The active fluid transport across the retinal pigment epithelium, mediated by a transcellular ion (sodium, chloride, bicarbonate) and water flux (Miller and Steinberg, 1977; Joseph and Miller,

1991; Pederson, 1994; Bialek and Miller, 1994; Marmor, 1999; Marmorstein, 2001; Stamer et al., 2003; Strauss, 2005), is important to maintain the volume and ionic composition of the extracellular space surrounding the photoreceptor segments and is the basis for the proper attachment of the neural retina to the retinal pigment epithelium (Meyer et al., 2002; Maminishkis et al., 2002; Strauss, 2005; Levin and Verkman, 2006). Pharmacological stimulation of the ion transport across the retinal pigment epithelium facilitates the subretinal fluid clearance and is a method to reattach the retina after retinal detachment (Marmor, 1990; Meyer et al., 2002; Maminishkis et al., 2002).

Because the extracellular space is highly convolute and extremely narrow in the plexiform (synaptic) layers (Reichenbach et al., 1988a), these layers constitute high-resistance barriers against the paracellular fluid movement, ion currents, and diffusion of large molecules (Tso and Shih, 1977; Xu and Karwoski, 1994; Antcliff et al., 2001). Therefore, the inner retinal water must be largely cleared into the blood by a transcellular transport through Müller cells (Figs. 40A, 68, 69A, 70, 71) (Bringmann et al., 2004, 2006; Reichenbach et al., 2007).

5.5.4.2 Retinal Water Channels

By facilitation of the bidirectional transmembrane water transport in dependence on osmotic gradients and hydrostatic pressure, AQP water channels are critically involved in the maintenance of the ionic and osmotic balance in the CNS including the retina (Agre et al., 2002; Verkman et al., 2008). Generally, AQPs are specifically expressed in membrane domains that mediate rapid and extensive fluid exchange. At present, 13 members of the AQP protein family (AQP0-12) have been identified in mammals which differ in their cellular localization and permeability for water, ions, and small non-charged solutes (Verkman and Mitra, 2000; Agre et al., 2002). AQPs belong to the two subgroups of pure water channels (AQPs 0, 1, 2, 4, 5, 6, 8) and aquaglyceroporins (AQPs 3, 7, 9, 10, 12). In addition to their role as water channels, aquaglyceroporins facilitate also the transmembrane transport of a variety of small solutes including glycerol, lactate, and urea, as well as of hydrogen peroxide (Ishibashi et al., 1994; Echevarria et al., 1996; Kuriyama et al., 1997; Tsukaguchi et al., 1998, 1999; Magni et al., 2006; Miller et al., 2010). For structural reasons, the intracellular AQPs 11 and 12 are categorized as an own subgroup (Ishibashi, 2006).

Gene transcripts of a diversity of AQP subtypes were described to be expressed in the retina. The human neuroretina contains transcripts of all mammalian AQP subtypes while the rat retina contains transcripts of all mammalian AQPs with the exception of AQPs 2 and 7 (Tenckhoff et al., 2005; Hollborn et al., 2011a, 2012a). AQP0 is the major intrinsic protein of lens fiber cells (Gorin et al., 1984). In the rat retina, AQP0 protein is localized to the nuclei, somata, and synaptic terminals of subpopulations of PKCα- and β-expressing rod bipolar and amacrine cells, as well as to

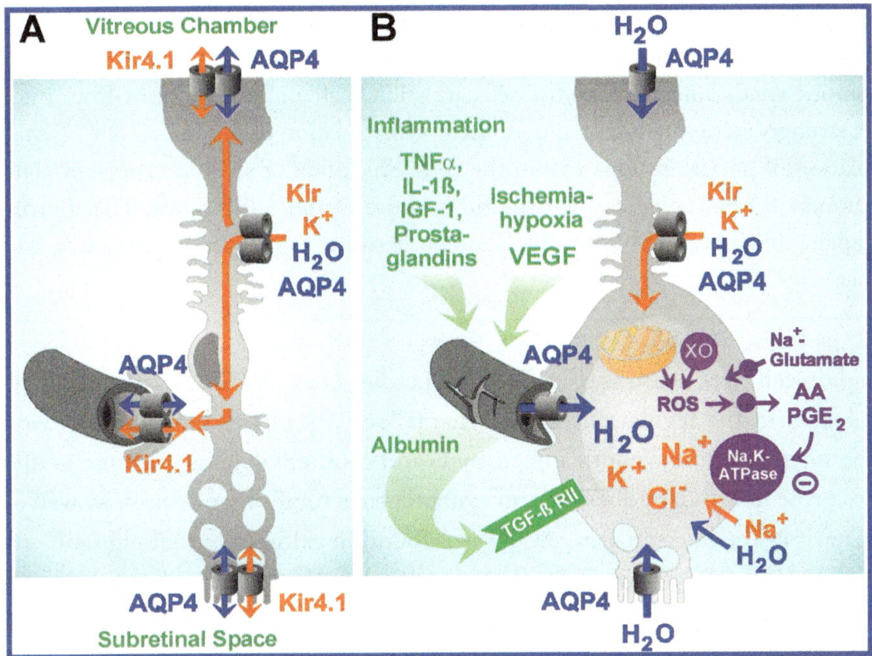

FIGURE 69: Mechanisms of osmotic Müller cell swelling. **A.** Under normal conditions, Müller cells mediate the fluid clearance from the retinal tissue into the blood mainly by a transcellular co-transport of water (facilitated by AQP4) and distinct osmolytes, predominantly potassium ions. The transglial potassium currents are facilitated by Kir channels, in particuler Kir4.1. **B.** Under pathological conditions, an increase in the intracellular osmotic pressure of Müller cells results in an osmotic gradient across the plasma membrane that pulls water into the Müller cells facilitated by AQP4 water channels. Ischemic-hypoxic and inflammatory conditions, e.g., in diabetic retinopathy, are associated with vascular leakage due to the action of inflammatory factors and VEGF. Vascular leakage results in serum influx into the retinal parenchyma. In the presence of osmotic gradients, extravasated serum albumin induces a swelling of Müller cells via activation of the TGF-β receptor type II (TGF-ß RII). Albumin is internalized by receptor-mediated endocytosis; endocytosis is associated with the generation of oxygen radicals and activation of PLA_2. Osmotic stress induces the production of reactive oxygen species (ROS) in the mitochondria and by xanthine oxidases (XO) and NADPH oxidases. ROS stimulate the production of arachidonic acid (AA) and prostaglandins (PGs) which inhibit the Na,K-ATPase. Inhibition of the ATPase results in a sodium influx which is associated with a water influx into the cells. In the normal healthy retina, the sodium influx can be compensated by a potassium efflux through Kir4.1 and (after autocrine activation of adenosine A_1 receptors) two-pore domain potassium channels. Müller cells

continued on next page

downregulate the expression of functional Kir4.1 channels and abrogate the swelling-inhibitory purinergic signaling cascade under pathological conditions. This impairs the compensatory efflux of potassium under hypoosmotic conditions. Because the cells are still capable to take up ions from the extracellular space through strongly rectifying Kir channels, the downregulation of functional Kir4.1 channels results in an accumulation of potassium ions within the cells. An influx of sodium via electrogenic glutamate uptake carriers may further enhance the osmotic pressure of the cell interior. The downregulation of Kir4.1 also impairs the resolution of osmotic gradients across the glio-vascular interface. Modified from Reichenbach et al. (2007).

---

nuclei of ganglion cell layer neurons (Fig. 72A,B) (Iandiev et al., 2007c; Fukuda et al., 2011). AQP0 is likely implicated in the regulation of the synaptic activity of rod bipolars, by mediating rapid water movements to facilitate synaptic ion currents and counterbalancing osmotic gradients. AQP0 may play also a role in cellular adhesion and synaptic structural organization, as well as in the osmotic homeostasis of the nucleoplasm. AQP3 was found in cultured retinal pigment epithelial cells (Hollborn et al., 2012b). AQP5 was described to be localized to Müller cells of the equine retina, in particular in their secondary processes (Fig. 72A), and to retinal pigment epithelial cells (Eberhardt et al., 2011; Hollborn et al., 2011a). In the retinal pigment epithelium, AQP5 expression is relatively specifically regulated by osmotic gradients and blood serum (Hollborn et al., 2011a). *In situ*, the hypoosmotic downregulation of AQP5 may decrease the water permeability of the retinal pigment epithelium and thus may inhibit the osmotic water influx into the retinal tissue, while the hyperosmotic upregulation of AQP5 may increase the water clearance across the retinal pigment epithelium when high blood osmolarity induces a breakdown of the outer blood-retinal barrier (Shirao and Steinberg, 1987; Orgül et al., 1993). Increased osmolarity also induces upregulation of AQP8 in retinal pigment epithelial cells (M. Hollborn, Leipzig, unpublished observation). AQP9 is confined to dopaminergic amacrine cells in the neuroretina (Fig. 72C) (Iandiev et al., 2006d; Hollborn et al., 2012a). AQP9-expressing (tyrosine hydroxylase-positive) and AQP1-expressing (tyrosine hydroxylase-negative) amacrine cells are different subpopulations of amacrines which differ in their soma size and morphology of the dendritic trees (Fig. 72Cc) (Iandiev et al., 2006d). In addition, AQP9 is expressed in the retinal pigment epithelium (Hollborn et al., 2011a, 2012a). (However, in another study, AQP9 was found widely distributed in the rat retina, and localized to glial cells, rod bipolars, amacrines, and retinal ganglion cells; Naka et al., 2010.) AQP9 is an aquaglyceroporin permeable to water and a wide variety of non-charged solutes including glycerol and lactate which serve as neuronal energy substrates (Kuriyama et al., 1997; Tsukaguchi et al., 1998, 1999). Retinal ischemia and increased intraocular pressure induce transcriptional upregulation of AQP9 in the retina (Hollborn et al., 2012a; Yang et al., 2013b). AQP9 may be a part of metabolic sensors constituted by dopaminergic amacrines (inner retina) and retinal pigment epithelial cells (outer retina), as

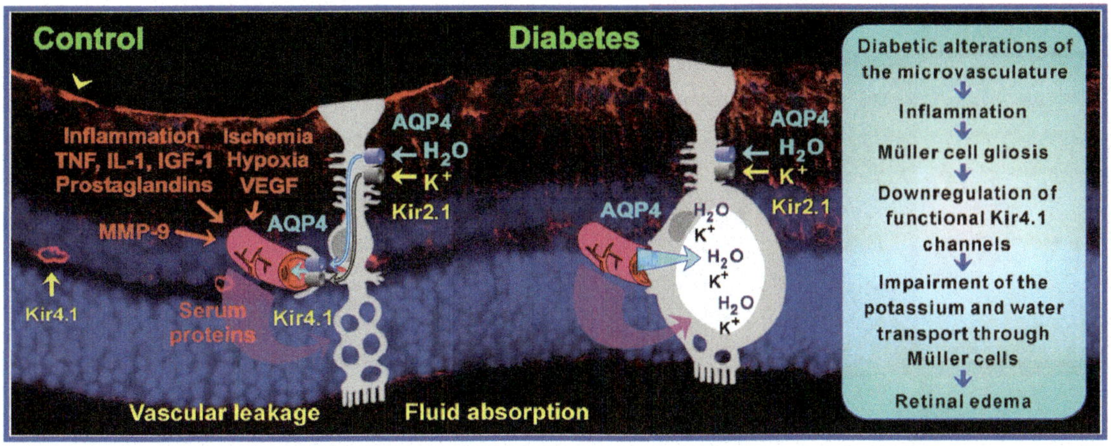

FIGURE 70: Disruption of Müller cell-mediated fluid clearance and (under conditions of osmotic imbalances) Müller cell swelling may contribute to the development of diabetic retinal edema. In diabetic retinopathy, the major potassium channel of Müller cells (Kir4.1), which is predominantly expressed around the retinal vessels and at the inner limiting membrane (*arrowhead*), is downregulated. This disrupts the water transport through the cells which is facilitated by water channels (AQP4) and coupled to potassium currents through potassium channels (Kir2.1, Kir4.1). Accumulation of potassium within the cells increases the intracellular osmotic pressure, resulting in water influx into the cells and cellular swelling.

suggested for catecholaminergic neurons of the brain stem (Badaut and Regli, 2004). The ischemia-induced upregulation of AQP9 in retinal pigment epithelial cells may prevent lactic acidosis and subretinal edema *in situ* (Hollborn et al., 2012a).

There is a conspicuous segregation of the expression of AQP1 and AQP4 in the rodent retina which reflects the two major water clearance regions (Fig. 68): AQP1 is predominantly expressed in the outer retina including the outer nuclear layer and the retinal pigment epithelium (Figs. 8E, 15A, 18A, 21A, 22A,B,D, 23C) while AQP4 is predominantly expressed by astrocytes and Müller cells in the inner retina from the inner limiting membrane to the outer plexiform layer (Figs. 8C, 9A, 15A, 18C, 19, 21B, 22A,C, 23B, 49).

5.5.4.3 Glial Expression of AQP1

AQP1 is normally localized to the retinal pigment epithelial cells, photoreceptor cells, and subpopulations of glycinergic and GABAergic amacrine cells (Figs. 8E, 21A, 72Cc) (Nagelhus et al., 1998; Kim et al., 1998b, 2002; Stamer et al., 2003; Iandiev et al., 2005a; Kang et al., 2005; Naka

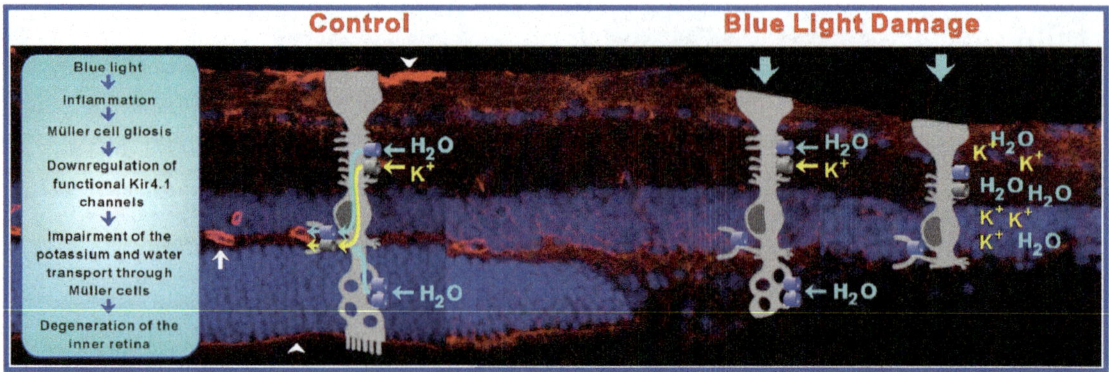

FIGURE 71: Putative involvement of Müller cell dysfunction in the degeneration of the inner retina after exposure to blue light. Excess illumination with blue light causes a degeneration of the photoreceptors and the pigment epithelium, resulting in local inflammation which induces Müller cell gliosis. The gliosis is associated with a redistribution of the Kir4.1 protein (*red*) from the prominent expression sites around the vessels (*white arrow*) and at the limiting membranes of the retina (*white arrowheads; left*). The redistribution and functional inactivation of Kir4.1 disrupts the transglial potassium and water flux (*middle*), resulting in dysfunctional potassium and water homeostasis within the retinal tissue. This contributes to edema development and neuronal degeneration in the inner retina, as indicated by the decrease in the thickness of the inner retina, in particular of the inner plexiform layer (IPL; *right*). Cell nuclei are *blue* stained. GCL, ganglion cell layer; INL, inner nuclear layer. Bar, 20 μm. The *image* is a composition of three images obtained from different areas of a light-injured rat retina. Modified from Iandiev et al. (2008a).

et al., 2010; Motulsky et al., 2010; Vogler et al., 2013b). The AQP1 immunolabeling of the outer neuroretina disappears along with the degeneration of photoreceptor cells in the *rds* mouse, after light damage of the retina, and in a transgenic rat model of inherited photoreceptor degeneration (Figs. 18A, 21A, 22D, 23C) (Iandiev et al., 2005a, 2008a,b; Vogler et al., 2013b). AQP1 in photoreceptor cells is likely involved in the maintenance of the osmotic balance necessary for the phototransduction process. In contrast to AQP4 which is a pure water channel, AQP1 is a channel for both water and cations (Yool et al., 1996) which can be gated by cyclic guanosine monophosphate (cGMP) (Anthony et al., 2000; Saparov et al., 2001). However, it remains to be proven whether AQP1 plays a role in the regulation of the photoreceptor excitability.

Transient retinal ischemia and diabetic retinopathy result in complex alteration in the retinal localization of AQP1. Normally, retinal glial cells do not express AQP1 (Figs. 8E, 13A, 21A, 22A,D). After transient ischemia and in the retina of diabetic rats, AQP1 is strongly expressed by glial cells in the nerve fiber/ganglion cell layers (Figs. 8E, 13C,D,E, 15A, 22A) (Iandiev et al.,

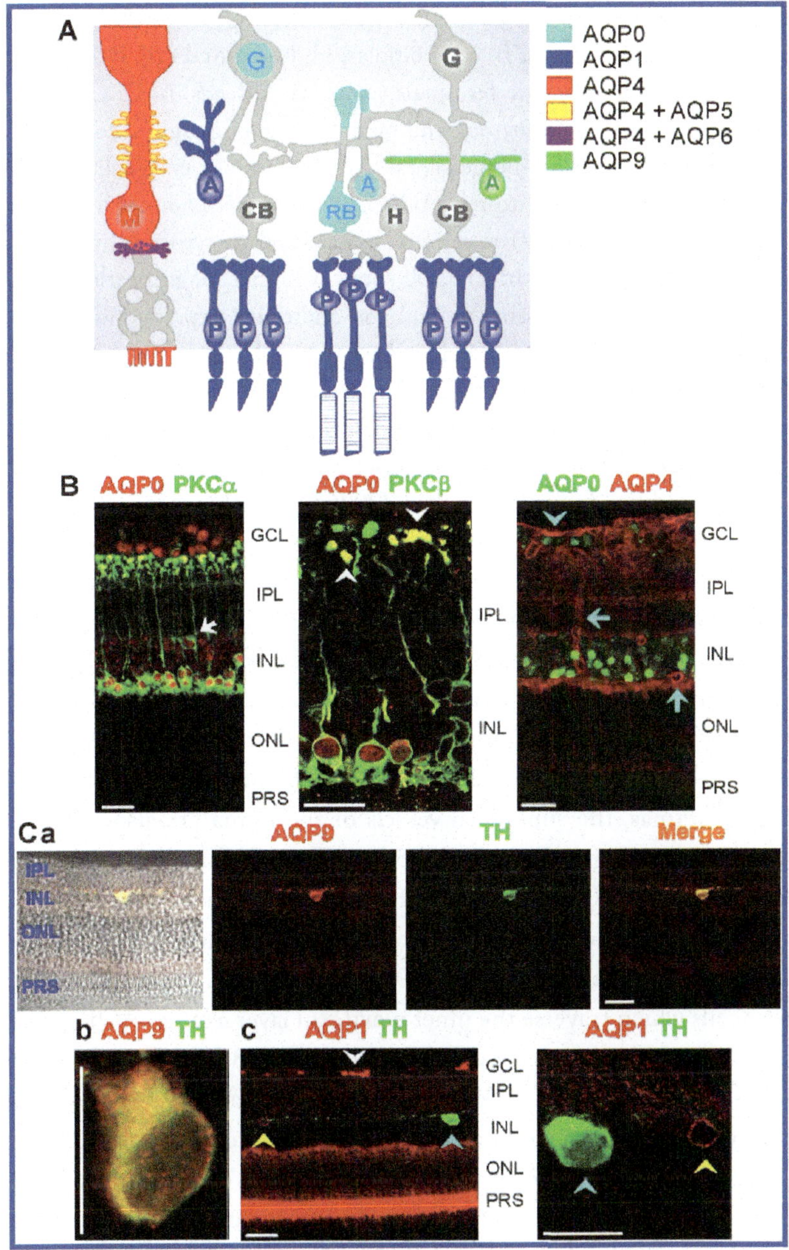

FIGURE 72: Retinal water channels. **A.** Schematic summary of the cellular localization of different AQP subtypes identified so far in the neuroretina of different species. AQP0 is localized to rod bipolar (RB), amacrine (A), and ganglion cells (G). AQP1 is localized to glycinergic amacrines and

continued on next page

photoreceptor cells (P). AQP4 is localized to retinal glial cells, AQP5 and AQP6 to Müller cells (M), and AQP9 to dopaminergic amacrines. CB, cone bipolar; H, horizontal cell. **B.** In the rat retina, AQP0 is localized to the nuclei and the synaptic terminals (*white arrowheads*) of PKCα and β expressing bipolar and distinct amacrine cells (*white arrow*), and by the nuclei of ganglion cell layer (GCL) neurons. Co-localization yielded a *yellow-orange* merge signal. AQP0 does not co-localized with AQP4 (*right*), suggesting that retinal glial cells do not express AQP0. *Blue arrowhead*, inner limiting membrane. *Blue arrows*, retinal vessels. **C. a.** AQP9 (*red*) is selectively localized to tyrosine hydroxylase (TH; *green*)-positive amacrine cells of the rat retina. **b.** The cell soma at higher magnification shows diffuse localization of AQP9 and TH in the cytoplasm (*yellow*) and additional expression of AQP9 in the plasma membrane where it is not co-localized with TH (*red* points). **c.** There is no overlap of AQP1 (*red*) and TH (*green*) immunoreactivities in rat retinal slices. *Blue arrowheads*, TH-expressing amacrine cell bodies. *Yellow arrowheads*, AQP1-expressing amacrine cell bodies. *White arrowhead*, AQP1-expressing red blood cells. INL, inner nuclear layer. IPL, inner plexiform layer; ONL, outer nuclear layer; PRS, photoreceptor segments. Bars, 20 μm. Modified from Iandiev et al. (2006d, 2007c).

2006a, 2007a; Fukuda et al., 2010). Upregulation of glial AQP1 was also observed during inherited (Fig. 23C) but not light-induced photoreceptor degeneration (Figs. 18A, 21A, 22D) (Iandiev et al., 2005a, 2008a, b; Vogler et al., 2013b). Normally, the vessels of the superficial vascular plexus of the retina (localized to the nerve fiber/ganglion cell layers) are surrounded by AQP4-containing glial membranes (Figs. 13C-E) (Iandiev et al., 2006a, 2007a; Qin et al., 2009a; Fukuda et al., 2010). In ischemic and diabetic retinas, the superficial vessels of the retina are also surrounded by AQP1-containing glial membranes (Figs. 8E, 13C-E, 15A, 22A, 23C) (Iandiev et al., 2006a, 2007a; Qin et al., 2009a; Fukuda et al., 2010). The vessels of the deeper vascular plexi (localized to the inner nuclear layer) remained surrounded by AQP4-containing glial membranes after ischemia and in diabetes (Figs. 15B, 22B) (Iandiev et al., 2006a, 2007a; Wurm et al., 2011a). In addition, inner stem processes of Müller cells which traverse the inner plexiform layer express AQP1 in the postischemic retina and during inherited photoreceptor degeneration (Figs. 23C, 72B) (Iandiev et al., 2006a; Vogler et al., 2013b). The redistribution of AQP4 from perivascular Müller cell processes is induced, at least in part, by AGEs/ALEs (Curtis et al., 2011). In the neuroretina and Müller cells of diabetic rats, the gene expression of AQP1 is elevated whereas the gene expression of AQP4 was found to be either unaltered, decreased, or increased compared to control (Gerhardinger et al., 2005; Qin et al., 2009a; Fukuda et al., 2010; Hollborn et al., 2011a; Curtis et al., 2011; Zhang et al., 2011b; Cui et al., 2012). The functional relevance of the alteration of the AQP subtype in glial membranes that surround the superficial retinal vessels is unclear. Possibly, the expression of AQP1 may represent a response of glial cells to facilitate the water clearance around leaky vessels and may represent a response of glial cells to osmotic imbalances across the glio-vascular interface which may be caused by various factors including impaired glial water transport after downregulation of perivascular Kir4.1 and alteration of the blood osmolarity due to liver and kidney diseases. The alteration in the type of perivascular AQPs was found to coincide with neuronal apoptosis in the ganglion cell and inner nuclear layers of the diabetic retina (Fukuda et al., 2010). An expression of AQP1 in retinal vascular endothelial cells supports the hypoxia-induced angiogenesis (Kaneko et al., 2008b), a characteristic of the progression of diabetic retinopathy to a proliferative state (see 5.11.8.).

High salt intake is a major cause of hypertension (Bringmann et al., 2014) which represents the main secondary risk factor of the development and progression of diabetic retinopathy to the neovascular stage (Kostraba et al., 1991; Klein et al., 1998; Kamoi et al., 2013). Hypertension aggravates retinal inflammation in experimental diabetes (Silva et al., 2007). High-salt diet and hypertension induce an increase in the retinal content of AQP4 and exacerbates the increase in the retinal content of AQP1 and the upregulation of AQP1 in glial cells around the superficial retinal vessels associated with experimental diabetic retinopathy (Qin et al., 2009a,b, 2012). This is associated with intracellular edema in retinal ganglion cells and mitochondrial swelling in glial cells (Qin et al., 2009a). Although the retinal expression of AQP1 protein is increased in response to retinal ischemia (Figs. 8E, 13C,D,E, 15A, 22A), the retinal gene expression of AQP1 is strongly decreased (Rehak et al., 2009, 2011; Köferl et al., 2014).

5.5.4.4 Glial Expression of AQP4 and AQP6

The major glial aquaporin in the retina expressed by astrocytes and Müller cells is AQP4 (Hasegawa et al., 1994; Frigeri et al., 1995; Patil et al., 1997; Nagelhus et al., 1998; Hamann et al., 1998; Li et al., 2002b). AQP4 is prominently localized to the inner retinal layers, whereas labeling of the outer retina (with exception of the outer plexiform layer) is faint (Figs. 8C, 15A,B, 18C, 19, 21B, 22A,C, 23B). Enriched AQP4 labeling is found in the ganglion cell/nerve fiber layers in glial membranes which abut the inner limiting membrane and which surround ganglion cell bodies, nerve fibers, and blood vessels (Figs. 13A-E, 18C, 19, 21B, 22A). In the inner plexiform layer, AQP4 is enriched in distinct sublaminae. In the outer plexiform layer, Müller cell membranes which surround the ribbon synapses contain AQP4 (Figs. 36C, 72A,B). Thus, AQP4 is localized in Müller cells in perisynaptic membrane domains (where the cells take up neuron-derived osmolytes such as potassium) as well as in perivascular and vitreous-abutting membrane domains (where the cells release neuron-derived osmolytes into the blood and vitreous) (Figs. 68, 69A). In membrane domains through which Müller cells release excess potassium, AQP4 and Kir4.1 potassium channels are colocalized (Nagelhus et al., 1999; Connors and Kofuji, 2006). The colocalization of Kir4.1 and AQP4 allows a bidirectional flux of potassium and water across the Müller cell membrane (Figs. 40A, 68, 69A, 71) (Nagelhus et al., 1999) which is involved in the resolution of osmotic gradients between the retina and extra-retinal fluid-filled spaces. In the fish retina, AQP4 was also described to be localized to cone photoreceptors and a GABAergic subpopulation of amacrine cells, in addition to Müller cells (Hombrebueno et al., 2012).

At the ultrastructural level, AQP4 is the main constituent of the orthogonal arrays of intra-membrane particles localized to Müller cell and astrocyte endfeet (Raviola, 1977; Wolburg and Berg, 1987, 1988; Gotow and Hashimoto, 1989; Richter et al., 1990; Yang et al., 1996b; Verbavatz et al., 1997). Astrocytes of the optic nerve head, which have no contact to the vitreous, do not show such arrays of particles (Berg-von der Emde and Wolburg, 1989). Whereas endfeet membranes of frog Müller cells lack these arrays of particles, such membranes contain the arrays in all other verte-brates investigated, including fish and urodeles (Berg-von der Emde and Wolburg, 1989; Wolburg et al., 1992; Wolburg, 1995). The density of the arrays varies with the size of vitreal endfeet mem-branes and is higher in Müller cells of the central retina compared to cells of the retinal periphery (Wolburg and Berg, 1987; Richter et al., 1990).

In addition to AQP4, Müller cells express AQP6 (Iandiev et al., 2011a; Hollborn et al., 2011a). AQP6 is selectively localized in Müller cell membranes which surround the ribbon synapses in the outer plexiform layer where it is colocalized with AQP4 (Fig. 36A–C) (Iandiev et al., 2011a). The different localization of AQP4 and AQP6 may suggest different functional roles of both AQPs in Müller cells. It has been shown that rat AQP6 has a low water permeability and functions pre-dominantly as pathway for small hydrophilic molecules such as glycerol and urea (Holm et al., 2004). In addition, AQP6 was suggested to be an anion channel with high permeability for nitrate (Yasui et al., 1999; Ikeda et al., 2002). It could be but remains to be proven that glial AQP4 medi-ates the water homeostasis around ribbon synapses whereas glial AQP6 delivers anion conductance (to maintain electroneutrality) and may have further functional roles involved in the homeostasis of the perisynaptic space and the regulation of vesicle filling and exocytosis, as well as in the glial delivery of the neuronal energy substrate glycerol to highly active synapses (Iandiev et al., 2011a).

Although the overall retinal distribution of AQP4 does not alter after ischemia and in dia-betic retinopathy (Figs. 8C, 15A, 19, 22A, B), both conditions are associated with distinct altera-tions in the retinal distribution of AQP4. The most prominent alteration is the redistribution of perivascular AQP4 from the vessels of the superficial vascular plexus and the appearance of AQP1 around the vessels (Figs. 8E, 13C–E) (Iandiev et al., 2006a, 2007a; Fukuda et al., 2010). In the ischemic and light-injured retina, glial AQP4 and AQP6 around the ribbon synapses of the outer plexiform layer disappear along with the degeneration of the synapses (Figs. 22B, 36D) (Iandiev et al., 2006a, 2011).

Under conditions associated with edema in the outer retina (e.g., after retinal light injury, which is associated with a degeneration of photoreceptor and retinal pigment epithelial cells, and in a rat model of inherited photoreceptor degeneration), Müller cell processes within the outer nuclear layer increase strongly their expression of AQP4 (Figs. 14B, 18C, 21B, 23B) (Iandiev et al., 2008a,b; Ren et al., 2010; Vogler et al., 2013b). In a mouse model of retinal bright white light damage (Fig. 18C), but not in a rat model of retinal blue light damage (Fig. 52), the upregulation of AQP4 in the outer retina is associated with an upregulation of Kir4.1 (Iandiev et al., 2008a,b). Under these conditions, Müller cells are also responsible for the osmohomeostasis of the outer nuclear layer. The outer retinal edema develops as a result of the opening of the outer blood-retinal barrier due to injury of the retinal pigment epithelium (Fuller et al., 1978; Putting et al., 1992) and the normo-tonic shrinkage of cells that undergo apoptosis. The volume decrease of apoptotic cells occurs via channel- and transporter-mediated efflux of osmolytes (potassium, sodium, chloride); the ion efflux creates an osmotic gradient that draws water out of the cells (Bortner et al., 1997; Yu et al., 1997; Szabo et al., 1998; Maeno et al., 2000).

Müller cells of patients with PVR and from animal models of ischemic-hypoxic retinopathies and glaucoma exhibit a strong downregulation of AQP4 (Tenckhoff et al., 2005; Dibas et al., 2008; Rehak et al., 2009, 2011; Drechsler et al., 2012; Köferl et al., 2014). AQP4 is a target for degrada-tion by the ubiquitin-dependent proteasome (Dibas et al., 2008). The downregulation of AQP4 may contribute to the osmotic swelling of Müller cells and the dysregulation of the retinal fluid clearance (see 5.5.5.2. and 5.11.9.1.2.). In other studies, retinal ischemia-hypoxia was found to in-crease the expression of AQP4 in astrocytes and Müller cells (Kaur et al., 2007; Zou et al., 2009).

5.5.4.5 Possible Coupling of Glial Water and Potassium Transport

Spatial buffering potassium currents through glial cells are believed to be not associated with a water flux (Orkand et al., 1966; Kofuji and Newman, 2004). On the other hand, it was suggested that the water transport through Müller cells is osmotically driven by transcellular spatial buffering potassium currents (Figs. 40A, 68) (Nagelhus et al., 1999; Bringmann et al., 2004, 2005; Binder et al., 2012). This assumption is based on the fact that AQP4 and Kir4.1 potassium channels are colocalized in Müller cell membranes that abut fluid-filled spaces outside the neuroretina, i.e., blood vessels, vitreous chamber, and subretinal space (Figs. 8C, 9A, 14A,B, 21B, 22A, 49) (Nagelhus et al., 1999; Binder et al., 2012). AQP4 is also localized to the perisynaptic membranes of Müller cells (Figs. 8C, 9A, 14A,B, 21B, 22A, 49) (Nagelhus et al., 1998) where other Kir channel subtypes, e.g., Kir2.1 (Figs. 7I, 8C, 12B, 55) and Kir4.1/5.1, mediate the passive potassium influx into Müller cells (Kofuji et al., 2002). By the coupling of potassium and water transport, Müller cells may de-hydrate the inner retina in dependence on the neuronal activity (Figs. 40A, 68, 69A) (Nagelhus et al., 1999; Bringmann et al., 2004, 2006; Reichenbach et al., 2007). The colocalization of AQP4 and Kir4.1 proteins also suggests that osmotic gradients between the retinal tissue and the blood and vitreous are compensated by bidirectional potassium and water fluxes through Müller cell membranes. Under various pathological conditions including retinal ischemia and inflammation, the protein expression of AQP4 is unaltered or even increased (Figs. 8C, 12A, 14A,B, 21B, 22A, 23B) whereas the protein expression of Kir4.1 is decreased (Figs. 8C,D, 23A, 70, 71) (Pannicke et al., 2004, 2006; Wurm et al., 2006a; Iandiev et al., 2006a,b, 2007a, 2008a; Liu et al., 2007; Vogler et al., 2013b; see 5.5.3.5.). The decrease of functional Kir4.1 channels disrupts the regular potassium and water transport through Müller cells and the homeostasis of osmotic imbalances between Müller cells and the spaces outside the neuroretina (Bringmann et al., 2004; Reichenbach et al., 2007; see 5.11.9.1.2.).

It has been shown, however, that the Kir4.1-mediated transmembrane potassium currents of Müller cells are not altered by deletion of AQP4 (Ruiz-Ederra et al., 2007; Pannicke et al., 2010), suggesting that AQP4 has (also) functional roles other than the support of spatial buffering potassium currents. Deletion of AQP4 does not alter the localization and activity of Kir4.1, suggesting that the expression of AQP4 and Kir4.1 proteins is independently regulated. The neuroretina of AQP4-null mice (Ma et al., 1997) does not contain gene transcripts and immunoreactivity of AQP4 (Fig. 9A) (Ruiz-Ederra et al., 2007; Pannicke et al., 2010). The osmotic water permeability is >4-fold reduced in Müller cells from AQP4-null mice compared to cells from wildtype mice (Ruiz-Ederra et al., 2007). Although the gene expression of Kir4.1 is slightly enhanced in the neuroretina of AQP4-null mice compared to the tissue of wildtype mice, the retinal Kir4.1 protein content and the retinal distribution of Kir4.1 protein are not different between retinas of knockout and wildtype mice (Fig. 9A) (Da and Verkman, 2004; Ruiz-Ederra et al., 2007; Pannicke et al., 2010). In addition, the GFAP labeling is not different between retinal slices from knockout and wildtype mice (Fig. 9A) (Pannicke et al., 2010), suggesting that Müller cells are not activated (see 5.11.3.). The potassium currents are not different between Müller cells from AQP4-null and wildtype mice (Ruiz-Ederra et al., 2007; Pannicke et al., 2010). The similar potassium currents in Müller cells from AQP4-null and wildtype mice do not support the assumption that the water transport through AQP4 is required for the maintenance of the potassium buffering currents through Müller cells (Ruiz-Ederra et al., 2007). However, Müller cells of AQP4-null mice were shown to display a delayed swelling under hypoosmotic conditions which was not observed in cells from wildtype mice (Fig. 9B,C) (Pannicke et al., 2010); the swelling induction was explained with an impairment of the potassium currents through Kir4.1 (see 5.5.5.1. and 5.11.9.2.3.). A similar delayed hypoosmotic swelling was described in primary brain astrocytes from AQP4-knockout mice (Benfenati et al., 2011). Whether the delayed osmotic swelling of Müller cells from AQP4-null mice is indicative of an impairment of transmembrane potassium currents remains to be determined by future investigations.

AQP4-null mice exhibit a mildly defective light-induced retinal signal transduction (Li et al., 2002b). This can be explained either with an impairment of the glial potassium clearance (Nagelhus et al., 1999; Bringmann et al., 2004) and/or with an impairment of the synaptic activity due to an impaired glial delivery of water (see 5.5.4.6.). An independent regulation of the expression of AQP4 and Kir4.1 is also suggested by the fact that in various retinopathies, the downregulation and redistribution of Kir4.1 channels is not accompanied by altered expression and distribution of AQP4 (with the exception of Müller cell membranes that surround the superficial retinal vessels) (Figs. 8C, 15A, 19) (Pannicke et al., 2004, 2006; Rehak et al., 2009; see 5.5.4.4.). α-Syntrophin (a protein of the dystrophin-associated protein complex) is required for the membrane anchoring of approximately 70% of the AQP4 protein in Müller cells while deletion of this protein has no effect on the membrane anchoring of Kir4.1 (Puwarawuttipanit et al., 2006; Enger et al., 2012). Deletion of the dystrophin gene product Dp71 in mice markedly reduces the retinal AQP4 level and has no effect on the level of Kir4.1, while both proteins display a dislocation in Müller cells (Dalloz et al., 2003; Fort et al., 2008; Sene et al., 2009). Differences in the PDZ domain-binding C-termini of Kir4.1 and AQP4 may facilitate the preferential binding of both proteins to different syntrophin isoforms. On the other hand, deletion of laminins β2 and γ3 induces a reduction in the expression and function of both Kir4.1 and AQP4 (Hirrlinger et al., 2011). In addition to differences in membrane anchoring, different transcriptional regulation of AQP4 and Kir4.1 (with a downregulation of Kir4.1 and no alteration or an upregulation of AQP4; Liu et al., 2007; Kaur et al., 2007) may contribute to the distinct regulation of both proteins under various pathological conditions.

5.5.4.6 AQP4-Mediated Support of Synaptic Activity

The localization of AQP4 in the perisynaptic membranes of Müller cells in the plexiform and ganglion cell layers (Figs. 13E, 19, 36C) suggests that the water transport through Müller cells supports the rapid ion flux associated with synaptic activity (Fig. 40B) (Bringmann et al., 2005). The assumption that the AQP4-mediated water flux through Müller cells is required for the synaptic excitability is supported by the fact that deletion of AQP4 in mice results in reductions of the electroretinogram b-wave (generated by ON bipolars; Stockton and Slaughter, 1989) and oscillatory potentials (originating in the inner plexiform layer; Karwoski and Kawasaki, 1991), but not of the a-wave (generated by photoreceptors; Smith and Hamasaki, 1994) when compared to wildtype control (Li et al., 2002b).

As indicated by the glutamate-induced neuronal cell swelling (see 5.5.1.1.), the synaptic ion flux is associated with a flux of a huge amount of water. However, the paracellular water flux is largely restricted in the plexiform (synaptic) layers (see 5.5.4.1.). Because the synapses are closely ensheathed by Müller cell membranes, the rapid water flux into activated synapses occurs predominantly from the Müller cell interior, and is facilitated by AQP4 in the perisynaptic glial membranes (Fig. 40B) (Bringmann et al., 2005). Inhibition of the transglial water transport (from the blood and vitreous through Müller cells into the synapses) should delay the ion movement into activated synapses, resulting in a lower level of neuronal activity and swelling. This will have two consequences: (i) under normal conditions, inhibition of the AQP4-mediated water flux will decrease the light-induced activity of inner retinal neurons (Li et al., 2002b); and (ii) under ischemic conditions, inhibition of the AQP4-mediated water flux will decrease the rate of glutamate-induced neuronal hyperexcitation and degeneration (Fig. 40C) (Bringmann et al., 2005). Indeed, it has been shown that deletion of AQP4 in mice protects against impaired retinal function and cell death after ischemia (Da and Verkman, 2004). Further research is required to determine the functional significance of the AQP4-mediated water transport for the neuronal activity in the retina under physiological and pathological conditions.

5.5.4.7 AQP4-Mediated Suppression of Retinal Inflammation

Deletion of AQP4 in mice is associated with an upregulation of inflammatory proteins and enzymes including IL-1β, IL-6, and inducible NO synthase, and with a downregulation of the cyclooxygenase-2 in the retina, while other inflammatory factors such as TNFα are unaltered in their expression (Pannicke et al., 2010). The reason of the altered expression of inflammatory proteins in the retina of AQP4-null mice is unclear and could be related to osmotic stress (that increases the activity of inflammatory enzymes such as PLA_2 and NO synthases; Lambert et al., 2006) or to alterations in protein-protein interaction followed by changes in gene expression. It is known, for example, that AQP4 and NO synthases are clustered by dystrophin (Thomas et al., 1998; Liu et al., 1999) and that the AQP4-containing macromolecular complex in glial membranes includes other proteins such as glutamate transporters (Hinson et al., 2008). Whether the downregulation of cyclooxygenase-2 is an adaptation to avoid overproduction of prostaglandins, which induce Müller cell swelling in the presence of osmotic gradients (see 5.11.9.2.3.), remains to be determined. Upregulation of proinflammatory proteins may represent also a neuroprotective response to osmotic stress. Different inflammatory factors including IL-6 and NO were shown to have neuroprotective effects (Kashii et al., 1996; Mendonca Torres and de Araujo, 2001; Sanchez et al., 2003; Inomata et al., 2003; Chong et al., 2008).

Knockdown of AQP4 was shown to exacerbate experimental diabetic retinopathy through aggravating retinal inflammation and edema (Cui et al., 2012). AQP4 knockdown results in increased leukostasis, vascular permeability, and retinal thickness, in expression of proinflammatory factors including IL-1β, IL-6, and ICAM-1, and in upregulation of VEGF and GFAP in the retina of diabetic rats (Cui et al., 2012). High glucose induces upregulation of AQP4 in Müller cells (Cui et al., 2012). It was suggested that the increased expression of AQP4 in diabetic animals may represent a compensatory response against diabetic retinal edema (Cui et al., 2012). Deletion of AQP4 was also shown to exacerbate experimental glaucoma (Luo et al., 2012).

5.5.5   MÜLLER CELL VOLUME REGULATION

In addition to the modulation of the neuronal activity (see 5.6.1.3. and 5.6.3.4.), retinal gliotransmitters have autocrine effects, i.e., they mediate the propagation of glial calcium waves (see 5.6.3.3.) and the autocrine regulation of the Müller cell volume under varying osmotic conditions (Uckermann et al., 2006; Wurm et al., 2008a). In addition, retinal gliotransmitters may be involved in the cell volume regulation of retinal neurons (see 5.5.5.5.). Neuronal activity is associated with rapid ion shifts between intra- and extracellular spaces. Sodium, chloride, and calcium ions flow into active neurons, and potassium ions are released from neurons and taken up by glial cells. Such ion shifts cause changes in the volume of neuronal cell structures, in particular of synapses, as well as changes in the osmotic balance in the tissue. Neuronal activity is associated with a swelling of neuronal cell bodies and synapses in the retina (see 5.5.1.1.); neuronal swelling results in a decreased extracellular space volume (Uckermann et al., 2004b). In addition, the ion flux into neurons (and that of potassium and sodium glutamate into Müller cells) decreases the osmolarity of the extracellular fluid (Dmitriev et al., 1999). In order to compensate the activity-dependent decreases in the extracellular space volume (which otherwise will cause neuronal hyperexcitation; Dudek et al., 1990; Chebabo et al., 1995), Müller cells should not swell (even when the extracellular fluid is hypoosmotic and when they take up neuron-derived osmolytes such as potassium and sodium-glutamate which both favor water influx and osmotic cell swelling), or even decrease their volume when the activated neurons swell. Indeed, it has been shown that the decrease in the extracellular space volume in retinal slices superfused with glutamate is lower than expected when only the swelling of neuronal cell bodies is considered (Uckermann et al., 2004b).

While retinal neurons display a rapid swelling of their cell bodies upon stimulation with glutamate (see 5.5.1.1.), glutamate does not induce a rapid swelling of Müller cells (Fig. 38B) (Vogler et al., 2013a). A swelling of Müller cells is only seen cells after prolonged (1 h) stimulation with glutamate (Casper et al., 1982; Izumi et al., 1996, 1999). Müller cells also do not display cellular swelling for up to 10–15 min when the extracellular fluid becomes hypoosmotic (Figs. 50A, 57D) (Uckermann et al., 2006; Hirrlinger et al., 2008; Lipp et al., 2009; Wurm et al., 2010; Brückner et al., 2012). This cell volume homeostasis is similar to that observed in protoplasmatic astrocyte somata in hippocampal slices (which display cell volume homeostasis for ~7 min under hypoosmotic conditions) but different to Bergmann glial cell somata in cerebellar slices which display immediate swelling in response to hypoosmotic stress (Hirrlinger et al., 2008). Similarly, astrocytes in cortical slices display immediate swelling followed by a regulatory volume decrease (Thrane et al., 2011). Apparently, different astrocytic cell types display distinct osmotic properties and volume-regulatory mechanisms. In addition, different mechanisms may be present in somata and processes of hippocampal astrocytes (Hirrlinger et al., 2008).

Generally, cells possess a number of adaptive mechanisms that allow them to survive varying osmotic conditions by restoration of the osmotic balance. The cell survival under anisoosmotic conditions is initially mediated by ion fluxes across the plasma membrane through ion channels and transporters and thereafter by cellular accumulation or release of small organic osmolytes such as glutamate, sorbitol, myo-inositol, and taurine. The homeostasis of the Müller cell volume under hypoosmotic conditions is mediated by various mechanisms including: (i) Kir4.1- and AQP4-mediated potassium and water transport; (ii) activation of an endogenous purinergic signaling cascade that prevents cellular swelling; and (iii) release of amino acid osmolytes such as taurine.

5.5.5.1 Kir4.1-Dependent Cell Volume Regulation

Müller cells display a highly efficient cell volume regulation which compensates for a decrease (but not an increase; Figs. 8I, 38B; Pannicke et al., 2004; Vogler et al., 2013a) of the extracellular osmolarity. The cell volume regulation largely depends on the activity of weakly rectifying Kir4.1 potassium channels. Inhibition of the Kir channel-mediated potassium efflux by barium ions causes an immediate swelling of Müller cell bodies under hypoosmotic stress (Figs. 50C,D, 57D,F,G, 61F) (Pannicke et al., 2004; Uckermann et al., 2006; Wurm et al., 2006a,b, 2008b, 2009b, 2010; Hirrlinger et al., 2008; Krügel et al., 2010; Brückner et al., 2012). There is a direct relation between the amplitude of the barium-blocked Kir currents and the severity of the hypoosmotic swelling of Müller cells (Fig. 57E) (Pannicke et al., 2004). The Kir channels of Müller cells display a high open probability between 0.8 and 0.9 around the resting membrane potential (Fig. 59C) (Newman, 1993; Ishii et al., 1997; Bringmann et al., 1999a,b). The high open probability allows a prompt bidirectional flux of potassium across the plasma membrane which compensates for the osmotic gradient. Rapid transmembrane potassium currents may explain the lack of Müller cell swelling under hypoosmotic conditions (Bringmann et al., 2005; Wurm et al., 2006a).

If the regulation of the Müller cell volume under varying osmotic conditions depends upon the transmembrane potassium currents through Kir channels, the cells should display an impaired cell volume regulation when they lack functional Kir4.1 channels, i.e., in the early postnatal stage before differentiation into mature cells (Figs. 46C, 58A, 59D, 61A, 63B) (Bringmann et al., 1999a, 2000a; Pannicke et al., 2002; Schopf et al., 2004; Wurm et al., 2006b), under various pathological conditions which are characterized by a downregulation of functional Kir4.1 channels (see 5.5.3.5.), and in cultured Müller cells (Kuhrt et al., 2008). Indeed, under these conditions, hypoosmotic stress induces a rapid swelling of Müller cells (Figs. 8I, 12M, 21E, 50A,B, 57F, 61C,E, 73A) (Pannicke et al., 2004, 2005b, 2006; Uckermann et al., 2006; Weuste et al., 2006; Wurm et al., 2006a,b, 2008a, b, 2011a; Iandiev et al., 2006b, 2008a; Kuhrt et al., 2008; Rehak et al., 2009; Wurm et al., 2009b; Krügel et al., 2010; Neumann et al., 2010). There is an inverse relation between the amplitude of Kir currents and the severity of osmotic cell swelling during the early postnatal stage (Figs. 58A, 61A,C) (Wurm et al., 2006b). Around the time of eye opening at the end of the second postnatal week, developing rat Müller cells begin to express Kir4.1 channels (simultaneously with AQP4 water channels; Fig. 49); this is associated with a steep increase of the potassium conductance (Fig. 58A, 61A) (Wurm et al., 2006b). Mature Müller cells display large Kir currents and no significant swelling in response to osmotic stress (Fig. 61F) whereas immature Müller cells in the first two postnatal weeks display small Kir currents and a significant osmotic swelling (Fig. 58A, 61A,C,E) (Wurm et al., 2006b). There is also an inverse relation between the pathological downregulation/inactivation of Kir4.1 channels and the severity of Müller cell swelling under hypoosmotic conditions (Figs. 12N) (Pannicke et al., 2004, 2005b, 2006; Wurm et al., 2006a, 2011a; Iandiev et al., 2008a; Wurm et al., 2011a; Grosche et al., 2012). Retinal ischemia and Kir channel-blocking barium ions induce a similar osmotic swelling of Müller cells (Fig. 57F) (Uckermann et al., 2006; Wurm et al., 2006a). In rat Müller cells, there is an inverse relation between the severity of osmotic swelling under control conditions and in the presence of Kir channel-blocking barium ions (Fig. 61C,D) (Pannicke et al., 2004; Wurm et al., 2006b). The induction of osmotic Müller cell swelling, which is not observed in cells from healthy control tissues, suggests that the rapid water transport across Müller cell membranes is altered when the cells become gliotic and downregulate Kir4.1. The downregulation of Kir4.1 channels will impair the retinal potassium and water homeostasis which may contribute to retinal degeneration and the development of retinal edema (see 5.11.5. and 5.11.9.1.2.). The proposed mechanism of glial cell swelling may have impact not only for the retina but also for the brain because a decrease of Kir currents was also found in reactive brain astrocytes (Schröder et al., 1999; D'Ambrosio et al., 1999; Köller et al., 2000; Hinterkeuser et al., 2000).

5.5.5.2 AQP4-Dependent Cell Volume Regulation

The water flux through AQP4 is implicated in the rapid volume regulation of Müller cells in response to osmotic stress. Müller cells of AQP4-null mice (Fig. 9A), but not of wildtype mice,

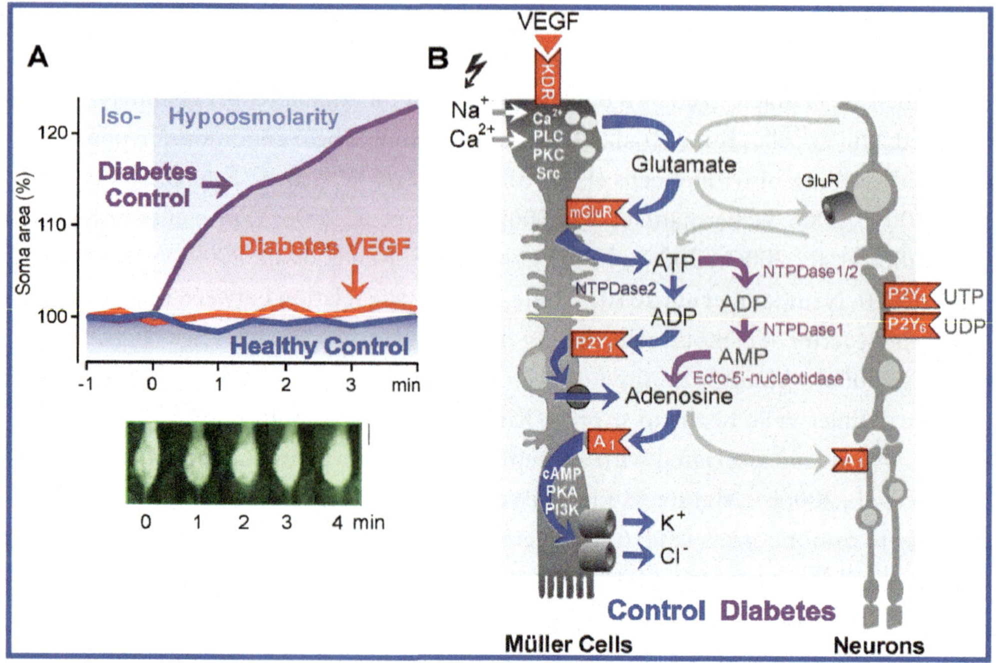

FIGURE 73: The release of the gliotransmitters glutamate, ATP, and adenosine is involved in the VEGF-induced prevention of osmotic soma swelling of Müller cells. **A.** Under hypoosmotic conditions, Müller cells in retinas of diabetic rats display a time-dependent swelling of their somata, a response not observed in Müller cells of control rats. The osmotic Müller cell swelling is prevented by VEGF (10 ng/ml). *Image above*, soma of a Müller cell before (*left*) and during (*right*) hypoosmotic exposure. Scale bar, 5 μm. **B.** Scheme of the autocrine glutamatergic-purinergic signaling cascade involved in the VEGF-induced inhibition of the osmotic swelling of rat Müller cells. Activation of KDR/flk-1 by VEGF induces a calcium-, phospholipase C (PLC)-, protein kinase C (PKC)-, and Src kinase-dependent exocytotic release of glutamate from Müller cells. Voltage-gated sodium channels mediate rapid fluctuations of the membrane potential required for the activation of voltage-gated calcium channels implicated in the exocytosis of glutamate-containing vesicles. Glutamate activates metabotropic glutamate receptors (mGluRs) that results in a calcium-independent release of ATP from Müller cells. ATP is extracellularly converted by the nucleoside triphosphate diphosphohydrolase-2 (NTPDase2) to ADP that activates $P2Y_1$ receptors, resulting in nucleoside transporter-mediated release of adenosine. Activation of A_1 adenosine receptors causes a cAMP-, protein kinase A (PKA)-, and phosphatidylinositol-3 kinase (PI3K)-dependent opening of potassium and chloride channels; the ion efflux equalizes the osmotic gradient across the plasma membrane and thus prevents water influx and cellular swelling under hypoosmotic stress conditions. In swollen cells, the ion efflux is associated with a water efflux, resulting in decreased cell volume. While the release of glutamate from Müller cells is calcium-dependent, all steps of the cascade after activation of mGluRs are calcium-independent. Neuron-derived glutamate and ATP may

activate the volume-regulatory signaling cascade in dependence on the neuronal activity. In the murine retina, activation of $P2Y_4$ and $P2Y_6$ receptors by UTP and UDP, respectively, might result in a release of neuronal ATP and glutamate that activate glial receptors. Müller cell-derived glutamate and adenosine may also activate neuronal glutamate receptors (GluR) and A_1 receptors, resulting in stimulation and inhibition, respectively, of neuronal activity. In the retinal parenchyma of diabetic rats, NTPDase1 (which hydrolyses ATP and ADP about equally well) is upregulated, and extracellular formation of adenosine contributes to the swelling-inhibitory effect of glutamate and ATP. Modified from Uckermann et al. (2006) and Wurm et al. (2008a,b).

display a swelling of their cell bodies under hypoosmotic conditions mediated by an influx of sodium ions (Fig. 9B,C), suggesting that Müller cells from AQP4-null mice are more sensitive to osmotic stress than cells from wildtype mice (Pannicke et al., 2010). In contrast, Müller cells from both wildtype and AQP4-null animals swell during hypoosmotic exposure in the presence of the Kir channel blocker barium chloride (Fig. 9B,C) (Pannicke et al., 2010). Müller cells of AQP4-null animals swell significantly later (by ~1 min) in the absence than in the presence of barium (Fig. 9B) (Pannicke et al., 2010). The reason for this delay in the swelling induction is unclear. It was suggested that during the early time period, the cell volume regulation is mediated by potassium efflux through Kir4.1; however, the concomitant water flux across the plasma membrane seems to be insufficient in cells from AQP4 null animals, resulting in a delayed swelling of the cells (Pannicke et al., 2010). Other possibilities are an effect of AQP4 deletion on the autocrine purinergic signaling which normally regulates Müller cell volume under hypoosmotic conditions (see 5.5.5.3.) and the presence of a low-level inflammation and enhanced oxidative stress level in the retina of AQP4-null mice (see 5.5.4.7.) which renders Müller cells more susceptible to osmotic stress. Oxidative stress and production of inflammatory lipid mediators by PLA_2 and cyclooxygenases are causative factors of the osmotic swelling of AQP4-null Müller cells (Pannicke et al., 2010). The role of AQP4 in the Müller cell volume homeostasis remains to be clarified.

5.5.5.3 Receptor-Dependent Cell Volume Regulation

Müller cells of the rodent retina possess a volume-regulatory endogenous glutamatergic-purinergic signaling cascade that inhibits cellular swelling under hypoosmotic conditions. This signaling cascade consists of the consecutive release of glutamate, ATP, and adenosine from Müller cells which activate mGluRs, purinergic $P2Y_1$, and adenosine A_1 receptors, respectively (Fig. 73B) (Uckermann et al., 2006; Wurm et al., 2008a, 2009b, 2010, 2011b; Krügel et al., 2010). ATP is extracellularly catabolized to ADP by the action of the ecto-ATPase (CD39L1, nucleoside triphosphate diphosphohydrolase-2, NTPDase2). ADP activates P2Y$_1$, which triggers the release of adenosine from Müller cells via nucleoside transporters (Uckermann et al., 2006; Wurm et al., 2006b, 2008a). Activation of this autocrine signaling cascade results in the opening of potassium and chloride channels in the Müller cell membrane; the ion efflux compensates the osmotic gradient across the plasma membrane and thus prevents the swelling of Müller cells under hypoosmotic conditions (Uckermann et al., 2006; Wurm et al., 2008a,b, 2009b, 2010). In swollen Müller cells, the ion efflux is associated with water efflux from the cells, resulting in a reduction in the cell volume (Fig. 50B) (Uckermann et al., 2006). The ion channel-activating action of adenosine is mediated by activation of the adenylyl cyclase, PKA, and PI3K (Uckermann et al., 2006; Wurm et al., 2008a, 2009b). Originally, adenosine A$_1$ receptors were described to interact mainly with G$_i$ proteins which inhibit the adenylyl cyclase (Fredholm et al., 2001). However, A$_1$ receptors have also been reported to interact with different G proteins (Baker and Hill, 2007), or even independent of G proteins (Tabata et al., 2007; Cao et al., 2007). In dependence on the receptor density, or in dependence on the adenosine concentration, A$_1$ receptors may couple to stimulating G proteins resulting in increased activity of the adenylyl cyclase (Cordeaux et al., 2000; Finkelberg et al., 2006; Baker and Hill, 2007). The type of the second messenger-activated potassium channels that open after activation of adenosine A$_1$ receptors is unclear. Because these channels are barium-insensitive, they are distinct from Kir channels and probably comprise two pore-domain potassium channels that are present in Müller cells (see 5.5.3.10.). Two pore-domain potassium channels mediate outward potassium currents (Fig. 55); therefore, opening of these channels may mediate the cell volume regulation under pathological conditions which are associated with an absence of the Kir4.1 channel-mediated outward potassium currents (Fig. 7A,B) (Pannicke et al., 2004). In Müller cells which express BK channels (see 5.5.3.8.), ATP-induced activation of BK channels (Fig. 64A,C) may contribute to the regulation of Müller cell volume under hypoosmotic conditions (Puro, 1991a). The autocrine purinergic signaling may also prevent the osmotic swelling of Müller cell compartments that lack Kir4.1 channels and that are electrotonically uncoupled from the Müller cell stem processes, e.g., of the thin perisynaptic processes (Kofuji et al., 2002).

The release of ATP is induced by activation of group I/II mGluRs (Uckermann et al., 2006; Wurm et al., 2008a, 2010; Krügel et al., 2010). The volume-regulatory cascade can be activated upstream of the vesicular release of glutamate (see 5.6.1.2.) by various different receptor ligands including VEGF (Fig. 73A), neuropeptide Y (NPY) (Fig. 50A–C), agonists of EGF and natriuretic peptide receptors, erythropoietin (Fig. 50D), sex steroids, osteopontin, and NGF (Uckermann et al., 2006; Weuste et al., 2006; Kalisch et al., 2006; Wurm et al., 2008a; Krügel et al., 2010; Neumann et al., 2010; Linnertz et al., 2011; Brückner et al., 2012; Slezak et al., 2012; Grosche et al., 2013; Wahl et al., 2013; Garcia et al., 2014). Some of the agonists such as erythropoietin and osteopontin werde found to trigger this cascade by inducing a release of VEGF from Müller cells via activation of JAK and ERK1/2 (Krügel et al., 2010; Wahl et al., 2013).

There are various differences in the cell volume-regulatory signaling cascade between Müller cells from rats and mice. First, whereas adenosine is released from rat Müller cells via nucleoside transporters (Uckermann et al., 2006; Wurm et al., 2008a), it is rather extracellularly formed by the ecto-5'-nucleotidase (CD73) in murine Müller cells (Wurm et al., 2009b, 2010). Second, whereas the swelling-inhibitory effect of ATP in rat Müller cells is calcium-independent, the effect of ATP (but not of adenosine) in murine Müller cells is calcium-dependent (Wurm et al., 2010). In retinal slices from wildtype mice, chelation of calcium with BAPTA/AM induces a rapid swelling of Müller cells under hypoosmotic conditions (Lipp et al., 2009). Müller cells in retinas of IP_3R2-deficient mice start swelling as soon as hypoosmotic exposure begins (Lipp et al., 2009). In retinal slices from IP_3R2-deficient mice, adenosine (but not ATP) prevents the osmotic swelling of Müller cells, suggesting that the autocrine $P2Y_1$ signaling is not functional (Wurm et al., 2010; Grosche et al., 2013). The reasons for the species differences remain to be determined.

In addition to the release of ATP induced by the activation of mGluRs, Müller cells also release ATP upon mechanical stimulation (Newman, 2001a,b, 2003b). It has been suggested that membrane stretch induced by osmotic pertubations as occurring during intense neuronal activity (Dmitriev et al., 1999) triggers the release of ATP from Müller cells (Fig. 43G) which, via autocrine activation of $P2Y_1$ and (in murine cells) intracellular calcium signaling, prevents the osmotic swelling of the cells (Wurm et al., 2010; Krügel et al., 2010). The assumption that Müller cells release ATP upon osmotic/mechanical stress is supported by the following facts: although osmotic stimulation does not usually induce a swelling of Müller cells, it induces a swelling when antagonists of $P2Y_1$ or adenosine A_1 receptors (or inhibitors of potassium and chloride channels) are present in the extracellular solution (Wurm et al., 2009b, 2010; Krügel et al., 2010, 2011). (A blockade of $P2Y_1$ or A_1 receptors results in oxidative stress [Krügel et al., 2011], a main factor which contributes to the induction of osmotic Müller cell swelling in response to osmotic pertubations; see 5.11.9.2.3.) Hypoosmotic stress does not induce a swelling of Müller cells in retinal slices from wildtype mice, whereas it induces an instantaneous swelling of Müller cells in retinal tissues of $P2Y_1$-, adenosine A_1 receptor-, and ecto-5'-nucleotidase-deficient mice (but not in retinal slices from $P2Y_{14}$-deficient mice) (Wurm et al., 2010). Thus, two different mechanisms may induce a release of ATP from Müller cells: glutamate receptor-dependent release and a receptor-independent release induced by osmotic membrane stretching. It cannot be ruled out that osmotic membrane stretch also induces a vesicular release of glutamate. Disruption of the calcium-dependent vesicular exocytosis of glutamate from Müller cells in bigenic BoNT/B mice resulted in a rapid swelling of Müller cells under hypoosmotic conditions (Fig. 74D) (Slezak et al., 2012). Müller cells of bigenic BoNT/B mice

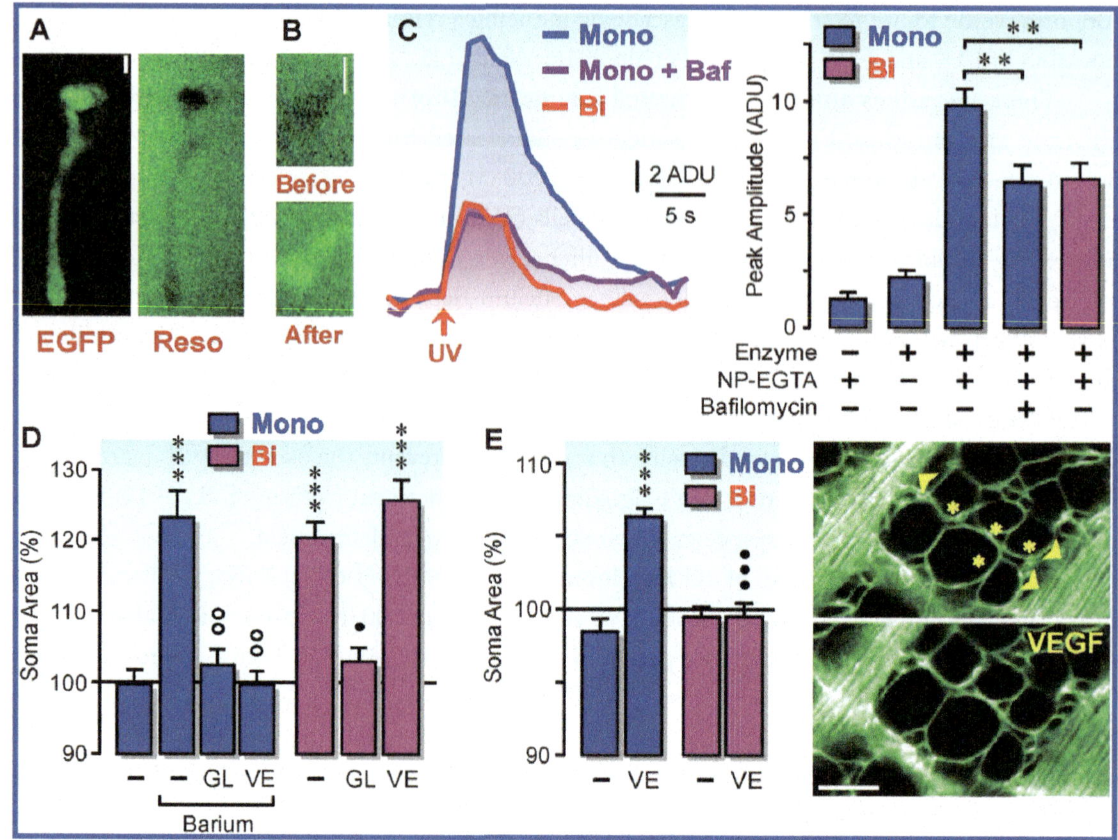

FIGURE 74: Neuronal and autocrine effects of Müller cell-derived glutamate released by calcium-dependent vesicular exocytosis in the mouse retina. The experiments were done with freshly isolated Müller cells (**A–C**), retinal slices (**D**), and retinal wholemounts (**E**) from mono- and bigenic BoNT/B mice. Bigenic BoNT mice expressed botulinum toxin B in glial cells where it cleaved vesicle-associated membrane proteins and thereby disrupted exocytosis. **A–C.** Detection of extracellular glutamate with an enzyme-based assay that resulted in the generation of resorufin. Müller cells were genetically labeled with enhanced green-fluorescent protein (EGFP). Shortly before the experiments, they were loaded with the calcium chelator NP-EGTA. The release of glutamate from the cells was evoked by UV light-induced uncaging of calcium from the chelator. **A.** Micrographs depicting intracellular EGFP (*left*) and extracellular resorufin (*right*) fluorescence in Müller cell acutely isolated from the retina of a bigenic animal. Resorufin was generated outside the cell as enzymes and substrates were added to the extracellular gel matrix. Scale bar, 5 μm. **B.** Higher-magnification micrographs showing resorufin fluorescence before and after UV stimulation above the endfoot of a Müller cell from a monogenic mouse. Scale bar, 5 μm. **C.** *Left:* Representative time course of the resorufin signal measured above the endfeet of acutely

isolated Müller cells. In cells from a monogenic mouse, the UV-induced fluorescence increase (*thick line*) was reduced by the inhibitor of the vesicular glutamate uptake, bafilomycin (200 nM; *thin line*), to an extent similar to that observed in Müller cells from a bigenic mouse (*dotted line*). ADU, analog-to-digital units. *Right:* Mean peak amplitude of the glutamate release from endfeet of isolated Müller cells from mono- and bigenic animals in the absence and presence of resorufin-generating enzymes, NP-EGTA, and bafilomycin, respectively. Note that Müller cells of bigenic mice released significantly ($P<0.01$) less glutamate when compared to cells from monogenic animals, and that bafilomycin decreased the glutamate release from Müller cells of monogenic mice. **D.** Mean cross-sectional area of Müller cell somata after superfusion for 4 min with a hypoosmotic solution (60% osmolarity), expressed in percent of the values measured before hypoosmotic challenge (100%). The data were recorded in the absence and presence of glutamate (GL; 1 mM) and vascular endothelial growth factor (VEGF; 30 ng/ml), respectively. Note that Müller cells of bigenic mice, but not cells of monogenic mice, displayed hypoosmotic swelling. Cells from monogenic mice swelled in the presence of barium chloride (1 mM). Glutamate prevented the hypoosmotic swelling of cells from both mono- and bigenic animals. VEGF prevented the swelling of cells from monogenic, but not from bigenic animals. **E.** *Left:* Mean cross-sectional area of neuronal somata in the ganglion cell layer measured in the absence and presence of VEGF (30 ng/ml; 15 min). VEGF induced neuronal swelling in retinas of monogenic, but not of bigenic mice. $**P<0.01$ $***P<0.001$, *vs.* monogenic mice control; $\bullet P<0.05$ *vs.* bigenic mice control; $\bullet\bullet\bullet P<0.001$ *vs.* monogenic mice VEGF; $\circ\circ P<0.01$ *vs.* monogenic mice barium control. *Right:* Representative micrograph of neuronal cell bodies (*) in the ganglion cell layer of a retina from a monogenic animal which swelled during superfusion of VEGF (30 ng/ml). Plasma membranes were visualized with a FM dye. *Arrowheads*, nerve fibers. Scale bar, 10 µm. Modified from Slezak et al. (2012).

---

display no vesicular but a non-vesicular calcium-dependent release of glutamate (Fig. 74C) (Slezak et al., 2012). Like Müller cells from control mice, cells from monogenic animals fail to swell under hypoosmotic conditions (Fig. 74D); this suggests that only the vesicular glutamate release is implicated in cell volume regulation.

In the retinas of $P2Y_1$-deficient mice, the cell volume-regulatory effect of $P2Y_1$ receptor activation is partially compensated by $P2Y_{13}$ receptors (Wurm et al., 2010). Because pharmacological inhibition of $P2Y_{13}$ receptors in the retina of wildtype mice does not prevent the osmotic swelling of Müller cells, $P2Y_{13}$ is probably upregulated in the retina of $P2Y_1$-deficient mice (Wurm et al., 2010). However, $P2Y_{13}$ receptors seem to be neither essential nor sufficient for the endogenous purinergic cell volume regulation because Müller cells of $P2Y_1$-deficient mice swell in the absence of exogenous ATP (Wurm et al., 2010). One can speculate that $P2Y_{13}$ receptors (in contrast to $P2Y_1$ receptors) are not localized in close proximity to the ATP release sites of Müller cells (Wurm et al., 2010).

Glutamate implicated in the cell volume regulation may be derived from Müller cells and retinal neurons (Uckermann et al., 2006; Wurm et al., 2008a, 2010). Thus, the swelling-inhibitory signaling cascade may be activated according to the neuronal activity, i.e, while glutamate induces a swelling of retinal neurons, it inhibits the swelling of Müller cells. This neuron-to-glia signaling may be involved in the regulation of the extracellular space volume and the neurovascular coupling (see 5.8.) under conditions of intense neuronal activity. In murine retinal slices, exogenous ATP, uridine 5'-triphosphate (UTP), and uridine 5'-diphosphate (UDP) inhibit the swelling of Müller cells whereas the swelling of isolated Müller cells is prevented by ATP but not by UTP or UDP (Wurm et al., 2010). This suggests that uracil nucleotides indirectly regulate the volume of Müller cells by activation of neuronal $P2Y_4$ and $P2Y_6$ receptors and neuron-to-glia signaling likely mediated by glutamate and ATP (Fig. 73B) (Newman, 2001a,b; Rillich et al., 2009).

5.5.5.3.1 Receptor-Dependent Cell Volume Regulation During Ontogenetic Development

The somata of immature Müller cells in the early postnatal rat retina swell upon hypoosmotic stimulation; the amplitude of the swelling decreases in the course of the differentiation of the cells to mature cells (Figs. 58A, 61C,E,F) (Wurm et al., 2006b). The decline in osmotic soma swelling is related to the increase in the Kir currents of Müller cells (Fig. 61A) and to the decrease in the somatic $P2Y_1$ receptor-mediated calcium responsiveness (Fig. 58A) (Wurm et al., 2006b, 2009a). Exogenous ATP acting at $P2Y_1$ receptors inhibits the osmotic swelling of immature Müller cells (Wurm et al., 2009a). These data suggest that immature Müller cells are incapable of releasing ATP upon osmotic/mechanical stimulation, whereas the swelling-inhibitory purinergic signaling cascade is effective after receptor stimulation. In the course of the postnatal differentiation, Müller cells attain the capacity to release ATP upon osmotic/mechanical stimulation; therefore, mature Müller cells are capable to effectively regulate their volume under hypoosmotic conditions. The data also suggest a developmental shift in the functional role of $P2Y_1$ receptors, from a mitogenic (see 5.10.2.4.) toward a cell volume-regulatory role (Wurm et al., 2009a). It is likely that the onset of the synaptic activity at the end of the first postnatal week (Johnson et al., 2003) induces these alterations in Müller cells (Wurm et al., 2009a). The changes in the neuronal activity after eye opening also influence these alterations because visual deprivation causes a delay in the postnatal maturation of the Kir channel expression and cell volume regulation in Müller cells (Wurm et al., 2006b).

Regulation of the cell volume by the activity of potassium and chloride channels is critically involved in cellular proliferation and migration (Voets et al., 1995; Rouzaire-Dubois and Dubois, 1998). Activation of $P2Y_1$ receptors induces proliferation of late retinal progenitor cells (see 5.10.2.4.). Because rapid cell shape alterations depend on transmembrane ion and water fluxes through potassium and chloride channels, and through AQPs (Eder, 2005; Saadoun et al., 2005;

Auguste et al., 2007; Wu et al., 2007), P2Y$_1$ receptor signaling may (in addition to mitogenic stimulation) also facilitate the osmotic cell shape alterations implicated in cellular proliferation and migration. The P2Y$_1$ receptor-mediated cell volume regulation may also support the extension of Müller cell processes that occurs during retinal development, induced in part by passive stretching of the retinal tissue due to the eye growth (Reichenbach et al., 1993b; Kuhrt et al., 2012).

5.5.5.3.2 Receptor-Dependent Cell Volume Regulation Under Pathological Conditions
The receptor-dependent regulation of the Müller cell volume may be especially important under pathological conditions that are associated with ionic and osmotic imbalances in the retinal tissue, with tissue stretching (caused by, for example, tractional forces which deform the retina in cases of retinal detachment and proliferative retinopathies; see 5.11.11.3.), and with an impaired volume regulation of Müller cells after downregulation of Kir4.1 channels (see 5.5.3.5.). Hypoosmotic conditions *per se* do not usually induce a swelling of Müller cells in slices of control retinas; however, in the presence of additional pathogenic agents such as hydrogen peroxide (which induces oxidative stress), inflammatory lipids such as arachidonic acid and PGE$_2$ or after inactivation of Kir4.1 channels by barium ions (see 5.5.3.2.), hypoosmotic challenge induces instantaneous swelling of Müller cells (Pannicke et al., 2004; Uckermann et al., 2005c). Osmotic swelling of Müller cells (without additional administration of pathogenic agents) was observed in animal models of various different retinopathies and in the detached human retina (see 5.11.9.2.2.).

Although hypoosmotic challenge induces Müller cell swelling under these pathological conditions, administration of various receptor ligands including VEGF, erythropoietin, glutamate, ATP, or adenosine inhibits the swelling of Müller cells (Uckermann et al., 2006; Wurm et al., 2011a,b; Krügel et al., 2010; see 5.5.5.3.). The swelling-inhibitory effect of receptor ligands suggests that the receptor-dependent release of ATP from Müller cells is functional under pathological conditions, whereas the release of ATP induced by osmotic membrane stretch is abrogated. The mechanism and the functional relevance of the abrogation of the osmotic/mechanical release of ATP are unclear. Such abrogation might prevent an excess release of glial ATP which would otherwise disturb regular neuronal information processing and may even induce neuronal death (see 5.6.3.4.). The abrogation of the mechanical stress-induced release of ATP from Müller cells might be also glio-protective, i.e., it avoids a cytotoxic calcium overload due to excess activation of P2Y$_1$ receptors by ATP. In addition, it prevents an excessive ATP-induced release of growth factors from the cells (see 5.11.10.3.). A further neuroprotective mechanism might involve the upregulation of NTPDase1 by Müller cells (see 5.5.5.3.3.). Both mechanisms may decrease the extracellular availability of ATP. A decrease in the extracellular ATP level may lead to a resensitization of P2Y receptors that were desensitized by ATP (Weick et al., 2005); the resensitization of P2Y receptors may contribute to the enhanced calcium responsiveness of Müller cells to P2Y activation under pathological conditions (see 5.10.2.5.). The increase of the calcium responsiveness upon purinergic receptor activation may also facilitate the osmotic cell shape alterations implicated in the proliferation and migration of reactive Müller cells.

5.5.5.3.3 Involvement of Ecto-Nucleotidases in Cell Volume Regulation In the retina, extracellular nucleotides are degraded by ecto-enzymes while adenosine is taken up through nucleoside transporters. Both retinal neurons and glial cells take up adenosine (Ehinger and Perez, 1984). Cultured rat Müller cells express mRNAs of nucleoside transporters (ENT1-2 and CNT1-2) which take up adenosine in a sodium-independent and concentration-dependent manner (Akanuma et al., 2013). The transporter-mediated uptake of adenosine is stimulated by ERK1/2 (Dos Santos-Rodrigues et al., 2011). In the rat retina, the purinergic cascade of swelling inhibition involves the extracellular degradation of ATP to ADP (both of which are agonists of P2Y$_1$ receptors; Abbracchio et al., 2006) and the release of adenosine from Müller cells mediated by nucleoside transporters (Fig. 73B) (Uckermann et al., 2006; Wurm et al., 2008a,b, 2009b). The failure of the extracellular formation of adenosine from ATP can be explained with the distribution of NTPDases in the retina.

Extracellular adenosine can be formed by phosphohydrolysis of adenosine 5'-monophosphate (AMP) through the action of the ecto-5'-nucleotidase. In addition to neuronal cell bodies in the ganglion cell and inner nuclear layers, Müller cells display immunoreactivity and histochemical activity of ecto-5'-nucleotidase (Fig. 75) (Kreutzberg and Hussain, 1982; Hussain and Baydoun, 1985; Braun et al., 1995; Iandiev et al., 2007b; Wurm et al., 2008b). However, extracellular adenosine formation is not involved in the glutamatergic-purinergic regulation of the Müller cell volume in the rat retina (Uckermann et al., 2006; Wurm et al., 2008b). On the other hand, an inhibitor of NTPDases (ecto-ATPases) blocked the glutamatergic-purinergic regulation of the Müller cell volume (Uckermann et al., 2006; Pannicke et al., 2006; Wurm et al., 2008b), suggesting the involvement of extracellular degradation of ATP to ADP (Fig. 73B).

There are various extracellular ATP-degrading ecto-enzymes including NTPDases and alkaline phosphatases. NTPDase1 (ecto-apyrase) and NTPDase2 (ecto-ATPase), as well as NTPDases 3 and 8, are capable of hydrolyzing nucleoside 5'-tri- and diphosphates such as ATP and ADP, albeit with considerably different substrate preferences. Whereas NTPDase1 hydrolyzes ATP and ADP to a similar extent (resulting in an immediate formation of the ecto-5'-nucleotidase substrate AMP), NTPDase2 preferentially hydrolyzes ATP to ADP, and only very slowly ADP to AMP (the ATP-to-ADP hydrolysis ratio is approximately 10:1; Failer et al., 2003). NTPDases 3 and 8 exhibit intermediate substrate preferences (Zimmermann, 2001).

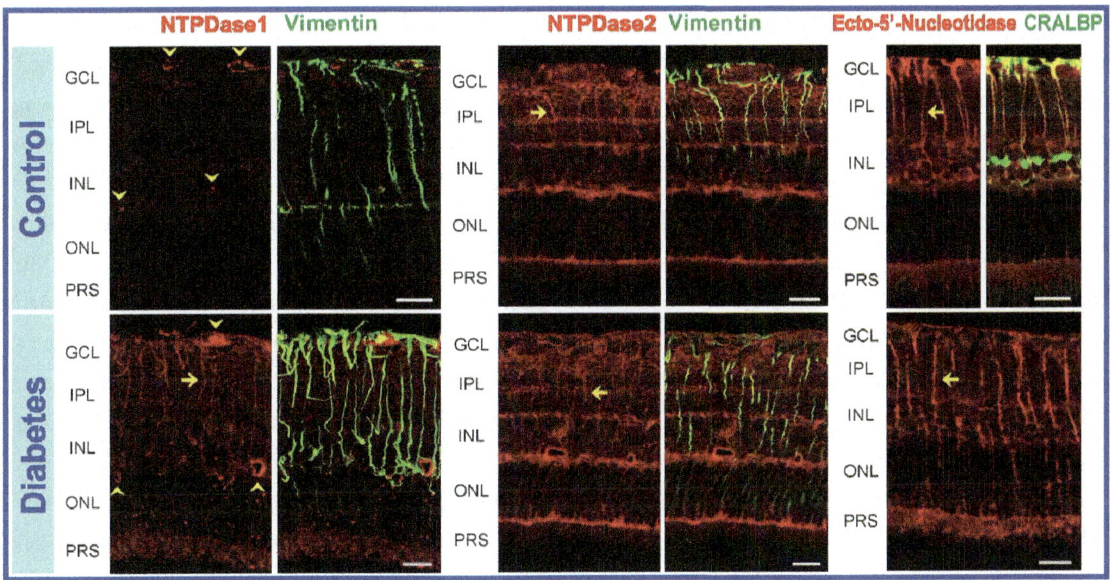

FIGURE 75: Immunolocalization of nucleotide-degrading ecto-enzymes in retinal slices from control (*above*) and diabetic rats (*below*). The slices were stained against the nucleoside triphosphate diphosphohydrolase-1 (NTPDase1), NTPDase2, and ecto-5'-nucleotidase, respectively (*red*). The slices were counterstained against the glial proteins vimentin and cellular retinaldehyde-binding protein (CRALBP), respectively (*green*). *Arrows*, Müller cell fibers traversing the inner plexiform layer (IPL). *Arrowheads*, blood vessels. Note that the immunolabeling of NTPDase1 is restricted to the blood vessels in the control retina, while in the retina of the diabetic animal, NTPDase1 immunoreactivity is also localized to Müller cell fibers. GCL, ganglion cell layer; INL, inner nuclear layer; ONL, outer nuclear layer; PRS, photoreceptor segments. Bars, 20 μm. Modified from Wurm et al. (2008b).

In human and rat retinas, two ATP-degrading ecto-enzymes are localized to different compartments: NTPDase1 is exclusively localized to the retinal vasculature, and NTPDase2 is localized to the retinal parenchyma, e.g., Müller cells (Fig. 75) (Lutty and McLeod, 1992; McLeod et al., 2006; Iandiev et al., 2007b; Wurm et al., 2008b). Alkaline phosphatase activity is virtually absent in the rat retina (Iandiev et al., 2007b). Ecto ATPase activity was also found in synaptic membranes (Puthussery and Fletcher, 2007), suggesting that both retinal neurons and glial cells express NTPDase2. The distribution of NTPDase1 and -2 proteins in the rat retina corresponds well with enzyme histochemical data obtained in slices of the mouse retina that showed that ADP is degraded solely in the vasculature but not in the retinal parenchyma, whereas ATP is hydrolyzed throughout the retinal tissue (Iandiev et al., 2007b). Apparently, rodent Müller cells express enzymes for the rapid extracellular degradation of ATP and AMP (NTPDase2 and ecto-5'-nucleotidase), but not of ADP (due to the absence of NTPDase1 and the very slow ADPase activity of NTPDase2). This explains the fact that inhibition of the ecto-5'-nucleotidase does not prevent the swelling-inhibitory effects of glutamate and ATP in rat Müller cells, because the substrate of adenosine formation (AMP) is not generated in sufficient quantity at the surface of the cells.

In experimental diabetic retinopathy in rats, there is an alteration in the source of extracellular adenosine that is involved in regulation of Müller cell volume (Fig. 73B) (Wurm et al., 2008b). The expression of NTPDase1 is increased in Müller cells of diabetic rats compared to control animals (Fig. 75) (Wurm et al., 2008b). In retinas from diabetic animals, glutamate induces both a transporter-mediated release of adenosine from Müller cells and the extracellular generation of adenosine from ATP by the consecutive action of the NTPDase1 and the ecto-5'-nucleotidase (Fig. 73B) (Wurm et al., 2008b). The upregulation of NTPDase1 suggests that the availability of extracellular adenosine is increased in the retina of diabetic animals compared to the retina of control animals. Increased levels of extracellular adenosine are neuro- (see 5.6.3.4.) and glioprotective (e.g., by preventing cytotoxic cell swelling). NTPDase1 may clear ATP that is excessively released from Müller cells under conditions associated with osmotic and mechanical stress.

5.5.5.4 Cell Volume Regulation by the Release of Organic Osmolytes

Müller cells have also a receptor-independent mechanism of osmoregulation that occurs via the transmembrane transport of amino acid osmolytes such as taurine, homotaurine, and myo-inositol (Adler, 1983; Faff-Michalak et al., 1994; Faff et al., 1996, 1997; El-Sherbeny et al., 2004). The release of amino acid osmolytes is particularly important in cultured Müller cells and Müller cells in diseased retinas; under these conditions, Müller cells lack functional Kir4.1 channels (see 5.5.3.5.) and cannot regulate their volume by osmotic ATP release (see 5.5.5.3.2.). This leads to a prompt swelling of Müller cells under hypoosmotic conditions and an impairment of Müller cell shrinkage when the osmolarity of the extracellular fluid is changed back to the normal level (Fig. 50A) (Uckermann et al., 2006). Extracellular ammonia, high extracellular potassium, and hypoosmotic media induce a swelling of cultured Müller cells and a subsequent (cAMP-dependent and -independent) release of taurine from the cells (Faff-Michalak et al., 1994; Faff et al., 1996, 1997). In the rat retina, taurine and homotaurine are localized mainly to Müller cells (Schulze and Neuhoff, 1983). The release of taurine may be mediated by sodium- and chloride-dependent taurine transporters and volume-regulated anion channels (Adler, 1983; Faff-Michalak et al., 1994; El-Sherbeny et al., 2004; Ando et al., 2012). Receptor agonists may modulate the taurine transport through PKA- and PKC-mediated regulation of the number of transporter molecules in the plasma membrane (Loo et al., 1996).

5.5.5.5 Müller Cell-Mediated Volume Regulation of Bipolar Cells

Müller cells may also regulate the volume of retinal neurons which lack an autocrine volume regulation under hypoosmotic conditions. Hypoosmolarity of the extracellular fluid or glutamate cause a swelling of bipolar cells (Fig. 38B); the hypoosmotic swelling results from a release of endogenous glutamate (Vogler et al., 2013a). Glutamate also induces a swelling of retinal ganglion cell somata (Figs. 3B, 39A,B) (Uckermann et al., 2004b; Wurm et al., 2008a; see 5.5.1.1.). The glutamate-induced swelling of bipolar cells is abrogated by the inhibitory neurotransmitters adenosine and GABA, but not by VEGF and ATP (Vogler et al., 2013a). It has been shown that exogenous NGF indirectly prevents the swelling of bipolar cells under hypoosmotic conditions by inducing a release of cytokines from Müller cells (Garcia et al., 2014). NGF acting at the tropomyosin-related receptor kinase A (TrkA) activates the glutamatergic-purinergic signaling cascade in Müller cells (see 5.5.5.3.). Activation of this signaling cascade triggers a release of bFGF and possibly further cytokines like GDNF and TGF-β from Müller cells; these cytokines act directly on bipolar cells (Garcia et al., 2014). Although bipolar cells express TrkA, NGF did not directly inhibit the swelling of bipolar cells (Garcia et al., 2014). This suggests that TrkA is coupled to cell volume-regulatory intracellular signaling cascades in Müller cells but not in bipolar cells, and that the neuroprotective effect of NGF in the retina (see 5.11.7.2.) is in part mediated by the prevention of the cytotoxic glial and bipolar cell swelling.

5.5.6 REMOVAL OF CARBON DIOXIDE AND REGULATION OF EXTRACELLULAR pH

Light-induced neuronal activity generates extracellular alkalinization in the retina of up to 0.1 units (Borgula et al., 1989; Oakley and Wen, 1989; Yamamoto et al., 1992) which is caused, for example, by activation of neurotransmitter receptors, the release of ammonia from neurons, and the uptake of protons by Müller cells through electrogenic glutamate transporters (Coles et al., 1996; Owe et al., 2006; Beart and O'Shea, 2007). This pH shift is balanced by an efflux of protons, e.g., from the photoreceptor terminals (DeVries, 2001), and by the consecutive action of the enzyme carbonic anhydrase and acid-base transporters of Müller cells (Parthe, 1981; Newman, 1996). Carbonic anhydrases convert carbon dioxide and water to bicarbonate and protons. Müller cells express a number of acid-base transport systems, including a sodium-bicarbonate cotransporter, a chloride-bicarbonate anion exchanger, and a sodium-proton exchanger (Fig. 76) (Sarthy and Lam, 1978; Newman and Astion, 1991; Newman, 1991, 1996, 1999; Kobayashi et al., 1994). The sodium-bicarbonate cotransporter and the anion exchanger are localized preferentially to the endfeet of the cells (Newman and Astion, 1991; Newman, 1991, 1996). The sodium-bicarbonate carrier transports three bicarbonate molecules along with one sodium ion (Newman, 1991). Because the

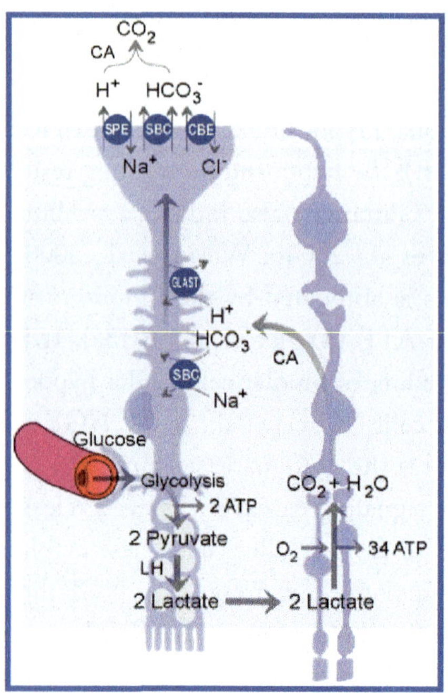

FIGURE 76: Carbon dioxide siphoning by Müller cells. The oxidative metabolism of retinal neurons and photoreceptors results in the formation of carbon dioxide and water from lactate/pyruvate which are in part produced in Müller cells. The carbonic anhydrase (CA) at the surface of Müller cells converts carbon dioxide and water into bicarbonate and protons which are taken up by the sodium-bicarbonate cotransporter (SBC) and the glutamate transporter GLAST, for example. Bicarbonate and protons are then preferentially released into the blood vessels and the vitreous by the concerted action of SBC, the chloride-bicarbonate exchanger (CBE), and the sodium-proton exchanger (SPE). LH, lactate dehydrogenase.

transporter is electrogenic, cell depolarization induced by increased extracellular potassium causes an influx of sodium and bicarbonate resulting in intracellular alkalinization in Müller cells and extracellular acidification; the efflux of acid equivalents buffers the light-induced extracellular alkalinization (Newman, 1996) and the glutamate transport-induced intracellular acidification (see 5.5.2.1.3.). Even the small depolarization-induced extracellular acidification generated by Müller cells may have a severe inhibitory effect on the synaptic transmission because, for example, an acidification of 0.05 units produces a 24% reduction in the synaptic transmission from photoreceptors to post-receptoral neurons (Barnes et al., 1993). The activity-dependent acid efflux from Müller cells represents a component of a negative feedback system which limits neuronal excitability and protects the neurons against overexcitation.

Oxidative degradation of glucose causes the formation of water and carbon dioxide (Fig. 76); both metabolic "waste products" are transported out of the retina through Müller cells. The retina is one of the most metabolically active tissues in the body and produces substantial amounts of carbon dioxide which must be removed to prevent tissue acidosis. By the removel of carbon dioxide, Müller cells also regulate the extracellular pH. Active neurons (in particular photoreceptors in the dark) release metabolic carbon dioxide which is rapidly hydrated to bicarbonate and protons by the enzyme carbonic anhydrase (Oakley and Wen, 1989). The soluble cytoplasmic carbonic anhydrase II (which constitutes 3% of the total protein of the chicken retina) is expressed by Müller cells and a subset of amacrine cells, while the membrane-bound carbonic anhydrase XIV is localized extracellularly on Müller cells, astrocytes, and vascular endothelia (Linser and Moscona, 1981; Kumpulainen et al., 1983; Linser et al., 1984; Vardimon et al., 1986; Palatroni et al., 1990; Newman, 1994; Ridderstråle et al., 1994; Ochrietor et al., 2005; Nagelhus et al., 2005). Bicarbonate is transported to the vitreous humor by sodium-bicarbonate cotransporters localized to the Müller cell endfeet (Fig. 76). The preferential localization of acid-base transport systems to Müller cell endfeet leads to a polarized "carbon dioxide siphoning" that augments the carbon dioxide transfer out of the retinal tissue (Newman, 1994). The membrane-bound carbonic anhydrase XIV is suggested to be the target of carbonic anhydrase inhibitors that enhance the subretinal fluid absorption in macular edema (Nagelhus et al., 2005). The recovery of intracellular pH following intracellular acidification of Müller cells is dependent on the sodium-proton exchanger.

5.5.7   METABOLIC SUPPORT OF PHOTORECEPTORS AND NEURONS

The retina has the highest metabolic demands of any tissue in the body, and the outer segments of the photoreceptors are the most metabolically active layer of the retina (Saari, 1987; Alder et al., 1990; Buttery et al., 1991; Linsenmeier et al., 1998; see 5.5.8.2.).

5.5.7.1   Glucose Metabolism

Photoreceptors and neurons of most mammalian retinas have an oxidative (or, at least, a mixed oxidative/glycolytic) energy metabolism while Müller cells rely mainly on (anearobic) glycolysis even if enough oxygen is available (Winkler, 1981; Poitry-Yamate et al., 1995; Wolburg et al., 1999). Because Müller cells lack the phosphoglucose isomerase-1, glycolysis proceeds entirely through the pentose phosphate pathway (Archer et al., 2004).

Glucose is crucial for the function of photoreceptors, retinal neurons, and glial cells. Exogenous glucose can be extracted from the retinal and choroidal circulation; endogenous glucose is generated from the breakdown of glycogen stores and by gluconeogenesis. Photoreceptors, retinal neurons, pigment epithelial cells, glial cells, and vascular endothelia express facilitative glucose transporters (GluT1-4), suggesting that they have the capability to transport exogenous glucose from the circulation (Kumagai et al., 1994; Watanabe et al., 1994; Nihira et al., 1995; Hosoya et al., 2008). In the brain, about half of the glucose leaving the capillaries crosses the extracellular space and directly enters neurons; the other half is taken up by astrocytes (Nehlig and Coles, 2007). Glucose transporters transfer also dehydroascorbic acid (vitamin C) across the blood-retinal barrier; vitamin C accumulates as reduced ascorbic acid in Müller cells (Woodford et al., 1983; Hosoya et al., 2008).

Müller cells are the "communicators" between vessels and neurons; they take up glucose from the circulation, metabolize glucose, and transfer monocarboxylates as energy substrates to neurons (see 5.5.7.2.). In the retina, the glucose uptake and metabolism occurs predominantly in the inner processes of Müller cells, localized to the inner plexiform and ganglion cell layers (Poitry-Yamate and Tsacopoulos, 1991; Poitry-Yamate et al., 2013) where glutamatergic signaling occurs and where rabbit Müller cells contain glycogen granula (see 5.2.). Müller cells may also take up extracellular lactate, transform it to glucose, and release it into the extracellular space, with no incorporation into glycogen (Goldman, 1990). Müller cells (as well as vascular endothelial cells and cone photoreceptors) also take up galactose (Keegan et al., 1985).

In the amphibian retina, the gluconeogenic pathway (synthesis of glucose from noncarbohydrates) is confined to Müller cells (Goldman, 1990). Glucagon and vasoactive intestinal peptide (VIP), or an increase of cAMP, stimulate gluconeogenesis, while VIP also inhibits the glycolytic flux (Goldman, 1990). In the rat retina, astrocytes, Müller cells, the inner segments of photoreceptors, and probably inner retinal neurons contain the muscle isozyme of fructose-1,6-bisphosphatase (Mamczur et al., 2010), an enzyme implicated in the regulation of gluconeogenesis. However, the activity of this enzyme in the rat retina is at least ten-fold lower than in other tissues which synthesize glycogen from non-carbohydrates, e.g., lungs and skeletal muscles, suggesting that gluconeogenesis does not play a significant role in retinal energy homeostasis but may be an auxiliary process enabling the removal of excess lactate and glutamate from the vicinity of neurons (Mamczur et al., 2010).

5.5.7.2 Supply of Monocarboxylates

The metabolization of glutamate in Müller cells is tightly coupled to the nutritive function of the cells; malfunction of the glutamate uptake and metabolism by Müller cells will also compromise the glia-mediated nutrition of retinal neurons. All retinal cells use glucose as primary energy substrate. In periods of intense neuronal activity (as in the dark), photoreceptors and neurons utilize monocarboxylates such as lactate and pyruvate as additional fuel for their oxidative energy metabolism. These monocarboxylates are formed in photoreceptors, and are derived from Müller cells (Poitry-Yamate and Tsacopoulos, 1991, 1992; Poitry-Yamate et al., 1995; Tsacopoulos and Magistretti, 1996; Winkler et al., 2000, 2003a,b, 2004a,b; Wood et al., 2005; Xu et al., 2007b). The neurotransmission in the retina is 80% faster in the dark than in the light; the increased neurotransmission is associated with an ~40% increase in aerobic glycolysis and an ~40% increase in the pyruvate consumption (Xu et al., 2007b). Half of the metabolic energy consumed in the retina (41% of oxygen uptake and 58% of glycolysis) is utilized to support the activity of the sodium-potassium-ATPase which maintains the dark current of photoreceptors and other cellular functions such as transmitter uptake (Ames et al., 1992). The metabolic interaction in periods of intense retinal activity has beneficial consequences for both photoreceptors (which survive the periods of metabolic stress associated with dark adaptation) and Müller cells (which are getting rid of the "unwarranted" acidic end product of their metabolism preventing them from acidotic damage).

The glycolytic metabolism of Müller cells produces various substrates for the oxidative metabolism of photoreceptors and neurons such as glutamine, lactate, pyruvate, alanine, and α-ketoglutarate (Fig. 44) (Poitry-Yamate et al., 1995; Kapetanios et al., 1998; Tsacopoulos et al., 1997a,b, 1998; Poitry et al., 2000; Xu et al., 2007b). The production of lactate in Müller cells is stimulated by glutamate (which also stimulates the uptake of glucose), ammonia, and potassium (Reichenbach et al., 1993a; Poitry-Yamate et al., 1995; Poitry et al., 2000; Marcaggi and Coles, 2001). Thus, agents released from activated neurons signal the neuronal energy requirements to Müller cells. Ammonia increases the formation of lactate by activating phosphofructokinase and inhibiting α-ketoglutarate dehydrogenase (Marcaggi and Coles, 2001).

In addition to the glutamine synthetase reaction, energy substrates are formed from glutamate in various other biochemical reactions such as transamination of pyruvate with glutamate to alanine and α-ketoglutarate, transamination of oxalacetate with glutamate to α-ketoglutarate and aspartate, and deamination of glutamate to α-ketoglutarate and ammonia (Fig. 44) (Tsacopoulos et al., 1997b; Poitry et al., 2000). By conversion to α-ketoglutarate, glutamate functions as a substrate for the tricarboxylic acid cycle in Müller cells (Kalloniatis and Napper, 2002; Ola et al., 2011b). Both the amidation of glutamate to glutamine and the oxidation of glutamate decreases the intracellular level of glutamate which is a precondition of an efficient glutamate uptake (Ola et al., 2011b). The conversion of glutamate to α-ketoglutarate is strongly reduced in Müller cells of diabetic rats; this results in increased glutamate levels in Müller cells which may contribute to the impaired glutamate uptake under diabetic conditions (Gowda et al., 2011; see 5.5.2.1.6.).

The transport of monocarboxylates through cellular membranes is facilitated by transport proteins. Müller cells, astrocytes, neurons, and retinal capillaries express different subtypes of monocarboxylate transporters (Bergersen et al., 1999; Gerhart et al., 1999; Chidlow et al., 2005; Martin et al., 2007; Ganapathy et al., 2008); loss of the transporters results in abnormal photoreceptor cell function and degeneration (Philp et al., 2003). Under culture conditions, inhibition of glucose transporters causes death of retinal glial cells, while inhibition of monocarboxylate transporters causes death of retinal neurons (Wood et al., 2005).

5.5.7.3 Glycogen and Creatine Metabolism

In the retina, glycogen synthesis from carbohydrates precursors, i.e., glyconeogenesis, might be a mechanism of metabolite and neurotransmitter (e.g., lactate and glutamate) removal during periods of high metabolic activity of retinal neurons and photoreceptors (Goldman and Witkovsky, 1987; Coffe et al., 2004). 11–15% of the glucosyl units in the glycogen of the amphibian retina are derived from C3 metabolites of the glycolytic pathway, presumably from lactate (Goldman, 1988). Glycogen is differentially distributed in retinas of various species. In the rabbit retina, glycogen particles are only present in Müller cells; in other species, Müller cells and subclasses of retinal neurons (ganglion cells, rod bipolars, distinct amacrines, the inner segments of photoreceptor cells) contain glycogen (Kuwabara and Cogan, 1961; Eichner and Themann, 1962; Newell and Kurimoto, 1963; Schabadasch and Schabadasch, 1972a; Johnson, 1977; Rhodes, 1984; Reichenbach et al., 1988a, 1993a; Niemeyer, 1997). Müller cells of the cat (vascularized retina) are filled uniformly with fine-grain glycogen throughout their whole cell bodies (Rungger-Brändle et al., 1996) while rabbit Müller cells (avascular retina) contain glycogen particles mainly in the inner part (Reichenbach, 1989; see 5.2.). In the rat retina, glycogen synthase is localized to Müller cells and the inner segments of photoreceptor cells (Pérezleón et al., 2013).

Glycogen is presumed to provide carbohydrate support to retinal neurons when the glucose supply of the tissue falls below its needs (Poitry-Yamate and Tsacopoulos, 1992; Poitry-Yamate et al., 1995). Short wavelength (blue) cone photoreceptors, distinct retinal neurons, and Müller cells express the brain isoform of glycogen phosphorylase (Reichenbach et al., 1993a; Pfeiffer et al., 1994; Nihira et al., 1995; Pfeiffer-Guglielmi et al., 2005; Rothermel et al., 2008). Glycogen is rapidly catabolized and resynthesized when the retina is stimulated by light (Schabadasch and Schabadasch, 1972b; Coffe et al., 2004) or during retinal ischemia-reperfusion (Johnson, 1977; Gohdo et al., 2001). Müller cells hydrolyze glycogen when they are exposed to elevated extracellular potassium, a signal that is involved in the regulation of neuronal-glial metabolic cooperation (Reichenbach et al., 1993a). The glycogen content of the rat retina is increased in response to high glucose, glutamate, and insulin (Pérezleón et al., 2013). Insulin increases the glycogen content of

Müller cells (Reichenbach et al., 1993a). Müller cells may produce insulin (Das et al., 1984, 1987) and have insulin receptors (see 5.10.10.; but see Fischer et al., 2009a).

In high-energy metabolic tissues like the retina, creatine and phosphocreatine play important roles in energy storage. Müller cells synthesize creatine; the creatine synthetic enzyme is colocalized with glutamine synthetase in the cells (Nakashima et al., 2005). The creatine transporter is localized to various cell types in the retina, including photoreceptors, amacrine, bipolar, and ganglion cells, blood vessels, and perivascular astrocytes, while Müller cells apparently lack this transporter (Acosta et al., 2005; Tachikawa et al., 2007).

5.5.7.4 Lipid Metabolism

The retina has the capacity both to synthesize cholesterol *de novo* and to take up blood-borne lipids (Fliesler and Keller, 1997). There is a lipid shuttle from Müller cells to neurons in supplying the needs of neurons for lipids, especially for the long axonal projection of retinal ganglion cells and the photoreceptor segments, as well as for synapse formation (Mauch et al., 2001). This shuttle involves both low- (LDL) and high-density lipoproteins (HDL). Circulating LDL enter the retina via the retinal pigment epithelium and Müller cells by a process mediated by LDL receptors which recognize ApoB (Tserentsoodol et al., 2006a). Müller cells and astrocytes synthesize ApoE and ApoJ which are assembled into cholesterol-rich lipoprotein particles (Boyles et al., 1985; Amaratunga et al., 1996; Shanmugaratnam et al., 1997; Kuhrt et al., 1997; Kurumada et al., 2007). These particles are secreted into the vitreous and subsequently taken up by retinal ganglion cells and transported centrally within the optic nerve (Amaratunga et al., 1996). Photoreceptor cells have receptors for ApoE (Kurumada et al., 2007); LDL receptors are localized to neurons and Müller cells (Tserentsoodol et al., 2006a). The ABCA1 transporter (responsible for the transport of ApoE and ApoA1, the major protein component of HDL) and the scavenger receptors SR-BI and SR-BII responsible for the HDL uptake are expressed by retinal neurons and photoreceptors (Tserentsoodolet al., 2006b).

Docosahexaenoic acid is required for the survival and differentiation of photoreceptors, for the renewal of their disc membranes, and to preserve the mitochondrial activity (Politi et al., 2001). Müller cells take up docosahexaenoic acid (Gordon and Bazan, 1990), incorporates it into phospholipids, and channels it to photoreceptors (Politi et al., 2001). Müller cells express fatty acid-binding and transfer proteins for the transport of docosahexaenoic acid and other fatty acids (Deguchi et al., 1992; Kingma et al., 1998). Fatty acids are considered to serve as a major energy source metabolized by fatty acid β-oxidation. The mitochondria of Müller cells and, to a lower level, restinal neurons contain fatty acid β-oxidation enzymes (Atsuzawa et al., 2010).

5.5.7.5 Metabolism of Toxic Compounds

Müller cells and photoreceptor cells express the sterol 27-hydroxylase (Lee et al., 2006) which is a mitochondrial P-450 enzyme that hydroxylates toxic oxysterols which are formed by photooxidation. Hydroxylation of cholesterol may also promote the efflux of cholesterol from the retina. The peroxisomes of Müller cells (Leuenberger and Novikoff, 1975; Beard et al., 1988; St Jules et al., 1992) may be involved in the metabolism of lipoproteins derived from photoreceptors. Müller cells express glutathione S-transferases (McGuire et al., 1996) which are involved in the detoxication of electrophilic xenobiotics. An increase in the expression of these enzymes may protect retinal neurons from environmental toxicants such as lead (McGuire et al., 1996, 2000). The immunoreactivity of the glutathione S-transferase, a biomarker of toxicant exposure, increases in Müller cells of mice exposed to aerosolized jet fuel; this finding has relevance for the Air Force personnel that clean and maintain fuel pods (McGuire et al., 2000).

Müller cells express the urea transporter UT3 (Berger et al., 1998). This transporter may mediate the equilibration of the retinal urea level by transport of excess urea into the blood vessels (Berger et al., 1998). UT3 expression is upregulated under pathological conditions (Berger et al., 1998), possibly as a result of increased urea levels during gliosis which is associated with increased polyamine formation (Biedermann et al., 1998).

5.5.8   SUPPORT OF PHOTORECEPTOR FUNCTION AND VIABILITY

In addition to the metabolic support (see 5.5.7.2.), the antioxidative support of photoreceptors under pathological conditions (see 5.5.2.1.15.), and the prosurvival effect of Müller cell-derived neurotrophic factors, growth factors, and cytokines (see 5.11.7.), Müller cells ensure the photoreceptor function and viability by various other functions. They protect the photoreceptors from the harmful effects of the circadian light exposure (see 5.5.8.2.), they promote the extension of rod photoreceptor neurites (Kljavin and Reh, 1991), they control the maturation of cone photoreceptor ribbon synapses (and prevent retinal degeneration) by the production of harmonin (Phillips et al., 2011), they contribute (in addition to retinal pigment epithelial cells) to the assembly of photoreceptor outer segments into stacked discs (Jablonski and Iannaccone, 2000), in part by the release of lactose and PEDF, and the production of isopropyl β-D-thiogalactoside, a permissive glycan (Jablonski et al., 1999; Wang et al., 2003, 2004, 2005b), and they phagocytize and degrade outer-segment disc shed from cone photoreceptors (Long et al., 1986). After retinal degeneration, photoreceptors might be regenerated from Müller cells (see 5.11.12.).

5.5.8.1 Recycling of Photopigments

The light-absorbing visual pigments in the photoreceptors (rhodopsin in rods, photopsins in cones) are composed of two molecular parts, an opsin protein and the chromophore 11-*cis* retinal (the aldehyde of vitamin A) (Reichenbach and Bringmann, 2012). Phototransduction is triggered by the photic conversion of 11-*cis* retinal to all-*trans* retinal which is subsequently reduced to all-*trans* retinol in the photoreceptor outer segments (Tsacopoulos et al., 1998). There are two retinoid or visual cycles that regenerate 11-*cis* retinal from all-*trans* retinol, the rod and the cone visual cycle (Muniz et al., 2007; Fleisch et al., 2008; Wang et al., 2009a; Fleisch and Neuhauss, 2010; Wang and Kefalov, 2011). While the rod-derived all-*trans* retinal is slowly (within 30-100 min) regenerated to 11-*cis* retinal by the retinal pigment epithelium, the cone-derived all-*trans* retinol is rapidly (within 5-12 min) processed in Müller cells. Müller cells convert all-*trans* retinol to 11-*cis* retinol which is subsequently oxidized to 11-*cis* retinal by a retinol dehydrogenase and released into the extracellular space for the uptake by cone photoreceptors (Das et al., 1992; Mata et al., 2002; Muniz et al., 2007). Retinal pigment epithelial and Müller cells express RDH10, an all-*trans* retinol dehydrogenase, in the microsomal fraction (Wu et al., 2004). RDH10 generates all-*trans* retinal which is the substrate for the photoisomerase retinal G protein-coupled receptor (RGR), an opsin found in pigment epithelial and Müller cells (Jiang et al., 1993; Pandey et al., 1994). RGR forms a complex with RDH5 (11-*cis* retinol dehydrogenase) that isomerizes all-*trans* retinal to 11-*cis* retinal, thus providing an alternate pathway to obtain *cis* retinoids in the visual cycle. In addition, Müller cells express dihydroceramide desaturase-1 as a retinol isomerase (Kaylor et al., 2013). The rapid supply of the cone chromophore through Müller cells is critical for extending the dynamic range of cones to bright light and for their rapid dark adaptation after light exposure (Wang et al., 2009a). However, the distinct pathways and enzymes implicated in the photopigment regeneration by Müller cells remain to be determined (Muniz et al., 2007).

Vitamin A (retinoids) are fat soluble molecules which need retinol binding proteins to be transfered in aqueous cytosolic and extracellular spaces. Müller cells express cellular retinol binding protein (CRBP), that binds all-*trans* retinol, and cellular retinal binding protein (CRALBP) (Figs. 49, 75, 77A,B) that binds 11-*cis* retinol and 11-*cis* retinal (Bunt-Milam and Saari, 1983; Bok et al., 1984; Eisenfeld et al., 1985). The zebrafish retina contains two CRALBP paralogs: CRALBP-A is exclusively expressed in the retinal pigment epithelium, and CRALBP-B is localized to Müller cells (Collery et al., 2008; Fleisch et al., 2008). The interphotoreceptor matrix, that surrounds the photoreceptor segments, contains the interphotoreceptor retinoid binding protein (IRBP) which transfers retinoids between cones and Müller cells, while the cone outer segments

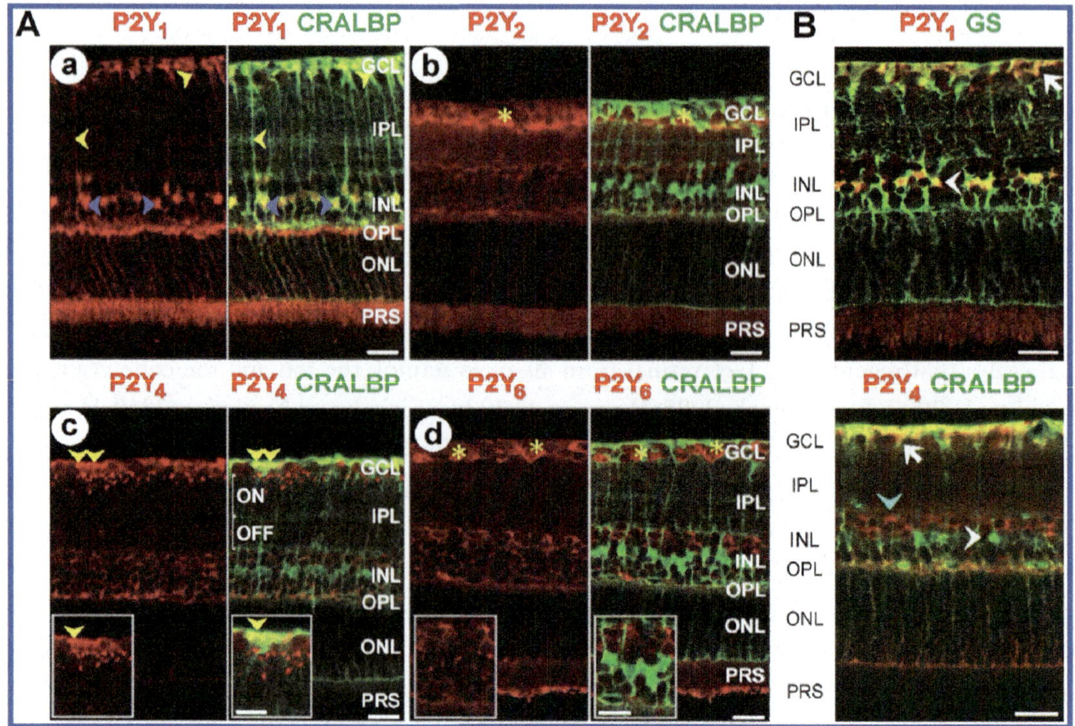

FIGURE 77: Subcellular localization of P2Y receptor proteins in rat (**A**) and murine (**B**) Müller cells. Retinal slices were costained against the glial cell markers glutamine synthetase (GS) and cellular retinaldehyde-binding protein (CRALBP), respectively; co-labeling yielded a *yellow-orange* merge signal. **A.** $P2Y_1$ and $P2Y_4$ receptor proteins, but not $P2Y_2$ and $P2Y_4$ receptor proteins, are localized to Müller cells of the rat retina. **a.** The $P2Y_1$ receptor protein (*red*) is enriched in Müller cell processes (*yellow arrowheads*) and somata (*blue arrowheads*). **b.** Müller cells do not display $P2Y_2$ immunoreactivity. Retinal ganglion cells (*asterisk*) and neuronal structures in the inner plexiform layer (IPL), inner nuclear layer (INL), and outer plexiform layer (OPL) display a faint staining. **c.** $P2Y_4$ receptor protein is enriched in the endfeet of Müller cells (*arrowheads*) and in perisynaptic glial membranes in the OPL. In addition, a band of globular structures, probably representing synapses of bipolar cells in the ON-sublamina (ON) of the IPL, is stained for this receptor subtype. **d.** The staining pattern of the $P2Y_6$ receptor protein is similar to that of $P2Y_2$ receptor protein. Retinal ganglion cells (*asterisks*) and neuronal somata in the INL display $P2Y_6$ immunoreactivity. The *insets* show the ganglion cell layer (GCL; **c**) and the INL (**d**) at higher magnification. **B.** Distribution of $P2Y_1$ and $P2Y_4$ receptor protein in slices of the murine retina. *Arrows*, Müller cell endfeet. *White arrowheads*, Müller cell somata. *Blue arrowhead*, $P2Y_4$-labeled amacrine cell soma. Note that Müller cell endfeet are immunoreactive for both $P2Y_1$ and $P2Y_4$ proteins, while Müller cell somata display immunoreactivity for $P2Y_1$, but not for $P2Y_4$ protein. $P2Y_4$ protein was also co-localized with CRALBP in the OPL and outer nuclear layer (ONL). GCL, ganglion cell layer; OFF, OFF-sublamina of the IPL; PRS, photoreceptor segments. Bars, 20 and 10 (*insets*) μm. Modified from Wurm et al. (2009a, 2010).

and the Müller cell microvilli have IRBP binding domains (Garlipp and Gonzalez-Fernandez, 2013). Müller cells synthesize components of the interphotoreceptor matrix such as laminin-β2 (Libby et al., 1997). Because CRALBP is also expressed by oligodendrocytes and in immature astrocytes during their developmental invasion of the retina (Saari et al., 1997; Johnson et al., 1997), it may have additional functions in addition to retinoid metabolism and visual pigment regeneration. Müller cells of distinct higher vertebrates also contain the cellular retinoic acid binding protein (CRABP) (Milam et al., 1990).

5.5.8.2 Circadian Protection of Photoreceptors

The glial production of neuroprotective factors such as bFGF and antioxidants is implicated in the protection of photoreceptors against the harmful effects of the circadian light exposure. The extremely high packing density of photoreceptor cells with their enormous energy demands to maintain the dark currents (Ames et al., 1992) makes the retina the organ of the body with the highest oxygen and glucose consumption per unit weight (Ames, 2000). Photoreceptors use 3–4 times more oxygen in the light-adapted state and 6–8 times more oxygen in the dark-adapted state than other neurons in the CNS, and are probably the cells of the body with the highest rate of oxidative metabolism (Alder et al., 1990; Linsenmeier et al., 1998). Oxygen is supplied to photoreceptors by the choriocapillaries. The choroidal blood flow shows little autoregulation in response to the oxygen requirements of photoreceptors (Bill and Sperber, 1990; Yu and Cringle, 2005). Therefore, the decrease of the oxygen consumption that occurs when photoreceptors go from a dark- to a light-adapted state causes a high increase of the oxygen tension in the outer retina (pO_2>30 mmHg; Yu and Cringle, 2001). Dark adaptation during the day decreases the oxygen tension especially in the synaptic layers and outer nuclear layer, where it reaches 0 mmHg (Linsenmeier, 1986; Ahmed et al., 1993).

Photoreceptors survive circadian periods of hyperoxia because retinal levels of antioxidants such as ascorbic acid, vitamin E, and glutathione are higher during light than in the dark (Penn et al., 1987), and because bFGF (a major neuroprotective factor of the retina; see 5.11.7.7.) is upregulated in the retina during the day, the time of higher oxygen exposure (Stone et al., 1999). Hypoxic states of photoreceptors in the dark are associated with an increase in the extracellular level of adenosine (which is, in addition to its neuromodulatory role, a neuroprotectant; see 5.6.3.4.); the increase in extracellular adenosine occurs by both a decrease in the transporter-mediated uptake of adenosine and an increase in the extracellular degradation of ATP released from neurons, astrocytes, and Müller cells (Ribelayga and Mangel, 2005).

5.6   REGULATION OF NEURONAL ACTIVITY BY GLIOTRANSMITTERS

There is a bidirectional signaling between retinal neurons and Müller cells, mediated by neurotransmitters (released from neurons) and gliotransmitters (released from Müller cells). Müller cells regulate the synaptic transmission mainly by the release of glutamate, ATP, and adenosine. Gliotransmitters have excitatory (glutamate, ATP) and inhibitory effects (adenosine) on neighboring neurons (Newman, 2003a, 2004a,b; Housley et al., 2009). Müller cells are involved in improving the retinal neuroplasticity, e.g., after exposure to stimulating environments or moderate corticosterone levels, via activation of ERK1/2-dependent signaling pathways (Matteucci et al., 2014). In addition to effects on retinal neurons, gliotransmitters of Müller cells have autocrine effects and mediate the propagation of intracellular calcium waves (see 5.6.3.3.) implicated, for example, in neurovascular coupling (see 5.8.). The autocrine actions of gliotransmitters also involve the regulation of the Müller cell volume in dependence on the neuronal cell volume and the extracellular osmolarity which both are altered during intense glutamatergic transmission (see 5.5.1.). Regulation of the Müller cell volume is of great importance for the prevention of neuronal hyperexcitability resulting from a decrease in the extracellular space volume (see 5.5.1.1.). In addition to the above-mentioned molecules, Müller cells release a variety of further neuroactive signaling molecules including D-serine, ACBP, retinoic acid, and NO. It is expected that the number of known molecules which mediate glia-to-neuron signaling in the retina will considerably increase in the future.

5.6.1   GLIAL RELEASE OF GLUTAMATE

5.6.1.1 Non-Vesicular Release of Glutamate

Under conditions of severe depolarization, Müller cells release glutamate via a reversal of the electrogenic glutamate transport; the non-vesicular, voltage-dependent release of glutamate from glial cells was found to contribute to the excitotoxic damage to neurons (Szatkowski et al., 1990; Billups and Attwell, 1996; Maguire et al., 1998; Zeevalk et al., 1998; Marcaggi et al., 2005). Severe depolarization of Müller cells may occur during pathological rises in extracellular potassium as observed, for example, in ischemia and glaucoma, and during opening of cation channels, e.g., ionotropic $P2X_7$ receptor channels (Pannicke et al., 2000a). During ischemia, which is associated with an energy failure that inhibits the activity of the sodium-potassium-ATPase, the reversed glutamate transport is caused by a reversal of the electrochemical gradients of the coupling ions (Kanai and Hediger, 2004; see 5.5.2.1.3.). Müller cells may also release aspartate, an agonist at NMDA receptors, via reversed action of glutamate transporters; glia-derived aspartate may contribute to the increase in extracellular aspartate and activation of NMDA receptors during ischemia (Marcaggi et al., 2005). However, also under normal conditions, some glutamate which was taken up by Müller cells might be transported back to neurons by the reversal of the glial glutamate transport (Pow et al., 2000). It has been shown that murine Müller cells may release glutamate by a calcium-dependent, non-vesicular mechanism (Fig. 74xB; see 5.6.1.2.) (Slezak et al., 2012). Whether a release of intracellular D-aspartate in exchange to extracellular L-glutamate via sodium-dependent EAATs as described for retinal neurons (Stutz et al., 2011) also occurs in Müller cells remains to be clarified.

Another mode of a non-vesicular glutamate release from Müller cells (but not neurons) is the transport via the electroneutral, sodium-independent, and chloride-dependent cystine-glutamate antiporter (system X_c^-) (Kato et al., 1993; Pow, 2001a; Tomi et al., 2003). This antiporter normally mediates an uptake of cystine in exchange for glutamate; cystine is used for the production of the antioxidant glutathione (Fig. 44; see 5.5.2.1.15.). Because this antiporter transports cystine using the transmembrane gradient of glutamate as the driving force (Bannai and Tateishi, 1986), the exchanger can also mediate a sodium-independent uptake of glutamate when the extracellular concentration of glutamate is high. Oxidative stress induces an increase in the expression of the cystine-glutamate antiporter in Müller cells (Mysona et al., 2009). This antiporter may contribute to the release of glutamate from Müller cells under oxidative stress conditions when an elevated production of glutathione (and, therefore, an increased uptake of cystine) is required (Kato et al., 1993; Pow, 2001a). It has been suggested that a significant proportion of the glutamate released from Müller cells during reperfusion after ischemia is mediated by the cystine-glutamate antiporter (Pow and Barnett, 2000); this might contribute to the excitotoxic damage of retinal neurons (in addition to the direct effects of glutathione on iGluRs; see 5.5.2.1.15.) (Pow, 2001a).

5.6.1.2 Vesicular Release of Glutamate

Müller cells also release glutamate via vesicular exocytosis. By measuring the cell volume regulation of freshly isolated Müller cells of the rodent retina, it has been demonstrated that Müller cells release glutamate which is part of an autocrine glutamatergic-purinergic signaling cascade that prevents the osmotic swelling of the cells (Fig. 73B; see 5.5.5.3.) (Wurm et al., 2008a; Linnertz et al., 2011; Brückner et al., 2012; Wahl et al., 2013). Secretion of glutamate from isolated Müller cells can be induced by activation of the VEGF receptor-2 with VEGF, and is likely mediated by calcium-dependent exocytosis of glutamate-containing secretory vesicles. The latter assumption is supported by the facts that inhibitors of vesicular exocytosis, vesicular glutamate transporters, and the vesicle-membrane ATPase prevent the effect of VEGF on the regulation of Müller cell volume (Wurm et al., 2008a; Brückner et al., 2012). Activation of phospholipase C (PLC), resulting in a release of calcium from intracellular stores, influx of calcium from the extracellular space, and activation of PKC and Src tyrosine kinases are involved in triggering the glutamate release from Müller cells (Fig. 78A) (Wurm et al., 2008a; Linnertz et al., 2011; Brückner et al., 2012). The VEGF-induced release of glutamate is not mediated by a reversal of glutamate transporters (Wurm et al., 2008a). Glutamate-containing vesicles are loaded by the activity of vesicular glutamate transporters (VGLUTs). Rat Müller cells were immunolabeled for VGLUT3 (Linnertz et al., 2011). In the lizard retina, glial somata contain VGLUT1 (Romero-Alemán et al., 2010). In addition to VEGF, various other receptor ligands (including neuropeptide Y, epidermal growth factor, natriuretic peptides, erythropoietin, endothelin-1, osteopontin, sex steroids, and NGF) inhibit the osmotic swelling of rat Müller cells via induction of vesicular glutamate release (Uckermann et al., 2006; Weuste et al., 2006; Kalisch et al., 2006; Krügel et al., 2010; Neumann et al., 2010; Linnertz et al., 2011; Wahl et al., 2013; Garcia et al., 2014). It is likely but remains to be proven that all stimuli which trigger an increase in the cytosolic free calcium level (receptor activation, electrical, and mechanical stimulation) may also induce a vesicular release of glutamate from Müller cells.

The vesicular release of glutamate is dependent on an influx of calcium from the extracellular space (Wurm et al., 2008a; Brückner et al., 2012). The influx of calcium is mediated by activation of transient (T-type) voltage-gated calcium channels (Krügel et al., 2010; Linnertz et al., 2011; Brückner et al., 2012). It has been shown electrophysiologically that Müller cells of various species display T-type and long-lasting (L-type) calcium currents upon membrane depolarization (see 5.9.1.). Müller cells of the rat were immunolabeled for the α_{1C} ($Ca_v1.2$) subunit of L-type channels and the α_{1G} ($Ca_v3.1$) subunit of T-type channels (Fig. 45F) (Linnertz et al., 2011). T-type voltage-gated calcium channels mediate low-threshold fast inactivating calcium currents (Fig. 45A-C). Rapid depolarization-hyperpolarization cycles are required for opening of the channels. Because blockers of voltage-gated sodium channels prevent the inhibitory effect of VEGF and of other receptor ligands on the osmotic swelling of Müller cells (Krügel et al., 2010; Linnertz et al., 2011; Brückner et al., 2012), activation of voltage-gated sodium channels is apparently involved in the agonist-induced release of glutamate from Müller cells. Müller cells of various species display currents through voltage-gated sodium channels (see 5.9.2.). Müller cells of the rat retina were immunolabeled for the $Na_v1.6$ subunit (Fig. 67xE) (Linnertz et al., 2011). It is suggested that, *in situ*, rapid membrane depolarization sufficient to activate voltage-gated sodium channels occurs preferentially in such membrane domains that do not contain Kir4.1 channels, and which are electrotonically uncoupled from Kir4.1-expressing membrane domains; such membrane domains are, for example, the fine side branches and glial membrane sheets that surround the synapses. The fact that blockers of

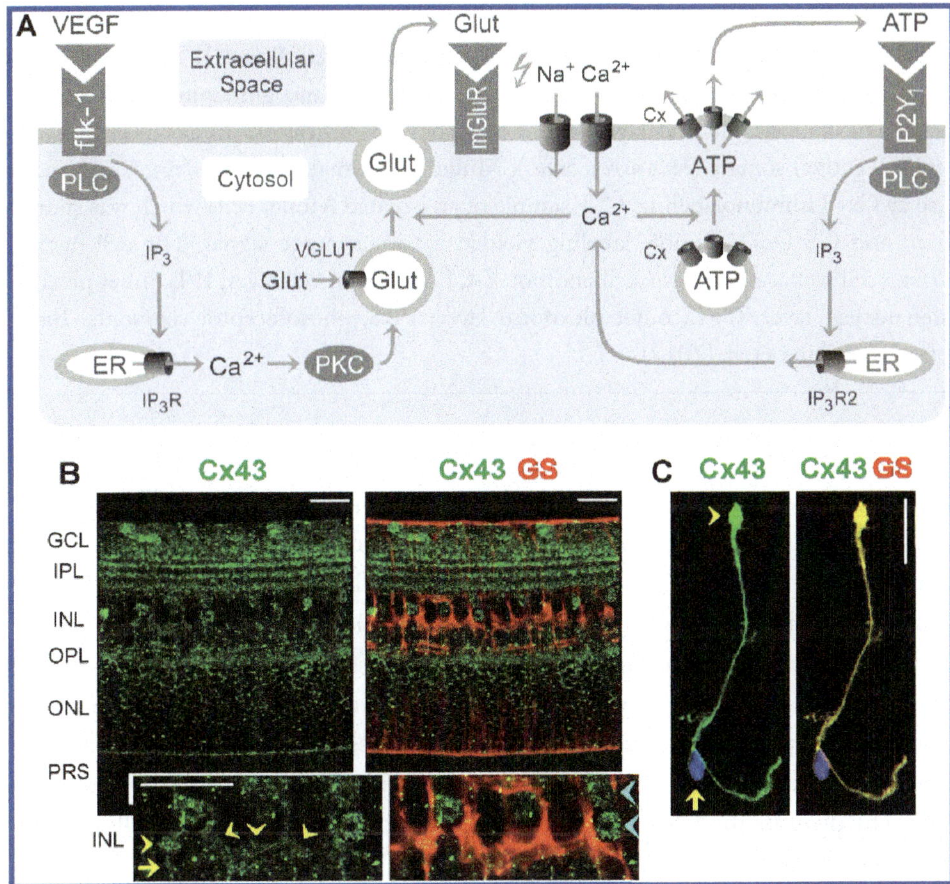

FIGURE 78: Murine Müller cells release glutamate by calcium-dependent vesicular exocytosis, while ATP is calcium-dependently released through connexin hemichannels. **A.** Hypothetical scheme of the intracellular signaling involved in the VEGF-induced release of glutamate and ATP from murine Müller cells. Activation of fetal liver kinase (flk)-1 by VEGF induces a phospholipase C (PLC)-mediated release of calcium from endoplasmic reticulum (ER) stores and activation of protein kinase C (PKC), resulting in exocytotic release of glutamate (Glut)-containing vesicles. These vesicles are loaded by the activity of vesicular glutamate transporters (VGLUTs). Activation of metabotropic glutamate receptors (mGluRs) by glutamate induces an activation of voltage-gated sodium and T-type calcium channels. The calcium influx from the extracellular space results in trafficking of connexin (Cx) hemichannel-containing vesicles towards the plasma membrane, fusion of vesicle and plasma membranes, and a release of ATP from the cells. Activation of P2Y₁ receptors by ATP results in a release of calcium from inositol 1,4,5-triphosphate

continued on next page

receptor type 2 (IP$_3$R2)-gated stores. The calcium release amplifies the release of ATP from Müller cells. **B, C.** Distribution of connexin 43 immunoreactivity in mouse retinal slices (**B**) and isolated Müller cells (**C**). **B.** The slice was stained against connexin 43 (Cx43; *green*) and glutamine synthetase (GS; *red*). The *insets* display the inner nuclear layer (INL) at higher magnification. In addition to Cx43-labeled neuronal (GS negative) somata (*blue arrowheads*), Müller cell somata (*yellow arrowheads*) and processes (*arrow*) display Cx43 immunolabeling. **C.** Example of an isolated Müller cells which was stained against Cx43 (*green*) and GS (*red*). Double labeling yielded a *yellow* merge signal. The cell nucleus is *blue* stained. *Arrow*, cell soma. *Arrowhead*, cell endfoot. GCL, ganglion cell layer; IPL, inner plexiform layer; ONL, outer nuclear layer; OPL, outer plexiform layer; PRS, photoreceptor segments. Bars, 20 μm. Modified from Brückner et al. (2012).

---

voltage-gated sodium channels (e.g., tetrodotoxin) inhibit the ligand-induced release of glutamate from Müller cells (Linnertz et al., 2011) may have impact for the interpretation of data obtained in retinal tissue preparations, i.e., blockers of the channels should be used with caution for the separation of glial and neuronal glutamatergic activities in retinal tissue preparations.

A calcium-dependent vesicular release of glutamate from Müller cells was also shown by using mono- and bigenic BoNT/B mice that express botulinum toxin B under the control of the glia-specific GLAST promoter (Slezak et al., 2007). In these mice, toxin activity in the retina is restricted to Müller cells where it cleaves all three subtypes of vesicle-associated membrane proteins and thereby disrupts the SNARE-dependent exocytosis. Murine Müller cells express vesicle-associated membrane proteins 2 and 3 (Roesch et al., 2008). In freshly isolated Müller cells from mono- and bigenic mice, calcium-dependent glutamate release was evoked by inducing intracellular calcium transients with UV-induced uncaging of calcium from a cell-permeable photolabile chelator (Fig. 74A,B) (Slezak et al., 2012). In comparison to the glutamate release from Müller cells of monogenic mice, the glutamate release from Müller cells of bigenic mice was reduced by approximately 40% (Fig. 74C) (Slezak et al., 2012). A pharmacological blocker of vesicular glutamate uptake reduced the calcium-induced glutamate release from cells of monogenic mice to the same extent as the toxin (Fig. 74C) (Slezak et al., 2012). The fact that the blocker or the toxin did not completely abolish the glutamate release (Fig. 74C) suggests that Müller cells release glutamate also by a calcium-dependent, non-vesicular mechanism (Slezak et al., 2012).

5.6.1.3 Neuronal Effects of Glial Glutamate

In addition to the cytotoxic effects of Müller cell-derived glutamate under pathological conditions (Szatkowski et al., 1990; Billups and Attwell, 1996; Maguire et al., 1998; Marcaggi et al., 2005), glutamate released from Müller cells may also modify the neuronal activity in the normal retina. In eyecup preparations of the rat, calcium waves in retinal glial cells induced by mechanical stimulation causes a release of glutamate that activates inhibitory interneurons (presumably GABA- and glycinergic amacrine cells) via activation of AMPA/KA and mGluRs; this results in decreases and increases of the light-induced spike activity in different subpopulations of neurons in the ganglion cell layer (Newman and Zahs, 1998).

Glutamate and VEGF induce a swelling of retinal ganglion cell somata in the rodent retina (Figs. 3B, 39A,B) (Uckermann et al., 2004b; Wurm et al., 2008a; see 5.5.1.1.). Because the effect of VEGF was inhibited by a blocker of AMPA/KA receptors and the gliotoxin iodoacetate (Fig. 39B), the effect of VEGF is likely mediated by inducing a release of glutamate from Müller cells and subsequent activation of neuronal iGluRs (Wurm et al., 2008a). The swelling of neuronal somata reflects glutamatergic excitation of the cells. The VEGF-induced glutamatergic regulation of retinal neurons was also investigated in retinal tissue preparations from monogenic and bigenic BoNT/B mice; in bigenic BoNT/B mice, the exocytotic glutamate release from Müller cells is disrupted (see 5.6.1.2.). As shown in Figure 74E, VEGF induced a swelling of retinal ganglion cells in retinas of monogenic, but not of bigenic BoNT/B mice (Slezak et al., 2012). These data suggest that only Müller cell-derived glutamate that was released via calcium-dependent vesicular exocytosis, but not glutamate liberated by calcium-dependent non-vesicular release, mediates the VEGF-induced glutamatergic excitation of retinal ganglion cells. The data also suggest that Müller cells, but not retinal neurons, possess VEGF receptors linked to a release of glutamate. In addition to neuronal effects, Müller cell-derived glutamate has also autocrine effects, e.g., the regulation of the glial cell volume (see 5.5.5.3.).

5.6.2   RELEASE OF D-SERINE

Müller cells are involved in setting the sensitivity of retinal ganglion and amacrine cells to light stimuli by the release of D-serine (Miller, 2004). D-Serine is an endogenous ligand of the glycine modulatory binding site of the NMDA receptor that must be occupied before glutamate can open the receptor channel. D-Serine activates the glycine binding site with a potency three-fold greater than glycine, and (because this site is normally not saturated) is required for the full activity of NMDA receptors in retinal ganglion cells (Stevens et al., 2003). NMDA receptors are intrinsic to retinal ganglion cells and most amacrine cells as well as horizontal cells in some species (O'Dell and Christensen, 1989; Dixon and Copenhagen, 1992). On the other hand, D-serine inhibits the activation of calcium-permeable AMPA receptors expressed by various types of retinal neurons including retinal ganglion cells (Daniels et al., 2012). D-serine is synthesized from L-serine by the serine racemase that is present in various types of retinal neurons and in astrocytes and Müller cells

(Stevens et al., 2003; O'Brien et al., 2005; Dun et al., 2008; Takayasu et al., 2008). Pharmacological blockade of the D-serine synthesis in the salamander retina, or deletion of the serine racemase in mice, result in a greatly reduced NMDA receptor component of the light-induced retinal ganglion cell responses (Stevens et al., 2010; Sullivan et al., 2011). The D-serine degrading enzyme D-amino acid oxidase was localized to Müller cells and rods of the frog retina (Beard et al., 1988).

The transmembrane transport of D-serine in Müller cells is likely mediated by the sodium-dependent neutral amino acid exchanger ASCT2 (O'Brien et al., 2005; Dun et al., 2007), coupled to a counter-movement of L-serine or L-glutamine (Ribeiro et al., 2002). The release of D-serine from Müller cells can be induced by activation of glutamate receptors (Oliet and Mothet, 2006; Sullivan and Miller, 2010). The coupling of the glutamine efflux to the D-serine uptake, and the glutamate-induced D-serine release, may regulate the extracellular D-serine concentration in dependence on the strength of the neuronal activity (Ribeiro et al., 2002). It cannot be ruled out that D-serine is released from Müller cells via exocytosis of secretory vesicles because it is located to vesicle-like structures within the cells (Diaz et al., 2007). NMDA receptors of cultured chick Müller cells and retinal neurons are structurally different, resulting in a 30-fold lower affinity for D-serine of Müller cell receptors compared to neuronal receptors (Lamas et al., 2005). In the human fetal retina, Müller cells express D-serine immunoreactivity shortly before the development of the first functional synapses at 12 weeks of gestation, suggesting a role of Müller cell-derived D-serine in the shaping of synaptogenesis (Diaz et al., 2007). Inflammatory conditions as occurring in experimental diabetic retinopathy induce an upregulation of the serine racemase in the retinal tissue; a higher retinal D-serine level may aggravate the glutamate-induced death of retinal ganglion cells observed under these conditions (Jiang et al., 2011). In cultured Müller cells, D-serine acting on NMDA receptors regulates the gene expression, the phosphorylation of the cAMP-responsive element-binding protein (CREB), and the expression of the immediate-early gene c-Fos (Lamas et al., 2007).

In addition to retinal ganglion cells, Müller cell endfeet express kynurenine aminotransferase (Rejdak et al., 2001, 2004, 2007) that is pivotal to the synthesis of kynurenic acid, an antagonist of the coagonist site of the NMDA receptor. This suggests that Müller cells may also inhibit NMDA receptor activation via the release of kynurenic acid.

5.6.3 GLIAL RELEASE OF PURINERGIC RECEPTOR AGONISTS

5.6.3.1 Release of ATP

Extracellular ATP acts as transmittter in the retina (Perez et al., 1988). Upon illumination of the retina or administration of a depolarizing high-potassium solution, neurons release ATP through a calcium-dependent mechanism (Perez et al., 1986; Santos et al., 1999; Newman, 2005). ATP was suggested to be coreleased from cholinergic neurons resulting in activation of an inhibitory glycinergic feedback loop (Neal and Cunningham, 1994). ATP modulates the uptake of GABA in the rat retina (Neal et al., 1998). In addition to neurons, ATP is released from retinal glial cells by receptor-dependent and -independent mechanisms. Osmotic gradients (Fig. 43G), mechanical or electrical stimulation, and receptor agonists such as ATP, dopamine, thrombin, and glutamate acting at group I/II mGluRs induce a release of ATP from rodent Müller cells (Fig. 73B) (Newman, 2001a,b, 2003b; Uckermann et al., 2006; Wurm et al., 2008a, 2010; Krügel et al., 2010; Linnertz et al., 2011). There is a species dependence in the mechanism of the ligand-induced ATP release from rat and murine Müller cells; whereas the glutamate-induced ATP release from rat Müller cells is not dependent on intracellular calcium signaling (Uckermann et al., 2006; Wurm et al., 2008a), the glutamate-induced ATP release from murine Müller cells is dependent on a release of calcium from IP_3R2-gated internal stores (Figs. 78A, 79A–C) (Lipp et al., 2009; Wurm et al., 2010; Brückner et al., 2012; see 5.5.5.3.). The calcium-independent glutamate-induced release of ATP from rat Müller cells is consistent with the fact that glutamate does not induce calcium responses in Müller cells of the rat (as well as of the rabbit and guinea pig; Fig. 17A,F) (Newman and Zahs, 1997; Uckermann et al., 2003, 2004b, 2006; Newman, 2005; Rillich et al., 2009). In contrast to rat Müller cells (Linnertz et al., 2011), the glutamate-induced release of ATP from murine Müller cells is inhibited by blockers of voltage-gated sodium and T-type voltage-gated calcium channels (Brückner et al., 2012). Because the release of ATP from murine Müller cells is suggested to be mediated by connexin hemichannels, in particular connexin 43 (Fig. 78B,C) (Janssen-Bienhold et al., 1998; Ball and McReynolds, 1998; Johansson et al., 1999; Zahs et al., 2003; Kihara et al., 2006; Kuo et al., 2008; Brückner et al., 2012; Kerr et al., 2010, 2012; Danesh-Meyer et al., 2012), calcium signaling was suggested to be involved in the trafficking of connexin hemichannel-containing vesicles towards the plasma membrane and/or in the calcium-dependent opening of connexin hemichannels (Fig. 78A) (Brückner et al., 2012). Further research is required to determine the different mechanisms of ATP release from rat and murine Müller cells. An exocytotic glutamate-induced release of ATP was also described in cultured avian Müller cells (Loiola and Ventura, 2011).

5.6.3.2 Release of Adenosine

The release of adenosine from rodent Müller cells is mediated by calcium-independent equilibrative nucleoside transporters (Uckermann et al., 2006; Wurm et al., 2008a; Linnertz et al., 2011; Brückner et al., 2012). In the murine retina, adenosine can be also extracellularly formed from ATP by the consecutive action of the ecto-ATPase (NTPDase2), ecto-apyrase (NTPDase1), and ecto-5'-nucleotidase (CD73) (Wurm et al., 2010). The rat parenchyma lacks an expression of NTPDase1

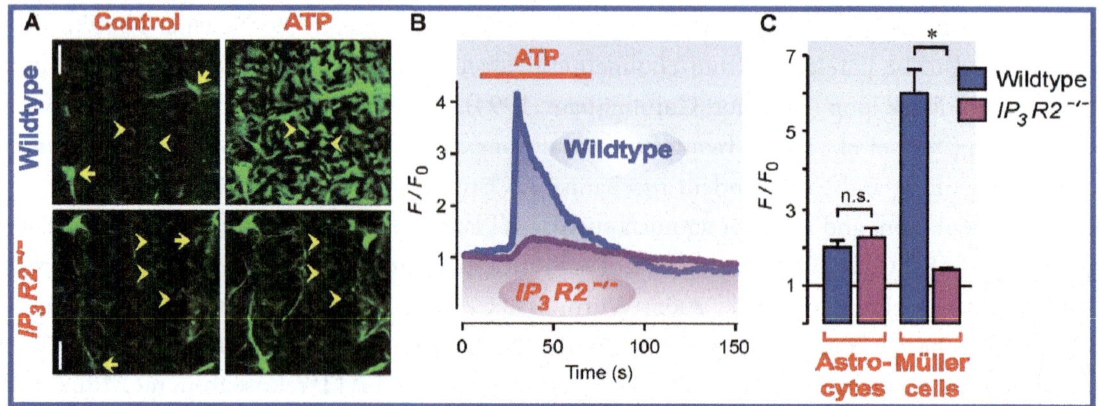

FIGURE 79: ATP-evoked calcium responses in murine Müller cells (but not in retinal astrocytes) depend largely on IP$_3$-receptor type 2 (IP$_3$R2)-gated internal stores. The calcium responses induced by ATP (50 µM) were recorded in astrocytic somata and Müller cell endfeet in the nerve fiber/ganglion cell layers of retinal wholemounts from wildtype and *IP$_3$R2$^{-/-}$* mice using the calcium-sensitive fluorescence dye Fluo4/AM. The dye was selectively taken up by glial cells. Astrocytes and Müller cell endfeet were distinguished according to their different morphology. The nerve fiber/ganglion cell layers contain the somata of fibrous astrocytes (*arrows*); multiple processes rise from each soma. Müller cell endfeet (*arrowheads*) fill the spaces between the unstained (*black*) ganglion cell somata. **A.** Examples of fluorescence records. The images were obtained before (*control*) and during the peak calcium response (*ATP*). Bars, 20 µm. **B.** Time dependence of the ATP-evoked calcium response in Müller cell endfeet. **C.** Mean peak amplitude of the ATP-evoked calcium response. *$P<0.001$. n.s., not significant. Modified from Lipp et al. (2009) and Wurm et al. (2010).

which forms the substrate of the ecto-5'-nucleotidase, AMP (Fig. 75) (Iandiev et al., 2007a; Wurm et al., 2008b). However, under pathological conditions such as experimental diabetic retinopathy, NTPDase1 is upregulated in the retinal parenchyma (Fig. 75), which allows the extracellular generation of adenosine from ATP (Fig. 73B) (see 5.5.5.3.3.).

5.6.3.3 Propagation of Glial Calcium Waves by Extracellular ATP Signaling

Autocrine/paracrine ATP signaling is involved in mediating the propagation of long-range calcium waves through the retinal glial cell network (Fig. 58D) (Newman and Zahs, 1997, 1998). The propagation of the waves from astrocytes to Müller cells, and among Müller cells, depends upon the release and extracellular diffusion of ATP, activation of P2Y$_1$ receptors (Li et al., 2001; Wurm et al., 2009a), and a release of calcium from internal stores (Fig. 17F) (Newman and Zahs, 1997; Newman, 2001a,b; Kurth-Nelson et al., 2009; Edwards and Gibson, 2010). Between astrocytes, the waves propagate by the spread of internal messengers (presumably IP$_3$) via gap junctions. The waves can be triggered in astrocytes and Müller cells by various stimuli including electrical and mechanical stimulation, and focal administration of neurotransmitters such as glutamate (Newman and Zahs, 1997, 1998). The waves propagate with 20–30 µm/s while ATP released from rat retinal glial cells propagates with a velocity of ~40 µm/s which is faster than the velocity of the calcium waves (Newman and Zahs, 1997, 1998; Newman, 2001a). The fact that the release of ATP precedes the elicitation of the calcium waves suggests that the release of ATP from rat Müller cells is calcium-independent.

In the rat retina, ATP-induced calcium responses are mainly restricted to the inner half of Müller cells, i.e., to processes that traverse the inner plexiform layer, and to the endfeet in the ganglion cell/nerve fiber layers; ATP induces very small calcium responses in the somata and outer processes of the cells (Fig. 58A,B) (Newman, 2005; Uckermann et al., 2006; Wurm et al., 2009a). This distribution coincides with the distribution of spontaneous calcium transients (Newman, 2005). In Müller cells of young postnatal rats, extracellular ATP induces calcium waves which start in the endfeet of the cells and propagate towards the somata and outer stem processes of the cells (Fig. 58C,D) (Wurm et al., 2009a). ATP-induced glial calcium waves that start in Müller cell endfeet were also found in the tiger salamander retina (Keirstead and Miller, 1997). Glial calcium waves may underlie an extraneuronal long-range signaling system that modifies neuronal activity (Newman and Zahs, 1998; Newman, 2004b), that mediate the neurovascular coupling (see 5.8.), and that may be involved in the activity-dependent regulation of the Müller cell volume (see 5.5.5.3.). The calcium waves may transmit volume-regulatory signals over long distances that prevent (via autocrine release of glutamate and purinergic receptors agonists) the swelling of the inner Müller cell processes and endfeet (Fig. 73B) when ganglion and bipolar cells enlarge their volume upon activation of glutamate receptors (Figs. 3B,E, 39A,B). Under pathological conditions, e.g., after local retinal detachment, glial calcium waves may spread via the release of ATP and growth factors (Fig. 54C), thus causing a spread of gliosis and retinal degeneration to larger retinal areas (see 5.11.5.).

Under constant light conditions, rat Müller cells generate spontaneous calcium transients by the release of calcium from internal stores (Newman, 2005). The transients have a duration of 2.5–6 s and are mediated by autocrine/paracrine ATP signaling (Newman, 2005). The calcium transients start within the inner and middle portions of the inner plexiform layer and propagate into the endfeet of Müller cells (Newman, 2005; Kurth-Nelson et al., 2009). Stimulation of the retina with flickering light, administration of ATP or adenosine, or antidromic stimulation of ganglion cells increases the frequency of the calcium transients in Müller cells (Newman, 2005). The effect of flickering light is mediated by a release of ATP from retinal neurons and activation of P2Y receptors on Müller cells (Newman, 2005). Amacrine cells are suggested to release ATP (Santos et al., 1999). The cholinergic starburst amacrine is a likely candidate that mediates the purinergic neuron-to-glia signaling because it may corelease ATP along with acetylcholine (Neal and Cunningham, 1994). The effect of antidromic activation of ganglion cells was explained with a release of ATP from ganglion cell axons or dendrites which have contact to other neurons (Newman, 2005). The increase in the frequency of the light-induced calcium transients in Müller cells is potentiated by adenosine, suggesting that this effect is augmented under pathological conditions such as ischemia and hypoxia when adenosine is rapidly released in the retina (Roth et al., 1997; Ribelayga and Mangel, 2005). Light-induced calcium responses are not observed in the soma or outer processes of Müller cells, nor in astrocytes (Newman, 2005).

Whereas in rat Müller cells, ATP-induced calcium responses are restricted to the inner processes and the endfeet of the cells (Fig. 58A,B), calcium-independent responses (such as $P2Y_1$ receptor-induced release of adenosine) are also present in the somata of the cells (Newman, 2005; Uckermann et al., 2006; Wurm et al., 2009a). This suggests that the functional coupling of $P2Y_1$ receptors (which are, in rodent Müller cells, localized to the endfeet, stem processes, and somata of the cells; Fig. 77A,B; Wurm et al., 2009a, 2010) to calcium-dependent and -independent intracellular effector molecules differs according to the subcellular region of the cells. Alternatively, the expression of various P2Y receptor subtypes coupled to different effector molecules in distinct subcellular regions might explain the different intracellular responses (Wurm et al., 2009a, 2010). $P2Y_4$ protein is localized to the endfoot, outer process, and perisynaptic membranes in the outer plexiform layer of rodent Müller cells, but not to the inner process and the somatic region of the cells (Fig. 77A,B) (Wurm et al., 2009a, 2010).

5.6.3.4 Neuronal Effects of Glial ATP and Adenosine

Glial calcium waves are associated with a modulation of the firing rate of neighboring neurons; the light-induced spike activity of ~50% of the neurons in the ganglion cell layer is decreased when the calcium waves reach the neurons while other neurons display excitation (Newman and Zahs, 1998). The inhibition of the light-induced spike activity could be caused by glutamate released from Müller cells (Newman and Zahs, 1998) or by Müller cell-derived ATP and adenosine (Newman, 2003b). In the latter scenario, Müller cell-derived ATP released into the inner plexiform layer was suggested to be converted extracellularly to adenosine; adenosine activates neuronal adenosine A_1 receptors which results in reduced spontaneous activity in a population of ganglion cell layer neurons (Newman, 2003b). Müller cell-derived adenosine may act as a negative feedback regulator of neurotransmission (Housley et al., 2009). This mechanism adapts the level of neuronal activity to the capacity of Müller cells to maintain retinal homeostasis and is also implicated in the protection of photoreceptor cells under dark-adapted conditions which are associated with hypoxic stress (see 5.5.8.2.).

Various neuronal cell types in the retina including ganglion, amacrine, and horizontal cells express purinergic P2 receptors (Greenwood et al., 1997; Santos et al., 1998; Taschenberger et al., 1999; Xia et al., 2012; Ho et al., 2014) and thus may respond also to ATP released from Müller cells. Müller cell-derived ATP (acting at neuronal $P2X_7$ receptors) may induce overstimulation and degeneration of photoreceptors (Puthussery and Fletcher, 2009) and retinal ganglion cells, for example, in glaucoma (Zhang et al., 2005c; Resta et al., 2007; Hu et al., 2010a). In chick and human retinas, where Müller cells express $P2X_7$ receptors, activation of glial $P2X_7$ receptors causes a membrane depolarization which impairs the uptake of glutamate (Fig. 47E); the resulting elevated extracellular glutamate level induces excitotoxic death of neurons (Pannicke et al., 2000a; Anccasi et al., 2013). Because Müller cells release ATP in response to mechanical stimulation (Fig. 43G) (Newman, 2001a,b, 2003b), excess ATP may be liberated from Müller cells under conditions associated with mechanical perturbations such as retinal detachment and elevated intraocular pressure (Resta et al., 2007; Zhang et al., 2007a; Reigada et al., 2008). Because adenosine acting at adenosine A_3 receptors inhibits the $P2X_7$ receptor-induced increases in calcium and apoptosis of retinal ganglion cells, the balance between extracellular ATP and adenosine levels determines the level of the ganglion cell death (Zhang et al., 2006a; Hu et al., 2010a). Thus, glial upregulation of NTPDase1 in the diseased retinal parenchyma (Fig. 75) may be neuroprotective because larger amounts of adenosine can be formed extracellularly from ATP by the consecutive action of NTPDase1 and ecto-5'-nucleotidase (Fig. 73B; see 5.5.5.3.3.). Müller cell-derived ATP may also regulate the motility of microglial cell processes (Wang and Wong, 2014; see 3.2.).

Release of adenosine is an important component of the retinal response to ischemia-hypoxia, including hypoxic states of photoreceptors in the dark (Roth et al., 1997; Ribelayga and Mangel, 2005). Adenosine has antiinflammatory effects, induces retinal hyperemia after ischemia, and protects neurons from glutamate toxicity by suppressing excitatory neurotransmission (Larsen and Osborne, 1996; Ostwald et al., 1997; Ghiardi et al., 1999; Clark et al., 2009; Housley et al., 2009). Activation of adenosine A_1/A_2 receptors, or ischemic preconditioning mediated by the release of endogenous adenosine and subsequent A_1 receptor activation, protects the retina from ischemic injury (Larsen and Osborne, 1996; Ghiardi et al., 1999; Sakamoto et al., 2004). The inhibitory effect of adenosine on the osmotic swelling of Müller cells (see 5.5.5.3.) and bipolar cells (see 5.5.5.5.) may contribute to its neuroprotective effect by preventing detrimental reductions of the extracellular space volume that otherwise will result in neuronal hyperexcitability (Dudek et al., 1990; Chebabo et al., 1995). Facilitated degradation of extracellular ATP/ADP by NTPDase1 may protect Müller cells from overstimulation of $P2Y_1$ receptors; this may avoid cytotoxic calcium overload without impairing the regulation of Müller cell volume.

5.6.4   RELEASE OF ACBP AND RETINOIC ACID

ACBP is expressed in Müller cells (Yanase et al., 2002). ACBP interacts with the $\alpha1$-subunit of the $GABA_A$ receptor, resulting in a reduction of receptor currents. GABAergic synaptic transmission is critical for the direction-selectivity of retinal ganglion cells. Horizontal optokinetic stimulation of the retina induces increased expression and phosphorylation of ACBP in Müller cells (Barmack et al., 2004; Qian et al., 2008). It has been suggested that Müller cells, depolarized by activated GABAergic amacrine cells, secrete ACBP into the inner plexiform layer (Barmack et al., 2004). This results in a decreased sensitivity of $GABA_A$ receptors located on ganglion cell dendrites which receive a GABAergic direction-selective signal from starburst amacrine cell axon terminals (Barmack et al., 2004). Thus, Müller cells may be implicated in the horizontal optokinetic reflex by providing a local negative feedback loop on the GABAergic transmission in neighboring retinal neurons. Cultured Müller cells secrete phosphorylated ACBP upon membrane depolarization or activation of PKC (Qian et al., 2008).

Müller cells are a source of all-*trans* retinoic acid (which does not participate in the visual cycle). Besides being a morphogenetic factor, retinoic acid also acts as a neuromodulator, via regulation of the gap junctional conductance and the synaptic transfer between photoreceptors and horizontal cells (Weiler et al., 2001; Dirks et al., 2004). Müller cells synthesize retinaldehyde and retinoic acid from retinol; retinoic acid is subsequently released into the extracellular space (Edwards et al., 1992). Müller cells express also aldehyde dehydrogenase-2 which oxidizes retinaldehyde to retinoic acid (McCaffery et al., 1991). The presence of retinoic acid receptors in inner retinal neurons (Fischer et al., 1999) suggest a role of retinoic acid in glia-to-neuron signaling.

5.6.5   PRODUCTION OF NO, CARBON MONOXIDE, AND HYDROGEN SULFIDE

In addition to retinal neurons, Müller cells express constitutive NO synthases (Yamamoto et al., 1993; Liepe et al., 1994; Huxlin, 1995; Kurenni et al., 1995; Djamgoz et al., 1996; López-Costa et al., 1997; Fischer and Stell, 1999; Ota et al., 1999; Haverkamp et al., 1999; Cao et al., 1999a; Kobayashi et al., 2000; Cao and Eldred, 2001). Under pathological conditions such as inflammation, ischemia, diabetes, and elevated hydrostatic pressure, Müller cells also express the inducible NO synthase and increase the expression of the neuronal NO synthase (Goureau et al., 1994, 1997, 1999; Goldstein et al., 1996; De Kozak et al., 1997; Cotinet et al., 1997a,b; Kobayashi et al., 2000; Tezel and Wax, 2000; Abu-El-Asrar et al., 2001; Mishra and Newman, 2010; Chen et al., 2013b). NO is an activator of the soluble guanylyl cyclase that produces cGMP (Knowles et al., 1989). In addition to photoreceptors, bipolar cells, and some amacrine and ganglion cells (Gotzes et al., 1998), guanylyl cyclases are expressed by Müller cells (Rambotti et al., 1999).

In the rat retina, NO is primarily produced in amacrine, bipolar, and Müller cells while carbon monoxide (which inhibits the soluble guanylyl cyclase activity) is produced by the heme oxygenase-2 in Müller cells (Kajimura et al., 2003). (However, another study found heme oxygenase-2 only in retinal neurons; Cao et al., 2000.) NO can readily diffuse out of Müller cells and activates neuronal guanylyl cyclases. NO closes NMDA receptor channels (Kashii et al., 1996) and increases calcium channel currents (Goldstein et al., 1996). NO activates cGMP-gated conductances in ganglion cells and photoreceptors (resulting in increased phototransduction), closes gap junctions in horizontal cells, and enhances the light-induced response of cholinergic amacrine cells (Koch et al., 1994; Ahmad et al., 1994; Goldstein et al., 1996; Pottek, 1997; Neal et al., 1997). The NO production by Müller cells is strongly increased during dark adaptation (Ye and Yang, 1996; Zemel et al., 1996). NO affects the contractile tone of Müller cells (Kawasaki et al., 1999) and regulates the neurovascular coupling in the retina (see 5.8.). Müller cells may also support the neuronal NO synthesis by the release of arginine which is taken up by neurons (Cossenza and Paes de Carvalho, 2000).

Retinal glial cells are the major source of NO under hypoxic conditions (Kashiwagi et al., 2003). In response to ischemia and inflammation, early in diabetic retinopathy, and after excitotoxic damage to the retina, Müller cells increase the expression of inducible NO synthetase (Goureau et al., 1994; Jacquemin et al., 1996; Kobayashi et al., 2000; Abu-El-Asrar et al., 2001, 2004a,b; Nakamichi et al., 2003). NO produced by Müller cells has both beneficial (see 5.11.1.1.) and detrimental effects in the diseased retina (see 5.11.1.2.). Cultured Müller cells express neuronal, endothelial, and inducible NO synthases and produce NO in response to cytokines, inflammatory factors, hypoxia, and elevated hydrostatic pressure; the inflammatory NO production is blocked by TGF-β (Liepe et al., 1994; Goureau et al., 1994, 1997, 1999; De Kozak et al., 1997; Cotinet et al., 1997b; Haverkamp et al., 1999; Kim et al., 1999; Cao et al., 1999a; Tezel and Wax, 2000; Kashiwagi et al., 2003). Excess NO production by Müller cells results in apoptotic death of neurons *in vitro* (Goureau et al., 1999; Tezel and Wax, 2000). *In vivo*, the susceptibility to develop endotoxin-induced uveitis is correlated with the extent of the production of TNF and nitrite by Müller cells, suggesting that Müller cell-derived NO is a causative factor of ocular inflammation (De Kozak et al., 1994; Cotinet et al., 1997b). The inherited retinal dystrophy observed in RCS rats was suggested to be caused by an abnormal release of TNF and NO from microglial and Müller cells in response to inflammatory stimulants (De Kozak et al., 1997; Cotinet et al., 1997a).

Hydrogen sulfide (H_2S) is a gaseous neuromodulator that is synthesized by transsulfuration enzymes such as cystathionine γ-lyase. In salamander retinas, this enzyme is localized to Müller cells, suggesting that Müller cells produce H_2S (Pong et al., 2007). The presence of the enzyme may also reflect a requirement for cysteine and glutathione synthesis via the transsulfuration pathway as a defense against oxidative stress (see 5.5.2.1.15.).

5.7 GLIAL FORWARD AND FEEDBACK REGULATION OF THE NEURONAL ACTIVITY

Repetitive light stimulation of the (avascular) guinea-pig retina (Fig. 80A,B) induces two different calcium responses in Müller cells: a slowly developing immediate response that occurs simultaneously over the whole length of Müller cell fibers, and rapid transient calcium responses which appear with a latency of ~3 min (Fig. 80C) (Rillich et al., 2009). The rapid responses originate in the Müller cell endfeet within the ganglion cell layer and propagate as waves through Müller cells toward the outer processes in the photoreceptor layer (Fig. 80D) (Rillich et al., 2009). The immediate slow response is induced by photoreceptor-to-glia signaling, and is mediated by an influx of calcium from the extracellular space (probably via Kir channels; Dallwig et al., 2000; Härtel et al., 2007) induced by zinc ions (which are released from photoreceptors; Wu et al., 1993; Qian et al., 1994; Redenti et al., 2007) and Müller cell hyperpolarization (Fig. 80E) (Rillich et al., 2009). The membrane hyperpolarization is induced by decreases of the subretinal potassium concentration and of the activity of electrogenic glutamate transporters due to the light-induced reduction of the photoreceptor activity (Rillich et al., 2009). The rapid responses are mediated by the release of calcium from intracellular stores and are partially dependent on the release of endogenous ATP (Fig. 80F) (Rillich et al., 2009). The data indicate that light stimulation of the guinea-pig retina causes glial activation by alterations of the membrane potential and by receptor-mediated mechanisms. The immediate calcium response, caused by membrane hyperpolarization (Fig. 80G), may be implicated in the glial support of the neuronal signal transfer from photoreceptors to ganglion cells (glial forward signaling) while the latter may constitute a glial feedback signaling from the ganglion cells to photoreceptors (Rillich et al., 2009). The glial forward signaling may include the opening of calcium-dependent potassium channels (to increase the potassium buffering capacity), as well as the calcium-dependent release of glutamate to prevent a hypoosmotic Müller cell swelling (Fig. 73B; see 5.5.5.3.); both supports the homeostasis of the extracellular space volume when activated neurons swell (see 5.5.1.1.). In addition, the hyperpolarization of Müller cells enhances

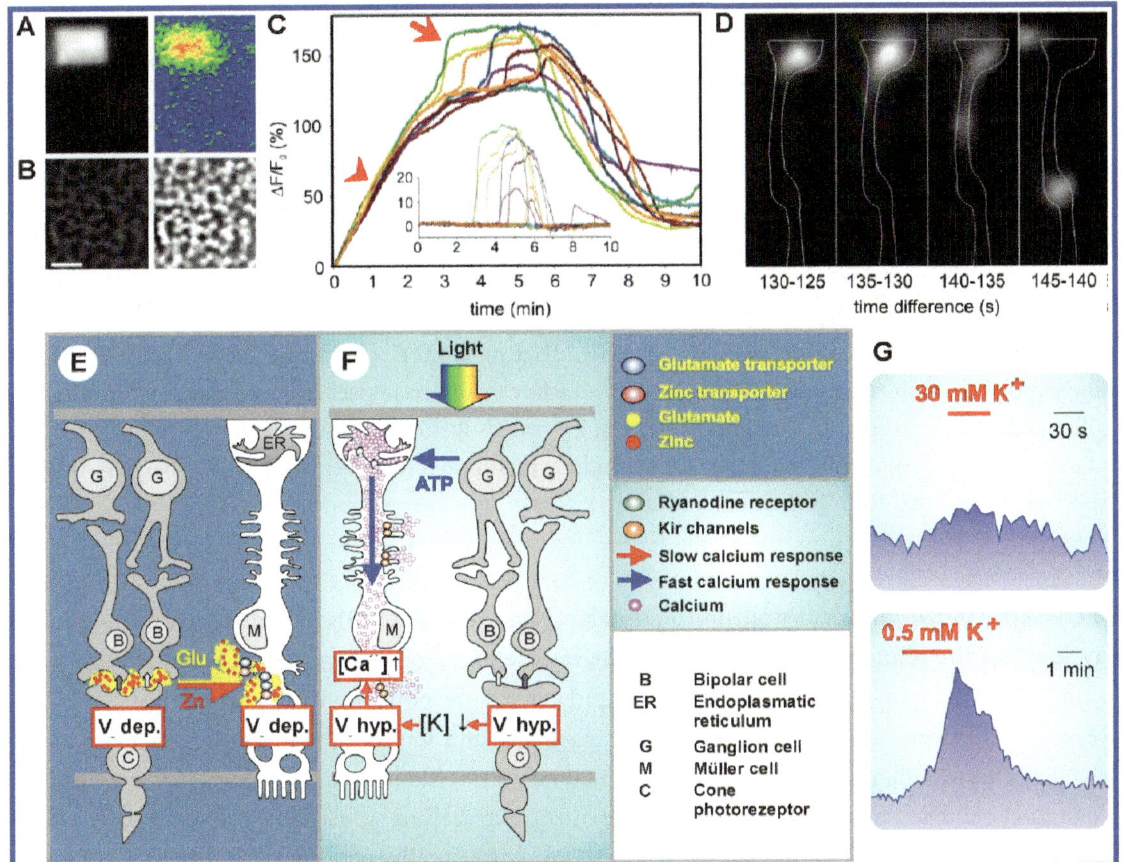

FIGURE 80: Neuronal activity, induced by repetitive light stimulation of the guinea-pig retina, is sensed by Müller cells. Light stimulation induces calcium responses in Müller cells. **A.** Müller cell calcium responses (*right part*) are confined to the area of the retinal wholemount which is illuminated (*left part*). **B.** Example of a calcium response in a retinal wholemount loaded with x-rhod-1. The focus of the images is in the inner nuclear layer which contains the somata of Müller cells. The images were obtained before (*left*) and after (*right*) a 3-min light stimulation. Bar, 25 μm. **C.** Time course of the light-induced calcium responses in Müller cells. The time-dependent calcium responses in 9 individual Müller cells during light stimulation are shown. The calcium response is composed of a slowly developing calcium rise (*arrowhead*) and (after a delay of ~3 minutes) fast calcium rises (*arrow*). The *inset* shows the fast calcium rises after subtraction of the slow responses. **D.** Example of the intracellular progression of the fast calcium rise in a retinal slice preparation. Shown are calculated differences of two fluorescence images in time intervals of 5 seconds each (ΔF) during the propagation of the fast calcium rise in one Müller

continued on next page

cell. The time points of the pictures are given as time after the onset of stimulation. **E, F.** Hypothetical scheme of the light-induced calcium responses in Müller cells. **E.** Dark-adapted retina. The release of glutamate and zinc in the dark results in a depolarization of the Müller cell membrane by the actions on the electrogenic glutamate and zinc transporters of Müller cells. **F.** Retina during light stimulation. The decrease of the extracellular potassium concentration around the photoreceptors along with the decreased glutamate and zinc concentration result in a hyperpolarization of the Müller cell membrane. The hyperpolarization induces the slow calcium rise by causing a calcium influx into Müller cells through Kir channels. The slow calcium rise may induce a release of calcium from the endoplasmatic reticulum by the action on ryanodine receptors, resulting in the fast calcium rise. Part of the fast calcium rise may also be induced by ATP released from retinal neurons and acting at P2Y receptors of Müller cells. **G.** Membrane hyperpolarization, but not depolarization, induces calcium responses in acutely isolated guinea-pig Müller cells. The cytosolic free calcium level was recorded during administration of a high (30 mM)- and a low (0.5 mM)-potassium solution which induce membrane depolarization and hyperpolarization, respectively. Modified from Rillich et al. (2009).

---

the efficiency of the glial neurotransmitter uptake (Figs. 34D, 47C,D). The glial feedback signaling may suppress the photoreceptor activity (by the release of adenosine from Müller cells) depending on the activity of retinal ganglion cells. The rapid calcium responses may in part be induced by the release of ATP from amacrine and ganglion cells (Neal and Cunningham, 1994; Newman, 2005) as well as from Müller cells (as a result of the osmotic/mechanical stress induced by the swelling of ganglion cell layer neurons and the decrease of the extracellular osmolarity). However, the functional relevance of the different calcium responses in Müller cells remains to be determined.

5.8   NEUROVASCULAR COUPLING

Because of the high metabolic activity of the retina (see 5.5.7.), the capability to regulate the local blood flow is an essential feature of the retina. The retina maintain a constant blood flow despite variations in perfusion pressure, blood gasses, and intraocular pressure, by intrinsic autoregulatory responses (Kur et al., 2012). Light stimulation dilates retinal arterioles producing blood flow increases, a response termed functional hyperemia (Newman, 2013). Multiple mechanisms contribute to functional hyperemia (Kur et al., 2012; Newman, 2013). Purinergic neuron-to-glia signaling and glial calcium waves are involved in the activity-dependent regulation of the blood flow rate in the superficial vascular plexus in dependence on the synaptic activity in the inner plexiform layer (Metea and Newman, 2006; Kurth-Nelson et al., 2009). In response to light, retinal neurons may release ATP in the inner plexiform layer which induces IP_3-mediated calcium responses in Müller cells

(Metea and Newman, 2006). The blood flow-regulatory signals transmit to the inner surface of the retina (where arterioles are localized) via propagation of glial calcium waves (Newman, 2005; Metea and Newman, 2006). These waves activate the calcium-dependent PLA_2 in glial cells; arachidonic acid metabolites are then produced which cause dilation (epoxyeicosatrienoic acids, prostaglandins) or constriction (20-hydroxyeicosatetraenoic acid) of arterioles (Metea and Newman, 2006; Mishra et al., 2011). Whether vasodilating or vasoconstricting responses are produced by glial cells is dependent on the production of NO; increased NO levels reduce vasodilation possibly by modulating the production of distinct arachidonic acid metabolites (Metea and Newman, 2006; Mishra and Newman, 2010). Oxygen decreases the light- and glia-induced vasodilation (Mishra et al., 2011). ATP and adenosine, which are released from both neurons and glial cells (Housley et al., 2009), induce constriction (Fig. 17E) and relaxation, respectively, of pericytes (Li and Puro, 2001; Peppiatt et al., 2006). In addition, lactate induces retinal vasodilation (Kur et al., 2012) while the potassium efflux from Müller cells apparently does not contribute to functional hyperemia (Metea et al., 2007). $GABA_A$ and $GABA_B$ receptors localized in perivascular Müller cell membranes may be implicated in the regulation of the retinal blood flow (Hinds et al., 2013).

5.9   FURTHER ION CHANNELS OF MÜLLER CELLS

In addition to potassium channels, Müller cells express other kinds of voltage- and second messenger-gated ion channels in their plasma membranes.

5.9.1   VOLTAGE-GATED CALCIUM CHANNELS

Müller cells from all species investigated so far (e.g., salamander, toad, rat, rabbit, guinea pig, man) express voltage-gated calcium channels (Newman, 1985b; Puro and Mano, 1991; Puro, 1994; Puro et al., 1996a; Bringmann et al., 2000b-d, f; Xu et al., 2002; Welch et al., 2005; Linnertz et al., 2011). In whole-cell records of cells from many species, however, the calcium channel-mediated currents are very small when calcium or barium ions are used as charge carriers. The detection of calcium channel-mediated currents can be improved when the extracellular solution does not contain divalent cations; under these conditions, sodium ions flow through the channels, and the amplitude of the currents is increased (Fig. 45A,B) (Bringmann et al., 2000b-d,f). The reason for the small amplitude of calcium currents is unclear. It has been hypothesized that, simultaneous to the membrane depolarization, the action of certain second messengers (formed after activation of growth factor or neurotransmitter receptors) is necessary to open the channels (Bringmann et al., 2000b). This assumption corresponds to findings in cultured astrocytes where calcium currents are usually undetectable but recordable after addition of neurotransmitters or agents that increase the intracellular cAMP level (MacVicar, 1984; Barres et al., 1989). Sodium currents through voltage-gated calcium channels may not be physiological. However, there are indications that under certain pathophysiological conditions, e.g., after lipid peroxidation, voltage-gated calcium channels of retinal cells may indeed become permeable to sodium ions (Agostinho et al., 1997).

In salamander Müller cells, depolarizing current pulses induce regenerative calcium spikes via activation of voltage-gated calcium channels (Newman, 1985b). High potassium-induced depolarization of the cells triggers a verapamil-sensitive rapid increase of the intracellular free calcium level throughout the length of the cells (Keirstead and Miller, 1995). In contrast, depolarization of dissociated Müller cells of the guinea pig with a high-potassium solution does not induce calcium responses in the cells (although the cells express voltage-gated calcium channels as observed in electrophysiological recordings). Instead, a membrane hyperpolarization by a low-potassium solution induces calcium responses in the cells (Fig. 80G) (Rillich et al., 2009). Such cytosolic calcium transients upon lowering of the extracellular potassium concentration to 2 mM or below were also found in brain astrocytes, and were suggested to be mediated by a calcium influx through Kir4.1 potassium channels (Dallwig et al., 2000; Härtel et al., 2007). In the postnatal development of the rabbit retina, the incidence of radial glial/Müller cells that display depolarization-induced calcium responses decreases with the maturation of Müller cells (Fig. 51) (Uckermann et al., 2002). These responses are induced (at least in part) by activation of autocrine/paracrine purinergic P2Y receptor signaling (Uckermann et al., 2002).

In whole-cell records, human Müller cells display both transient (T-type) and long-lasting (L-type) calcium channel currents (Fig. 45B). T-type currents are low threshold voltage-activated (LVA) currents, i.e., the threshold of activation of the currents with a depolarizing pulse is low. Calcium currents through LVA channels activate at potentials positive to -60 mV, and maximal currents are observed at -30 mV (Fig. 45C) (Bringmann et al., 2000b,g). L-type currents are high threshold voltage-activated (HVA) currents; these currents activate at potentials positive to -30 mV and have their maximal amplitude at 0 mV (Fig. 45C) (Bringmann et al., 2000b). Human Müller cells express regularly both LVA and HVA currents, whereas Müller cells of adult rabbits express regularly LVA currents, but only a subpopulation of the cells (~25%) display also HVA currents (Bringmann et al., 2000d). Human Müller cells in culture have L-type calcium channels composed of α_{1D}, α_2, and β_3 subunits (Puro et al., 1996a). Activation of the channels results in opening of calcium-activated potassium (BK) channels (Puro et al., 1996a). Acutely isolated human Müller cells display immunoreactivities for different types of the pore-forming subunits of L-type channels, including α_{1C} and α_{1D} (Fig. 45G). Müller cells of the rat express the α_{1C} subunit of L-type and the α_{1G} subunit of T-type voltage-gated calcium channels (Fig. 45F) (Linnertz et al., 2011). Chicken Müller cells express α_{1C} and perhaps α_{1D} subunits (Firth et al., 2001). Müller cells of the tiger salamander have HVA channels which are distributed over the entire membrane of the cells, and express $\alpha_{1A, B, C, D}$ subunits (Welch et al., 2005).

The expression of voltage-gated calcium channels in rabbit Müller cells alters in the course of the ontogenetic development. In the rabbit retina, proliferation of late progenitor cells occurs up to postnatal days 4 (central retina) and 10 (peripheral retina), respectively (Fig. 51) (Schnitzer, 1990; Reichenbach et al., 1991a; Sharma and Ehinger, 1997). The differentiation of immature radial glial cells into mature Müller cells occurs between the postnatal days 6 and 20, as indicated by the developmental increase of the Kir currents (Fig. 51) (Bringmann et al., 1999a). Immature radial glial/Müller cells of the rabbit express only LVA channels; HVA currents are observed solely in mature Müller cells after postnatal day 20 (Bringmann et al., 2000d). The amplitude of LVA currents increases during the first postnatal week and remains constant after postnatal day 6 (when the light-induced ganglion cell activity begins; Fig. 51) (Bringmann et al., 2000d). This means that immature and mature rabbit Müller cells have similar numbers of LVA channels. The density of LVA currents decreases during the postnatal maturation of Müller cells (Fig. 51) (Bringmann et al., 2000d). This may suggest that the increase of the plasma membrane area of developing Müller cells (as reflected by the increase of the cell membrane capacitance; Fig. 51) is not associated with an increase in the expression of LVA channels. The early and sole expression of LVA calcium channels suggests that these channels are involved in the regulation of the proliferation of late progenitor cells as well as of the differentiation of Müller cells, e.g., of the outgrowth of glial side branches and perisynaptic membrane sheets. The different expression patterns of LVA and HVA channels in developing and mature rabbit Müller cells suggest that the two channel types have different functional roles.

The expression of voltage-gated calcium channels in human Müller cells alters in the course of aging and under pathological conditions. In correlation with the age of human subjects, the density of the HVA currents increases while the Kir currents decrease (Fig. 45D) (Bringmann et al., 2000b, 2003c). In Müller cells of patients with PVR, both LVA and HVA currents display a substantial reduction in their amplitudes (Bringmann et al., 2000b). The membrane conductance of Müller cells from patients with PVR and PDR is characterized by an almost full absence of Kir currents (Figs. 45E, 46B–D, 56B), a severe increase of voltage-dependent sodium currents, and an enhanced activity of BK channels (Fig. 60B) (Reichelt et al., 1997a; Francke et al., 1996, 1997; Bringmann et al., 1999b; see 5.11.10.2.). Because of the high expression of voltage-dependent sodium channels, single action potential-like discharges can be induced by large depolarizing current steps in Müller cells of patients with PVR (Fig. 67C) (Francke et al., 1996). All of these alterations favor rapid fluctuations of the membrane potential that will enhance the activity of voltage-gated calcium channels. The downregulation of voltage-gated calcium channels in Müller cells of patients with PVR may protect the cells from cytotoxic calcium overload (Bringmann et al., 2000b).

Voltage-gated calcium channels play a crucial role in Müller cell proliferation which commonly occurs in response to retinal injury (see 5.11.10.). The growth factor- and nucleotide-induced proliferation of cultured Müller cells of the guinea pig is inhibited in the presence of blockers of T- and L-type calcium channels (Kodal et al., 2000). bFGF, but not PDGF, increases the amplitude of L-type calcium currents in cultured human Müller cells; the bFGF-induced proliferation of the cells depends upon the activity of L-type calcium channels (Puro and Mano, 1991; Uchihori and Puro, 1991). Elevation of the free cytosolic calcium level is required for various steps of the cell cycle, and activation of voltage-gated calcium channels may result in a higher transcription rate and exocytotic release of growth factors which stimulate the proliferation of Müller cells in autocrine and paracrine fashions. In cultured Müller cells of the guinea pig, the release of growth factors from the cells, and the activation of MMPs that induce a release of membrane-bound growth factors, occur downstream of the calcium responses (see 5.11.10.3.). It has been shown that electrical stimulation of cultured Müller cells enhances the transcription of neurotrophic factors such as IGF-1 and BDNF; this effect is mediated by a calcium influx through L-type calcium channels (Sato et al., 2008a, b). IGF-1 stimulates the proliferation of cultured Müller cells (Ikeda and Puro, 1995; Ikeda et al., 1995). It was suggested that voltage-gated calcium and BK channels work together to mediate the sustained calcium influx from the extracellular space required for the mitogen-induced Müller cell proliferation (see 5.11.10.2.).

In Müller cells of the healthy rodent retina, activation of voltage-gated calcium channels is implicated in the exocytotic release of glutamate; this release is stimulated by various receptor ligands and is implicated in the autocrine regulation of the cellular volume (see 5.5.5.3.). Activation of T-type voltage-gated calcium channels is also involved in mediating the glutamate-induced release of ATP from murine Müller cells (see 5.6.3.1.). Apparently, voltage-gated calcium channels have similar roles in differentiated and proliferating Müller cells: they mediate the calcium influx into the cells necessary for the exocytotic release of gliotransmittes such as glutamate and the secretion of growth factors from Müller cells. In addition, activation of voltage-gated calcium channels is implicated in the phagocytotic activity of Müller cells (Mano and Puro, 1990).

5.9.2   VOLTAGE-GATED SODIUM CHANNELS

Müller cells of a variety of animal species express neuron-type voltage-dependent sodium channels that generate, upon depolarizing voltage steps, fast transient, inwardly directed sodium currents which are sensitive to tetrodotoxin and saxitoxin (Fig. 67A). In human cells, the currents activate at voltages positive to –60 mV, peak at –20 mV, and reverse close to the equilibrium potential of sodium ions (Fig. 67B). Müller cells of tiger salamanders and guinea pigs do not have such currents, independent of age and retinal pathology (Newman, 1985b; Chao et al., 1994a,b). Müller cells of the cat, dog, horse, zebra, and baboon, and a subpopulation of primate Müller cells, display voltage-dependent sodium currents (Chao et al., 1993, 1994b, 1997; Reichelt et al., 1997c; Han et al., 2000). Rabbit Müller cells may display such currents under pathological conditions. Only a small fraction (~3%) of Müller cells of the adult rat retina display small tetrodotoxin-sensitive sodium currents when recorded in the whole-cell mode of the patch-clamp technique (Wurm et al., 2006b) while approximately 50% of Müller cells of the adult murine retina have such currents (Pannicke et al., 2002). One third of Müller cells of the healthy human retina investigated display voltage-gated sodium currents; the incidence of cells with these currents increase up to ~90% under pathological conditions (Francke et al., 1996; Reichelt et al., 1997a). In addition, the amplitude of the currents in human Müller cells increase under pathological conditions; Müller cells derived from patients with proliferative retinopathies show action potential-like discharges upon administration of depolarizing currents (Fig. 67C) (Francke et al., 1996). This capability may reflect the dedifferentiation of Müller cells and likely the transdifferentiation of the cells into progenitor/neuron-like cells in the course of proliferative gliosis (see 5.11.10.2. and 5.11.12.). The activity of voltage-gated sodium channels produces rapid fluctuations of the membrane potential that supports the opening of voltage-gated calcium channels; the calcium influx is required for the Müller cell proliferation (see 5.11.10.2.) and for the exocytotic release of growth factors and gliotransmitters such as glutamate from Müller cells (see 5.6.1.2.). Activation of voltage-gated sodium channels is also required for the glutamate-induced release of ATP from murine Müller (see 5.6.3.1.).

The presence of voltage-dependent sodium currents is differentially regulated in the course of the ontogenetic development of Müller cells from various species. While the incidence of murine Müller cells that display such currents increases in the course of retinal development (Pannicke et al., 2002), the incidence of rat Müller cells with such currents rapidly decreases (Fig. 67D) when the Kir currents display a steep developmental increase after postnatal day 14 (Fig. 61A) (Wurm et al., 2006b). The reason for this species difference is unclear. Interestingly, Müller cells of the adult rat retina display immunoreactivity for $Na_v1.6$ (Fig. 67E), and tetrodotoxin prevents the VEGF-induced inhibition of the osmotic swelling of Müller cells isolated from the adult rat retina which is mediated by the exocytotic release of glutamate (Fig. 73B) (Linnertz et al., 2011). (Rodent Müller cells may also express the tetrodotoxin-resistant channel $Na_v1.9$; O'Brien et al., 2008.) These data suggest that Müller cells of the mature rat retina express voltage-gated sodium channels which are implicated in the agonist-induced exocytosis of glutamate. However, these channels are not activable by membrane depolarization alone; instead, additional intracellular messengers (which are formed after receptor activation) are necessary to activate the channels. These second messengers are absent during electrophysiological whole-cell recordings. On the other hand, in immature

Müller cells of the rat, these channels may be activable solely by membrane depolarization, and likely mediate (in association with other channels such as K_A channels; Fig. 67D) rapid fluctuations of the membrane potential which enhance the open probability of voltage-gated calcium channels. Thus, the decrease in the incidence of Müller cells in the developing rat retina that display voltage-gated sodium currents (Fig. 67D) may reflect an alteration in channel gating rather than a downregulation of channel proteins. However, the functional significance and activation parameters of voltage-gated sodium channels in Müller cells remain to be further elucidated.

5.9.3 EPITHELIAL SODIUM CHANNELS

Müller cells have α-epithelial sodium channels (ENaCα) (Brockway et al., 2002; Deliyanti et al., 2014). The expression of ENaCα in Müller cells is increased by activation of mineralocorticoid receptors with aldosterone, by activation of angiotensin type 1 receptors, and by high salt (Golestaneh et al., 2001; Deliyanti et al., 2014). ENaCα may play a role in the regulation of the extracellular sodium concentration and in the regulation of the cell volume under varying osmotic conditions. The expression of ENaCα in Müller cells is increased in ischemic retinopathy and reduced by a low-salt diet, likely via a downregulation of angiotensin type 1 and mineralocorticoid receptors (Deliyanti et al., 2014).

5.9.4 CATION CHANNELS

Müller cells may express several kinds of non-selective cation channels. In bovine and human Müller cells, blood serum (but not plasma) activates calcium-permeable cation channels that is followed by a delayed activation of an outward potassium conductance; both conductances are also activated by serum-derived molecules such as lysophosphatidic acid (Kusaka et al., 1998, 1999). Cultured human Müller cells express calcium-permeable cation channels which are activated by cytosolic calcium; the open time of the channels is increased during administration of bFGF (Puro, 1991b). The opening of these channels provides a pathway for the influx of calcium from the extracellular space at the resting membrane potential.

Müller cells have calcium-permeable, store-operated channels which are activated after depletion of internal calcium stores, e.g., upon activation of metabotropic receptors (Moll et al., 2002; Da Silva et al., 2008). Although the molecular identity of store-operated channels is not well established, several members of the cation-permeable transient receptor potential canonical (TRPC) channel family may be candidate store-operated channels and may contribute to the receptor- and store-operated capacitative calcium entry. Cultured mouse Müller cells express TRPC1 and TRPC6; these channels are activated after stimulation of muscarinic M1 receptors (Da Silva et al., 2008). In the chicken retina, TRPC4 is localized to Müller cells and neurons (Crousillac et al., 2003).

Cultured human Müller cells have stretch-activated calcium-permeable cation channels; activation of the channels results in an increased activity of BK channels (Puro, 1991a). The efflux of potassium ions through BK channels (which is associated with an efflux of cell water) was suggested to be a mechanism to decrease the volume of Müller cells after cell swelling (Puro, 1991a).

cGMP activates cGMP-gated cation channels in bovine and human Müller cells that results in membrane depolarization, calcium influx, and activation of BK channels (Kusaka et al., 1996). NO donors induce currents that are similar to those activated by cGMP (Kusaka et al., 1996). The presence of calcium-permeable cGMP-gated non-selective cation channels was also described in freshly isolated Müller cells of the bullfrog; these channels open upon activation of the natriuretic peptide receptor-A (Cao and Yang, 2007) that is coupled to the guanylyl cyclase. The calcium-binding protein S-100B stimulates a membrane-bound guanylyl cyclase in Müller cells at high calcium concentrations (Rambotti et al., 1999).

5.9.5   CHLORIDE CHANNELS

Normally, the chloride conductance of Müller cell membranes is very low (Newman, 1985a). However, pharmacological investigations suggest that Müller cells of the rat express second messenger-gated chloride channels; opening of the channels and an efflux of chloride ions are implicated in the equalization of the osmotic gradient across Müller cell membranes under hypoosmotic conditions (Fig. 73B; see 5.5.5.3.). These channels are activated after stimulation of adenosine A_1 receptors and subsequent activation of the adenylyl cyclase, PKA, and PI3K. Müller cells of the tiger salamander express calcium-activated chloride channels which are activated upon a depolarization-induced calcium influx through voltage-gated calcium channels (Welch et al., 2006).

5.10   RECEPTOR EXPRESSION BY MÜLLER CELLS

There is a bidirectional dialogue between Müller cells and retinal neurons (Newman, 2004a); neuronal activity and neurotransmitter release modulate the function of Müller cells and, in turn, Müller cells can modify the neuronal extracellular environment and, more directly, the synaptic transmission (see 5.6.). Receptors expressed by Müller cells play functional roles in the bidirectional signal transfer between retinal neurons and glial cells. Transmitter molecules released from neurons such as glutamate, GABA, and ATP activate receptors expressed by Müller cells resulting in activation and functional changes of Müller cells such as alterations in the membrane conductance, cellular depolarization, and intracellular calcium responses. Cytosolic calcium rises may trigger the release of neuroactive substances from Müller cells (such as glutamate, ATP, and adenosine) that influence the synaptic activity (see 5.6.) and regulate the Müller cell volume under conditions of osmotic imbalances associated with neuronal activity (see 5.5.5.3.). Activation of Müller cells may also result in alterations of the homeostatic functions of Müller cells that influence the neuronal activity.

Generally, there are metabotropic receptors (which are coupled to intracellular second messenger systems) and ionotropic receptors (which represent ligand-gated ion channels). Müller cells may express both kinds of receptors. However, there are species-dependent variations in the expression of distinct receptor subtypes. Whereas metabotropic purinergic P2Y and possibly mGluRs are commonly expressed by Müller cells, ionotropic receptors are solely expressed in Müller cells of distinct species. Even Müller cells of one animal may vary in their expression of receptors, i.e., receptors may be expressed in distinct subpopulations of Müller cells from one retina.

It should be noted that many data regarding the receptor expression in Müller cells were obtained in cultured cells. These data must be interpreted with caution because cultured Müller cells are known to differ from cells *in situ* in important aspects; for example, cultured Müller cells dedifferentiate and lose their Kir channels (Kuhrt et al., 2008; Wurm et al., 2009b), change their receptor expression (Small et al., 1991), undergo a fibroblastic transdifferentiation (Guidry, 1996, 2005, 2009; see 5.11.11.2.), or even a transdifferentiation into a neuron-like phenotype (Kubrusly et al., 2005; see 5.11.12.). However, results obtained in cultured cells may reflect properties of glial dedifferentiation, proliferation, and transdifferentiation in reactive gliosis *in situ* (see 5.11.).

5.10.1 GLUTAMATE RECEPTORS

Glutamate is the most important excitatory neurotransmitter in the retina, acting in the vertical axis composed by photoreceptor, bipolar, and ganglion cells (Reichenbach and Bringmann, 2012). In addition, glutamate is a gliotransmitter and can be released from Müller cells by various mechanisms (see 5.6.1.). Excitatory amino acids (glutamate and aspartate) exert their action through the activation of specific ionotropic and metabotropic receptors. iGluRs are ligand-gated cation channels; the direction of the receptor currents reverses at the equilibrium potential of cations (0 mV); therefore, activation of the receptors causes a depolarization of the cells. mGluRs are G protein-coupled receptors linked to second messenger systems, for example phosphoinositide hydrolysis and release of calcium from intracellular stores, inhibition or activation of the adenylyl cyclase, and activation of phosphodiesterases.

5.10.1.1 iGluRs

There are three major families of iGluRs called NMDA, AMPA, and KA receptors. Native receptors of all of these families are tetrameric assemblies comprising more than one type of subunit. NMDA receptors may be composed of NR1, NR2, and possibly NR3 subunits. While NR1 is essential for the formation of functional channels, NR2 and NR3 play modulatory roles. Glutamate binds to the NR2 subunit while the glycine-binding site is on the NR1 subunit. AMPA receptors are composed of GluR1-4 subunits, and KA receptors are composed of GluR5-7 and KA-1 and 2 subunits.

The AMPA receptor subunit GluR4 is localized on Müller cells of the goldfish and frogs (Yazulla and Studholme, 1999; Vandenbranden et al., 2000b; Vitanova, 2007). Müller cells of the cat express immunoreactivity for the AMPA receptor subunit GluR2 which is increased after retinal detachment (Lewis et al., 1999a). GluR4 was immunohistochemically localized to Müller cells in slices of the rat retina (Peng et al., 1995). Activation AMPA receptors induces the release of D-serine from murine retinal glial cells (Sullivan and Miller, 2010). Frog and turtle Müller cells display immunoreactivities of NR1, NR2C, and NR2D subunits (Vitanova, 2012). Müller cells of the cat express NR2A subunits (Goebel et al., 1998), while Müller cells of the rat show immunoreactivities of NR1, NR2A, and NR2B subunits (Gründer et al., 2000) and express mRNA for NMDA receptor subunits (Pannicke et al., 1999). NMDA receptor agonists induce a release of VEGF from cultured rat Müller cells (Cervantes-Villagrana et al., 2010), suggesting that NMDA receptors exert a tonic inhibition on VEGF secretion contributing to the antiangiogenic role of Müller cells (see 5.11.8.). However, freshly dissociated Müller cells of the rat do not have functional iGluRs, as indicated by the fact that receptor agonists (KA, NMDA) do not induce membrane currents when recorded in the whole-cell mode of the patch-clamp technique (Fig. 48A) (Felmy et al., 2001; Pannicke et al., 2005a). A lack of alterations in the membrane conductance upon administration of iGluR agonists was also observed in whole-cell records of Müller cells from tiger salamanders, mice, guinea pigs, and rabbits (Brew and Attwell, 1987; Schwartz and Tachibana, 1990; Sarantis and Attwell, 1990; Reichenbach et al., 1997; Pannicke et al., 2002; Uckermann et al., 2004b). Acutely dissociated human Müller cells display NMDA-induced currents when recorded in the perforated-patch configuration of the patch-clamp technique (Puro et al., 1996b). The reason for the absence of KA- and NMDA-evoked membrane currents in whole-cell records of freshly isolated rat Müller cells is unclear. It could be that in Müller cells (in contrast to neurons) iGluRs are not activated by agonist binding alone but that coactivation by distinct intracellular second messengers is required to open the channels. These second messengers may be washed out from the cytosol after establishment of the whole-cell configuration of the patch-clamp technique.

Functional iGluRs are regularly found in cultured Müller cells. Cultured human Müller cells express NMDA receptors and the NR1 subunit (Uchihori and Puro, 1993; Puro et al., 1996b). Activation of the receptors inhibits the Kir currents by ~50%; this effect is mediated by an influx of calcium from the extracellular space (Puro, 1996; Puro et al., 1996b). Cultured Müller cells of young postnatal rats express NMDA receptors (Taylor et al., 2003). Here, NMDA receptor activation results in altered activity of the transcription factor downstream regulatory element antagonist modulator (DREAM), a decrease in the NMDA receptor level, an increase in the secretion of neurotrophic factors such as BDNF, NGF, neurotrophins-3 and -4, and GDNF, sustained activation of the tropomyosin-related kinase B (TrkB) by BDNF, and upregulation of the glutamate transporter (GLAST) protein (Taylor et al., 2003; Chavira-Suárez et al., 2008). It has been suggested that the decrease in the NMDA receptor level and the sustained activation of TrkB serve as protective mechanisms for the Müller cell survival, while the secretion of neurotrophic factors and the upregulation of GLAST may protect retinal neurons from glutamate toxicity (Taylor et al., 2003). Cultured Müller cells of the rabbit express AMPA/KA receptors that mediate a calcium influx from the extracellular space (Minei, 2002). Glutamate induces an exocytotic release of ATP from cultured avian Müller cell by activation of both AMPA/KA and NMDA receptors (Loiola and Ventura, 2011). Cultured Müller cells are normally resistant to neurotoxic levels of glutamate (up to 1 mM) (Uchihori and Puro, 1993; Kitano et al., 1996; Heidinger et al., 1998). This resistance has been ascribed (at least in part) to a lower affinity of Müller cell's AMPA receptors compared to neuronal receptors (Kawasaki et al., 1996) and the expression of glutamate transporters and glutamine synthetase that rapidly detoxify glutamate.

Cultured chick Müller cells express NMDA (NR1, NR2) and AMPA/KA receptors (GluR1,4,5) (Lopez-Colome et al., 1993; Lopez et al., 1994, 1997, 1998). Activation of the receptors results in an increase in AP-1 DNA binding activity (Lopez-Colome et al., 1995). The expression of GluR4 is decreased after treatment with glutamate acting at group I mGluRs (Lopez et al., 1998). NMDA receptors are coupled to the phosphoinositide cascade, entry of calcium, and activation of PKC (Lopez-Colome et al., 1993; Lamas et al., 2005, 2007). Activation of AMPA/KA receptors results in cytosolic calcium responses (Wakakura and Yamamoto, 1994).

Activation of NMDA receptors (for example, by the tripeptide glycine-proline-glutamate which is a cleavage product of IGF-1) stimulates the proliferation of cultured Müller cells (Uchihori and Puro, 1993; Ikeda et al., 1995; see 5.11.10.5.). In addition to being a mitogen, glutamate also has antiproliferative effects in Müller cells. Activation of mGluRs inhibits the growth factor-induced proliferation of cultured Müller cells (Ikeda and Puro, 1995; see 5.11.10.6.). In adult mice, subretinal administration of subtoxic levels of glutamate or α-aminoadipic acid (a glutamate analogue acting selectively in glial cells) causes Müller cell dedifferentiation, proliferation, migration, and transdifferentiation into neurons and photoreceptors (Takeda et al., 2008; see 5.11.12.).

5.10.1.2. mGluRs

Müller cells express mGluRs which are coupled to calcium-dependent or calcium-independent intracellular signaling pathways. There is a species variability in the coupling of mGluR activation to intracellular calcium responses in Müller cells. In the absence of extracellular calcium, agonists of group I/III mGluRs induce calcium waves in Müller cells acutely dissociated from the salamander retina; the waves are mediated by a release of calcium from intracellular stores (Keirstead and Miller, 1997). The increase in the cytosolic free calcium level oftenly begins in the outer ends of the cells, moves through the cells, and occurs 7–70 s later in the endfeet (Keirstead and Miller, 1997). Such waves can be also induced by elevated potassium, ATP, as well as caffeine and ryanodine (Keirstead and Miller, 1997). While glutamatergic agonists induced such waves only in a subpopulation of Müller cells, nearly all cells investigated displayed such waves in response to ATP (Keirstead and Miller, 1997). The calcium waves in Müller cells were suggested to provide an extraneuronal pathway for signals to be relayed from the outer to the inner retina (Newman and Reichenbach, 1996; see 5.6.3.4.). Müller cells of the tiger salamander have calcium-activated potassium channels (Newman, 1985b); an increase in the cytosolic free calcium level will enhance the potassium buffering capacity of the cells. The mechanism for the propagation of the calcium waves in Müller cells of the tiger salamander is unclear. In salamander and rat Müller cells, antibodies against IP_3 receptors labels most strongly the outer region of the cells (Peng et al., 1991). Glutamate transporters are localized preferentially to the outer region of salamander Müller cells (Brew and Attwell, 1987), and it may be possible that mGluRs are also more densely distributed in this region (Keirstead and Miller, 1997).

In rat Müller cells, glutamate and agonists of group I/II mGluRs are ineffective in inducing cytosolic calcium responses (Newman and Zahs, 1997; Newman 2005) but potentiate the calcium responses triggered by other stimuli (Newman and Zahs, 1997). However, glutamate induces a calcium-independent release of ATP from rat Müller cells; this effect is implicated in the autocrine regulation of Müller cell volume (see 5.5.5.3.). Pharmacological investigation of the cell volume regulation revealed the presence of the mGlu1 receptor subtype (belonging to the group I mGluRs) and of group II mGluRs in rat Müller cells (Uckermann et al., 2006; Wurm et al., 2008a). In retinas of rabbits and guinea pigs, glutamate induces cytosolic calcium responses in neurons but not Müller cells (Fig. 17A,B) (Uckermann et al., 2003, 2004b; Rillich et al., 2009).

A subpopulation of acutely isolated Müller cells of the human retina (~30% of cells investigated) was shown to respond to extracellular glutamate with transient increases in the intracellular free calcium level (Fig. 48B) and BK currents (Figs. 43A, 64D,E), suggesting the presence of mGluRs (Bringmann et al., 2002a). The BK current responses were always delayed by 10–60 seconds after beginning of glutamate exposure (Fig. 43A); similar long latencies of glutamate-induced calcium responses were observed in Müller cells of the tiger salamander (Keirstead and Miller, 1997). The delayed responses are different from the ATP-induced BK current responses; ATP induces instantaneous increases of the BK currents in virtually all human Müller cells investigated

(Fig. 43A,B,D,G) (Bringmann et al., 2002a). It cannot be ruled out that glutamate induces a release of ATP (see 5.6.3.1.) which subsequently induces the calcium response. The glutamate-induced increase of the BK currents may be associated with a transient activation of a calcium-activated cation conductance (Fig. 43A) (Bringmann et al., 2002a).

Cultured chicken Müller cells express mGluR1 and mGluR5 (Lopez et al., 1998). Activation of the receptors elicit calcium responses and activation of PKC and ERK1/2 (Lopez-Colome et al., 1993; Lopez et al., 1998; Lopez-Colome and Ortega, 1997).

5.10.2 PURINERGIC RECEPTORS

In the retina, the purines ATP and adenosine act as neuro- and gliotransmitters (see 5.6.3.), and purinergic signaling is involved in mediating the bidirectional neuron-glia signaling (Newman, 2004a; Housley et al., 2009). Purinergic signaling plays a crucial role in many of the homeostatic functions of Müller cells, and in gliotic responses under pathological conditions (Housley et al., 2009). In the retina, photoreceptors, most neurons, glial cells, the microvasculature, and pigment epithelial cells express P1 (adenosine) and P2 (nucleotide) receptors (Housley et al., 2009). Adenosine receptors are subdivided into four subtypes ($A_{1, 2A, 2B, 3}$); all of which couple to G proteins. P2 receptors (which primarily recognize adenine and uracil tri- and diphosphates) comprise two families, ionotropic P2X and G protein-coupled P2Y receptors. P2X receptors (which are ATP-gated ion channels) are subdivided into seven subtypes ($P2X_{1-7}$); P2Y receptors comprise at least eight subtypes ($P2Y_{1, 2, 4, 6, 11, 12, 13, 14}$) (Burnstock, 2007). ATP is an agonist of $P2Y_{1, 2, 4, 11}$ receptors and, to a lesser extent, $P2Y_6$ receptors (Fields and Burnstock, 2006). Some P2Y receptor subtypes show greater sensitivity to adenine ($P2Y_{1, 11}$) or uracil nucleotides ($P2Y_{2, 4, 6}$) (Fields and Burnstock, 2006).

In the retina, purines are tonically released in the dark; this release increases with neuronal activity (Perez et al., 1986). ATP is liberated from neurons in a calcium- and/or pannexin-dependent manner (Perez et al., 1986; Santos et al., 1999; Xia et al., 2012), and from glial and pigment epithelial cells by calcium-independent and -dependent mechanisms (Newman, 2001a, b; Mitchell, 2001; Pearson et al., 2005; Uckermann et al., 2006; Wurm et al., 2010; see 5.6.3.1.). Adenosine may be released from Müller cells via nucleoside transporters (Uckermann et al., 2006) but is also formed enzymatically from ATP by ecto-nucleotidases in the extracellular space, at least under pathological conditions (Newman, 2003b, 2004b; Ribelayga and Mangel, 2005; see 5.5.5.3.3. and 5.6.3.2.). ATP contributes to fast excitatory neurotransmission by activation of P2X receptors, and has a neuromodulatory role, acting at P2Y receptors on neuronal and glial cells (see 5.6.3.4.). Adenosine suppresses the excitatory neurotransmission in the retina by various mechanisms including inhibition of presynaptic voltage-dependent calcium channels which results in reduced transmitter release (see 5.6.3.4.). Müller cells of all animal species investigated so far express multiple P2Y receptor subtypes, while the expression of functional P2X receptors seems to be restricted to Müller cells of distinct species. In the retinas of most animal species investigated so far, the expression of functional P2X receptors is restricted to neurons.

5.10.2.1 Adenosine Receptors

Müller cells in the rat express adenosine A_1, A_{2A}, and A_{2B} receptors; activation of the receptors potentiates the light-induced calcium responses of Müller cells (Newman, 2005). In another study, activation of A_2, but not A_1, receptors was found to induce calcium responses in rat Müller cells, via the release of calcium from intracellular stores (Li et al., 2001). Adenosine also induces calcium responses in a subpopulation of monkey Müller cells (Pannicke et al., 2005c). In Müller cells of tiger salamanders, skates, rabbits (Fig. 63A), and man, adenosine does not induce calcium responses (Malchow and Ramsey, 1999; Francke et al., 2002; Bringmann et al., 2002a; Uckermann et al., 2002; Uhlmann et al., 2003; but see Liu and Wakakura, 1998). In the rat retina, Müller cells (in addition to inner nuclear and ganglion cell layer neurons) express immunoreactivity for adenosine A_1 receptors (Iandiev et al., 2007b). In these cells, activation of the receptors by endogenously released adenosine is implicated in the purinergic signaling cascade which inhibits the swelling of the cells under hypoosmotic conditions (see 5.5.5.3.). In cultured rat Müller cells, adenosine acting at A_{2A} receptors was described to decrease the expression of GLAST and glutamine synthetase (Yu et al., 2012).

5.10.2.2 Ionotropic P2X Receptors

In addition to calcium responses induced by activation of metabotropic receptors, Müller cells may sense the neuronal activity by alterations of the membrane potential upon activation of receptor channels (Bringmann et al., 2006). Human, *Macaca*, and chick Müller cells (but not Müller cells of other mammalian species investigated so far) express ionotropic $P2X_7$ receptors which are ligand-gated cation channels (Pannicke et al., 2000a, 2005c; Felmy et al., 2001; Bringmann et al., 2001, 2002a,b; Francke et al., 2002; Uckermann et al., 2002; Anccasi et al., 2013; Ishii et al., 2003b). In the rodent retina, the expression of $P2X_7$ receptor protein is restricted to neuronal and microglial cells (Brändle et al., 1998; Wheeler-Schilling et al., 2001a; Innocenti et al., 2004; Franke et al., 2005; Vessey and Fletcher, 2012). Although gene transcripts of $P2X_{3, 4, 5}$ receptors, and of $P2X_4$ immunoreactivity, were reported to be present in rat Müller cells (Jabs et al., 2000; Ho et al., 2014), purinergic receptor agonists do not induce alterations in the plasma membrane conductance which would indicate the presence of functional P2X receptors (Felmy et al., 2001; Bringmann et al., 2001). In addition, Müller cells of mice, guinea pigs, rabbits, and pigs do not express functional P2X receptors, as suggested by the absence of changes in the intracellular free calcium level and the membrane conductance upon administration of exogenous ATP (Liu and Wakakura, 1998; Bringmann et al., 2001; Francke et al., 2002). Müller cells of lower vertebrates (frog, turtle) may express various P2X receptor subtypes (Vitanova and Kupenova, 2014).

$P2X_7$ receptors are non-selective cation channels which are permeable for sodium, potassium, and calcium ions. Activation of $P2X_7$ receptors by ATP or BzATP (a more specific $P2X_7$ receptor agonist) in human Müller cells results in membrane depolarization, calcium influx from the extracellular space, sustained activation of BK channels, and calcium release from thapsigargin-sensitive intracellular stores (Fig. 43B,C,E,F) (Pannicke et al., 2000a; Bringmann et al., 2001, 2002a). The $P2X_7$-induced depolarization of the cells is balanced by the hyperpolarization caused by the potassium flux through the BK channels. The currents through $P2X_7$ receptor channels are increased when the extracellular fluid contains low concentrations of divalent cations (Pannicke et al., 2000a); thus, light-induced reductions in extracellular calcium will facilitate the gating of $P2X_7$ receptor channels in Müller cells. In contrast to the $P2X_7$ receptors of immune cells such as retinal microglia (Innocenti et al., 2004), prolonged activation of $P2X_7$ receptors in Müller cells does not result in the formation of large pores in the plasma membrane (Pannicke et al., 2000a).

5.10.2.3 Metabotropic P2Y Receptors

G protein-coupled P2Y receptors are linked to different intracellular signaling pathways in Müller cells, for example to phosphoinositide hydrolysis and release of calcium from intracellular stores (which is followed by a second phase of calcium influx from the extracellular space) (e.g. $P2Y_{1,2,4}$) or to a calcium-independent mechanism of transporter-mediated release of adenosine ($P2Y_1$). The former second messenger pathway is involved in the propagation of intra- and intercellular calcium waves (see 5.6.3.3.) and the purinergic stimulation of Müller cell proliferation (see 5.11.10.3.), the latter in the autocrine regulation of the Müller cell volume (see 5.5.5.3.).

Müller cells express various P2Y receptor subtypes. In cells of the tiger salamander, the gene expression of $P2Y_{1,2,4,6,11,13}$ receptors was described (Reifel Saltzberg et al., 2003). P2Y receptor agonists induce a release of calcium from intracellular stores; the increase in the cytosolic free calcium level in response to P2Y receptor agonists occurs first in the outer region and later in the endfoot in most salamander Müller cells (Keirstead and Miller, 1997; Reifel Saltzberg et al., 2003). Extracellular ATP also induces calcium-independent morphological alterations of salamander Müller cells (Innocenti et al., 2001).

Cultured Müller cells of the guinea pig express, among others, $P2Y_{1, 2, 4}$ receptors (Weick et al., 2005). In the endfeet of rabbit Müller cells, calcium responses can be induced by ATP, ADP (a selective agonist of $P2Y_1$ receptors), and UTP (an agonist of $P2Y_{2, 4}$ receptors), but not by UDP (an agonist of $P2Y_6$ receptors) (Figs. 25, 63A,C), suggesting the presence of $P2Y_{1, 2, 4}$ receptors (Uhlmann et al., 2003). Human and rat Müller cells contain gene transcripts of $P2Y_{1, 2, 4, 6}$ receptors (Pannicke et al., 2001; Fries et al., 2004b, 2005). In rat Müller cells, calcium responses can be induced by various P2Y agonists including ATP, ADP, UTP, and UDP (Figs. 17C–E, 58B,C; Fig. 17F) (Li et al., 2001; Wurm et al., 2009a). In the rodent retina, $P2Y_1$ and $P2Y_4$ receptor proteins are localized to Müller cells with different subcellular distribution; while the $P2Y_1$ receptor protein is enriched in Müller cell processes and somata, the $P2Y_4$ receptor protein is enriched in Müller cell endfeet and perisynaptic Müller cell membranes in the outer plexiform layer (Fig. 77A, B) (Wurm et al., 2009a, 2010). In the rat retina, $P2Y_2$ and $P2Y_6$ proteins are localized to ganglion cell layer and inner nuclear layer neurons, but not to Müller cells (Fig. 77A) (Wurm et al., 2009a). In contrast to rodent Müller cells, porcine Müller cells have predominantly $P2Y_2$ and $P2Y_4$ receptors, and to a lower level $P2Y_1$ receptors (Fig. 81) (Iandiev et al. (2006b).

The predominant P2 receptor subtype that induces calcium responses in Müller cells is $P2Y_1$ (Newman and Zahs, 1997; Li et al., 2001; Wurm et al., 2009a). $P2Y_1$ receptors, ryanodine receptors, and PLC-β1 are present in close spatial proximity in caveolae or lipid rafts which accelerates the $P2Y_1$ receptor-mediated calcium release from intracellular stores (Krishnan and Chatterjee, 2013). In murine Müller cells, purinergic calcium responses are mainly induced by $P2Y_1$ receptors coupled to IP_3R2-gated intracellular stores (Figs. 78A, 79A-C) (Lipp et al., 2009; Wurm et al., 2010; Brückner et al., 2012). In the retina of IP_3R2-deficient mice, Müller cells show a large reduction of the amplitude of ATP-induced calcium responses compared to cells from wildtype mice (Fig. 79A–C) (Lipp et al., 2009). In contrast, the ATP-induced calcium responses in murine retinal astrocytes do not depend on IP_3R2-gated internal stores (Fig. 79A–C) (Wurm et al., 2010). It is known that retinal astrocytes express IP_3R1 and 3, but not IP_3R2 (Kuo et al., 2008).

In human Müller cells, a release of calcium from IP_3-gated intracellular stores is induced by various nucleotides including ATP (Fig. 48B), ADP, UTP, UDP, guanosine 5'-triphosphate, and inosine 5'-triphosphate (Bringmann et al., 2002a). The increase of the cytosolic free calcium level results in activation of BK and cation channels (Figs. 64A–C, 66) (Bringmann et al., 2002a). The cation conductance is mediated by calcium-activated cation channels (Fig. 66) (Puro, 1991b); clamping the cytosolic calcium at a low level or a depletion of intracellular calcium stores by IP_3 before P2Y receptor activation abolish these currents (Fig. 66) (Bringmann et al., 2002a). In Müller cells of the rabbit, extracellular ATP, ADP, and UTP (but not UDP) induce calcium responses and

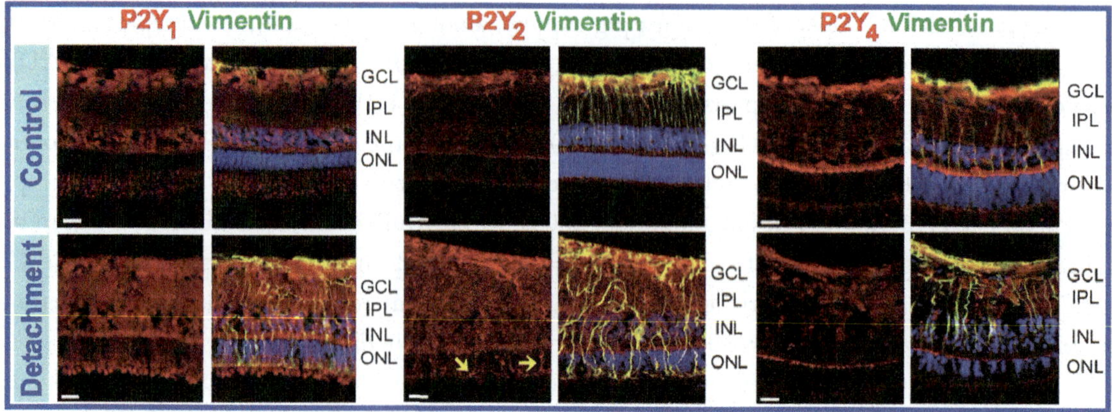

FIGURE 81: Experimental retinal detachment increases the glial P2Y protein expression in the porcine retina. The retinal slices were derived from an attached control retina (*above*) and from a detached retina 7 days after surgery (*below*). The slices were immunostained for P2Y$_1$, P2Y$_2$, and P2Y$_4$ receptor proteins (*red*), and counterstained for the glial marker vimentin (*green*). Co-localization of the proteins yielded a *yellow* merge signal. The *arrows* indicate vimentin-positive fibers in the outer retina that were also stained for P2Y$_2$ protein. GCL, ganglion cell layer; INL, inner nuclear layer; IPL, inner plexiform layer; ONL, outer nuclear layer. Bars, 20 μm. Modified from Iandiev et al. (2006b).

activation of BK currents, but not of cation currents (Fig. 63D) (Francke et al., 2002, 2003; Uhlmann et al., 2003).

The incidence of Müller cells that respond to P2Y receptor activation with intracellular calcium responses varies between mammalian species. In rabbit and porcine retinas, only a small subpopulation of Müller cells (~10% of the cells) responds to exogenous ATP with an increase in the cytosolic free calcium level (Figs. 12F, 25, 63B,C,G, 82B) (Francke et al., 2002, 2003; Uckermann et al., 2002, 2005a; Uhlmann et al., 2003; Iandiev et al., 2006b). On the other hand, nearly every Müller cell examined from tiger salamanders, guinea pigs (Fig. 17A,B), rodents (Figs. 17C–F), and man display calcium responses upon activation of P2Y receptors (Li et al., 2001; Bringmann et al., 2002a; Reifel Saltzberg et al., 2003; Uckermann et al., 2004b, 2006; Wurm et al., 2009a, 2010). In the guinea-pig retina, exogenous ATP induces calcium responses in Müller cells but not in neuronal cells whereas glutamate induces calcium responses in neurons but not Müller cells (Fig. 17A,B) (Uckermann et al., 2004b). A similar absence of ATP-induced calcium responses in neurons and their presence in Müller cells was found in the rabbit and rat retina (Fig. 17F) (Uckermann et al., 2003).

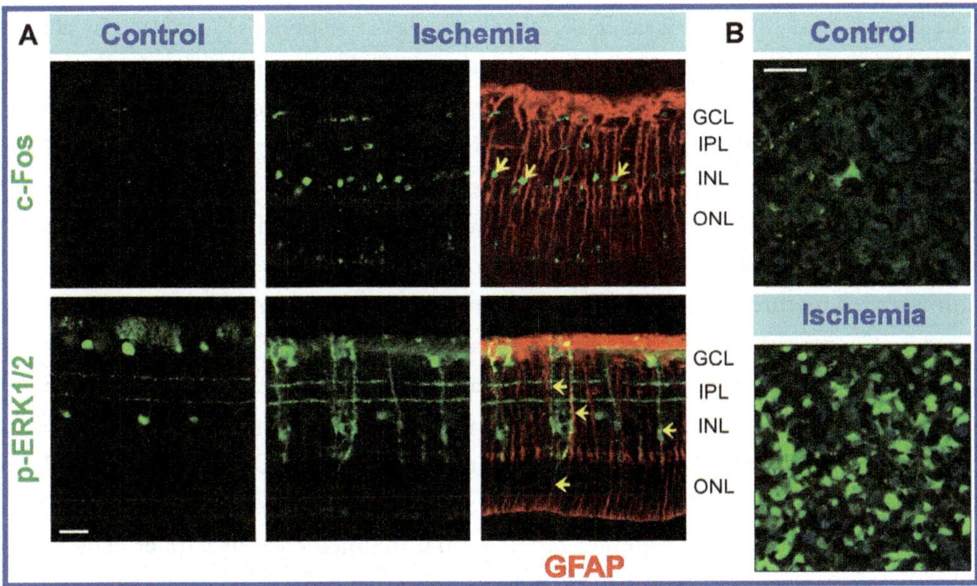

FIGURE 82: Müller cell reactivity in the ischemic porcine retina. Tissues from control retinas and from retinas 3 days after a 1-h transient retinal ischemia were investigated. **A.** Upregulation of c-Fos (*above*) and phosphorylation of extracellular signal-related kinases 1/2 (p-ERK1/2; *below*) after ischemia. Retinal slices were co-stained against GFAP. While c-Fos is not expressed in the control retina, c-Fos is expressed in Müller cell nuclei in the postischemic retina (*arrows*). In the control retina, p-ERK1/2 is present in some cell nuclei in the ganglion cell layer (GCL) and inner plexiform layer (INL) as well as in two distinct bands in the inner plexiform layer (IPL). After ischemia, distinct Müller cells contain p-ERK1/2 protein in their cytosol (*arrows*). **B.** Ischemia-reperfusion increases the P2Y receptor-mediated calcium responsiveness in the Müller cell endfeet of retinal wholemounts. The calcium responses were recorded 1 min after beginning of the administration of ATP (200 µM). ONL, outer nuclear layer. Scale bars, 20 µm. Modified from Wurm et al. (2011a).

5.10.2.4 Involvement of Purinergic Receptors in the Ontogenetic Development

Purinergic signaling is involved in the early eye formation and retinal development. In *Xenopus laevis* larvae, ADP, extracellularly formed from ATP, induces the expression of the eye field transcription factors, Pax6, and Rx1, which are required for the eye development (Massé et al., 2007). In the chick, activation of P2Y$_2$ and P2Y$_4$ receptors by ATP or UTP stimulates the proliferation of early retinal progenitors (Sugioka et al., 1999; Pearson et al., 2002, 2005), and activation of P2Y$_1$ receptors by ATP or ADP stimulates the proliferation of late glial/bipolar progenitors (Sanches et al., 2002; Nunes et al., 2007; Franca et al., 2007). The latter response is mediated by activation of PKC and ERK1/2 (Sanches et al., 2002; Nunes et al., 2007). The division of progenitor cells in the ventricular zone of the chick retina is stimulated by ATP released from the retinal pigment epithelium (Pearson et al., 2004, 2005). In the murine retina, P2Y$_1$ signaling is apparently involved in the proliferation of early and late progenitors (Pannicke et al., 2014).

In the rodent and rabbit retina, radial glial (immature Müller) cells are generated from the late progenitor cells during the first week after birth (Young, 1985; Cepko et al., 1996); the differentiation of immature to mature Müller cells occurs mainly during the second and third postnatal weeks, as indicated by the expression of the major membrane conductance of differentiated cells, i.e., currents through Kir channels (Bringmann et al., 1999a, b, 2000a; Felmy et al., 2001; Uckermann et al., 2002; Wurm et al., 2006b). Mature Müller cells have large Kir currents, while progenitor cells and immature Müller cells have very small or no Kir currents (Figs. 46A,C, 51, 58A, 61A, 62, 63B).

The postnatal differentiation of Müller cells is associated with changes in the ATP-induced calcium responsiveness. In the developing rabbit retina, the incidence of Müller cells that display ATP-induced calcium responses, and the amplitude of the responses, decrease strongly with the postnatal age; these decreases are closely related to the increase of the Kir currents (Fig. 63B) (Uckermann et al., 2002). Immature Müller cells in the postnatal rabbit retina respond to membrane depolarization (induced by high extracellular potassium) with an increase in the cytosolic calcium level (Uckermann et al., 2002). This response is mediated by a release of calcium from internal stores and a calcium influx from the extracellular space through voltage-gated calcium channels (Bringmann et al., 2000d; Uckermann et al., 2002). The release of calcium from internal stores is induced by ATP, which is released from retinal cells in a calcium-independent manner, and subsequent activation of P2Y receptors on immature Müller cells (Uckermann et al., 2002). The percentage of cells that display depolarization-induced calcium responses decreases strongly in the course of the postnatal differentiation of Müller cells (Uckermann et al., 2002). Mature Müller cells exhibit calcium responses upon membrane hyperpolarization rather than depolarization (Fig. 80G; see 5.7.).

In developing Müller cells of the rat, ATP-induced calcium responses are differentially regulated in the endfeet and somata (Wurm et al., 2009a). The incidence of Müller cell somata that display ATP-induced calcium responses (Fig. 58A) decreases in the course of the postnatal development, as does the amplitude of the somatic response (Fig. 58B) (Wurm et al., 2009a). On the other hand, almost all Müller cell endfeet display ATP-induced calcium responses with similar amplitudes at all postnatal stages and in adult animals (Fig. 58B) (Wurm et al., 2009a). The decrease in the incidence of responding Müller cell somata is related to the increase of the Kir currents and the decrease of the osmotic soma swelling observed under hypoosmotic conditions (Fig. 58A) (Wurm et al., 2006b). Both Kir channels and autocrine purinergic signaling have been implicated in the inhibition of the osmotic swelling of Müller cell somata (see 5.5.5.1. and 5.5.5.3.). In immature Müller cells of the rat, ATP-induced calcium responses are triggered in the endfeet of the cells and propagate as a wave toward the somata and the outer processes (Wurm et al., 2009a). In later developmental stages and in cells from adult animals, the waves stop at the inner stem process-soma border, and the ATP-induced calcium responses are restricted to the inner stem process and the endfeet of the cells (Newman, 2005; Uckermann et al., 2006; Wurm et al., 2009a).

The $P2Y_1$ receptor is the principal P2Y receptor subtype that induces intracellular calcium responses and mediates cell volume regulation upon administration of ATP in immature and mature rat Müller cells (Wurm et al., 2009a). Müller cells express $P2Y_1$ receptors at all postnatal ages and in adult animals (Wurm et al., 2009a). In contrast, unequivocal $P2Y_4$ immunolabeling of rat Müller cells was found at postnatal day 20 and thereafter, but not in immature Müller cells (Wurm et al., 2009a). The $P2Y_4$ receptor agonist UTP induces small calcium responses solely in the endfeet of mature Müller cells, but not in immature cells (Wurm et al., 2009a). Immature Müller cells also show no immunolabeling for $P2Y_2$ and $P2Y_6$ receptors (Wurm et al., 2009a).

5.10.2.5 Increase of Purinergic Calcium Responses Under Pathological Conditions

In the retinas of mature healthy rabbits and pigs, only small subpopulations of Müller cells exhibit calcium responses upon activation of P2Y receptors (Figs. 12F, 25, 63B,C,G, 82B) (Francke et al., 2002, 2003; Uckermann et al., 2002, 2005a,b; Uhlmann et al., 2003; Iandiev et al., 2006b; Wurm et al., 2011a). However, the calcium responsiveness of Müller cells to P2Y receptor activation increases under pathological conditions. The incidence of Müller cells that show P2Y-induced calcium responses and activation of BK channels is elevated after transient retinal ischemia and retinal detachment, in experimental dispase-induced retinopathy, and in proliferative retinopathies (Figs. 12F,G, 63B,C,G, 82B) (Francke et al., 2002, 2003; Uhlmann et al., 2003; Uckermann et al., 2003, 2005a; Iandiev et al., 2006b; Wurm et al., 2011a). The increase of the purinergic calcium responsiveness is related to the decrease of the Kir currents (Fig. 63B,H) and thus is proportional to the severity of gliosis. Because the expression level of Kir channels is an indicator of the differentiation degree of Müller cells (Bringmann et al., 2000a), both the decrease of the Kir currents and the increase of the P2Y receptor-induced calcium responsiveness indicate a dedifferentiation of the cells under pathological conditions, supporting the proliferation (see 5.11.10.2.) and other gliotic alterations of the cells such as upregulation of GFAP (see 5.11.3.2.). Because $P2Y_1$ receptor-deficient mice display a significant weaker decrease of the Kir currents upon transient retinal ischemia than wildtype mice (Pannicke et al., 2014), upregulation of the purinergic calcium signaling might be involved in triggering reactive gliosis. The increased P2Y receptor responsiveness may be also involved in the regulation of the cell shape and volume (see 5.5.5.3.) associated with cellular migration and proliferation. Müller cells of patients with PVR display an increase of the calcium-activated cation currents induced by activation of P2Y receptors (Bringmann et al., 2002a). Müller cells of patients with PVR also exhibit a greater density of cation currents through $P2X_7$ receptor channels when compared to cells from donors without eye disease (Bringmann et al., 2001). The increase in the amplitude of $P2X_7$ receptor-mediated cation currents is correlated to the decrease of the Kir currents and other signs of gliosis (Bringmann et al., 2001). $P2X_7$ receptors are suggested to play a role in the induction of proliferative gliosis (see 5.11.10.3.). In the rat retina, the spontaneous calcium waves in the glial cell network display an age-dependent increase in the wave frequency; this is likely induced by an increased release of ATP from retinal cells (Kurth-Nelson et al., 2009).

The mechanisms underlying the increase of the P2Y receptor-induced calcium responsiveness of Müller cells under pathological conditions are unclear. Such mechanisms may involve an increased expression of P2Y receptor proteins (Fig. 81) (Iandiev et al., 2006b; Ward and Fletcher, 2009), increases in the expression (Fig. 11A) and activity of BK channels (Fig. 60B) (Bringmann et al., 1999b, 2007) resulting in a prolongation of the P2Y-induced calcium responses (Fig. 83C; see 5.11.10.2.), a resensitization of P2Y receptors by the action of growth factors (see 5.11.10.3.), an increased expression of ryanodine receptors (Huang et al., 2011d), and/or a change in the amount of ATP released from retinal cells. The increased P2 receptor-induced responses of Müller cells may be involved in the induction of gliotic alterations including the upregulation of glial intermediate filaments, cellular hypertrophy, proliferation, and migration, and downregulation/inactivation of Kir4.1 channels (Franke et al., 2001; Uhlmann et al., 2003; Iandiev et al., 2006b). This assumption is supported by the fact that administration of suramin (which inhibits the binding of nucleotides and growth factors to their receptors) inhibits the decrease of the Kir currents and the hypertrophy (but not the increase of the ATP-induced calcium responses) of Müller cells after experimental retinal detachment (Fig. 54C) (Uhlmann et al., 2003). Rabbit Müller cells that display ATP-induced BK current responses after experimental retinal detachment also show a reduction of their Kir currents, while non-responding cells show no such decrease (Uhlmann et al., 2003). However, further research is required to determine the mechanisms and the relevance of purinergic signaling in the induction of Müller cell gliosis.

5.10.3 GABA RECEPTORS

Ionotropic $GABA_A$ and $GABA_C$ receptors are ligand-gated chloride channels while $GABA_B$ receptors are metabotropic, G protein-coupled receptors. Using electrophysiological recordings of the whole-cell membrane currents, the expression of ionotropic GABA receptors in Müller cells was found to be strikingly species-dependent. Müller cells derived from different species such as the

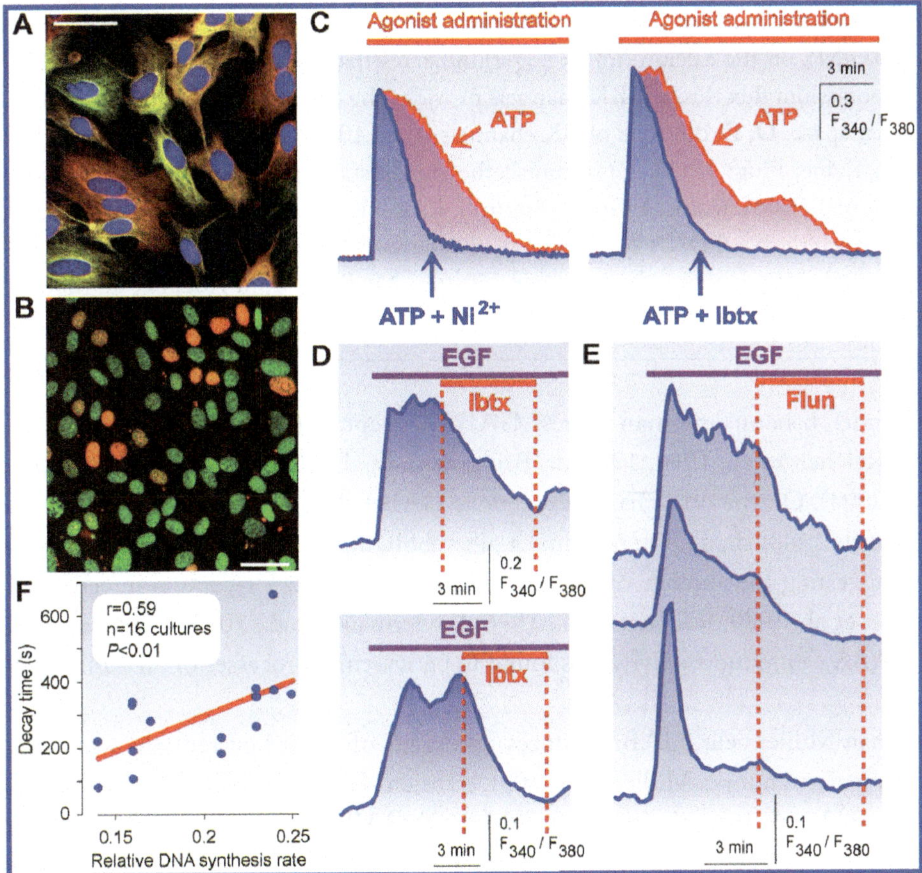

FIGURE 83: The activities of BK and voltage-gated calcium channels are required for the mitogen-induced calcium responses and the proliferation of Müller cells. The data were obtained in cultures of guinea-pig Müller cells. **A.** Cultured Müller cells were immunostained against vimentin (*red*) and GFAP (*green*). Co-labeling yielded a *yellow-orange* merge signal. Cell nuclei are *blue* stained. **B.** Determination of the DNA synthesis rate (a marker of the proliferation rate) using BrdU immunolabeling (*red*). All cell nuclei were labeled with acridin orange (*green*). BrdU-labeled cell nuclei display a *yellow-orange* merge signal. **C.** The potassium flux through BK channels prolongs the P2Y-induced calcium response of Müller cells. Calcium imaging experiments were carried out in cultured Müller cells of the guinea pig. The cytosolic calcium response evoked by ATP (500 µM) consists of a transient release of calcium from IP₃-gated intracellular stores followed by a calcium influx from the extracellular space. The calcium influx is abrogated in the presence of nickel ions (40 µM; *left*) which blocks E/R-type and T-type

continued on next page

voltage-gated calcium channels. The abrogating effect of the selective blocker of BK channels, iberiotoxin (Ibtx; 100 nM), on the calcium influx (*right*) indicates that the membrane hyperpolarization produced by the potassium flux through BK channels provides the driving force for the calcium influx from the extracellular space. **D, E.** Blockers of BK channels (Ibtx; 100 nM; **D**) and of voltage-gated calcium channels (flunarizine; Flun; 1 µM; **E**) diminish the steady-state rise of the cytosolic free calcium induced by epidermal growth factor (EGF; 200 ng/ml). Examples of 2 and 3 cells, respectively, are shown. **F.** Relation between the basal DNA synthesis rate of cultured Müller cells and the decay time of the ATP (500 µM)-induced calcium response. Scale bars, 50 µm. Modified from Kodal et al. (2000) and Moll et al. (2002).

---

skate, salamander, baboon, and man express $GABA_A$ receptors (Malchow et al., 1989; Qian et al., 1993, 1994; Reichelt et al., 1996, 1997a,b; Bringmann et al., 2002a; Zhang et al., 2003a; Biedermann et al., 2004). On the other hand, exogenous GABA does not induce membrane currents in Müller cells of the goldfish, mouse, rat, guinea pig, rabbit, pig, and the cynomolgus monkey *Macaca fascicularis*, suggesting the absence of functional ionotropic GABA receptors in cells of these species (Malchow et al., 1989; Reichelt et al., 1996; Biedermann et al., 2002; Pannicke et al., 2005c). However, $GABA_A$ immunoreactivity was found in perivascular processes of rat Müller cells (Hinds et al., 2013).

In human Müller cells, GABA induces two kinds of inward currents in a subpopulation of enzymatically isolated human Müller cells: a fast, transient $GABA_A$ receptor current and a sustained current mediated by electrogenic (sodium-dependent) GABA transporters (Fig. 34A,C) (Reichelt et al., 1997a; Bringmann et al., 2002a; Biedermann et al., 2004; see 5.5.2.2.1.). The direction of the currents through $GABA_A$ receptor channels reverses at the equilibrium potential of chloride ions (approximately −30 mV; Fig. 34E) (Biedermann et al., 2004); therefore, opening of the receptor channels results in a depolarization of the cells (Malchow et al., 1989). The current-voltage relation of perforated-patch $GABA_A$ receptor currents (Fig. 34E) suggests that human Müller cells have an intracellular chloride concentration of ~37 mM (Biedermann et al., 2004). The receptor currents are increased by known modulators of $GABA_A$ receptor channels such as pentobarbital, diazepam, and zinc ions (Fig. 34F) (Qian et al., 1996; Reichelt et al., 1997b; Biedermann et al., 2004). Zinc ions are released from the synaptic terminals of photoreceptor cells (Wu et al., 1993; Qian et al., 1994; Redenti et al., 2007). $GABA_A$ receptors are localized across the whole plasma membrane of human Müller cells (Fig. 34B) (Biedermann et al., 2004). The GABA-induced chloride currents in human Müller cells are totally suppressed by bicuculline; this excludes the possibility that the cells also express functional $GABA_C$ receptors (Biedermann et al., 2004). Similarly, Müller cells of the skate do not express functional $GABA_C$ receptors (Qian et al., 1996). $GABA_A$ receptors may have different functional roles; they may be involved in the buffering of extracellular pH (because the receptor channels are also permeable for bicarbonate), and a chloride efflux through the receptor channels may stimulate the GABA uptake by the cells (which is driven by a cotransport of sodium and chloride ions; see 5.5.2.2.1.) and may compensate the decrease of the extracellular chloride concentration caused by the chloride influx into activated neurons. The GABA-induced depolarization of the cells may activate voltage-gated potassium, sodium, and calcium channels, resulting in activation of Müller cells and a release of gliotransmitters. $GABA_A$ receptors in perivascular Müller cell processes may be implicated in the regulation of the retinal blood flow (see 5.8.). However, the functional roles of $GABA_A$ receptors in Müller cells remain to be determined. Müller cells of bullfrog and rat retinas were described to express metabotropic $GABA_B$ receptors (Zhang and Yang, 1999; Hinds et al., 2013) while guinea-pig Müller cells have no functional $GABA_B$ receptors (Biedermann et al., 1994). In cultured postnatal Müller cells, GABA induces the expression of neuronal proteins (Ramírez et al., 2012).

5.10.4 GLYCINERGIC RECEPTORS

Glycine receptors (GlyRs) are ligand-gated chloride channels. Müller cells of the bullfrog retina express functional GlyRs (Du et al., 2002) and the subunits $GlyR\alpha1$ and $GlyR\beta$ (Lee et al., 2005). GlyRs were not found in Müller cells of rats, mice, and primates (Greferath et al., 1994; Wässle et al., 1998; Haverkamp and Wässle, 2000; Lin et al., 2000; Haverkamp et al., 2003). In human Müller cells, glycine does not induce alterations of the membrane conductance (Bringmann et al., 2002a), suggesting the absence of glycine receptors and transporters.

5.10.5 CHOLINERGIC RECEPTORS

Focal administration of carbachol onto astrocyte somata initiates calcium waves in the network of astrocytes and Müller cells of the rat retina (Newman and Zahs, 1997). In a small subpopulation of human Müller cells, acetylcholine causes delayed and small BK current increases, suggesting the expression of acetylcholine receptors coupled to a release of calcium from internal stores (Bringmann et al., 2002a). Acetylcholine (but not nicotine) induces calcium responses in a subpopulation of cultured rabbit Müller cells, via activation of muscarinic M_1 receptors (Wakakura et al., 1998). Acetylcholine also induces calcium responses in a subpopulation of Müller cells of the tiger salamander but not of the skate (Malchow and Ramsey, 1999). Cultured chicken Müller cells express muscarinic and nicotinic receptors, and the $\beta2$-nicotinic receptor subunit, but not choline acetyltransferase (Kubrusly et al., 2005). Cultured mouse Müller cells have M_1 and M_4 receptors; M_1

receptor activation results in a release of calcium from internal stores and subsequent calcium influx from the extracellular space through TRPC channels (Da Silva et al., 2008).

5.10.6 CATECHOLAMINERGIC RECEPTORS

Retinal glial cells express α_{2A}-, α_{2B}-, and β-adrenergic receptors (Woldemussie et al., 2007). Epinephrine and norepinephrine induce inward currents and an increase in the input resistance in Müller cells of the tiger salamander (Henshel and Miller, 1992). In human Müller cells, epinephrine and serotonin do not induce alterations of the membrane conductance (Bringmann et al., 2002a). Systemic or intravitreal administration of α_2-adrenergic agonists in rats elicits phosphorylation of ERK1/2 and an increase of GFAP in Müller cells (Peng et al., 1998). In cultured Müller cells, activation of α_2-adrenergic receptors triggers activation of ERK1/2 which is mediated by an autocrine transactivation of EGF receptors (Harun-Or-Rashid et al., 2014). In tissue preparations of the rat retina, norepinephrine induces calcium responses in a small fraction of Müller cells (Li et al., 2001), and focal administration of phenylephrine onto astrocyte somata initiates calcium waves in the network of astrocytes and Müller cells (Newman and Zahs, 1997). Norepinephrine stimulates the production and release of BDNF by cultured rat Müller cells (Seki et al., 2005). Activation of β-adrenergic receptors in Müller cells reduces the expression and formation, respectively, of various inflammatory molecules like PGE_2, TNF, IL-1ß, and inducible NO synthase (Walker and Steinle, 2007). Activation of β_2-adrenergic receptors counteracts the downregulation of the insulin receptor signaling in Müller cells under hyperglycemic conditions (Walker et al., 2011). Activation of β_2-adrenergic receptors inhibits the high glucose-induced apoptosis of Müller cells via a mechanism involving the insulin receptor substrate-1 and phosphorylation of the insulin receptor and of Akt (Walker et al., 2011, 2012). Müller cells of the bullfrog but not rat retina express 5-hydroxytryptamine 2A receptors (Han et al., 2007).

5.10.7 DOPAMINERGIC AND HISTAMINERGIC RECEPTORS

Müller cells of amphibians, rats, and guinea pigs express dopamine D_2 receptors (Muresan and Besharse, 1993; Biedermann et al., 1995). Müller cells of the tiger salamander respond to dopamine with an activation of an inward current and an increase in the input resistance (Henshel and Miller, 1992). In Müller cells of the guinea pig, activation of D_2 receptors results in a closure of Kir channels (Biedermann et al., 1995). In human Müller cells, dopamine does not induce alterations of the membrane conductance (Bringmann et al., 2002a). In tissue preparations of the rat retina, focal ejection of dopamine to glial cells triggers calcium responses in Müller cells resulting in a release of ATP from the cells (Newman, 2003b). Müller cells of the goldfish display immunolabeling for D_1

receptors (Mora-Ferrer et al., 1999). Cultured chick Müller cells express D_1 receptors; activation of the receptors stimulates the adenylyl cyclase activity (Kubrusly et al., 2005). In addition, cultured chick, murine, and monkey Müller cells can express the machinery for the dopamine synthesis and release (Kubrusly et al., 2008; Stutz et al., 2014). In the murine retina, Müller cells express the histamine receptor 2 while amacrine and retinal ganglion cells express the histamine receptor 1 (Greferath et al., 2009).

5.10.8 VEGF RECEPTORS

VEGF operates primarily through two tyrosine kinase receptors, the type 1 receptor (fms-like tyrosine kinase-1, flt-1) and the type 2 receptor (kinase insert domain-containing receptor/fetal liver kinase-1, KDR/flk-1) (Ferrara et al., 2003). In the human retina, VEGF is expressed by vascular endothelial cells, all major classes of neurons, astrocytes, and Müller cells (Amin et al., 1997; Famiglietti et al., 2003). VEGF receptor-1 is localized to pericytes (Witmer et al., 2002), and VEGF receptor-2 is expressed by blood vessels, astrocytes, Müller cells, and retinal ganglion cells (Stone et al., 1995a; Stitt et al., 1998). Under pathological conditions, Müller cells may also express VEGF receptor-1 (Anderson et al., 2008). In the rodent retina, Müller cells express both types of VEGF receptors (Vinores et al., 2001).

In rodent Müller cells, activation of the VEGF receptor-2 results in an exocytotic release of glutamate that is involved in the autocrine regulation of the cell volume (see 5.5.5.3.). This effect is dependent on the activation of PLC, a release of calcium from intracellular stores, an influx of calcium from the extracellular space, and activation of the PKC and of Src tyrosine kinases (Fig. 78A) (Wurm et al., 2008a; Linnertz et al., 2011; Brückner et al., 2012). In addition, activation of voltage-gated sodium and calcium channels is implicated in the VEGF-induced exocytotic release of glutamate (see 5.6.1.2.).

Glial cells in epiretinal membranes of patients with proliferative retinopathies and cultured human Müller cells express VEGF receptors-1 and -2 (Chen et al., 1997b; Eichler et al., 2004b). Activation of the receptors suppresses the release of PEDF from the cells (Eichler et al., 2004b). Hypoxia increases the expression of VEGF receptors in Müller cells (Eichler et al., 2004b).

5.10.9 THROMBIN RECEPTORS

In tissue preparations of the rat retina, thrombin induces calcium responses in Müller cells which results in a release of ATP from the cells (Newman, 2003b). Thrombin inhibits the Kir currents and stimulates the proliferation of cultured human Müller cells (Puro et al., 1990; Puro and Stuenkel, 1995). The inhibition of the Kir currents is mediated by a release of calcium from intracellular stores (Puro and Stuenkel, 1995). On the other hand, in whole-cell records of freshly isolated human Müller cells, thrombin does not induce alterations of the membrane conductance (Bringmann et al., 2002a).

5.10.10 FURTHER PEPTIDERGIC RECEPTORS

Müller cells express different subtypes of FGF receptors including FGF receptor 1, 2, and 3 (see 5.11.7.7.). bFGF stimulates the ganglioside production (Hicks et al., 1996), Müller cell proliferation (see 5.11.10.4.1.), and induces a release of VEGF and HGF from the cells (see 5.11.8. and 5.11.10.4.4.).

Müller cells express the erythropoietin receptor (Fig. 50E) (Krügel et al., 2010) which is a potent neuroprotective factor in the retina (Grimm et al., 2002, 2004; Zhu et al., 2008; McVicar et al., 2011; see 5.11.7.9.). Erythropoietin activates the swelling-inhibitory glutamatergic-purinergic signaling cascade by inducing a release of VEGF from Müller cells (Krügel et al., 2010; see 5.5.5.3.). The swelling-inhibitory effect of erythropoietin may contribute to the neuroprotective action. Erythropoietin attenuates the reactive gliosis in the diabetic retina and promotes the production of neurotrophic factors like BDNF and CNTF in Müller cells via activation of ERK1/2 and Akt signaling pathways (McVicar et al., 2011; Hu et al., 2011). Müller cells express the receptor $\alpha2\delta1$ for thrombospondins-1 and -2 (Huang et al., 2013a) implicated in the inhibition of pathological neovascularization (see 5.11.8.).

The retinal level of natriuretic peptides such as ANP is increased after transient ischemia-reperfusion (Kalisch et al., 2006). Müller cells and neurons of the rat retina express ANP, brain NP (BNP), and C-type NP (CNP) (Cao et al., 2004). Bullfrog Müller cells express the natriuretic peptide receptor-A; activation of the receptor induces the opening of a non-selective cation conductance likely mediated by calcium-permeable cyclic nucleotide-gated cation channels (Cao and Yang, 2007). In rat Müller cells, ANP induces a glutamatergic-purinergic signaling cascade of autocrine regulation of the Müller cell volume (see 5.5.5.3.) which is mediated by the activation of different subtypes of natriuretic peptide receptors (Kalisch et al., 2006). The effects of natriuretic peptide receptor activation are mediated by the actions of PLC and PKC, and an influx of calcium from the extracellular space; the intracellular calcium response is likely induced by cGMP (Kalisch et al., 2006).

NPY is expressed in the rat retina by neuronal, vascular, microglial, and Müller cells, and in the toad retina by amacrine and Müller cells (Zhu and Gibbins, 1996; Alvaro et al., 2007). NPY is released in the retina in response to light (Bruun and Ehinger, 1993) and is increasingly expressed under hypoxic and oxidative stress conditions (Yoon et al., 2002). Cultured Müller cells, as well as other types of cultured retinal glial and neuronal cells, express the NPY Y_1 and Y_2 receptors (Santos-Carvalho et al., 2013). Müller cells in retinas of patients with PVR and glial cells in epiretinal fibroproliferative membranes express NPY Y_1 receptors; this is not the case in healthy control retinas (Cantó Soler et al., 2002a). NPY inhibits the osmotic swelling of Müller cells observed under osmotic stress conditions (Uckermann et al., 2006). This effect is mediated by activation of NPY Y_1 receptors that induces activation of a glutamatergic-purinergic signaling cascade (see 5.5.5.3.). In cultured Müller cells of the guinea pig, NPY has both antiproliferative (at low concentrations) and proliferative effects (at higher concentrations) (Milenkovic et al., 2004). The mitogenic effect is mediated by activation of NPY Y_1 receptors, ERK1/2, and partially of the p38 MAPK, PI3K, and PDGF and EGF receptor tyrosine kinases (Milenkovic et al., 2004). NPY Y_1 and P2Y receptors share partially common signal transduction pathways in cultured Müller cells (Milenkovic et al., 2004).

Cultured Müller cells of chicks and rats have receptors for VIP and glucagon that, upon activation, induce an increase of cAMP (Koh et al., 1984; Koh and Roberge, 1989). In amphibian Müller cells, VIP and glucagon stimulate the gluconeogenesis and inhibit the glycolysis (Goldman, 1990). Cultured rat and chicken Müller cells have PAC1 receptors for PACAP (Kubrusly et al., 2005; Seki et al., 2006). PACAP stimulates the production of cAMP and IL-6 in the cells (Nakatani et al., 2006; Seki et al., 2006). Arginine-vasopressin (AVP) increases the protein synthesis in cultured Müller cells (Reichelt et al., 1989). Müller cells express angiotensin II type 1 and 2 receptors, and angiotensin II and its bioactive metabolite Ang-(1-7) (Kurihara et al., 2006; Senanayake et al., 2007; Downie et al., 2009; Semba et al., 2014a). Under inflammatory conditions, endogenous angiotensin II induces GFAP in Müller cells through activation of STAT3 (Kurihara et al., 2006). Inhibition of angiotensin II type 1 receptors suppresses the lipopolysaccharide-induced expression of the inducible NO synthase in Müller cells (Semba et al., 2014a). A low salt diet decreases the expression of angiotensin II type 1 receptors (Deliyanti et al., 2014). In addition, Müller cells express angiotensin-converting enzyme (Wheeler-Schilling et al., 2001b) which converts angiotensin I into the physiologically active angiotensin II, and which inactivates a number of peptides, e.g., substance P.

Rat and human Müller cells express the somatostatin receptors sst1 and sst2 (Helboe and Møller, 1999, 2000). Topical administration of somatostatin prevents glial activation and the downregulation of GLAST induced by diabetes mellitus (Hernández et al., 2013). Müller cells have insulin receptors which have roles in metabolic and functional mechanisms, and in cellular survival; the expression of insulin receptors is decreased in diabetes (Naeser, 1997; Gosbell et al., 2002; Walker et al., 2012; Fischer et al., 2009a). Insulin may also activate IGF-1 receptors expressed by Müller cells (Charkrabarti et al., 1991; Layton et al., 2006). Müller cells express endothelin-B receptors (Iandiev et al., 2005b) and the receptor Gnai2 (Roesch et al., 2008) that mediates the signaling from the endothelin-B receptor. Retinal light damage and inherited photoreceptor degeneration increases the expression of these receptors in Müller cells; endothelin-2 released from photoreceptors may function as a stress signal that activates Müller cells *in situ* (Rattner and Nathans, 2005). Activation of endothelin receptors was also implicated in the development of PVR (Iribarne et al., 2008).

Müller cells express the apelin receptor APJ and produce apelin (Wang et al., 2012c). Apelin is upregulated under hypoxic conditions, stimulates Müller cells viability and migration, and prevents Müller cells apoptosis (Wang et al., 2012c). Müller cells express the Wnt receptors Frizzled-4 and -5 (Liu and Nathans, 2008; Seitz et al., 2010). Deletion of Frizzled-5 in mice is associated with a late-onset progressive retinal degeneration which is apparent at 6 months of age (Liu and Nathans, 2008). Activation of Frizzled-4 by Norrin activates the Wnt/β-catenin signaling pathway in Müller cells resulting in increased expression of neurotrophic growth factors like bFGF, LIF, PEDF, BNDF, and CNTF (Seitz et al., 2010). Müller cells also express neogenin and its ligand repulsive guidance molecule A; both proteins are upregulated under inflammatory conditions (Schnichels et al., 2012). In addition, Müller cells express the (pro)renin receptor; activation of this receptor may have neuroprotective effects (Wilkinson-Berka et al., 2010).

5.10.11 STEROID HORMONE RECEPTORS

Müller cells express progesterone receptors (Li et al., 1997a). In cultured porcine Müller cells, the membrane-associated progesterone receptor component 1 is localized to the plasma membranes and microsomes (Swiatek-De Lange et al., 2007). Progesterone induces alterations in the morphology of the cells, a calcium influx and subsequent PI3K-mediated phosphorylation of PKC and ERK1/2, as well as a PKC-dependent activation of VEGF expression and secretion (Swiatek-De Lange et al., 2007). 17β-Estradiol protects cultured Müller cells from oxidative stress-induced apoptosis through alterations in the gene expression (Li et al., 2006). Sex steroids such as 17β-estradiol, estriol, progesterone, and testosterone inhibit the osmotic Müller cell swelling in postischemic and diabetic retinal tissues (Neumann et al., 2010). The effect of progesterone is mediated by activation of the endogenous glutamatergic-purinergic signaling cascade that inhibits the osmotic swelling of Müller cells (see 5.5.5.3.). The effects of progesterone and testosterone were apparent at nanomolar concentrations while 17β-estradiol and estriol inhibit the swelling at micromolar concentrations (Neumann et al., 2010). The dose dependencies suggest that the effects of 17β-estradiol and estriol are mediated by receptor-independent mechanisms (see 5.11.9.4.) while the effects of progesterone and testosterone are mediated by specific receptors.

Müller cells express glucocorticoid receptors (Gorovits et al., 1994; Gallina et al., 2014). In salamander Müller cells, glucocorticoid receptors colocalize with the glutamine synthetase in the cytoplasm and are also present in the mitochondria (Psarra et al., 2003). The selective localization of glucocorticoid receptors in Müller cells (Gorovits et al., 1994) is responsible for the cell-specific expression of proteins like glutamine synthetase (Grossman et al., 1994; see 5.5.2.1.11.). The expression of glucocorticoid receptors in Müller cells is upregulated after retinal injury (Gallina et al., 2014). Activation of glucocorticoid receptors inhibits the formation of Müller stem cells (see 5.11.12.) and antagonizes the bFGF/MAPK signaling in Müller cells (Gallina et al., 2014). Steroid hormones regulate also the mitochondrial metabolism such as the glutamate-induced increase of mitochondrial NADH (Psarra et al., 2003). Müller cells also express mineralocorticoid receptors (Mirshahi et al., 1997; Deliyanti et al., 2014). Activation of these receptors by aldosterone increases the expression of ENaCα (Golestaneh et al., 2001). A low salt diet reduces the expression of ENaCα in Müller cells (Deliyanti et al., 2014).

5.10.12 RECEPTORS FOR EXTRACELLULAR MATRIX COMPONENTS

Müller cells express various receptors for extracellular matrix components including all four integrin subunits (α1, α2, α3, β1) that comprise the collagen-binding receptors, as well as α-dystroglycan, a central member of the membrane-associated dystrophin-glycoprotein complex (Schmitz and Drenckhahn, 1997; Hering et al., 2000; Moukhles et al., 2000; Guidry et al., 2003; Méhes et al., 2005). This complex forms a bridge between the extracellular matrix towards the cytoskeleton; dystrophin binds to subplasmalemmal actin filaments as well as to a plasma membrane anchor, β-dystroglycan, which is associated on the external side with the extracellular matrix receptor α-dystroglycan that binds to the basal lamina proteins laminin and agrin (Schmitz and Drenckhahn, 1997). Müller cells express distinct glycosylated isoforms of α-dystroglycan in apposition to the basal laminae of the inner limiting membrane and blood vessels, as well as in processes that enwrap the synapses in the ganglion cell and inner plexiform layers (Moukhles et al., 2000). In addition, β-dystroglycan and dystrobrevin are expressed in membrane domains that contact basement membranes (Blank et al., 1997; Koulen et al., 1998; Ueda et al., 1998, 2000). Dystroglycans of Müller cells may participate in organizing synapses and may be important for the adhesion of Müller cells to the extracellular matrix molecule laminin as a component of the basement membranes around the vessels and in the inner limiting membrane (Fig. 8B). Laminin induces a clustering of α-dystroglycan and of intracellular protein components of the dystroglycan-containing complex, such as syntrophin, in the Müller cell membrane (Noel et al., 2005). Given that syntrophin binds utrophin and Dp71 which in turn bind to the actin cytoskeleton in Müller cells (Claudepierre et al., 2000), the interaction of laminin with the dystroglycan-containing complex may have also roles in the stabilization of their radial architecture. The transduction of signals from the extracellular matrix towards the cytoskeleton is also involved in the laminin-1-induced stimulation of the migration and path-searching activity of Müller cells (Méhes et al., 2002, 2005).

Müller cells express various other cell surface adhesion/receptor molecules such as N-cadherin, cadherin-11, neuron cell adhesion molecule, CD44, and CD81 (Bartsch et al., 1990; Duguid et al., 1991; Kuppner et al., 1993; Chaitin et al., 1994; Rich et al., 1995; Nishina et al., 1997; Kuhrt et al., 1997; Clarke et al., 1998; Chaitin and Brun-Zinkernagel, 1998; Krishnamoorthy et al. 2000; Honjo et al., 2000a). The transmembrane adhesion molecule CD44 is prominently expressed at the outer limiting membrane of the rodent retina, i.e., in the microvilli of Müller cells (Chaitin et al., 1994; Kuhrt et al., 1997; Shinoe et al., 2010; Wahl et al., 2013). Retinal injury and disease stimulates the production of CD44 by reactive glial cells (see 5.11.2.7.). Müller cells *in vitro* express the neural cell recognition molecule F11 (Willbold et al., 1997a) which is a multifunctional protein that interacts with L1/Ng-CAM, Nr-CAM, tenascin-C, tenascin-R, and receptor protein tyrosine phosphatase-β.

5.10.13 OTHER RECEPTORS OF MÜLLER CELLS

Goldfish Müller cells express cannabinoid type 1 and 2 receptors (Yazulla et al., 2000) while monkey Müller cells express the type 2, but not the type 1 receptor (Bouskila et al., 2012, 2013). In cultured Müller cells of mice, type 1 sigma receptors are localized to the nuclear and endoplasmic reticulum membranes (Ola et al., 2001; Jiang et al., 2006). The binding activity of the receptors is increased under oxidative-nitrosative stress. Deletion of sigma receptor 1 in mice results in upregulation of key genes involved in endoplasmatic reticulum stress in Müller cells (Ha et al., 2014). Salamander Müller cells express the multifunctional ectoenzyme CD38 which converts NAD^+ into the intracellular calcium-mobilizing second-messenger cyclic ADP-ribose; NAD^+ triggers intracellular calcium waves that depends on the activation of ryanodine receptors, (Esguerra and Miller, 2002).

Melatonin is a cytoprotective agent against hyperglycemic injury of Müller cells (Jiang et al., 2012c). In addition to its function as a direct free radical scavenger, melatonin elicit cellular signaling pathways via activation of the membrane receptors MT1 and MT2; high glucose induces upregulation of the receptors (Jiang et al., 2012c). Melatonin activates Akt and inhibits the production of VEGF in Müller cells (Jiang et al., 2012c).

Lysophosphatidic acid (LPA) acting at G protein-coupled receptors activates a non-specific, calcium-permable cation conductance in cultured bovine and human Müller cells (Kusaka et al.,

1998). However, in freshly isolated human Müller cells, LPA does not induce alterations in the membrane conductance (Bringmann et al., 2002a). In the rat retina, LPA induces calcium responses in Müller cells resulting in a release of ATP from the cells (Newman, 2003b). In cultured Müller cells, LPA stimulates actin polymerization and cell spreading (Santos-Bredariol et al., 2006). Cultured Müller cells were suggested to express the sphingosine-1-phosphate/endothelial differentiation gene family receptor (Esche et al., 2010). Sphingosine-1-phosphate induces calcium responses via a release from internal stores and an influx across the plasma membrane, and stimulates Müller cell migration but not proliferation (Esche et al., 2010). Müller cell endfeet express the inositol 1,3,4,5-tetrakisphosphate receptor (IP_4R); IP_4 may function as a transmitter in the retina (Kreutz et al., 1997).

Müller cells express the pattern recognition receptor RAGE which recognizes, among other molecules, AGEs (Soulis et al., 1997; Hammes et al., 1999; Barile et al., 2005; Tezel et al., 2007a; Wang et al., 2008; Zong et al., 2011). AGEs are formed during oxidative stress and hyperglycemia; the levels of AGEs and AGE receptors in the retina increase with age, in diabetic retinopathy, and in the course of glaucoma (Hammes et al., 1999; Barile et al., 2005; Harada et al., 2006; Tezel et al., 2007a; Zong et al., 2010). AGEs induce the production and secretion of proinflammatory cytokines such as VEGF and MCP-1 in Müller cells (Hirata et al., 1997; Harada et al., 2006; Zong et al., 2010). In addition, Müller cells express receptors for different inflammatory factors like IL-1β (Liu et al., 2012a).

Müller cells express the low-density lipoprotein-related protein (LRP1; CD91) (Birkenmeier et al., 1996; Sánchez et al., 2006) which is a multifunctional receptor for α2-macroglobulin and ApoE. α2-Macroglobulin, an acute-phase response protein associated with inflammation, forms complexes with proteinases and binds different cytokines and growth factors; binding to α2-macroglobulin results in inhibition of the growth factor action. In PVR retinas, the gene expression of LRP1 is enhanced compared with control retinas (Hollborn et al., 2004c). In retinas of rats with ischemia-induced neovascularization or diabetes, and in the vitreous and retinas of human subjects with neovascular glaucoma or PDR, the expression of LRP1 and α2-macroglobulin is increased (Luna et al., 2003; Gerhardinger et al., 2005; Sánchez et al., 2006; Barcelona et al., 2010). The protease activated form of α2-macroglobulin induces expression of GFAP, cell migration, and proMMP-2 activation in cultured Müller cells which is mediated by a mechanism involving LRP1, activation of JAK/STAT3, and MT1-MMP (Barcelona et al., 2011, 2013). LRP1 is also involved in the lipid shuttle from Müller cells to neurons.

Müller cells express a retina-specific nuclear receptor which interacts with the promoter of the CRALBP gene in the presence of the retinoic acid receptor and/or retinoid X receptor (Chen et al., 1999b). Activation of the retinoic acid receptor-α induces upregulation of GDNF and down-regulation of VEGF in Müller cells (Nishikiori et al., 2007). Furthermore, Müller cells express receptors for neurotrophic (see 5.11.7.) and growth factors (see 5.11.10.4.).

5.11 MÜLLER CELL GLIOSIS

Diseases and injuries of the retina are associated with a reactive gliosis which is a complex response involving the interplay of all three kinds of retinal glial cells, i.e., Müller cells, astrocytes, and microglia (Bringmann and Reichenbach, 2001; Garcia and Vecino, 2003; Bringmann et al., 2006). Reactive gliosis includes morphological, biochemical, and physiological changes of Müller cells; these responses vary with the type and severity of the insult. Activation of Müller cells is associated with a downregulation of the LIM homeodomain transcription factor Lhx2 which, under normal conditions, actively maintains Müller cells in a nonreactive state (De Melo et al., 2012). Deletion of Lhx2 from mature Müller cells leads to the induction of reactive gliosis in the absence of retinal injury (De Melo et al., 2012).

Retinal gliosis has both protective and detrimental effects (Bringmann et al., 2009b; Bringmann and Wiedemann, 2012). Gliosis is thought to represent a cellular attempt to protect the tissue from further damage, to preserve tissue function, to promote tissue repair, and to limit tissue remodeling (Bringmann et al., 2009b; Reichenbach and Bringmann, 2010; Bringmann and Wiedemann, 2012). Müller cells may dedifferentiate to progenitor-like cells, and a subsequent (restricted) transdifferentiation to cells with neuronal phenotype may participate in tissue regeneration (see 5.11.12.). However, dedifferentiated Müller cells also quit supporting the neurons and contribute to neurodegeneration (Bringmann and Reichenbach, 2001; Bringmann et al., 2009b). A better understanding of this "Janus face" of Müller cell gliosis is a precondition for the development of new therapeutic approaches for the treatment of a variety of retinal diseases.

5.11.1 THE "JANUS FACE" OF MÜLLER CELL GLIOSIS

5.11.1.1 Protective Effects of Müller Cell Gliosis

Early after tissue injury, gliosis is neuroprotective and is thought to be a cellular attempt to limit the severity of the tissue damage. The protective and regenerative responses of Müller cells involve, among others, the buffering of elevated potassium levels (see 5.5.3.), the uptake of excess glutamate which is neurotoxic especially to the inner retina (see 5.5.2.1.), the release of antioxidants (see 5.5.2.1.15.), the production of neurotrophic factors, growth factors, and cytokines that protect photoreceptors and neurons from cell death (see 5.11.7.), the restoration of the blood-brain barrier (see 5.11.9.1.1.), and the inhibition of neovascularization (see 5.11.8.).

One of the most relevant factors released from Müller cells under hypoxic conditions is VEGF (Aiello et al., 1995; Drescher and Whittum-Hudson, 1996a; Amin et al., 1997; Eichler et al., 2000, 2004a; Yafai et al., 2004). VEGF supports the survival of vascular endothelial cells, photoreceptors, neurons, and Müller cells, and restricts the glucose- and oxidative stress-induced damage of retinal vessels (Yamada et al., 1999; Saint-Geniez et al., 2008; Foxton et al., 2013). The protective effects of VEGF also include vasodilation, revascularization, inflammation, glial cell proliferation, and neurogenesis (Krum and Khaibullina, 2003; Yasuhara et al., 2004; Storkebaum et al., 2004), as well as inhibition of the cytotoxic swelling of Müller cells (see 5.5.5.3.).

Müller cells protect neuronal cells from glutamate and NO toxicity, in particular by glutamate uptake (see 5.5.2.1.1.) and subsequent detoxification via the synthesis of glutamine (see 5.5.2.1.9.) and the antioxidant glutathione which is rapidly released from Müller cells and provided to neurons (see 5.5.2.1.15.). Protection from oxidative-nitrosative stress is also achieved by the production and release of further antioxidants (see 5.5.2.1.15.). The expression of the inducible NO synthase under pathological conditions (see 5.6.5.) results in enhanced NO production by Müller cells. NO increases the retinal perfusion by dilating blood vessels, prevents platelet aggregation, and protects neurons from glutamate toxicity via closure of NMDA receptor channels (Kashii et al., 1996; Goldstein et al., 1996).

Regenerative responses of Müller cells involve the phagocytosis of exogenous substances, cell fragments (Fig. 53E,F), serum proteins (Fig. 21C), and hemoglobin (Friedenwald and Chan, 1932; Inomata, 1975; Rosenthal and Appleton, 1975; Miller and Oberdorfer, 1981; Ehrenberg et al., 1984; Bellhorn, 1984; Mano and Puro, 1990; Stolzenburg et al., 1992; Büchi, 1992; Nishizono et al., 1993; Egensperger et al., 1996; Marín-Teva et al., 1999c; Thanos, 1999; Crafoord et al., 2000; Francke et al., 2001b; Chang et al., 2006; Kaur et al., 2007; Zou et al., 2009). Inflammatory factors like IL-1ß and TNFα cause an increased vesicular transport of serum proteins through vascular endothelia; these proteins are accumulated in pericytes, perivascular microglia, and Müller cells, suggesting that these cells act as secondary barriers to extravasated serum proteins (Claudio et al., 1994). In addition, Müller cells can directly kill bacteria through the production of antimicrobial peptides and reactive oxygen and nitrogen species (Shamsuddin and Kumar, 2011; Kumar et al., 2013a).

5.11.1.2 Detrimental Effects of Müller Cell Gliosis

Reactive gliosis also contributes to neurodegeneration and impedes tissue repair and regular neuroregeneration after retinal injury. Reactive Müller cells may dedifferentiate which results in a disruption of the regular glial-neuronal interactions and retinal degeneration. The downregulation of proteins involved in specific Müller cell functions such as glycolysis, transmitter recycling (glutamine synthetase; see 5.5.2.1.12.), spatial potassium buffering (Kir channels; see 5.5.3.5.), carbon dioxide siphoning (carbonic anhydrase; see 5.5.6.), visual pigment cycling (CRALBP; see 5.5.8.1.), and water clearance (AQPs; see 5.5.4.) disrupts the glio-neuronal interaction and the retinal acid-base, ion, and osmohomeostasis, and contributes to the development of edema (see 5.11.9.), neuronal hyperexcitation, and glutamate toxicity which is a major cause of neuronal degneration (see 5.5.2.1.6.). The impairment of the supportive functions of Müller cells increases the susceptibility of neurons to stressful stimuli in the diseased retina. Under ischemic conditions, Müller cells may enter a state which conserves metabolic energy by downregulation of ATP-consuming molecular components (e.g., Kir channels [see 5.5.3.1.], glutamine synthetase, etc.) that are not required for the survival of Müller cells but crucially involved in neuronal survival and activity. It could be that Müller cells functionally uncouple from neurons in order to enhance their own survival (Francke et al., 2005). However, gliotic alterations of Müller cells might be also caused by a disturbed communication between glial cells and neurons. By forming scar tissues (see 5.11.2.6.), reactive Müller cells impede regenerative processes that inhibits a regular regeneration of the retinal tissue.

Activated Müller cells have also more direct cytotoxic effects by the release of soluble factors such as the proinflammatory cytokines TNFα, IL-1β, and MCP-1 (De Kozak et al., 1994, 1997; Drescher and Whittum-Hudson, 1996a; Cotinet et al., 1997a,b; Yuan and Neufeld, 2000; Tezel and Wax, 2000; Hollborn et al., 2008; Liu et al., 2012a). The cytotoxic effects of reactive Müller cells contribute to retinal degeneration in various retinopathies, e.g., diabetic retinopathy (Roth, 1997; Goureau et al., 1999; Koeberle and Ball, 1999; Tezel and Wax, 2000; Bringmann et al., 2006). MCP-1 promotes the infiltration of blood-derived immune cells and subsequent photoreceptor apoptosis (Cuthbertson et al., 1990; Nakazawa et al., 2006b, 2007a). Excess production of NO by Müller cells and the formation of free nitrogen radicals results in protein nitrosylation which has toxic effects in surrounding neurons (Goureau et al., 1994, 1999; De Kozak et al., 1994, 1997; Kashii et al., 1996; Goldstein et al., 1996; Oku et al., 1997; Cotinet et al., 1997b; Kobayashi et al., 2000; Kashiwagi et al., 2001; Du et al., 2004; Zou et al., 2009; Chen et al., 2013b). The increase of the NO production by Müller cells under hyperglycemic conditions causes the diabetic loss of functional hyperemia (Mishra and Newman, 2010) and stimulates the production of cytotoxic prostaglandins by the cyclooxygenase-2 (Du et al., 2004). Prostaglandins are implicated in the pathological angiogenesis and retinal cell death (Sennlaub et al., 2003; Wilkinson-Berka, 2004), and in the induction of cytotoxic Müller cell swelling (see 5.11.9.2.2.). NO has been also implicated in the development of uveoretinitis, glaucoma, and photoreceptor degeneration (De Kozak et al., 1994, 1997; Chen et al., 2013b). An enhanced poduction of polyamines (that coactivate NMDA receptors) by Müller cells after upregulation of arginase I (the rate limiting enzyme for the polyamine biosynthesis) contributes to the excitotoxic damage of retinal neurons (Pernet et al., 2007).

In diabetic retinopathy, Müller cells are activated by inflammatory factors like IL-1β which are produced by the vascular endothelium in response to hyperglycemia (Liu et al., 2012a). Activated Müller cells contribute to leukostasis and vessel occlusion in the diabetic retina. In the course of diabetes, capillary leukostasis and thrombosis, and hyperplasia of endothelial cells result in capillary nonperfusion, ischemia, and the development of acellular vessels (Barouch et al., 2000; Boeri et al., 2001). Müller cells of diabetic animals increase the expression of the intercellular adhesion molecule ICAM-1 (Gerhardinger et al., 2005). NF-κB, which induces the expression of ICAM-1, is activated in vascular endothelial cells, pericytes, and retinal glial cells in diabetes (Shelton et al., 2007). High glucose induces NF-κB activation and ICAM-1 expression in Müller cells (Wang et al., 2010b). Conditional disruption of VEGF in Müller cells reduces diabetic leukostasis (Wang et al., 2010b). Thrombi consist of fibrin, platelets, and leucocytes in the early stage of their formation, and glial cells and macrophages are involved in the later stage (Ishibashi, 2000). Hypertrophied Müller cell processes grow into the vascular lumen where they form glial scars which cause further vessel occlusion (Bek, 1997, 1998).

It is noteworthy that the same gliotic response may have both deleterious and beneficial effects. It has been shown, for example, that deletion of $P2Y_1$ receptors (which mediate, among others, the calcium responses of Müller cells that are increased under pathological conditions; see 5.10.2.3. and 5.10.2.5.) is associated with an increased survival of amacrine cells after retinal ischemia-reperfusion while the ischemic death of photoreceptor cells is more pronounced (Pannicke et al., 2014). The same gliotic response or glial factor may also exert biphasic effects, depending on the time or level of gliotic alterations; dysregulation or overstimulation of protective glial responses may result in detrimental effects. For instance, the induction of acute-phase proteins (e.g., of antioxidant proteins and iron-binding proteins like transferrin; Picard et al., 2008) in Müller cells of diabetic rats and during inflammation represents an adaptive response to defend the tissue from damage (Gerhardinger et al., 2005). On the other hand, persistent overexpression of acute-phase proteins, e.g., of ceruloplasmin and transferrin, may contribute to tissue damage via inducing endothelial dysfunction and angiogenesis (Cappelli-Bigazzi et al., 1997; Carlevaro et al., 1997). VEGF is one of the factors released by activated Müller cells under hypoxic and inflammatory conditions (Aiello et al., 1995; Drescher and Whittum-Hudson, 1996a; Amin et al., 1997; Eichler et al., 2000, 2004a; Yafai et al., 2004; see 5.11.8.). Although low concentrations of VEGF have prosurvival effects (see 5.11.1.1.), overproduction of VEGF exacerbates retinal disease progression by inducing inflammation (Ishida et al., 2003), vascular leakage (see 5.11.9.1.1.), and neovascularization (see 5.11.8.). High concentrations of VEGF cause endothelial cell hyperplasia resulting in capillary non-perfusion, and induce other vascular features characteristic for diabetic retinopathy including vessel dilation and tortuousity, vascular leakage, focal hemorrhages, microaneurysms, and preretinal neovascularization

(Tolentino et al., 2002). Furthermore, proinflammatory cytokines produced by Müller cells such as IL-1β, IL-6, and TNFα (Roberge et al., 1988; Drescher and Whittum-Hudson, 1996b; De Kozak et al., 1997; Cotinet et al., 1997a,b; Vinores et al., 2001; Yoshida et al., 2001; Nakamura et al., 2003; Nakatani et al., 2006; Seki et al., 2006; Hauck et al., 2007; Cheng et al., 2013) have both beneficial (Mendonca Torres and de Araujo, 2001; Diem et al., 2001; Sanchez et al., 2003; Inomata et al., 2003; Namekata et al., 2008; Chong et al., 2008; Chidlow et al., 2012; Perígolo-Vicente et al., 2013; Leibinger et al., 2013) and detrimental effects in the retina (Maruo et al., 1992; Luna et al., 1997; De Kozak et al., 1997; Tezel and Wax, 2000; Shen and Xu, 2009; Shen et al., 2010b, 2011b). In addition, Müller cell-derived growth factors such as IGF-1 and bFGF have beneficial and detrimental effects in the retina (Arroba et al., 2011; Villacampa et al., 2013; see 5.5.2.1.13. and 5.11.7.7.). Another example of an overstimulated protective response of Müller cells is the phagocytosis of blood-borne factors and cells in cases of vitreal hemorrhage. It has been suggested that a main mechanism that leads to epiretinal membrane formation is the phagocytosis of hemoglobin and damaged erythrocytes, which adhere at the vitreal surface of the retina, by processes of Müller cells that extend through holes in the inner limiting membrane (see 5.11.11.3.).

5.11.2 CHARACTERISTICS OF MÜLLER CELL GLIOSIS

5.11.2.1 Unspecific and Specific Müller Cell Responses

Müller cell gliosis is characterized by specific and unspecific responses to pathogenic stimuli; the former are dependent and the latter are independent on the kind of the stimulus. Müller cells show (at least) three important unspecific gliotic responses: cellular hypertrophy (Figs. 8H, 12C,J, 15A), proliferation (see 5.11.10.), and upregulation of intermediate filaments (see 5.11.3.). The upregulation of GFAP is the most sensitive non-specific response to retinal disease and injury, and can be used as "retinal stress" indicator, i.e., as a universal early cellular marker for retinal injury and Müller cell activation (Bignami and Dahl, 1979; Bringmann and Reichenbach, 2001; Lewis and Fisher, 2003). Another non-specific Müller cell response is the activation of ERK1/2 which is observed in animal models of most retinopathies including retinal detachment, ischemia-reperfusion (Figs. 8A, 82A), uveitis, glaucoma, and optic nerve transection (Geller et al., 2001; Akiyama et al., 2002; Takeda et al., 2002; Tezel et al., 2003; Galan et al., 2014; Joly et al., 2014b).

A prominent example of a specific gliotic response is the alteration in the expression of the glutamine synthetase. After loss of major glutamate-releasing neurons, for example, after photoreceptor degeneration induced by light or retinal detachment, the expression of the glutamine synthetase in Müller cells is reduced (see 5.5.2.1.12.). An enhanced expression of this enzyme is observed during hepatic retinopathy when its activity is required to detoxify the tissue from elevated levels of ammonia (see 5.5.2.1.14.).

5.11.2.2 Heterogeneity of Müller Cell Responses

Not all Müller cells of a retina may respond to a pathogenic stimulus in the same way. Such a heterogeneity between neighboring Müller cells in the same region of the retina in respect to gliotic alterations was found, for example, in the chick (Fischer and Reh, 2003). In regions of the chick retina where Müller cell proliferation occurs in response to NMDA-induced retinal injury, ~65% of the Müller cells reentered the cell cycle, while the remaining 35% do not (Fischer and Reh, 2003). Müller cells which increase their expression of GFAP in response to injury do not reenter the cell cycle while cells that fail to increase their expression of GFAP proliferate (Fischer and Reh, 2003). In retinas of diabetic rats, there is a substantial variation among Müller cells of one retina in the downregulation of functional Kir channels (Fig. 15C) (Pannicke et al., 2006). There are also species and time dependencies in Müller cell responses. In most mammalian species investigated, retinal detachment results in Müller cell proliferation and hypertrophy (Fig. 12C, J) and an increase in the expression of GFAP and vimentin (Fig. 11A, 12A, 33B; see 5.11.5.); these alterations were not observed after detachment of the cone-dominant ground squirrel retina (Linberg et al., 2002). Slow degeneration of the retina (as observed in *rds* mice and RCS rats with slowly developing inherited photoreceptor degeneration, or after Borna virus infection) cause less dramatic changes in Müller cells than rapid degenerations (Felmy et al., 2001; Iandiev et al., 2006e).

5.11.2.3 "Conservative" and Massive Gliosis

Increasingly severe retinal insults result in greater degrees of functional and biochemical changes of Müller cells that was described as "conservative" or non-proliferative gliosis (Fig. 62) (Bringmannn et al., 2000a). Such gliosis is characterized by an upregulation of GFAP, cellular hypertrophy, a moderate or no decrease of Kir currents which is associated with a slight membrane depolarization (by ~10 mV), a moderate transient or no proliferation of Müller cells (Fisher et al., 1991; Geller et al., 1995; Härtig et al., 1995; Kacza et al., 2000; Inman and Horner, 2007), and a decrease in the expression of proteins and enzymes associated with normal functions such as glutamine synthetase, CRALBP, and carbonic anhydrase (Lewis et al., 1994; Lieth et al., 1998; Joly et al., 2008). A moderate or no decrease of the Kir currents was observed in animal models of various retinopathies such as Borna disease virus-induced retinitis, inherited photoreceptor degeneration, damage to the optic tract, and bright white light-induced retinal degeneration (see 5.5.3.5.). Downregulation of the

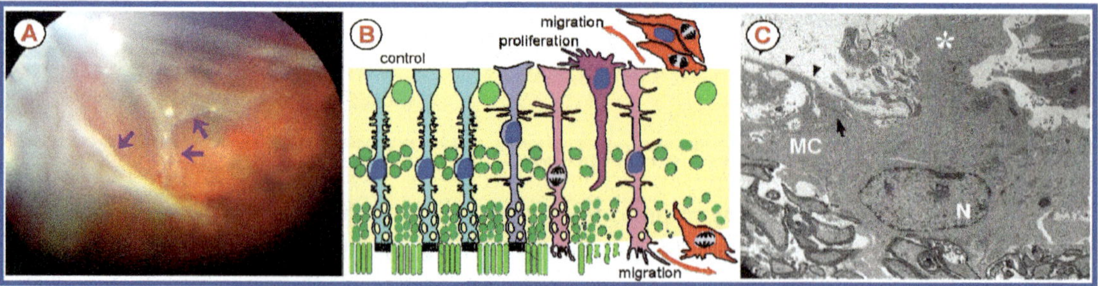

FIGURE 84: Müller cell reactivity in proliferative vitreoretinopathy (PVR). **A.** Ophthalmoscopic image of an experimentally induced PVR in the rabbit eye. Note the large, folded cellular masses on the vitreal surface of the retina (*arrows*). **B.** Schematic drawing of increasing degrees of Müller cell reactivity (from *left* to *right*). Müller cells re-enter the proliferation cycle, migrate out of the neural retina, and participate in the formation of periretinal fibrocellular membranes. **C.** Transmission electron micrograph of a reactive Müller cell (MC) of the rabbit retina which migrate through a hole in the inner limiting membrane (*arrowheads*) into the vitreous body (*asterisk*). The nucleus (N) of the Müller cell is translocated to the innermost retinal layer. Modified from Bringmann et al. (2006).

transcription factor Lhx2 in Müller cells leads to the induction of hypertrophic but not proliferative gliosis (De Melo et al., 2012).

The most severe insults induce yet another level of Müller cell response described as "massive" or proliferative gliosis (Bringmannn et al., 2000a). Expression of proteins associated with normal physiologic support of retinal neurons cease, the Kir conductance of Müller cell membranes decreases dramatically (to approximately 5% of control; Figs. 46A–D, 56B, 63B), which is associated with a depolarization of the cells by 30–40 mV (Figs. 46A,B,D, 60B), and the cells begin a phase of seemingly uncontrolled proliferation, forming masses of cells referred to as "gliotic scar" within the retina and on the subretinal and epiretinal surfaces (Fig. 84A–C; see 5.11.11.). In epiretinal scar tissues, Müller cells change their phenotype and transdifferentiate into contractile myofibrocytes (Guidry, 1996, 2005, 2009; see 5.11.11.2.). A possible trigger for the transition from "conservative" to "proliferative" gliosis is the breakdown of the blood-retinal barrier (see 5.11.9.1.1.), resulting in increases of the retinal and vitreal contents of growth factors, cytokines, and inflammatory factors, and infiltration of blood-derived cells (see 5.11.11.3.). Proliferative gliosis is clearly detrimental to the retina while "conservative" gliosis might be helpful, e.g., through the secretion of neurotrophic factors (see 5.11.7.) and an increased expression of glutamate transporter proteins in pathologies associated with increased retinal glutamate (Reichelt et al., 1997a; see 5.5.2.1.6.).

5.11.2.4 Resistance and Susceptibility of Müller Cells to Pathogenic Stimuli

Retinal neurons and photoreceptor cells are highly susceptible to various forms of injury and disease including insufficient blood supply. By contrast, Müller glial cells are strikingly resistant to ischemia, anoxia, hypoglycemia, elevation of the hydrostatic pressure, and increased extracellular glutamate concentration (Anderson and Davis, 1975; Shay and Ames, 1976; Kitano et al., 1996; Silver et al., 1997; Stone et al., 1999; Baptiste et al., 2002; Kashiwagi et al., 2004). Müller cells survive most retinal injuries and diseases, and remain available as players in the pathogenic events. There is no degeneration of Müller cells even after virus-induced loss of most retinal neurons (Pannicke et al., 2001). One reason for this relative insusceptibility to injury is their specialized energy metabolism which depends to 80–90% on glycolysis (aerobically and anaerobically); thus Müller cells can reliably switch to anaerobic glycolysis in the presence of insuffcent oxygen supply and withstand even long-lasting anoxia (Poitry-Yamate et al., 1995; Winkler et al., 2000). As long as oxygen is available, Müller cells are also resistant to the absence of glucose because other substrates such as lactate, pyruvate, glutamate or glutamine can be metabolized to generate energy substrates by the tricarboxylic acid cycle, a pathway that is normally non-dominant (Tsacopoulos et al., 1998; Winkler et al., 2000). Under these conditions, the carbon skeleton of glutamate enters the tricarboxylic acid cycle as α-ketoglutarate (Fig. 44) (Kalloniatis and Napper, 2002). Short periods of glucose deprivation (45–60 min; Johnson, 1977) can be compensated by the glycogen deposits in Müller cells (Kuwabara and Cogan, 1961; Magalhães and Coimbra, 1972; Reichenbach et al., 1988a, 1999; Gohdo et al., 2001). However, the extent of glycolysis and mitochondrial respiration differ in Müller cells of avascular and vascularized retinas. Müller cells of avascular retinas (e.g., of guinea pigs and rabbits) contain only a few mitochondria at their distal-most end, directed towards the choroid as the only oxygen source (Figs. 31, 34J, L; see 5.2.). The mitochondrial energy production of these cells can be blocked over hours without measurable effects on energy-consuming functions such as the maintenance of the very negative plasma membrane potential whereas the cells rapidly depolarize when the anaerobic glycolysis is blocked (Reichenbach et al., 1999). Müller cells of vascularized retinas contain many mitochondria which are distributed along the entire length of the cells probably due to a suffcent oxygen availability throughout the tissue (Fig. 35B; see 5.2.). When the mitochondrial energy production of such cells (from rats) is blocked, their plasma membranes slowly depolarize, suggesting that these cells cannot be completely resistant to anoxia (A. Reichenbach, unpublished results). The plasma membranes of these cells also depolarize more rapidly when the anaerobic glycolysis is blocked.

The resistance of Müller cells to pathogenic stimuli was also attributed to their high antioxidant content (see 5.5.2.1.15.), their capacity to proliferate and regenerate, a downregulation of iGluRs in response to excess glutamate (Lopez et al., 1998; Taylor et al., 2003), a lower affinity of Müller cell's AMPA receptors compared to neuronal AMPA receptors (Kawasaki et al., 1996), the presence of glutamate transporters and glutamine synthetase that detoxify excess glutamate (see 5.5.2.1.), and the prosurvival effect of insulin signaling (Walker et al., 2012; Küser-Abali et al., 2013). Under pathological conditions, Müller cells enhance the expression of αB-crystallin which functions as a stress-inducible molecular chaperone involved in the defensive response to the stress of apoptotic photoreceptor cell death (Jones et al., 1998). In addition, a sustained autocrine activation of receptors for neurotrophic factors was implicated in the Müller cell survival under pathological conditions (Giardino et al., 1998; Taylor et al., 2003). For instance, hyperglycemic conditions induce an upregulation of GDNF and its receptors in Müller cells (Zhu et al., 2012). GDNF inhibits the apoptosis of Müller cells as well as the degeneration of photoreceptors and neurons, in part via upregulation of neurotrophic and growth factors such as bFGF, BDNF, and osteopontin (see 5.11.7.3.). Müller cell survival is also enhanced by autocrine VEGF and apelin signaling (Saint-Geniez et al., 2008; Wang et al., 2012c). On the other hand, reduced levels of neurotrophic factors like BDNF are a characteristic of the diabetic retina (Seki et al., 2004; Sasaki et al., 2010; Ola et al., 2013). Reduced BDNF levels contribute to oxidative stress and neurodegeneration, and impair the neuron-supporting functions of Müller cells by decreasing their glutamate uptake and metabolism (see 5.5.2.1.13.).

There are various pathological conditions which are associated with Müller cell degeneration. Apoptotic or edematous degeneration of Müller cells was observed, for example, during long-term exposure to high ammonia (see 5.5.2.1.14.), under hyperglycemic conditions and in retinas of diabetic animals, after retinal ischemia and retinal detachment (Fig. 54B), and in retinas of animals which were fed with a cholesterol-enriched diet (Hammes et al., 1995; Reichenbach et al., 1995d; Faude et al., 2001; Gwon et al., 2004; Kusner et al., 2004; Xi et al., 2005; Trivino et al., 2006; Fort et al., 2011; Küser-Abali et al., 2013). Hyperglycemia induces Müller cell apoptosis via nuclear translocation of the glyceraldehyde-3-phosphate dehydrogenase, inactivation of the Akt survival pathway, upregulation of the thioredoxin-interacting protein, and increased activity of the salt-inducible kinase which negatively modulates the insulin-dependent survival pathway (Kusner et al., 2004; Xi et al., 2005; Devi et al., 2012; Küser-Abali et al., 2013). The high glucose-induced accumulation of glyceraldehyde-3-phosphate dehydrogenase in Müller cell nuclei is mediated by IL-1β (Yego et al., 2009). In addition, TNFα was shown to decrease the tyrosine phosphorylation of the insulin receptor and Akt, and to increase the phosphorylation of the insulin receptor substrate-1, in high-glucose conditions, resulting in increased death of Müller cells (Walker et al., 2011). Extravasated modified lipoproteins such as highly oxidized glycated LDL may contribute to the induction of Müller cell apoptosis via enhanced levels of oxidative and endoplasmic reticulum stress (Wu et al., 2012). In addition, ALEs were shown to induce Müller cell apoptosis at high concentrations (Yong et al., 2010). Taurine may prevent the hyperglycemic apoptosis of Müller cells (Zeng et al., 2010a).

5.11.2.5 Primary Müller Cell Injuries

There are cases in which Müller cells are suggested to be the primary targets of pathogenic agents, e.g., hepatic retinopathy (see 5.5.2.1.14.), amyloid-β peptide-induced retinal degeneration (Walsh et al., 2002), in the presence of autoantibodies against Müller cells or CRALBP (Peek et al., 1998; Deeg et al., 2007), after intake of organophosphate pesticides (Uga et al., 1977), and methanol-induced retinal toxicity (Garner et al., 1995). Methanol poisoning results in retinal toxicity in humans and non-human primates (but not rodents) and is mediated by its metabolite formate which is toxic to the mitochondria resulting in degeneration of the retinal ganglion cell axons (Baumbach et al., 1977). Formate is detoxified to carbon dioxide by a two-step oxidation process that is ATP- and folate-dependent. The sensitivity of the primate retina to methanol/formate toxicity was ascribed to the limited capacity to oxidize formate due to the low amount of retinal folate (Martinasevic et al., 1996). Because the enzymes for formate detoxification are preferentially localized in Müller cells (Martinasevic et al., 1996), they are the primary target for the methanol/formate-induced retinal toxicity (Garner et al., 1995). Müller cells take up folate, a vitamin also necessary for cell proliferation, via the proton-coupled folate transporter and folate receptor-α (Umapathy et al., 2007; Bozard et al., 2010, 2012).

Müller cell dysfunction or degeneration has been also suggested as a primary cause for the visual loss in Müller cell sheen dystrophy, retinoschisis, macular hole formation, and macular telangiectasia (MacTel) type 2 (Condon et al., 1986; De Jong et al., 1991; Kirsch et al., 1996; Kellner et al., 1998; Gass, 1999; Sugiyama et al., 2006; Powner et al., 2010). Far more than 100 different mutations were described to cause retinitis pigmentosa. Although most mutations in hereditary retinal dystrophies are related to photoreceptors and/or the retinal pigment epithelium, there are also mutations in Müller cell proteins underlying photoreceptor degeneration. In an autosomal recessive retinitis pigmentosa, a mutation of the gene encoding CRALBP was described (Maw et al., 1997). The mutant protein lacks the ability to bind 11-cis-retinaldehyde resulting in a disruption of retinal vitamin-A metabolism (Maw et al., 1997). Mutations in the human Crumbs homologue-1 (Crb1) gene cause retinal blinding diseases such as Leber congenital amaurosis and retinitis pigmentosa. The Crb1 transmembrane protein localizes in Müller cells at the subapical region near the adherens junctions between Müller and photoreceptor cells (Van Rossum et al., 2006). Crb1 regulates the number and size of Müller cell's apical microvilli; a disturbance in the formation of the villi results in degeneration of photoreceptor and pigment epithelial cells, and subsequent choroidal neovascularization (Van de Pavert et al., 2007).

5.11.2.6 Glial Scar Formation

Retinal injury triggers hypertrophy, proliferation, and migration of Müller cells (Figs. 12C, J, 84A–C) resulting in a formation of a glial scar that fills retinal breaks and that replaces degenerated neurons, photoreceptors, retinal pigment epithelial cells, and blood vessels (Foos and Gloor, 1975; Burke and Smith, 1981; Hara et al., 2000). Glial scarring is associated with the formation of new tissues above both surfaces of the neuroretina (Figs. 53C, 84A–C). Periretinal glial membranes (see 5.11.11.) can be supposed to represent a kind of glial scar that protects the neuroretina from further damage by pathogenic factors present in the vitreous and in the injured retinal pigment epithelium (Bringmann and Wiedemann, 2009). The formation of neovascular epiretinal membranes in PDR and of neovascular subretinal membranes in wet AMD can be considered as an attempt to reoxygenize ischemic retinal areas. However, periretinal membranes contribute to further tissue damage, by the development of subretinal edema as occurring in wet AMD, by inducing retinal detachment and retinal folds due to the contraction of preretinal membranes (see 5.11.11.), by the impairment of the oxygen and nutrient supply of ischemic retinal areas from the vitreal humor, and by the impairment of the exchange of ions across the inner retinal surface which is important, for example, for retinal potassium buffering (see 5.5.3.).

Following photoreceptor degeneration after retinal detachment or during aging, Müller cell processes grow through the outer limiting membrane into the subretinal space (Fig. 53C) (Fan et al., 1996; Lewis and Fisher, 2000; Francke et al., 2001b; Fisher and Lewis, 2003). The growth of subretinal Müller cell processes occurs in association with cone photoreceptors (Lewis and Fisher, 2000). After reattachment of detached retinas, the process extension of Müller cells into the subretinal space is inhibited, and Müller cells and their processes translocate to the vitreal retinal surface where they form preretinal membranes as in PVR (Fisher and Lewis, 2003; see 5.11.11.). In AMD, retinal glial cells form membranes between the vitreous humor and the inner limiting membrane (Ramírez et al., 2001). Subretinal choroidal neovascular membranes (formed in wet AMD) are composed of vascular endothelial cells, retinal pigment epithelial cells, Müller cells, macrophages, and lymphocytes; the membranes oftenly adhere to the neuroretina by a gliotic band of hypertrophied and displaced Müller cells (Kimura et al., 1999). In cases of geographic atrophy, the degenerated retinal pigment epithelium is substituted by Müller cell processes (Wu et al., 2003), and Müller cells extend processes into the choroid through gaps in Bruch's membrane (Sullivan et al., 2003).

Glial scars within and at the margin of the injured tissue are one reason for the failure of retinas of warm-blooded vertebrates to regenerate whereas retinas of cold-blooded vertebrates such as fishes and amphibians retain the capability of full regeneration also in adults (see 5.11.12.1.). Apparently, gliotic Müller cells simultaneously promote and inhibit tissue repair processes in the injured retinas of higher vertebrates, i.e., distinct remodeling events of neuronal processes and synapses are supported by Müller cells whereas other regeneration processes are inhibited resulting in aberrant tissue repair (see 5.11.5.).

5.11.2.7 Prevention of Retinal Regeneration

In higher vertebrates, the ongoing regeneration processes in the injured retina are dysregulated due to the absence of a permissive environment for a regular regeneration (see 4.2. and 5.11.12.). Müller cell processes that form a fibrotic layer in the subretinal space (Fig. 53C) inhibit the regeneration of deconstructed photoreceptor segments after reattachment of detached retinas (Anderson et al., 1986; Fisher and Lewis, 2003; Francke et al., 2005; see 5.11.5.). Hypertrophied Müller cell processes that fill the spaces left by retracted photoreceptor synapses in the outer plexiform layer prevent a regular regeneration of the disconnected synaptic contacts (Erickson et al., 1983; Anderson et al., 1986; Lewis and Fisher, 2000; Sethi et al., 2005). After optic nerve crash, hypertrophied Müller cell and astrocytic processes infiltrate nerve fiber bundles, and surround and intrude into ganglion cell somata (Barron et al., 1986).

The non-permissive environment for tissue remodeling and regeneration is caused by the increased stiffness of gliotic Müller cells which inhibits neurite growth (see 5.5.1.3.) and provided by inhibitory extracellular matrix and cell adhesion molecules (chondroitin sulfate proteoglycans such as neurocan and versican, and the hyaluronan-binding glycoprotein CD44) and repulsive guidance molecules that are increasingly expressed on the surface of reactive micro- and macroglial cells (Silver, 1994; Canning et al., 1996; Normand et al., 1998; Fawcett and Asher, 1999; Inatani et al., 2000; Sellés-Navarro et al., 2001; Inatani and Tanihara, 2002; Fisher and Lewis, 2003; Busch and Silver, 2007; Singhal et al., 2008; Siddiqui et al., 2009; Schnichels et al., 2012; see 4.2.). These molecules bind a variety of extracellular matrix and cell adhesion proteins and are chemical inhibitors of axonal growth and neuronal regeneration, and thus prevent the functional regeneration of the tissue (Ponta et al., 2003). Both neurocan and CD44 are expressed in the normal retina, and injury stimulates the production of these proteins by reactive glial cells (Chaitin et al., 1994, 1996; Kuhrt et al., 1997; Chaitin and Brun-Zinkernagel, 1998; Krishnamoorthy et al. 2000; Jones et al., 2000; Zhang et al. 2003b; Wahl et al., 2013). The increased expression of chondroitin sulfate proteoglycans creates regenerative boundaries in the injured mature retina. In the developing retina, these molecules constitute developmental boundaries which control the pathfinding of growing ganglion cell axons, for example (Silver, 1994; Oster et al., 2004).

The non-permissive environment for tissue remodeling and regeneration prevents also the migration and integration of neural grafts and transplanted stem cells (Johnson et al., 2010). It has been proposed that attempts to reduce the glial hypertrophy and to remove the glial barrier for neuronal regeneration by degradation of inhibitory extracellular matrix molecules (with chondroitinase or MMPs), or of their hyaluronan-expressing targets (with hyaluronidase), support the regular retinal regeneration after injury, as well as the integration of transplanted exogenous cells into the tissue (Silver, 1994; Moon et al. 2003; Fisher and Lewis, 2003; Francke et al., 2005; Zhang et al. 2007b; Tucker et al., 2008; Bull et al., 2008; Singhal et al., 2008; Siddiqui et al., 2009). An elevated expression of MMPs (which is associated with a decrease in the deposition of inhibitory extracellular matrix molecules) supports the migration and integration of transplanted photoreceptors in retinal explant cultures (Tucker et al., 2008). The inhibitory effects of chondroitin sulfate proteoglycans are mediated by the Rho GTPase and Rho kinase; blockade of these molecules may be helpful for the reestablishment of a permissive environment for neurite growth (Monnier et al., 2003).

Glial scar formation may be also a reason for the failure of visual recovery after implantation of an electronic device into the subretinal space. Müller cell responses to retinal electronic implants involve upregulation of GFAP (Pardue et al., 2001; Tamaki et al., 2008) and downregulation and redistribution of Kir4.1 (I. Iandiev, Leipzig, unpublished data), suggesting an inflammatory reactivation of Müller cells. The glial scar tissue may function as an electrical barrier between the implant and retinal neurons.

5.11.2.8 Promotion of Retinal Remodeling

The glial inhibition of tissue remodeling is incomplete (Jones et al., 2012). Neurite sprouting and neuronal migration to ectopic sites were observed in AMD, retinal detachment (see 5.11.5.), PVR, and experimental diabetic retinopathy (Gastinger et al., 2001). However, the reparative processes in the injured mammalian retina proceed in a dysregulated fashion, resembling in part the developmental plasticity. Hypertrophied Müller cell processes function as guiding structures for neuronal migration and aberrant sprouting of neuronal cell processes (Marc et al., 2003). After photoreceptor degeneration, hypertrophied Müller cell processes form a scar tissue between the neuroretina and the pigmented epithelium; neurons migrate along the glial surfaces to ectopic sites (Jones et al., 2003). Slowly developing inherited rod photoreceptor degeneration triggers the reorganization of the cone mosaic into an orderly array of rings; within the rings, remodeled Müller cell processes envelope cones (Lee et al., 2011b; Zhu et al., 2013). In retinas of aged albino rats which suffer from a light-induced degeneration of photoreceptor and pigment epithelial cells, Müller cells extend processes into the choroid through gaps in the Bruch's membrane, and neuronal somata and processes migrate along the remodeled processes of Müller cells into the choroidal region (Sullivan et al., 2003). A similar glial rearrangement and displacement of neurons was found in retinas of patients with AMD (Sullivan et al., 2003). Aberrant axon extension and neurite sprouting along Müller cell fibers occur also after retinal detachment (Charteris et al., 2002; Lewis et al., 2004). The remodeling in the first-, second-, and third-order neurons of detached retinas may represent an attempt to reestablish synaptic connectivity (Sethi et al., 2005). Ganglion cell neurites grow into human epiretinal membranes in association with glial cells, suggesting that glial cells have a permissive role in neurite growth into extra-retinal tissues (Lesnik Oberstein et al., 2008).

5.11.3 UPREGULATION OF INTERMEDIATE FILAMENTS

A heterogeneous group of proteins form 10 nm-diameter intermediate filaments as a component of the cytoskeleton. In the course of retinal development, retinal progenitor cells and immature Müller cells express the intermediate filaments vimentin and nestin (Schnitzer, 1988b; Walcott and Provis, 2003; Fischer and Omar, 2005; Xue et al., 2006b; Valamanesh et al., 2013). Nestin cannot form filaments on its own but requires vimentin as polymerization partner. As maturation proceeds, Müller cells downregulate nestin, and mature Müller cells express predominantly vimentin (Figs. 11A, 31, 32, 33A,B, 75) while retinal astrocytes express predominantly GFAP and less vimentin (Figs. 6A,B, 14D, 15A, 21B, 85) (Dixon and Eng, 1980; Dahl and Bignami, 1982; Molnar et al., 1984; Shaw and Weber, 1984; Eisenfeld et al., 1984; Pixley et al., 1984; Björklund et al., 1985; Schnitzer, 1985, 1988b; Tuccari et al., 1986; Penn et al., 1988; Davidson et al., 1990; Scherer and Schnitzer, 1989, 1991; Sarthy et al., 1991; Chien and Liem, 1995; Osborne and Larsen, 1996; Grosche et al., 1997; Li et al., 2002a; Powner et al., 2010; Zayit-Soudry et al., 2010; Valamanesh et al., 2013). In the human retina, three populations of astrocytes are distinguishable: vimentin$^+$/GFAP$^+$, vimentin$^-$/GFAP$^+$, and vimentin$^+$/GFAP$^-$ (Pérez-Alvarez et al., 2008). If Müller cells in a mature retina of higher vertebrates express GFAP, this expression is restricted to the endfeet and inner stem process of the cells (Figs. 12A) and to cells located at the ora serrata and around the optic nerve (Bromberg and Schachner, 1978; Erickson et al., 1987; Vaughan et al., 1990; De Raad et al., 1996; Karim et al., 1996). In retinas of lower vertebrates (fish, amphibians) which show a lifelong growth (see 5.11.12.1.) and which lack retinal astrocytes (see Ch. 2), Müller cells express GFAP (Bignami, 1984; Nona et al., 1989; Vaughan and Lasater, 1990; Mitashov et al., 1995; Koke et al., 2010; Arenzana et al., 2011). In newts, GFAP is also expressed by retinal progenitor cells (Mitashov et al., 1995). Astrocytes of optic nerves in many fish express cytokeratins and not GFAP (Koke et al.,

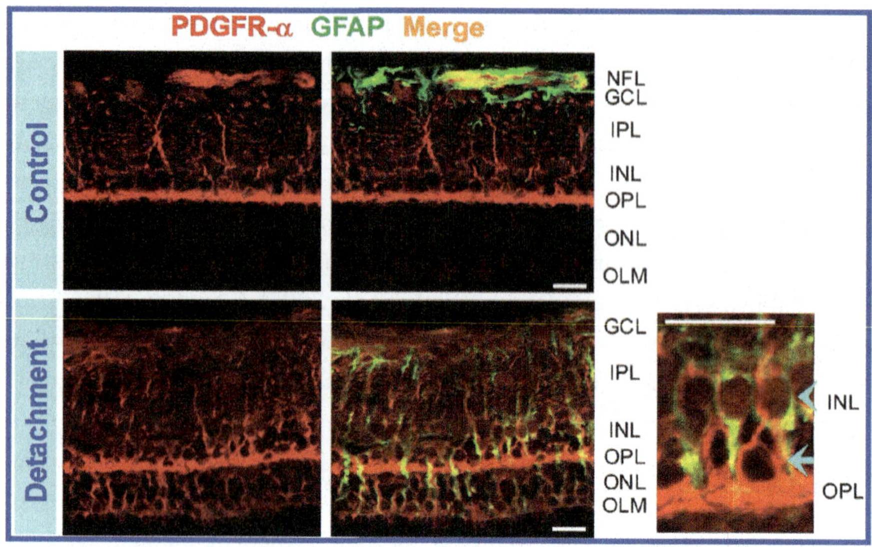

FIGURE 85: Localization of the PDGF receptor-α protein in the porcine retina. The slices were co-immunostained against the glial marker GFAP and were derived from a control retina (*above*) and a retina which was experimentally detached from the pigment epithelium for 7 days (*below*). The *small image* at right displays the inner nuclear layer (INL) at higher magnification. Note that bipolar cell somata (*arrow*) as well as Müller cell somata (*arrowhead*) and processes express PDGF receptor-α protein. GCL, ganglion cell layer; IPL, inner plexiform layer; NFL, nerve fiber layer; OLM, outer limiting membrane; ONL, outer nuclear layer; OPL, outer plexiform layer. Scale bars, 20 μm. Unpublished results (I. Iandiev, Leipzig).

2010). In the healthy adult retina, nestin expression is restricted to blood vessels (Fig. 14C,E) (Xue et al., 2011a; but see Wohl et al., 2011). The constitutive expression of GFAP in (a subpopulation of) retinal astrocytes and the absence of GFAP in Müller cells of higher vertebrates can be explained with the fact that the GFAP gene is activated by different control elements in Müller cells and astrocytes (Verderber et al., 1995). In addition, astrocytes and Müller cells express desmin (Dahl and Bignami, 1982). Müller cells in culture downregulate GFAP and vimentin, while α-smooth muscle actin becomes the major cytoskeletal protein (Hui et al., 1988; Sramek et al., 1989; McGillem et al., 1998; McGillem and Dacheux, 1999; Guidry, 2005; Abrahan et al., 2009). This alteration in the cytoskeletal protein expression reflect the transdifferentiation of proliferating Müller cells into myofibrocytes (see 5.11.11.2.). In addition to retinal glial cells, horizontal cells may express vimentin (Dräger, 1983; Vaughan and Lasater, 1990). However, the expression of glial intermediate filaments in horizontal cells is extremely species-variable (Shaw and Weber, 1984).

In response to virtually any insult, Müller cells increase the expression of the intermediate filaments GFAP, vimentin, nestin, and synemin (Figs. 12A, 14A-E, 21B, 24, 33A,B, 53A–C) (Bignami and Dahl, 1979; Molnar et al., 1984; Eisenfeld et al., 1984; Björklund et al., 1985; Tuccari et al., 1986; Penn et al., 1988; Lewis et al., 1989; Sarthy and Fu, 1989; Davidson et al., 1990; Scherer and Schnitzer, 1991; Osborne et al., 1991; Erickson et al., 1992; Humphrey et al., 1993; Huxlin et al., 1995; Reichenbach et al., 1995d; De Raad et al., 1996; Osborne and Larsen, 1996; Blanks et al., 1996; Grosche et al., 1997; Bringmann and Reichenbach, 2001; Sabbatini et al., 2001; Lewis and Fisher, 2003; Ramírez et al., 2006; Anderson et al., 2008; Luna et al., 2010; Hirrlinger et al., 2010; Roesch et al., 2012; Xu et al., 2013; Valamanesh et al., 2013). After acute retinal inhury, increased GFAP expression of Müller cells remains detectable for at least one month while the GFAP mRNA is only present for a few days, suggesting that the GFAP protein in Müller cells has a long lifetime similar to that of astrocytes despite different gene control elements (Humphrey et al., 1997). In Müller cells of the detached human retina, vimentin and GFAP proteins were found in the same filaments (Okada et al., 1990). The reexpression of nestin by reactive Müller cells in the mature retina, e.g., in diabetic retinopathy (Fig. 15A), inherited retinal degeneration, and after neurotoxic injury, optic nerve transection, retinal detachment, and laser injury (Lieth et al., 1998; Barber et al., 2000; Rungger-Brändle et al., 2000; Ooto et al., 2004; Xue et al., 2006a, b; Kohno et al., 2006; Chang et al., 2007; Luna et al., 2010; Kumar and Zhuo, 2010), may reflect a dedifferentiation of the cells, toward becoming neurogenic progenitor cells (Fischer and Omar, 2005; Goel and Dhingra, 2012; see 5.11.12.). After retinal detachment, nestin is localized to the foremost processes of those Müller cells that grew into the subretinal space, as well as in proliferating Müller cells (Luna et al., 2010).

Intermediate filaments stabilize the hypertrophied Müller cell processes and may be involved in signal transduction cascades underlying reactive gliosis (see 5.11.3.3.). The filaments provide resistance to mechanical stress; after retinal detachment, the absence of GFAP and vimentin results in a shearing of the Müller cell endfeet away from the rest of the retina or even in a separation of the endfeet from the retina (Lundkvist et al., 2004; Verardo et al., 2008). Following retinal detachment, Müller cell nuclei migrate to the outer retina, undergo mitosis, and reside in subretinal glial scars (Fig. 53C) (Lewis et al., 2010). It was suggested that the Müller cell nuclei use vimentin filaments as a "track" for migration into the outer retina (Lewis et al., 2010).

Upregulation of intermediate filaments in Müller cells is a very sensitive and early "retinal stress" indicator. Retinal ischemia-hypoxia causes increases in gene and protein expression of GFAP in Müller cells within 1–3 h (Kim et al., 1998a; Kaur et al., 2007). In experimental glaucoma, the expression of nestin and GFAP is induced within 2 h of elevated intraocular pressure (Xue et al., 2006a). In the rat retina, GFAP appears in Müller cells 4–5 h after axotomy of the ganglion cells; increased GFAP spread out in a declining wave over the whole dorsoventral retina within one day

(Seiler and Turner, 1988). Oxygen therapy in experimental retinal detachment, beginning one day after the onset of detachment, preserves the photoreceptor segments and inhibits neurite sprouting, but does not affect the increased expression of GFAP and vimentin in Müller cells (Lewis et al., 2004).

5.11.3.1 Intermediate Filaments are Crucial for Glial Scarring

Upregulation of intermediate filaments is a crucial step for the gliotic response. Mice deficient in GFAP and vimentin exhibit fewer morphologic changes in glial cells and less glial scarring after injury compared to wildtype mice (Pekny et al., 1999; Kinouchi et al., 2003; Wilhelmsson et al., 2004). Subretinal glial scar formation after retinal detachment is greatly reduced in mice deficient for GFAP and vimentin (Nakazawa et al., 2007b; Verardo et al., 2008). In these mice, the shearing of Müller cell endfeet away from retinal ganglion cells results in aberrant neurite sprouting (Verardo et al., 2008). The absence of GFAP and vimentin leads also to improved integration of retinal transplants (Kinouchi et al., 2003). In an animal model of hypoxia-induced neovascularization, the absence of GFAP and vimentin resulted in a less frequent growth of newly formed vessels from the retina into the vitreous cavity (Lundkvist et al., 2004). The absence of GFAP and vimentin also attenuates various reactive responses of Müller cells upon retinal detachment including activation of ERK1/2 and c-Fos, and induction of MCP-1 (Nakazawa et al., 2007b). The decreased Müller cell reactivity is associated with attenuated monocyte infiltration and photoreceptor apoptosis (Nakazawa et al., 2007b). Apparently, inhibition of intermediate filament expression under stress conditions (e.g., by administration of a soluble TGF-β receptor II; Hisatomi et al., 2002a) may represent a method to attenuate glial scar formation, to limit photoreceptor degeneration, and to provide a permissive environment for the integration of retinal transplants (Kinouchi et al., 2003).

5.11.3.2 Cellular Signaling Involved in Upregulation of Intermediate Filaments

Several factors and signaling pathways were described to induce or inhibit the upregulation of intermediate filaments. The diabetic upregulation of GFAP in Müller cells is inhibited by melatonin, an aldose reductase inhibitor, and an angiotensin II receptor blocker, suggesting that oxidative stress, the polyol pathway, and the renin-angiotensin system contribute to the progression of Müller cell gliosis (Asnaghi et al., 2003; Baydas et al., 2004; Qin et al., 2012). In addition, activation of the AGE receptor results in upregulation of GFAP in Müller cells (Zong et al., 2010).

Intraocular injection of insulin and bFGF induces intermediate filament expression in Müller cells (Lewis et al., 1992; Fischer and Omar, 2005). Release of endogenous bFGF is a very early event in the injured retina and occurs within minutes after retinal detachment, for example (Geller et al., 2001; see 5.11.5.). Activated α2-macroglobulin, CNTF, LIF, angiotensin II, and meteorin induce GFAP expression in Müller cells through the JAK/STAT3 signal transduction pathway (Peterson et al., 2000; Wang et al., 2002b; Fischer et al., 2004c; Kurihara et al., 2006; Bürgi et al., 2009; Lee et al., 2010; Kirsch et al., 2010; Barcelona et al., 2011; Xue et al., 2011b). TGF-β increases the expression of GFAP in Müller cells via activation of TGF-β receptor II and Smad4 (Hisatomi et al., 2002a). Exogenous BDNF or GDNF reduce the proliferative response of Müller cells, the upregulation of GFAP, and the glial scar formation in the subretinal space after retinal detachment (Lewis et al., 1999a,b; Wu et al., 2002). On the other hand, BDNF does not reduce the expression of GFAP in Müller cells after optic nerve crush (Chen and Weber, 2002). Calcium influx, activation of calpains, and elevated histone acetylation are implicated in the upregulation of glial intermediate filaments (Du et al., 1999; Wang et al., 2012a). Insulin and IGF acting through the IGF receptor-1 reverse the upregulation of GFAP in cultured Müller cells (Layton et al., 2006). The 5′ flanking region of the mouse GFAP gene contains a putative AP-1 binding site and a cAMP responsive element (CRE) (Kaneko et al., 1994), implying a role of the AP-1 complex (c-Fos and c-Jun) and CREB in the expression of the GFAP gene (Sarid, 1991). Activation of ERK2 is involved in the phosphorylation of CREB and induction of c-Fos.

5.11.3.3 Cellular Signaling Mediated by Intermediate Filaments

Vimentin-null mice display a defective wound repair which was attributed to the loss of the vimentin-associated signaling complexes involved in cell motility (Eckes et al., 2000). Downregulation of soluble vimentin and GFAP inhibits Müller cell proliferation and induces a cell cycle arrest at G_0/G_1 (Bargagna-Mohan et al., 2010). On the other hand, upregulation of GFAP is associated with a stimulation of the growth of new neurites from retinal ganglion cells (Toops et al., 2012b). Intermediate filament proteins provide a pathway for the information transfer from the cell periphery to the cell nucleus (Traub, 1985; Paramio and Jorcano, 2002; Chang and Goldman, 2004). In neurons, calpain cleavage products of newly synthesized vimentin interact with ERK1/2 and transport phosphorylated ERK1/2 to the peri-nucleus space along microtubule tracks; this action is implicated in the injury-induced neurite growth (Perlson et al., 2004; Helfand et al., 2005). The formation of phosphorylated ERK1/2-vimentin complexes is favored near the site of injury owing to a high concentration of calcium, and the complexes are dissociated in the region of the cell soma where the calcium level is low (Perlson et al., 2004). Vimentin can also be associated with other signaling molecules including cdc42, Rac1 and PLA_2 (Paramio and Jorcano, 2002). GFAP interacting with S-100 calcium-binding proteins is involved in mediating the injury-induced distribution shift of neurotransmitter transporters (Kim et al., 2003). However, the signal transduction events induced by intermediate filament proteins in Müller cells remain to be elucidated.

5.11.4 NETWORK OF REACTIVE GLIOSIS

Müller cell gliosis is a component of a complex retinal response to pathogenic stimuli which may include a local inflammatory response characterized by activation of microglia (see 3.3.), breakdown of the blood-retinal barrier (see 5.11.9.1.), and immigration of blood-derived leukocytes into the retinal tissue and subretinal space. The infiltration of leukocytes into the retinal parenchyma (which contributes to the NO-mediated death of retinal ganglion cells; Neufeld et al., 2002) must be approved by astrocytes and Müller cells because their processes tightly envelop the vessels. Molecules from inflammatory cells, platelets, and the plasma activate Müller cells, and Müller cells may express a wide variety of inflammation- and immune response-related factors and enzymes (Fig. 12H–J; see 5.11.6.2.). The initiation of (at least, certain steps or forms of) Müller cell gliosis requires an interaction between microglial and Müller cells (Fig. 24; see 5.11.4.). Müller cells play an active role in photoreceptor cell degeneration, e.g., after retinal detachment, by producing cytokines and chemokines such as MCP-1 and the fractalkine receptor CX3CR1 (Chan et al., 2005) that recruit phagocytotic monocytes/macrophages and microglia to the site of injury; monocytes/macrophages and microglia release oxygen free radicals and toxic cytokines that induce photoreceptor apoptosis (Cuthbertson et al., 1990; Nakazawa et al., 2006b, 2007a). A similar recruitment of blood-derived macrophages into the retinal tissue was observed after experimental blue light injury of the retina (Fig. 21A) (Iandiev et al., 2008a). On the other hand, the early expression of antioxidants such as heme oxygenase by Müller cells after injury decreases the infiltration of macrophages into the retinal tissue, resulting in reduced tissue damage and enhanced Müller cell survival (Arai-Gaun et al., 2004). Activated microglia, in part via a release of NGF, BDNF, and CNTF (see 3.6.), may induce upregulation of neuroprotective factors like bFGF, GDNF, and LIF in Müller cells (see 5.11.7.); this signaling is part of a microglia-Müller cell-photoreceptor network that serves to increase the survival of photoreceptor cells (Harada et al., 2002a; Wang et al., 2011).

5.11.5 MÜLLER CELL-MEDIATED SPREAD OF RETINAL DEGENERATION—RETINAL DETACHMENT

Retinal detachment is a major cause of vision loss. The neural retina may become separated from the pigment epithelium during trauma or incomplete posterior vitreous detachment (traction retinal detachment), inflammatory eye diseases (exudative detachment), in the presence of retinal holes and tears (rhegmatogenous detachment), neovascular or age-related macular degeneration, and high myopia. After surgical retinal reattachment in cases of local detachment, functional defects have also been localized to such areas of the visual field which correspond to retinal regions which had not been detached (Chisholm et al., 1975; Nork et al., 1995; Sasoh et al., 1997). These observations in human subjects suggest that, in addition the detached retinal areas, the surrounding non-detached retina also degenerates.

The cause for this spread of degeneration from detached into attached retinal areas, which may impair the recovery of visual acuity after reattachment surgery, is unclear. It has been suggested that the retinal degeneration in the non-detached retina is, at least in part, caused by Müller cell gliosis (Francke et al., 2005). Disturbed homeostasis mechanisms normally maintained by Müller cells may underlie the degeneration of both the detached and attached retinal areas. In animal models of local retinal detachment, a spread of gliosis into non-detached retinal areas was observed which was associated with a spread of retinal degeneration (Fig. 54A,B) (Faude et al., 2001; Francke et al., 2005; Iandiev et al., 2006b; Wurm et al., 2006a). The spread of gliosis involves both microglia (Figs. 10C, 12D,E) and Müller cell activation (Fig. 12A) and is a time-dependent process (Fig. 12K) (Francke et al., 2001a; Iandiev et al., 2006b; Wurm et al., 2006a). The Müller cell responses observed in the peri-detached retina include upregulation of vimentin and GFAP (Fig. 12A), cellular hypertrophy (Fig. 12C), alteration in the localization of the Kir4.1 protein (Fig. 12A), decrease of Kir currents (Fig. 12K,L), plasma membrane depolarization (Fig. 12K), cellular swelling under hypoosmotic conditions (Fig. 12M,N), increase of ATP-induced calcium responses (Fig. 12F,G), and upregulation of the expression of inflammation- and immune response-related genes such as MCP-1 (Iandiev et al., 2006b; Wurm et al., 2006a; Hollborn et al., 2008). A similar spread of microglia activation and Müller cell gliosis was found following focal light damage and laser photocoagulation lesions (Burns and Robles, 1990; Humphrey et al., 1993; Humphrey and Moore, 1996). The uniform alteration of various parameters of gliosis in dependence on the distance from the local detachment (Fig. 12C,E) may suggest a continuous spread of degeneration from the detached to the surrounding non-detached tissue. However, in a rabbit model of focal retinal detachment, a "patchy" pattern of degeneration in the attached retinal areas surrounding the focal detachment was observed (Fig. 54B) (Faude et al., 2001); this may rather disclose a continuous spread of degeneration from the detached to the non-detached tissue.

Retinal detachment causes initial damage to the photoreceptor outer segments (Fig. 53D), resulting in photoreceptor deconstruction and apoptotic death of photoreceptor cells (Machemer, 1968; Erickson et al., 1983; Anderson et al., 1983; Chang et al., 1995; Cook et al., 1995; Hisatomi et al., 2002b; Fisher and Lewis, 2003; Zacks et al., 2003; Fisher et al., 2005). Distinct structural and biochemical rearrangements in various retinal layers such as synaptic remodeling, anomalous sprouting of neurites into ectopic sites, degeneration of inner retinal neurons, and the presence of edema in the inner retinal tissue may contribute to the persistent reduction of visual acuity (Lewis et al., 1998; Faude et al., 2001; Fisher and Lewis, 2003). Müller cells are rapidly activated after experimental retinal detachment. Within minutes of detachment, they show increased protein phosphorylation, for example, of the FGF receptor-1 and of ERK1/2, as well as increased production of transcription factors (Geller et al., 2001). The immediate phoshorylation of the FGF receptor-1 in experimentally detached retinas (Geller et al., 2001) suggests that bFGF, possibly released from cones (Lewis et al., 1992) or Müller cells (Fig. 42E,F) (Lindqvist et al., 2010), is one of the major signaling molecules which initiates Müller cell activation and proliferation. Müller cell gliosis might be also caused (directly or indirectly) by the detachment-induced hypoxia, because Müller cell proliferation and hypertrophy were shown to be reduced by oxygen supplementation (Lewis et al., 1999a). The decrease of the Kir currents (Figs. 7D,E, 12K,L, 46A) and the increase of the purinergic calcium responsivenss (Fig. 63C) of Müller cells are intiated within 3 h of detachment (Fig. 63B) (Francke et al., 2001a; Uckermann et al., 2003; Uhlmann et al., 2003; Iandiev et al., 2006b). Within one day of detachment, Müller cells begin to proliferate and increase their expression of vimentin and GFAP (Figs. 11A, 12A, 20A, 53A) (Fisher et al., 1991; Lewis et al., 1994, 1995; Jackson et al., 2003). Also, within one day of detachment, Müller cells (in addition to other retinal cells) upregulate the expression of inflammation- and immune response-related genes such as MCP-1, TNFα, and IL-1β, as well as antioxidants such as metallothioneins and lysozyme, and blood coagulation-related proteins such as tissue factor (Nakazawa et al., 2006b; Hollborn et al., 2008). The detachment-induced proliferation of Müller cells is transient and peaks at 3–4 days of detachment (Erickson et al., 1990; Fisher et al., 1991; Fisher and Lewis, 2003). At this time point, Müller cell hypertrophy (Fig. 12C) and increased expression of bFGF (Fig. 33B) are obvious (Geller et al., 2001). The hypertrophied Müller cell processes fill the spaces left by dying photoreceptors and grow into the subretinal space (Fig. 53C) (Fisher et al., 1991; Lewis and Fisher, 2000; Iandiev et al., 2006b; Cebulla et al., 2012). The nuclei of many Müller cells migrate to the outer retina, undergo mitosis, and reside in subretinal glial scars (Lewis et al., 2010; Cebulla et al., 2012). (A similar interkinetic nuclear migration of Müller cells was found after retinal ischemia-reperfusion and during inherited photoreceptor degeneration [Kim et al., 1998a; Phillips et al., 2010]; in cases of retinal ganglion cell axon degeneration and PVR, the nuclei of Müller cells are displaced to the nerve fiber layer [Ramírez et al., 2006; see 5.11.11.3.].) The development of a subretinal fibrosis by outgrowing Müller cell processes (Fig. 53C) inhibits the regeneration of outer photoreceptor segments after successful reattachment (Anderson et al., 1986). Hypertrophied side branches of Müller cells which grow into the plexiform layers (Fig. 53B) inhibit the reformation of synaptic contacts which are disconnected (Erickson et al., 1983). The expression of Müller cell proteins which are involved in homeostatic functions of Müller cells and in glio-neuronal interactions such as glutamine synthetase, CRALBP, and carbonic anhydrase are downregulated in detached retinas (Marc et al., 1998b; Lewis et al., 1999a; Fisher and Lewis, 2003).

Photoreceptor cells begin to degenerate during the first day of experimental detachment (Fig. 54A), with a maximum degeneration occuring around three days, and it continues to some extent as long as the retina remains detached (Hisatomi et al., 2001, 2002b; Rex et al., 2002). The photoreceptor cell loss is a major cause of an irreversible vision loss even after reattachment (Isernhagen and Wilkinson, 1988; Nork et al., 1995), because of the failure to regenerate. The vulnerability of photoreceptor cells has been explained mainly by hypoxia and nutrient deprivation caused by detachment which leads to an increased distance between the choriocapillaris and the neural retina (Mervin et al., 1999; Linsenmeier and Padnick-Silver, 2000). Photoreceptor cell degeneration can be also observed (with smaller incidence and after longer time periods) in the surrounding non-detached retinal tissue (Fig. 54A,B) (Faude et al., 2001). However, there is an apparent difference in the mode of photoreceptor cell death between detached and peri-detached tissues. In the detached retina, photoreceptor cells degenerate from outside to inside. Detachment disrupts the contact between the outer segments and the pigment epithelium which results in collapse and disappearance of the outer segments within hours and days of detachment whereas the inner segments and cell bodies degenerate considerably later or may survive for longer time periods (Fig. 54A) (Foulds, 1963; Kroll and Machemer, 1969; Erickson et al., 1983; Faude et al., 2001). In the attached tissue surrounding the focal detachment, there are groups of adjacent photoreceptor cells which are in the process of degeneration (Fig. 54B) (Faude et al., 2001). These cells die from inside to outside; they show swollen cell bodies with disorganized chromatin and swollen mitochondria within the inner segments, while the outer segments, as well as the connection between inner and outer segments, appeared relatively well preserved (Fig. 54B) (Faude et al., 2001). This atypical or inversed degeneration patterns, which has been found in both rods and cones, suggests that in the non-detached tissue, the support of the photoreceptor cells by the neural retina, likely by Müller cells, is disturbed, and that the photoreceptor degeneration is most probably not caused by a functional disturbance of retinal pigment epithelial cells or by a disruption of the oxygen and nutrient supply from the choroid (Francke et al., 2005). The photoreceptor degeneration in the detached retina is known to occur primarily by apoptosis (Chang et al., 1995; Cook et al., 1995), and it was shown that there is a certain level of caspase activation also in the attached tissue surrounding a focal detachment, albeit at lower level (Zacks et al., 2003).

MCP-1 is rapidly upregulated in Müller cells after detachment (Nakazawa et al., 2006b) both in the detached and peri-detached retina (Hollborn et al., 2008). It has been suggested that the production of this chemokine by Müller cells plays a critical role in photoreceptor degeneration after retinal detachment. MCP-1 promotes photoreceptor apoptosis (Nakazawa et al., 2006b), probably due to its capability to recruit phagocytotic monocytes/macrophages and microglial cells to the injured area that release oxygen free radicals and cytotoxic cytokines (Cuthbertson et al., 1990;

Nakazawa et al., 2007a; see 3.3. and 3.5.). Mice deficient for the intermediate filaments GFAP and vimentin display an attenuation of the detachment-induced reactive responses of retinal glial cells (activation of ERK1/2 and c-Fos, induction of MCP-1) and, as a consequence, a decrease of monocyte infiltration and photoreceptor apoptosis (Nakazawa et al., 2007b). There are further mediators of immune responses which are implicated in the regulation of inflammation and photoreceptor apoptosis (Lohr et al., 2006), and which are rapidly upregulated in Müller cells after detachment, for example, lysozyme (Hollborn et al., 2008).

After retinal detachment, the inner retinal tissue shows distinct disorganization such as degeneration of single ganglion cells and anomalous sprouting of enlarged lateral branches from the hypertrophied Müller cell bodies into the plexiform layers (Fig. 53B) (Francke et al., 2001a,b; Fisher and Lewis, 2003). The detachment-induced degeneration and disorganization of the inner retina was suggested to be mediated, at least in part, by the impaired glial glutamate recycling resulting from the reduced glutamine synthetase activity (see 5.5.2.1.12.) which, together with an increase in extracellular potassium, will aggravate neurotoxicity. Excitotoxicity is one factor underlying the morphologic and biochemical alterations in the inner retina after detachment (Marc et al., 1998b; Fisher and Lewis, 2003). A decreased uptake of potassium by Müller cells in the outer retina may cause hyperexcitation and calcium overload of photoreceptor cells, resulting in apoptosis. In addition, detached retinas are characterized by an edematous cystoid degeneration, reflecting extracellular edema (Figs. 20A–C, 54A) (Arruga, 1936; Faude et al., 2001; Francke et al., 2005). The localization of the cystoid spaces depends on the vascularization of the retina. In the vascularized human and porcine retinas, the cysts develop predominantly in the outer plexiform and inner nuclear layers (Fig. 20A–C) (Arruga, 1936; Hagimura et al., 2000; Francke et al., 2005). A similar localization of cystoid spaces was observed in the ischemic rat retina (Fig. 19) (Rehak et al., 2009). In the avascular rabbit retina, edematous cysts are present in the nerve fiber and ganglion cell layers (Fig. 54A) (Faude et al., 2001). Intra- and extracellular edema in the inner retinal layers (e.g., of the Müller cell endfeet abutting the inner limiting membrane) have been described to be an early alteration (within one day) of the experimentally detached pig retina; the intracellular edema is associated with mitochondrial swelling (Jackson et al., 2003). Similarly, experimental detachment of the primate retina causes edematous swelling and cystoid degeneration of the inner retinal layers (Machemer, 1968; Machemer and Norton, 1969). It has been suggested that the cystoid degeneration reflects extracellular edema (Francke et al., 2005). The morphological deformation of ganglion cells which surround the cysts (Faude et al., 2001) suggests that the death of single ganglion cells is, at least in part, caused by mechanical injury due to the cysts.

The presence of edematous cysts is not restricted to the detached retina but is also observed in the surrounding attached tissue, several millimeters distant from the detachment (Fig. 54A) (Faude et al., 2001). The cysts in the non-detached inner retina are colocalized with groups of atypically dying photoreceptor cells (Fig. 54A); retinal portions without cysts also do not contain degenerating photoreceptors (Faude et al., 2001). The colocalization may suggest that both phenomenons are causally related. In addition to extracellular edema, there are also single Müller cells or small groups of Müller cells in the detached and neighboring non-detached tissues which show signs of degeneration, apparently due to intracellular edema (Fig. 54B) (Faude et al., 2001). The bodies, nuclei, and mitochondria of the cells are swollen, and photoreceptor cell somata enveloped by the cells are in the process of degeneration (Fig. 54B) (Faude et al., 2001). The degeneration of swollen Müller cells is associated with a disruption of the inner limiting membrane (Fig. 54B) (Faude et al., 2001), an early event in the pathogenesis of PVR (see 5.11.11.3.).

After retinal detachment, Müller cells show an early downregulation of functional Kir channels (Figs. 7D, 12K,L, 46A, 63B) (Francke et al., 2001a; Uhlmann et al., 2003; Iandiev et al., 2006b; see 5.5.3.5.). In addition to Müller cells of the detached areas, also cells in the surrounding non-detached retina display a downregulation of functional Kir channels, albeit during a longer time period (Fig. 12K,L) (Francke et al., 2001a; Uhlmann et al., 2003; Iandiev et al., 2006b). Another characteristic feature of gliotic Müller cells in the detached retina is the increase of their intracellular calcium responsiveness to stimulation of purinergic P2Y receptors (Fig. 12F,G, 63B, C) (Francke et al., 2002, 2003; Uckermann et al., 2003; Uhlmann et al., 2003; Iandiev et al., 2006b; see 5.10.2.5.). The increase of the calcium responsiveness is not restricted to the detached retina but is also observed in the non-detached tissue (Fig. 12G) (Iandiev et al., 2006b). Because P2Y receptor activation stimulates the proliferation of Müller cells (see 5.11.10.3.), it was suggested that, in addition to the alteration of the Kir currents (see 5.11.10.2.), the enhanced responsiveness to ATP may contribute to the proliferation of Müller cells in the detached retina (Bringmann et al., 2003a). A relation between the increased P2Y receptor responsiveness and the downregulation of functional Kir channels has been suggested based upon the observations that cells in detached retinas which respond to ATP display significantly smaller Kir currents (Uhlmann et al., 2003; a phenomenon also observed in an animal model of early PVR; Fig. 63H), and that Müller cells of $P2Y_1$ receptor-deficient mice display a weaker decrease of Kir currents upon transient retinal ischemia than wildtype mice (Pannicke et al., 2014). Inhibitory effects of suramin on the downregulation of the Kir conductance and the cell hypertrophy (Uhlmann et al., 2003) may be explained by the inhibitory action of this agent on P2Y and growth factor receptor signalings.

Müller cell gliosis may contribute to the atypical or inversed photoreceptor cell degeneration and the cyst formation in the attached tissue surrounding a focal detachment (Francke et al., 2005). Because the contact between the pigment epithelium and the photoreceptors is not disturbed in the attached tissue (which is reflected by the well-preserved outer segments; Fig. 54A), the atypical photoreceptor cell degeneration is likely not mediated by deprivation of oxygen and nutrient supply from the choroid (as it has been suggested to be the cause for the photoreceptor cell degeneration in the detached tissue; Lewis et al., 2004). A spread of damage caused by hyperoxia from the detached into the attached tissue (Stone et al., 1999) is also unlikely because the photoreceptor cell degeneration in the attached tissue is a "patchy" and not a continuous phenomenon; there are groups of dying photoreceptor cells which are surrounded by retinal tissue without any sign of degeneration (Fig. 54A, B). The inversed mode of photoreceptor cell degeneration in the attached tissue (from inside to outside; Fig. 54A) suggest that the support of the photoreceptor cells by the neural retina, i.e., by Müller cells, is disturbed (Francke et al., 2005). The downregulation of glial Kir channels indicates that the glial homeostasis mechanisms are disturbed not only in the detached but also in the non-detached retina (Fig. 12K,L) (Francke et al., 2001a; Uhlmann et al., 2003; Iandiev et al., 2006b). A decreased uptake of neuronally released potassium and glutamate by Müller cells in the outer retina may cause overexcitation and intracellular calcium overload of photoreceptor cells resulting in apoptosis which is associated with an alteration of the chromatin morphology, cellular swelling, and swelling of mitochondria in the inner segments (Fig. 54A,B). On the other hand, the outer segments are preserved due to the unaltered contact to the pigment epithelial cells (Fig. 54A).

The atypical photoreceptor cell degeneration in the attached retinal tissue surrounding a focal detachment is associated with the presence of edematous cysts in the inner retina (Fig. 54A) (Faude et al., 2001; Francke et al., 2005). The downregulation of functional Kir4.1 channels in Müller cells (Fig. 11B) should disturb the retinal potassium clearance and the resolution of osmotic gradients between the fluid-filled extra-retinal spaces and the retinal parenchyma, resulting in extracellular and Müller cell edema (see 5.11.9.1.2. and 5.11.9.2.3.). In vascularized retinas, Kir4.1 channels and the highest membrane potassium conductance are localized in Müller cell membrane domains which envelop the blood vessels in the inner nuclear layer and in endfeet membranes which abut the vitreous body (Fig. 7B,E,G,H, 15A,B,D; see 5.5.3.3.). In contrast, Müller cells of non-vascularized retinas, e.g., of guinea pigs and rabbits, display the highest potassium conductance in the endfeet membranes (Fig. 7C,D), and the cells release excess potassium predominantly into the vitreous (see 5.5.3.3.). There is an apparent spatial relation between the potassium secretion sites of Müller cells and the locations of edematous cysts in vascularized and non-vascularized retinas. In vascularized retinas, the edematous cysts are mainly located in the inner nuclear and outer plexiform layers (Figs. 19, 20A–C) (Rehak et al., 2009) where the vessels of the deepest vascular plexus are located (see 2.1.). In non-vascularized retinas, the edematous cysts are localized in the nerve fiber/ganglion cell layers (Figs. 54A) (Faude et al., 2001). (However, human and porcine Müller cells display their largest potassium conductance in endfeet membranes [Fig. 7E] while edematous cysts are predominantly localized to the inner nuclear and outer plexiform layers [Fig. 20A–C].) When the release of excess potassium is disturbed, potassium accumulates within Müller cells and in the retinal interstitium. The accumulation of potassium causes a high osmotic pressure of the retinal tissue (see 5.11.9.1.2.). The only borders to extra-retinal spaces which display stable low potassium levels (and relatively low osmotic pressure) are the Müller cell membrane domains contacting the vessels and the vitreous. The strong osmotic gradient across these borders pulls water into Müller cells (and subsequently, into the retinal interstitium) at these sites. It was suggested that the downregulation of functional Kir channels in Müller cells causes or contributes to both the cyst formation in the inner retina and the photoreceptor cell degeneration in the outer retina; water accumulates in the retinal tissue where excess potassium is normally extruded into extra-retinal spaces, and the disruption of the potassium clearance currents may strongly and long-lasting depolarize the photoreceptor cells which results in intracellular calcium overload and apoptosis (Fig. 40D) (Francke et al., 2005). The potassium accumulation due to the downregulation of Müller cell's Kir4.1 channels may be more extracellularly or intracellularly; in the first case, cysts develop in the retinal tissue (Fig. 20A–C); in the second case, Müller cells swell (Fig. 12M,N) and die (Fig. 54B) (Francke et al., 2005). The downregulation of functional Kir4.1 channels may also cause the degeneration of the inner retina, e.g., the apoptotic death of retinal ganglion cells and the decrease in the thickness of the inner plexiform layer (Thanos et al., 2001; Iandiev et al., 2008a), after retinal light injury which initially induces a degeneration of the outer retina (Fig. 71)

The spread of retinal gliosis from the detached into the surrounding non-detached tissue might be mediated by the diffusion of soluble factors including extracellular ATP (see 5.6.3.1.), growth factors such as bFGF (see 5.11.7.7.), inflammatory and immune mediators (see 5.11.6.2.), as well as by migrating activated microglia (Figs. 10C; 12D,E; see 3.3.). Retinal detachment is associated with mechanical stress of the tissue; mechanical deformation of glial cell membranes is an important stimulus which induces a glial release of ATP (see 5.6.3.1.), glial calcium waves (see 5.6.3.3.), and an induction of bFGF in the cells (Fig. 42E,F; see 5.5.1.4.). The bidirectional stimulation loop between ATP and growth factors in Müller cells (with enhanced growth factor release upon stimulation by ATP, and an increased sensitivity of P2Y receptors induced by growth factors; see 5.10.2.5. and 5.11.10.3.) may exacerbate the intraretinal release of soluble factors which diffuse from the detached into attached portions of the retina, and which may induce gliosis in some Müller cells far distant from the local detachment (Fig. 54C) (Francke et al., 2005).

Attached retinal areas display a "patchy" pattern of photoreceptor degeneration, edematous cysts, and edematous Müller cells which are surrounded by apparently normal Müller cells (Fig. 54A,B) (Faude et al., 2001). It was described that the decrease of the Kir currents of Müller cells after detachment is highly variable; there are cells with a strong decrease and cells with small or no alteration (Fig. 46A) (Francke et al., 2001a; Uhlmann et al., 2003; Iandiev et al., 2006b). A similar heterogeneity was observed in cells from attached retinal areas distant from detachment (Uhlmann et al., 2003; Iandiev et al., 2006b) and in other retinal diseases associated with a decrease of the Kir currents in Müller cells (Fig. 15C) (Pannicke et al., 2006). One may assume that groups of degenerating photoreceptor cell nuclei are enveloped by single Müller cells or small groups of Müller cells which show a relatively strong downregulation of the Kir conductance (Fig. 54C). Thus, both phenomenons of retinal degeneration in the attached tissue surrounding a focal detachment (cysts in the inner layers and atypical photoreceptor cell death in the outer layers) may be caused by single (or small groups of) Müller cells which display strong features of gliosis. The cause why Müller cells may display stronger or smaller signs of gliosis is unclear. It was suggested that different expression levels of functional P2Y receptors may be involved in determination of the severity of gliosis (Francke et al., 2005). The expression level of functional P2Y receptors is inversely related to the Kir current amplitude (Fig. 63B,H; see 5.10.2.5.), suggesting that the receptor expression level varies with the severity of gliosis in individual Müller cells. Interestingly, it has been reported that glial calcium responses in the murine retina (which are mediated by P2Y receptor signaling; see 5.6.3.3.) occur simultaneously in small groups of Müller cells which contain 2–6 cells (Agulhon et al., 2007). The heterogeneity of P2Y receptor expression (which may be also the case in regard to other types of receptors, e.g., of growth factors) may underlie the "patchy" pattern of Müller cell gliosis and degeneration in attached retinal areas. Small groups of gliotic or degenerating Müller cells may be formed when one strongly gliotic cell induces gliotic alterations in the neighboring cells (Fig. 54C) (Francke et al., 2005).

5.11.6 IMMUNOMODULATORY ROLE OF MÜLLER CELLS

Müller cells play an active role in retinal immune and inflammatory responses. Although essential for innate immunity against pathogens, inflammation is also a cause of unspecific tissue destruction. The retina is an immune-privileged tissue and thus is extremely sensitive to inflammatory damage (Kumar et al., 2013a; see 3.). Müller cells respond to pathogens and inflammatory factors released from infiltrating blood-borne immune cells and activated microglia, act as immunocompetent cells, and are a source of inflammatory factors (Caspi and Roberge, 1989; Roberge et al., 1991; Drescher and Whittum-Hudson, 1996a,b). Müller cells express various different receptors of inflammatory cytokines including gp130, the common signal transducer of the IL-6 family of cytokines (Echevarria et al., 2013), and other receptors implicated in the regulation of the innate immunity, for example, programmed cell death-1 (PD-1) (Sham et al., 2012). PD-1 recognizes PD ligands released, for example, by macrophages and dendritic cells upon stimulation with lipopolysaccharide and GM-CSF.

5.11.6.1 Antigen Presentation

Under normal conditions, microglial cells but not Müller cells express MHC class I and II molecules (Zhang et al., 1997; but see 3.3.2.). However, Müller cells (in addition to neurons) express the immunoproteasome that generates peptides for MHC class I occupancy (Ferrington et al., 2008). Oxidative stress, increased intraocular pressure, inflammatory mediators such as IFN-γ, retinal laser photocoagulation, or contact to activated lymphocytes cause an upregulation of MHC class II molecules in Müller cells (Kim et al., 1987; Roberge et al., 1988; Richardson et al., 1996; Drescher and Whittum-Hudson, 1996a; Tezel et al., 2007b; Gallego et al., 2012). *In vitro*, Müller cells act as immune suppressor cells which inhibit antigen presentation. Müller cells suppress the antigen- and IL-2-driven proliferation of T-helper lymphocytes, through a cell-cell-contact-dependent mechanism (Caspi and Roberge, 1989; Roberge et al., 1991). Inhibition of T-cell proliferation by Müller cells restricts the severity of autoimmune uveoretinitis (Chan et al., 1991). However, when the immune suppressive action of Müller cells is inhibited, they display the capacity to efficiently function as antigen-presenting cells for T-helper cells, via processing of antigens to immunogenic forms and the presentation of the processed antigens on MHC class II molecules (Roberge et al., 1988). Antigen presentation by retinal glial cells was suggested to be a cause for the activation of the immune system in glaucoma, for example (Tezel et al., 2007b).

5.11.6.2 Müller Cell-Derived Inflammatory and Immune Response-Related Factors

Hypoxia induces expression of inflammatory factors and enzymes like IL-1β, TNFα, and cyclooxygenase-2 in Müller cells (Fig. 12H–J) (Hangai et al., 1995; Li et al., 2012). In diabetic retinopathy, Müller cell gliosis is triggered by IL-1β produced by vascular endothelial cells (Liu et al., 2012a). After breakdown of the blood-retina barrier, Müller cell gliosis can be triggered by extravasated immunoglobulin G (Fig. 21C) (Chu et al., 1999) acting at their Fcγ receptors (Tripathi et al., 1991) and by blood-derived immune cells such as IFN-γ-producing T-lymphocytes. IFN-γ facilitates the immunogenic function of Müller cells. It induces the expression of MHC class I and II molecules (Mano et al., 1991) and ICAM-1 (Elner et al., 1992; Drescher and Whittum-Hudson, 1996a) which regulates a number of leukocyte functions including diapedesis and migration. Expression of ICAM-1 in Müller cells is also induced during the wound healing response after retinal laser photocoagulation and upon stimulation with IL-1β; the expression of ICAM-1 around infiltrated cells may regulate the migration of macrophages and activated T cells (Elner et al., 1992; Richardson et al., 1996). In addition, IFN-γ induces the expression of NO synthases in Müller cells (Goureau et al., 1994). Hypoxia and hyperglycemia stimulates the expression of glutaredoxin in Müller cells; glutaredoxin catalyzes the deglutathionylation of the IκB kinase resulting in translocation of NF-κB into the Müller cell nuclei where it induces the expression of proinflammatory factors such as ICAM-1 and IL-6 (Shelton et al., 2007, 2009).

TLRs recognize microbial and endogenous molecular patterns that function as danger signals. Human Müller cells express TLRs 1-10 (Kumar and Shamsuddin, 2012), while murine Müller cells express TLRs 2-5 (Lin et al., 2013b). After stimulation with TLR agonists and in response to retinal detachment and ocular infections, Müller cells increase the expression of TLRs (Hollborn et al., 2008; Shamsuddin and Kumar, 2011; Kumar and Shamsuddin, 2012). Via activation of TLR2, Gram-positive bacteria induce activation of the NF-κB, ERK1/2, and p38 MAPK signaling pathways, and the transcriptional expression and secretion of proinflammatory cytokines (TNFα, IL-1β, IL-6, IL-8, MIP-2), chemokines (IL-8), and antimicrobial peptides (LL-37) from Müller cells (Shamsuddin and Kumar, 2011; Kumar and Shamsuddin, 2012; Lin et al., 2013b). Infection of Müller cells with Gram-negative bacteria or fungal pathogens also stimulate the secretion of TNFα and IL-6 from Müller cells (Kumar et al., 2013a). Bacterial-challenged Müller cells produce neurotrophins (Kumar et al., 2013a) which increase the survival of retinal neurons in the presence of infectious agents (see 5.11.7.). Müller cells also regulate the innate immune response through NOD-like receptors which up- and downregulate inflammatory responses (Kumar et al., 2013a).

Lipopolysaccharide induces the expression of the inducible NO synthase in Müller cells via activation of the TLR4-apoptosis signal-regulating kinase 1 pathway (Semba et al., 2014a). In response to virus exposure, inflammatory stimulants such as IL-1β, and AGEs, and after downregulation of PEDF, Müller cells express and secrete IFN-α, -β, and -γ, and the proinflammatory cytokines IL-1β, IL-6, and TNFα (De Kozak et al., 1994; Drescher and Whittum-Hudson, 1996a, b, 1997; Cotinet et al., 1997b; Tezel and Wax, 2000; Vinores et al., 2001; Yoshida et al., 2001; Nakamura et al., 2003; Nakatani et al., 2006; Seki et al., 2006; Zhang et al., 2006c; Hauck et al., 2007; Liu et al., 2012a). TNFα has both neuroprotective (Diem et al., 2001) and cytotoxic effects, and was suggested to mediate the retinal ganglion cell death (Tezel and Wax, 2000), uveoretinitis, and inherited photoreceptor degeneration (De Kozak et al., 1994, 1997). IL-6 was shown to protect retinal ganglion cells and photoreceptors from cell death (Mendonca Torres and de Araujo, 2001; Sanchez et al., 2003; Inomata et al., 2003; Chong et al., 2008). Under pathological conditions and in response to TNFα, Müller cells are a source of IL-8 and express IL-8 receptors (Yoshida et al. 2004a; Goczalik et al., 2005, 2008). IL-8 induces cytosolic calcium responses in Müller cells (Goczalik et al., 2005, 2008). IL-8 is a proinflammatory chemokine involved in the recruitment of neutrophils to sites of inflammation. Müller cell-derived IL-8 may participate in the development of retinal inflammation, and activation of IL-8 receptors may induce gliotic responses such as cellular dedifferentiation, proliferation, and migration.

Other factors that regulate retinal tissue inflammation and local immunity are macrophage migration inhibitory factor (which is constitutively expressed by astrocytes and Müller cells; Matsuda et al., 1997), IL-1 (which is produced by Müller cells; Roberge et al., 1988), MCP-1 (which is induced in Müller cells by TNFα and after retinal detavchment; Yoshida et al. 2004a; Hollborn et al., 2008), other components of the chemokine system such as Xcr1 and Cxcl16 (Roesch et al., 2008), as well as lysozyme and allograft inflammatory factor-1 (Hollborn et al., 2008). Müller cells and astrocytes express the receptors for the complement factors C3a and C5a, and the complement-regulatory proteins CD55 and CD59 (Vogt et al., 2006; Cheng et al., 2013). PGE_2 and hyperglycemia increase the expression of the C5a receptor (Cheng et al., 2013). Activation of the C5a receptor induces production of IL-6 and VEGF in Müller cells (Cheng et al., 2013). In glaucomatous eyes, Müller cells increase the expression of the complement component 1q (C1q) before the extensive death of retinal ganglion cells, suggesting that Müller cell-derived complement may play a role in the pathogenesis of glaucoma (Stasi et al., 2006).

Müller cell-derived inflammatory factors are also involved in the breakdown of the blood-retinal barrier (see 5.11.9.1.1.) and the pathogenesis of proliferative retinopathies (see 5.11.11.). In the normal retina, cyclooxygenases 1 and 2 are expressed in microglia, astrocytes, distinct amacrine cells, and retinal ganglion cells, and in the outer plexiform layer (Fig. 12H, J) (Ju and Neufeld, 2002). Following ischemia and hypoxia, Müller cells also express cyclooxygenase-2 (Fig. 12H–J); inhibition of this enzyme reduces the retinal infiltration of hematogenous cells (Ju et al., 2003; Li et al., 2012). The vitreal level of IL-6 was proposed to be a predictive risk factor for the development of postoperative PVR (Kon et al., 1999; Limb et al., 1991). Infiltrating cells, retinal glial cells, and pigment epithelial cells are possible sources of IL-6, IL-1ß, TNFα, and IFN-γ in the vitreous of patients with PVR (Roberge et al., 1988; Benson et al., 1992; De Kozak et al., 1994; Drescher and Whittum-Hudson, 1996a, b; Cotinet et al., 1997b; El-Ghrably et al., 2001; Sappington et al., 2006; Li et al., 2012).

The devastating effects of long-term retinal inflammation may be restricted by antiinflammatory factors. Endocannabinoids inhibit the production of proinflammatory cytokines and increase the production of antiinflammatory mediators in activated but not resting Müller cells by activation of various intracellular signaling pathways (Krishnan and Chatterjee, 2012).

5.11.7 MÜLLER CELL-DERIVED NEUROPROTECTIVE FACTORS

Under pathological conditions, Müller cells are capable to protect photoreceptors and retinal neurons from cell death through various mechanisms including buffering of elevated potassium levels (see 5.5.3.), uptake of excess glutamate (see 5.5.2.1.), and the release of antioxidants (see 5.5.2.1.15.).

Another mechanism is the secretion of neurotrophic factors, growth factors, and cytokines. Various neurotrophic and growth factors, or combinations of the factors, are known to promote the survival of photoreceptors and inner retinal neurons (Sievers et al., 1987; LaVail et al., 1992). Receptors for BDNF, neurotrophin-3, GDNF, neurturin, CNTF, PEDF, HGF, and FGFs have been localized to photoreceptors and/or inner retinal neurons (Plouët et al., 1988; Mascarelli et al., 1989; Raymond et al., 1992; Jelsma et al., 1993; Meyer-Franke et al., 1995; Matsushima et al., 1997; Cellerino and Kohler, 1997; Fontaine et al., 1998; Suzuki et al., 1998; Fuhrmann et al., 1999; Nag and Wadhwa, 1999; Pease et al., 2000; Di Polo et al., 2000; Harada et al., 2000, 2002b, 2003; Kinkl et al., 2002; Valter et al., 2003, 2005; Delyfer et al., 2005b; Miotke et al., 2007; Agarwal et al., 2007; Blanco et al., 2008; Hu et al., 2010b; Ren et al., 2012; Shen et al., 2012a,b; Rhee et al., 2013; Wong et al., 2014). Likewise, photoreceptor protection in response to LIF can be directly mediated by activation of STAT3 in photoreceptors (Ueki et al., 2008). It has been shown that the simultaneous action of various trophic factors is required to effectively promote the survival of photoreceptors (Ogilvie et al., 2000). Rod photoreceptors are capable to synthesize FGFs (Li et al., 1997b; Noji et al., 1990). Systemic administration of α_2-adrenergic agonists, retinal vein occlusion or retinal laser photocoagulation in rats elicits gene expression of bFGF in the inner photoreceptor segments (Wen et al., 1996; Matsushima et al., 1997; Xiao et al., 1998). Thus, the survival of photoreceptors and inner retinal neurons mediated by growth and neurotrophic factors is, at least in part, mediated by a direct autocrine effect of the factors.

However, part of the neurotrophic rescue of photoreceptor and neuronal cells is proposed to be indirect, mediated by interaction of neurotrophic factors with Müller cells that in turn release factors (in particular bFGF) that act directly on photoreceptors and retinal neurons (Wen et al., 1995; Wexler et al., 1998; Wahlin et al., 2000, 2001; Zack, 2000; Harada et al., 2000, 2002a; Garcia and Vecino, 2003; Yi et al., 2007; Fischer et al., 2009a; Saito et al., 2009; Seitz et al., 2010; Xia et al., 2011; Rhee et al., 2013; Wong et al., 2014; Semba et al., 2014b). Müller cells are also implicated in the regeneration of the injured retinal pigment epithelium by the release of neurotrophins (Machalińska et al., 2013). Under different *in vivo* and *in vitro* conditions, Müller cells produce various neuroprotective factors including bFGF, NGF, BDNF, neurotrophins-3 and -4, CNTF, IGF-1, GDNF, osteopontin, LIF, HGF, and PEDF (Chakrabarti et al., 1990; Gao and Hollyfield, 1992; Dicou et al., 1994; Cao et al., 1997a,b; Neophytou et al., 1997; Harada et al., 2000; Walsh et al., 2001; Taylor et al., 2003; Garcia et al., 2003; Eichler et al., 2004b; Hollborn et al., 2004b; Seki et al., 2005; Morimoto et al., 2005; Avwenagha et al., 2006; Zhang et al., 2006b; Wilson et al., 2007; Joly et al., 2007; Ghazi-Nouri et al., 2008; Douglas et al., 2009; Zhou et al., 2012; Yang et al., 2012; Unterlauft et al., 2012; Wahl et al., 2013; Machalińska et al., 2013; Garcia et al., 2014).

Generally, neurotrophins (NGF, BDNF, neurotrophins-3 and -4/5) control the neuronal survival via two types of receptors: the Trk family of high-affinity tyrosine kinase receptors transmit primarily prosurvival signals while the low-affinity $p75^{NTR}$ receptor transmits mainly antisurvival signals (Casaccia-Bonnefil et al., 1999; Ali et al., 2008; Coassin et al., 2008; Lebrun-Julien et al., 2009b; Bai et al., 2010a). However, activation of $p75^{NTR}$ was shown to have either pro- or antisurvival effects in the retina, in dependence on the experimental model studied (Wexler et al., 1998; Harada et al., 2000, 2002a). $p75^{NTR}$ binds all neurotrophins with similar affinity and ensures the specificity of each neurotrophin. Müller cells express both Trk and $p75^{NTR}$ (Schatteman et al., 1988; Yan and Johnson, 1988; Chakrabarti et al., 1990; Carmignoto et al., 1991; Hopkins et al., 1992; Radeke et al., 1993; Hu et al., 1998; Wexler et al., 1998; Vecino et al., 1998; Wahlin et al., 2000; Harada et al., 2000a, 2002, 2003; Oku et al., 2002; García et al., 2003, 2014; Garcia and Vecino, 2003; Valter et al., 2003; Sarup et al., 2004). In the rat retina, $p75^{NTR}$ is localized to Müller cells but not bipolar or ganglion cells (Hu et al., 1998; Wexler et al., 1998; Ding et al., 2001; Garcia et al., 2014).

5.11.7.1 BDNF and Neurotrophin-3

The survival of rods and cones, as well as the regeneration of the injured retinal pigment epithelium, is dependent on Müller cells (Gaudin et al., 1996; Picaud et al., 1998; Dubois-Dauphin et al., 2000; Balse et al., 2005; De Melo et al., 2012; Machalińska et al., 2013; Byrne et al., 2013). TrkB signaling in Müller cells, but not in retinal ganglion and amacrine cells, was shown to be critically involved in neural protection and regeneration during retinal degeneration (Harada et al., 2011). The truncated isoform of TrkB in Müller cells is implicated in the BDNF-mediated photoreceptor protection against light damage (Saito et al., 2009). In the murine neuroretina, Müller, amacrine, and retinal ganglion cells express the TrkB receptor for BDNF, neurotrophin-3, and neurotrophin-4/5, whereas photoreceptors do not (Rohrer et al., 1999; Saito et al., 2009; Harada et al., 2011; Shen et al., 2012b). Exogenous BDNF induces c-Fos expression and phosphorylation of ERK1/2 in these cells (Rohrer et al., 1999). Likewise, BDNF cannot exert its effect directly on most photoreceptors of the rodent retina because they do not express receptors for BDNF (Rickman and Brecha, 1995; Ugolini et al., 1995; Rohrer et al., 1999; Wahlin et al., 2000, 2001; Asai et al., 2007); though TrkB is expressed on green-red cones (Di Polo et al., 2000; Grishanin et al., 2008) they represent less than 1% of all photoreceptors in the rat retina (Szél and Röhlich, 1992). It has been proposed that BDNF released from Müller cells increases the CNTF and bFGF production in Müller cells; both factors enhance the photoreceptor survival. BDNF was also suggested to promote the survial of bipolar cells through activation of p75^{NTR} on Müller cells and subsequent secretion of bFGF from Müller cells which directly rescues bipolar cells (Wexler et al., 1998). Müller cell-derived BDNF and neurotrophin-3 stimulate the growth of retinal ganglion cell axons by the induction of the intramembraneous proteolysis of p75^{NTR} and inactivation of Rho (Douglas et al., 2009), and is involved in the regeneration of the injured retinal pigment epithelium (Machalińska et al., 2013).

Retinal ischemia, light-induced or inherited retinal degeneration, and ocular hypertension are associated with an increase in Müller cell expression of p75^{NTR} and TrkC, and induction of TrkC expression by photoreceptor cells (Tomita et al., 1998; Harada et al., 2000; Rudzinski et al., 2004; Nakamura et al., 2005). Neurotrophin-3 mediates its protective effect on photoreceptor cells by binding on TrkC receptors of photoreceptors and Müller cells; the latter event results in an increased release of bFGF from Müller cells (Harada et al., 2000). However, it was shown that glaucoma induces upregulation of the truncated TrkC.T1 receptor isoform in retinal glial cells; activation of the receptor stimulates the glial production of TNFα which contributes to the death of retinal ganglion cells (Bai et al., 2010b). Selective Müller cell ablation results in a reduced retinal expression of mature neurotrophin-3 and upregulation of pro-neurotrophin-3 which induces photoreceptor degeneration by activation of p75^{NTR} (Shen et al., 2013). The upregulation of pro-neurotrophin-3 and p75^{NTR} in the retina of RCS rats can be attenuated by systemic erythropoietin which inhibits photoreceptor apoptosis (Shen et al., 2014b).

5.11.7.2 NGF

In the rat retina, NGF is expressed by astrocytes and ganglion, Müller, and pigment epithelial cells (Chakrabarti et al., 1990; Douglas et al., 2009; Garcia et al., 2014). Rat Müller cells express the receptors of NGF, TrkA and p75^{NTR}, while bipolar cells express TrkA but not p75^{NTR}, and ganglion cells express NGF, TrkA, and p75^{NTR} (Garcia et al., 2014). NGF acting at TrkA protects retinal neurons from excitotoxicity (Kokona et al., 2012). NGF delays retinal cell degeneration in animal models of inherited retinitis pigmentosa, diabetic retinopathy, glaucoma, retinal ischemia, retinal detachment, and optic nerve transection (Carmignoto et al., 1989; Siliprandi et al., 1993; Hammes et al., 1995; Lenzi et al., 2005; Sun et al., 2007; Colafrancesco et al., 2011). NGF was shown to trigger a release of bFGF and futher cytokines from Müller cells; Müller cell-derived cytokines rescue bipolar cells from osmotic swelling (Garcia et al., 2014; see 5.5.5.5.). NGF is a potent antioxidant which reduces oxidant-induced apoptosis of Müller cells (Giardino et al., 1998). However, NGF was also suggested to have antisurvival effects in the retina, by decreasing the production of bFGF in Müller cells which results in increased photoreceptor apoptosis (Harada et al., 2000; Nakamura et al., 2005). Absence of p75^{NTR} attenuates light-induced photoreceptor apoptosis (Harada et al.,

2000). It has been suggested that NGF may represent a promising agent for the treatment of degenerative retinal diseases such as glaucoma and age-related macular degeneration (Lambiase et al., 2011). However, NGF may have also TrkA-dependent detrimental effects in the retina including promotion of retinal and choroidal neovascularization, and of Müller cell proliferation (Ikeda and Puro, 1994; Steinle and Granger, 2003; Liu et al., 2010).

5.11.7.3 GDNF and Neurturin

In the rat retina, GDNF is localized to photoreceptor cells while neurturin is localized to second- and third-order neurons (Harada et al., 2003). In addition, GDNF and neurturin are expressed by Müller cells and astrocytes (Igarashi et al., 2000; Machalińska et al., 2013). In the normal retina, the receptors for GDNF and neurturin, GFRα1 and 2, are mainly expressed in the photoreceptor cell layer (Harada et al., 2002b, 2003; Koeberle and Ball, 2002). However, other evidence has reported GFR expression in retinal ganglion cells, Müller cells, and photoreceptors (Koeberle and Ball, 2002; Delyfer et al., 2005a); the discrepancies may be related to differences between animal strains (Harada et al., 2003). In the porcine retina, GDNF receptors GFRα1 and RET (as well as the receptors for artemin and neurturin, GFRα2 and GFRα3) are localized to Müller cells but not photoreceptors; in addition, retinal ganglion cells express GFRα2 and GFRα3 (Hauck et al., 2006). Hyperglycemic conditions, injury to the retinal pigment epithelium, and activated microglia induce upregulation of GDNF and its receptors in Müller cells (Nishikiori et al., 2007; Wang et al., 2011; Zhu et al., 2012; Machalińska et al., 2013). Glial cells in epiretinal PDR membranes increase the expression of the receptor for neurturin, GFRα2, and decrease the expression of the receptor for GDNF, GFRα1 (Harada et al., 2002b).

GDNF inhibits the apoptosis of Müller cells as well as the degeneration of photoreceptors and neurons, in part via upregulation of neurotrophic and growth factors such as bFGF, BDNF, and osteopontin (Frasson et al., 1999; Harada et al., 2003; Delyfer et al., 2005a; Hauck et al., 2006; Koeberle and Bähr, 2008; Del Río et al., 2011; Wang et al., 2011; Zhu et al., 2012). GDNF induces phosphorylation of ERK1/2 in the perinuclear region of Müller cells, resulting in transcriptional upregulation of bFGF that in turn supports photoreceptor survival (Harada et al., 2003; Hauck et al., 2006). Light-induced photoreceptor degeneration results in upregulation of GFRα2 in Müller cells, suggesting that neurturin protect photoreceptors by utilizing both direct and indirect (via Müller cells) pathways (Harada et al., 2003). GDNF and neurturin protect retinal ganglion cells from glutamate-induced apoptosis by enhancing the glutamate uptake in the retina through upregulation of GLAST and GLT-1 (Koeberle and Bähr, 2008). Likewise, GDNF protects photoreceptors from apoptosis by upregulation of the glial glutamate transporter GLAST (Delyfer et al., 2005a). In cultured Müller cells (that express both GFRα1 and GFRα2), GDNF increases the gene expression of BDNF, bFGF, and GDNF, while neurturin increases the gene expression of neurturin (Harada et al., 2003).

5.11.7.4 Osteopontin

GDNF induces the expression and secretion of osteopontin from Müller cells (Del Río et al., 2011). In the neuroretina, osteopontin is localized to retinal ganglion cells and activated microglia, as well as to Müller cells (Ju et al., 2000; Hikita et al., 2006; Chidlow et al., 2008; Del Río et al., 2011; Deeg et al., 2011; Wahl et al., 2013). In addition to the interactions with extracellular matrix components, osteopontin is a ligand of CD44 receptor variants and cell surface integrins (Weber et al., 1996; Giachelli and Steitz, 2000). CD44 and integrins are localized to Müller cells, and retinal injury and disease stimulates the production of CD44 by reactive glial cells (see 5.11.2.7.). Retinal osteopontin is upregulated in experimental glaucoma and protects retinal ganglion cells from death (Birke et al., 2010). By stimulation of the production of neuroprotective cytokines in Müller cells, osteopontin exerts a prosurvival effect in photoreceptor cells and reduces the level of apoptosis in the retina of retinal degeneration-1 mice (Del Río et al., 2011). Osteopontin also prevents the osmotic swelling of Müller cells (but not bipolar cells), by activation of the cell volume-regulatory glutamatergic-purinergic signaling cascade (Wahl et al., 2013; see 5.5.5.3.).

5.11.7.5 CNTF

CNTF is a member of the IL-6 family of cytokines. CNTF enhances the survival of retinal ganglion and photoreceptor cells, and stimulates the growth of retinal ganglion cell axons (Fischer et al., 2004a; Ikeda et al., 2004; Zhang et al., 2005e; Leaver et al., 2006; Miotke et al., 2007; Pease et al., 2009; Shen et al., 2012; Chidlow et al., 2012; Rhee et al., 2013). Conditional ablation of Müller cells in transgenic mice results in photoreceptor apoptosis which is prevented by exogenous CNTF (Shen et al., 2012). Constitutive expression of CNTF prevents photoreceptor death; however, it also suppresses visual function (Liang et al., 2001; Bok et al., 2002; Schlichtenbrede et al., 2003), at least in part via induction of Müller cell gliosis and retinal inflammation (Xue et al., 2011b). In the rat retina, CNTF is localized to astrocytes, Müller cells, and the pigment epithelium (Kirsch et al., 1997; Walsh et al., 2001); the retinal CNTF level increases after optic nerve transection and excitotoxic retinal degeneration (Honjo et al., 2000b; Nakamichi et al., 2003; Sarup et al., 2004). In the light-stressed rat retina and after ischemia or transcorneal electrical stimulation, CNTF and bFGF are selectively upregulated in Müller cells (Ju et al., 1999; Joly et al., 2007; Ni et al., 2009).

CNTF interacts with a tripartite receptor complex consisting of two single-pass membrane spanning receptor subunits (gp130 and LIFRβ) and an additional ligand-specific α receptor (Ip, 1998). gp130 is expressed by photoreceptors, astrocytes, Müller cells and retinal ganglion cells (Echevarria et al., 2013; Rhee et al., 2013). Exogenous CNTF initially signals through gp130 in Müller cells, which subsequently triggers the production of neuroprotective factors that require gp130 in rod photoreceptors for the prevention of cell death (Rhee et al., 2013). The expression of the CNTF receptor-α in photoreceptor cells is species-dependent; the receptor is expressed by non-rodent, but not rodent rods and cones (Beltran et al., 2005). Retinal ganglion cell perikarya and axons express the CNTF receptor-α, at least after optic nerve transection (Sarup et al., 2004). However, the downregulation of the receptors from axons renders retinal ganglion cells unresponsive to CNTF; this contributes to regenerative failure and death after optic nerve transection, while the appearance of the receptors on glia promotes glial scarring (Miotke et al., 2007). Intravitreal injection of axokine (an analog of CNTF) into the rat eye results in a translocation of activated STAT3 into the nuclei of Müller cells, astrocytes, and ganglion cells, but not in photoreceptors, suggesting that CNTF protects photoreceptors via activation of Müller cells (Peterson et al., 2000). Another member of the IL-6 family of cytokines, oncostatin M, which protects photoreceptors, also induces STAT3 phosphorylation in Müller cells but not in photoreceptors (Xia et al., 2011). CNTF causes a shift of retinal glial cells toward a more neuroprotective phenotype which is characterized, for instance, by a more efficient buffering of excess glutamate (Van Adel et al., 2005). Hydrocortisone stimulates the regeneration of transected retinal ganglion cell axons by inducing CNTF and glutamine synthetase in Müller cells (Toops et al., 2012a). In murine Müller cells, CNTF regulates the expression of various different genes such as cytokines, growth factors, G-protein coupled receptors, transporters, and ion channels, leading to the activation of signaling networks associated with the induction of gliosis, cell proliferation, and inflammatory response (Xue et al., 2011b). In the fish retina, CNTF stimulates the the proliferation of Müller cells via activation of STAT3 (Kassen et al., 2009).

5.11.7.6 Endothelin-2 and LIF

In the murine retina, endothelin-2 is mainly expressed in photoreceptor cells (Joly et al., 2008) and the receptor for endothelin-2 is predominantly localized to Müller cells and astrocytes (Rattner and Nathans, 2005). Injured photoreceptors produce endothelin-2 which activates Müller cells, as indicated by the increased expression of GFAP and the decrease in glutamine synthetase; activated Müller cells produce and release bFGF to support the survival of photoreceptors (Rattner and Nathans, 2005; Joly et al., 2008). It was shown that the endothelin-2-mediated photoreceptor protection is part of a LIF-controlled intrinsic retinal signaling system that involves photoreceptors and Müller cells (Joly et al., 2008; Bürgi et al., 2009). A subset of Müller cells react to photoreceptor injury with the production of LIF; LIF induces endothelin-2 in photoreceptors and activates Müller cells (Joly et al., 2008; Agca et al., 2013). Activated microglia induce upregulation of LIF in Müller cells which provides neuroprotection to photoreceptor cells (Wang et al., 2011). CNTF increases the expression of LIF and endothelin-2 which positively promotes the Müller cell and photoreceptor interactions (Rhee et al., 2013). CNTF/LIF also enables retinal ganglion cells to survive axotomy and regenerate axons under inflammatory conditions (Leibinger et al., 2012). It has been shown that, in addition to Müller cells, cone photoreceptors are capable to produce LIF under pathological conditions (Schaeferhoff et al., 2010).

5.11.7.7 bFGF

bFGF is a major neuroprotective factor in the retina (Sievers et al., 1987; Faktorovich et al., 1990, 1992; Wen et al., 1995; Liu et al., 1998) that acts via increased phosphorylation of CREB and subsequent upregulation of its prosurvival transcriptional targets (O'Driscoll et al., 2008). Müller cells are a major source of bFGF in the normal and diseased retina (Hageman et al., 1991; Raymond et al., 1992; Kostyk et al., 1994; Wen et al., 1995; Amin et al., 1997; Li et al., 1997b; Cao et al., 1997b; Xiao et al., 1998; Johansson et al., 2010). In the rat retina, bFGF is present in astrocytes, Müller cells, ganglion cells, pigment epithelial cells, and blood vessels (Morimoto et al., 1993; Walsh et al., 2001; Humphrey et al., 1997). After light stress, the cytoplasm of photoreceptor cells also contains bFGF (Walsh et al., 2001). In addition to light injury, mechanical injury to the retina (Fig. 42E,F), ischemic-hypoxic conditions (Fig. 33A) induced, for example, by retinal detachment (Fig. 33B), and inherited photoreceptor degeneration cause an increase of retinal bFGF (Miyashiro et al., 1988; Wen et al., 1995; Gao and Hollyfield, 1995a,b, 1996; Cao et al., 1997a; Matsushima et al., 1997; Guillonneau et al., 1998; Geller et al., 2001; Kruchkova et al., 2001; Lindqvist et al., 2010; Yafai et al., 2013). The production and release of bFGF by Müller cells is stimulated by inflammatory factors such as IL-1, TNFα, and prostaglandins, and by growth factors and neurotrophins like VEGF, bFGF, BDNF, NGF, and CNTF (Cao et al., 1997b; Cheng et al., 1998; Harada et al., 2002a; Yoshida et al., 2004a; Yafai et al., 2013; Garcia et al., 2014).

In the chick retina, exogenous bFGF activates ERK1/2, p38 MAPK, CREB, and c-Jun exclusively in Müller cells (Kruchkova et al., 2001; Fischer et al., 2009a). Additional (previous) retinal injuries like mechanical stress (Faktorovich et al., 1990; Silverman and Hughes, 1990) and preconditioning with bright light (Liu et al., 1998) protect photoreceptors from degeneration because these stimuli cause an upregulation of bFGF and CNTF in Müller cells (Wen et al., 1995; Liu et al., 1998). Likewise, argon laser photocoagulation slows photoreceptor degeneration in RCS rats by induction of bFGF in retinal blood vessels, Müller cells, and astrocytes (Chu et al., 1998). In addition to the prosurvival activity, bFGF may have also harmful effects such as stimulation of aberrant vessel growth (see 5.11.8.), induction of Müller cell proliferation (see 5.11.10.4.1.), and exacerbation of the glutamate-induced neurotoxicity through downregulation of the glutamine synthetase (see 5.5.2.1.12. and 5.5.2.1.13.).

5.11.7.8 Prostaglandins

Although prostaglandins, in particular PGE_2, are implicated in detrimental inflammatory processes such as cytotoxic swelling of Müller cells (see 5.11.9.2.3.) and development of retinal edema (see 5.11.9.1.1.), they have also neuroprotective effects. Müller cells are one source of prostaglandins, at least under pathological conditions (Fig. 12H-J) (Wurm et al., 2006a). PGE_2 elicits a wide range of biological actions through binding to E-prostanoid receptors (EP1-4 receptors) which are G-protein coupled cell surface receptors (Narumiya et al., 1999; Sugimoto and Narumiya, 2007). The EP3 receptor subtype is localized to Müller cells and most types of neurons in the porcine retina (Zhao and Shichi, 1995), to Müller cells and the nerve fiber layer in the human retina (Schlötzer-Schrehardt et al., 2002), and to astrocytes in the mouse retina (Sennlaub et al., 2003). In the rat retina, EP1-4 receptors are associated with various types of neurons particularly located in the inner retina; after an ischemic insult and in culture, EP2 and EP3 are also increasingly expressed in Müller cells (Osborne et al., 2009). Activation of EP2 protects from apoptotic death of retinal cells *in vitro* and blunts the detrimental influence of ischemia-reperfusion to the retina *in vivo* (Andrade da Costa et al., 2009; Osborne et al., 2009). PGE_2 stimulates the proliferation, dedifferentiation, and stem cell-like properties of Müller cells (see 5.11.12.3.).

5.11.7.9 Other Neuroprotective Factors

Müller cells are the main source of erythropoietin in the retina (Fu et al., 2008); erythropoietin rescues retinal ganglion cells after chronic ocular hypertension (Fu et al., 2008). In response to ocular hypertension, Müller cells increase the production of erythropoietin, and retinal ganglion cells, amacrine and bipolar cells increase the expression of erythropoietin receptors (Fu et al., 2008). The inhibitory effect on the osmotic swelling of Müller cells (see 5.5.5.3.) may contribute to the neurprotective action of erythropoietin.

In response to inflammatory stimulants, ischemia, and elevated hydrostatic pressure, Müller cells produce TNFα (De Kozak et al., 1994; Drescher and Whittum-Hudson, 1996b; Cotinet et al., 1997b; Tezel and Wax, 2000). Although TNFα is a cytotoxic factor that contributes to the death of retinal ganglion cells (Tezel and Wax, 2000), it may also prevent the death of retinal ganglion cells after axotomy of the optic nerve *in vivo* and of ganglion cells *in vitro* (Diem et al., 2001). Other Müller cell-derived factors that support photoreceptor survival are IGFBP-5 and CTGF (Hauck et al., 2008). CTGF and LIF are rapidly upregulated in the retinal tissue after experimental retinal detachment, while IGFBP-5 is downregulated (Hollborn et al., 2008). Müller cells are a main source of VEGF (see 5.11.1.1.) and PEDF (see 5.11.8.) which have neurotrophic and neuroprotective functions (Cayouette et al., 1999; Cao et al., 1999b, 2001; Ogata et al., 2001; Takita et al., 2003; Liljekvist-Soltic et al., 2008; Unterlauft et al., 2012; see 5.11.1.1.).

Müller cells are a source of the antiapoptotic protein B cell lymphoma oncogene protein (Bcl)-2, e.g., after retinal light damage and optic nerve transection (Chen et al., 1994, 2003b; Grosche et al., 1995; Härtig et al., 1995; Sharma, 2001; Näpänkangas et al., 2003; Schuetz et al., 2003). Bcl-2 activates endogenous free radical-scavenging activities and protects photoreceptors and ganglion cells from apoptotic cell death (Chen et al., 1996; Zack, 2000). However, overexpression of Bcl-2 in Müller cells of transgenic mice leads to early postnatal apoptotic Müller cell death resulting in retinal dysplasia, photoreceptor apoptosis, retinal degeneration, and proliferation of the retinal pigment epithelium (Dubois-Dauphin et al., 2000).

Müller cells are one source of Dickkopf (Dkk)-3 (Nakamura et al., 2007). Dkk3 is a positive regulator of Wnt signaling and protects against apoptosis by reducing caspase activity. In response to photoreceptor degeneration, the Wnt signaling pathway is activated in Müller cells (Yi et al., 2007; Liu et al., 2013b). Like neurotrophins, Wnt ligands protect photoreceptors and retinal ganglion cells from death by both direct effects in the cells and indirectly by activation of the canonical Wnt signaling pathway in Müller cells (Yi et al., 2007, 2012; Fragoso et al., 2011). Similarly, the neuroprotective effects of Norrin in retinal ganglion cells and phoreceptors is indirectly mediated by activation of Frizzled-4 in Müller cells that activates the Wnt signaling pathway and increases the expression of neurotrophic factors like bFGF, LIF, PEDF, BNDF, and CNTF (Seitz et al., 2010; Braunger et al., 2013). Müller cells may also protect photoreceptors and neurons from apoptosis by the release of ApoE and α2-macroglobulin (Hayashi et al., 2007), the expression of the adhesion molecule on glia (AMOG; the β2-subunit of the sodium-potassium-ATPase) (Molthagen et al., 1996), the secretion of IL-6 (Yoshida et al., 2001) which is protective for retinal ganglion cells and photoreceptors (Mendonca Torres and de Araujo, 2001; Sanchez et al., 2003; Inomata et al., 2003; Chong et al., 2008), and by the release of galectins (Maldonado et al., 1999; Uehara et al., 2001).

5.11.7.10 Neurotrophic Signaling

Activation of ERK1/2 and c-Fos in Müller cells (Figs. 8A, 82A) are important steps in the mechanism which rescues retinal neurons from death (Peng et al., 1998; Rohrer et al., 1999; Akiyama et al., 2002; Nakazawa et al., 2008; Kassen et al., 2009; Rhee et al., 2013). BDNF, CNTF, and bFGF induce ERK1/2 and c-Fos activation in cells of the inner rodent retina, in particular Müller cells, but not in photoreceptor cells or retinal neurons (Wahlin et al., 2000, 2001; Fischer et al., 2009a; Hu et al., 2011). Intravitreal administration of the excitotoxin NMDA results in activation of ERK1/2 and c-Fos induction in Müller cells within 1 h (Nakazawa et al., 2008). Phosphorylated ERK1/2 is shuttled into the Müller cell nuclei where it induces increased transcription of bFGF mRNA, for example (Hauck et al., 2006). Deletion of ERK1 is associated with a higher rate of NMDA-induced apoptotic neuronal cell death in the retina (Nakazawa et al., 2008).

5.11.8 GLIAL REGULATION OF RETINAL NEOVASCULARIZATION

In addition to cataract and glaucoma, neovascular retinopathies such as wet AMD, PDR, retinopathy of prematurity and those stemming from retinal vein occlusion are the leading cause of low vision and blindness in industrialized countries (Gilbert et al., 1997; Friedman et al., 2004; Kempen et al., 2004; Klein, 2007). Regenerative responses in the ischemic retina involve the promotion of neovascularization. Neovascularization is induced by hypoxia and/or insulin deficiency (diabetes mellitus) that prevents a sufficient glucose uptake by retinal glial cells. Neovascularization is an attempt to regenerate the blood supply of ischemic-hypoxic retinal areas; however, the vessel growth proceeds in an unregulated fashion and causes secondary damage to the retinal tissue (Penn et al., 2008; Cheung et al., 2010; Carmeliet and Jain, 2011). PDR is characterized by the growth of fibrovascular tissues from the retina into the vitreous while wet AMD is characterized by the growth of subretinal neovascular membranes (choroidal neovascularization). Müller cells contribute to both preretinal and choroidal neovascularization (see 5.11.2.6. and 5.11.11.). In RCS rats with inherited retinal dystrophy, vascularization of the retinal pigment epithelium is preceded by migration and proliferation of Müller cell processes in the subretinal space where they contact the pigment epithelium; later, pigment epithelial cells enveloped the subretinal vessels which had lost their perivascular Müller cell sheath (Roque and Caldwell, 1990, 1991). There are also cases of intraretinal neovascularization which are permitted or induced by Müller cells: in patients with retinal angiomatous proliferation, a subform of wet AMD, neovascularization starts in the outer plexiform layer, progresses to the subretinal space, and anastomoses with choroidal vessels (Hartnett et al., 1996; Yannuzzi et al., 2001; Gass et al., 2003). Usually, the growing blood vessels are "leaky" whereas normally the neural retina is isolated from the blood by blood-retinal barriers (Campochiaro, 2000; see 2.1.).

The vessel growth is promoted by proangiogenic cytokines. VEGF is the most relevant angiogenic factor released in the retina under ischemic and inflammatory conditions, e.g., from Müller cells (D'Amore, 1994; Miller et al., 1994; Aiello et al., 1995; Drescher and Whittum-Hudson, 1996a; Pe'er et al., 1996; Vinores et al., 1997; Schlingemann and van Hinsbergh, 1997; Amin et al., 1997; Brooks et al., 1998; Behzadian et al., 1998; Jingjing et al., 1999; Eichler et al., 2000, 2001, 2004a, 2006; Witmer et al., 2003; Famiglietti et al., 2003; Yafai et al., 2004; Hollborn et al., 2004a,b, 2005; Bai et al., 2009; Yang et al., 2009; Huang et al., 2011a; Cheng et al., 2013; Krause et al., 2014). Although VEGF is constitutively expressed in the retina and ensures the survival of retinal cells (see 5.11.1.1.), overproduction of VEGF exacerbates retinal disease progression by inducing vascular leakage and neovascularization (see 5.11.1.2.). Following ischemia-hypoxia, VEGF is induced primarily in Müller cells, in addition to other cell types such as astrocytes, ganglion, amacrine, pigment epithelial, and vascular endothelial cells (Pierce et al., 1995; Dorey et al., 1996; Robbins et al., 1997; Vinores et al., 2000; Zou et al., 2009; Watkins et al., 2013). In addition, invading macrophages express VEGF (Krause et al., 2014). In PDR, the vitreal and subretinal concentration of VEGF is enhanced (Gao et al., 2001; Ogata et al., 2002a; Duh et al., 2004), and VEGF is increasingly expressed in Müller cells, astrocytes, and retinal neurons (Amin et al., 1997; Abu-El-Asrar et al., 2004b). The expression of VEGF in Müller cells precedes the neovascularization in the diabetic retina, at times when there is no anatomical evidence of retinal malperfusion (Amin et al., 1997). VEGF is localized to many cells in epiretinal membranes of diabetic patients, including glial cells (Chen et al., 1997b; Armstrong et al., 1998). In experimental choroidal neovascularization, Müller cells are activated by blood-derived macrophages as indicated by the induction of c-Fos and activation of ERK1/2 (Caicedo et al., 2005a, b), and increased expression of VEGF is detected in macrophages, migrating retinal pigment epithelial cells, and Müller cells (Ishibashi et al., 1997). In very low-density lipoprotein receptor (VLDLr) knockout mice, an animal model of retinal angiomatous proliferation, activation of Müller cells contributes to the strong expression of VEGF in the lesion area (Li et al., 2007a).

Müller cells express and release VEGF in response to hypoxia and inflammatory factors like prostaglandins (Hata et al., 1995; Behzadian et al., 1998; Cheng et al., 1998; Brooks et al., 1998; Eichler et al., 2000, 2004b; Caldwell et al., 2003; Yafai et al., 2004; Foulds et al., 2010; Yanni et al., 2010; Cheng et al., 2013; Campochiaro, 2013). Retinal ischemia causes activation of HIF-1α predominantly in neuronal cells and of HIF-2α predominantly in glial cells (Mowat et al., 2010). The effect of hypoxia on the VEGF expression in Müller cells is in part mediated by the hypoxic upregulation of cyclooxygenase-2, production of PGE_2 (that acts at EP_2 and/or EP_4 receptors) and activation of PKA (Yanni et al., 2010). In addition, various growth factors and cytokines, for example bFGF, heparin-binding epidermal growth factor-like growth factor (HB-EGF), HGF, and TGF-β, stimulate the expression and secretion of VEGF from Müller cells (Behzadian et al., 1998; Hollborn et al., 2004a, b, 2005). The high glucose-induced accumulation of AGEs in the diabetic retina (see 5.10.13.) contributes to the induction of VEGF (Hirata et al., 1997; Ishibashi, 2000). PGE_2 and high glucose induces upregulation of the complement C5a receptor in Müller cells; activation of the receptor stimulates the production of VEGF (Cheng et al., 2013).

The balance between angiogenic factors, in particular VEGF, and antiangiogenic factors such as PEDF is thought to be essential for the angiogenic homeostasis in the retina (Gao et al., 2001; Spranger et al., 2001; Ogata et al., 2002a; Duh et al., 2002, 2004). PEDF is expressed in the neuroretina by neurons and glial cells (Aymerich et al., 2001; Eichler et al., 2004b). A decrease of the vitreal PEDF level was suggested to be a predictor of the progression of diabetic retinopathy to PDR (Boehm et al., 2003). The decrease of the retinal PEDF level is at least partially responsible for the increase of the VEGF expression and the subsequent neovascularization in diabetic retinopathy (Zhang et al., 2006b). PEDF decreases also the expression of inflammatory factors like TNFα in Müller cells (Zhang et al., 2006c). PEDF inhibits angiogenesis by inducing apoptosis in vascular endothelial cells of newly formed vessels (Volpert et al., 2002; Chen et al., 2006) and inhibiting the (VEGF-induced) proliferation of retinal vascular endothelial cells (Yafai et al., 2007). Müller cells express PEDF; a decrease of the PEDF expression is associated with an upregulation of VEGF in the cells (Tombran-Tink et al., 2004; Eichler et al., 2004b; Zhang et al., 2006b; Li et al., 2006; Yafai et al., 2007; Yang et al., 2012). High glucose, inflammatory conditions, and (mild) hypoxia decrease the expression of PEDF by Müller cells (Mu et al., 2009; Eichler et al., 2004b; Hauck et al., 2007; Lange et al., 2008); the effect of hypoxia is mediated (at least in part) by VEGF (Eichler et al., 2004b). Strong or prolonged hypoxia induces an increase of the PEDF expression in Müller cells (Lange et al., 2008; Yang et al., 2012; Unterlauft et al., 2012), likely to protect the cells from death. The expression of PEDF in Müller cells is also regulated by soluble factors released from vascular endothelial cells (Yafai et al., 2007) and in response to 17β-estradiol and retinoic acid (Tombran-Tink et al., 2004; Li et al., 2006).

Reciprocal changes of VEGF and PEDF, however, were also found in retinal detachment and PVR (Su et al., 2000; Ogata et al., 2002b), suggesting that additional angiogenic factors are required for the development of neovascular diseases. The synergistic action of further proangiogenic factors is required for the angiogenic effect of VEGF (Castellon et al., 2002). In addition to VEGF, heparin-binding growth and inflammatory factors such as bFGF, PDGF, IGF-1, HGF, and TNFα, as well as angiopoietin-2 and MMPs promote pathological angiogenesis (D'Amore, 1994; ; Miller et al., 1994; Soubrane et al., 1994; Perry et al., 1995; Frank et al., 1996; Paques et al., 1997; Mori et al., 2002a; Umeda et al., 2002; Simó et al., 2006).

Among the angiogenic factors released from Müller cells under hypoxic conditions, bFGF and VEGF seem to play the key roles in the stimulation of abnormal vascular growth (Yafai et al., 2013). bFGF is rapidly released in the retinal tissue under ischemic-hypoxic conditions. Müller cells are a major source of bFGF (see 5.11.7.7.), e.g., in diabetic fibrovascular membranes (Yafai et al., 2013). bFGF induces (synergistically with VEGF) extracellular proteolysis and proliferation and migration of vascular endothelial cells (Yan et al., 2001; Yafai et al., 2013). The effects of bFGF are in part mediated by the stimulation of the secretion of VEGF from Müller and vascular cells (Stavri et al., 1995; Amin et al., 1997), and VEGF as well as inflammatory factors like IL-1 and TNFα trigger a release of bFGF from Müller cells (Yafai et al., 2013). Thus, the well-known angiogenic effect of TNFα might be in part mediated by stimulation of the secretion of bFGF from Müller cells. High-mobility group box-1, an endogenous ligand of TLR4 and RAGE, induces the production of proinflammatory factors in retinal glial cells that contributes to neurodegeneration and neovascularization in the ischemic retina (Dvoriantchikova et al., 2011; He et al., 2013).

The interaction of inflammatory cells with retinal glial cells is thought to be critical for the development of neovascular retinal diseases (Yoshida et al., 2003). In the presence of an inflammatory environment, activated macrophage/microglia produce angiogenic factors such as TNFα that stimulate the expression of angiogenic molecules like MCP-1, IL-8, and bFGF in macroglial cells (Yoshida et al., 2004a). The angiogenic effect of TNFα is mediated in part through the activation of the nuclear transcription factor NF-κB; retinal glial cells surrounding microvessels are immunopositive for NF-κB (Yoshida et al., 1998, 1999). There are further angiogenic factors produced by retinal glial cells. In diabetic retinopathy and other ischemic-hypoxic retinal diseases, cyclooxygenase-2 is induced in astrocytes and Müller cells (Fig. 12H–J); inhibition of this enzyme prevents neovascularization by upregulation of thrombospondin-1 (Sennlaub et al., 2003). Other vasoactive factors which are produced by Müller cells are renin and angiotensin II (Datum and Zrenner, 1991; Rong et al., 1994; Berka et al., 1995; Fletcher et al., 2005; Senanayake et al., 2007), netrin-4 (Lange et al., 2012), plasminogen activators and activator inhibitor (Schacke et al., 2002), and MMPs (Behzadian et al., 2001; Milenkovic et al., 2003). The action of MMPs allows endothelial cells to penetrate their underlying basement membrane, and eliminates the contact inhibition which normally blocks endothelial cell proliferation (Matrisian, 1990; Castilla et al., 1999).

However, the role of Müller cells in the pathogenesis of retinal neovascular diseases is incompletely understood. In the healthy retina, Müller cells provide a permanent angiostatic condition. Conditional ablation of Müller cells in transgenic mice results in intraretinal neovascularization

(Shen et al., 2012). Neovascular membranes are thought to be formed to reoxygenate the ischemic retinal tissue. However, neovascularization in PDR is misdirected, i.e., newly formed vessels grow towards the posterior surface of the vitreous, but not into the ischemic retinal tissue. Preretinal vessels originates mainly from the superficial veins and venules and not from intraretinal vessels (Tolentino et al., 2002). The reasons for the change from retinal to vitreal neovascularization are unclear and may include the vitreo-retinal gradient of angiogenic factors, the inhibition of retinal revascularization by NO and semaphorin-3A (Sennlaub et al., 2001; Joyal et al., 2011), alterations of the biomechanical properties of Müller cells (see 5.5.1.3.), and the growth-inhibitory effects of gliotic Müller cells provided by inhibitory extracellular matrix molecules (see 5.11.2.7.).

Under both normoxic and hypoxic conditions, Müller cells also provide an antiproliferative environment for vascular endothelial cells by the release of soluble antiangiogenic factors such as PEDF, thrombospondins-1 and -2, prolactin, TGF-β2, and possibly BMPs (Eichler et al., 2001, 2004a, b; Yafai et al., 2007, 2014a, b; Rivera et al., 2008; Huang et al., 2013a). Müller cell-derived soluble factors modulate the gene expression of vascular endothelial cells resulting in upregulation of the antiangiogenic plasminogen activator inhibitor 1 (PAI-1) and downregulation of the pro-angiogenic inhibitor of DNA binding 2 (Id2) (Abukawa et al., 2009). In spite of the observation that hypoxia enhances the expression of VEGF and downregulates the expression of PEDF and TGF-ß in Müller cells, conditioned media of Müller cells grown under hypoxic conditions inhibit rather than stimulate the proliferation of vascular endothelial cells (Eichler et al., 2001, 2004b; Yafai et al., 2004). The angiostatic effect of Müller cells is in part mediated by the hypoxic upregulation of thrombospondin-1 (Eichler et al., 2004a; Yafai et al., 2014a). However, the angiostatic *vs.* angiogenic effects of reactive Müller cells depend on the duration of hypoxia. Under short-term hypoxic conditions, Müller cells provide an angiostatic environment while under long-term hypoxic conditions, Müller cells increasingly secrete factors, in particular bFGF, that stimulate the proliferation of vascular endothelial cells (Yafai et al., 2013).

5.11.9 RETINAL EDEMA

The development of retinal edema is an important complication of various retinal, ocular, and systemic diseases including inherited defects and traumatic, ischemic-hypoxic, and inflammatory injuries such as uveitis, ocular tumors, diabetic retinopathy, retinal artery occlusion, artherosclerotic vascular disorders, neovascular AMD, and hypertension, and it may be iatrogenically induced by intraocular operations, in particular cataract surgery. In uveitis and non-proliferative diabetic retinopathy, retinal edema is the major cause of visual deterioration (Bresnick, 1983; Rothova et al., 1996; Fong et al., 2004; Larsen et al., 2005; Joussen et al., 2007). Wet AMD is associated with intra- and subretinal fluid accumulation from neovascular choroidal blood vessels which is an important cause of decreased vision in this condition (Bressler et al., 2001). By the compression of retinal neurons, nerve fibers, and blood vessels, edema aggravates tissue ischemia and contributes to the functional impairment and degeneration of retinal neurons. Edema is characterized by accumulation of water predominantly in the macular tissue resulting in thickening of the tissue. Macular edema may be diffuse or cystoid; the latter is characterized by the development of intraretinal fluid-filled cysts around the fovea (Irvine, 1976). In cystoid edema, the fluid accumulation causes cell displacement and splitting of the perifoveal retina predominantly in the inner nuclear and Henle fiber layers (Fig. 20B,C); the fluid-filled compartments are spanned by the trunks of Müller cell fibers (Wolter, 1981; Nork et al., 1987; Marshall, 1991; Antcliff and Marshall, 1999). In neovascular AMD, fluid accumulation occurs in the subretinal space resulting in functional impairment of photoreceptors and serous macular detachment.

Water may accumulate in retinal cells (intracellular or cytotoxic edema resulting in cellular swelling; Fig. 26A,D) and interstitial spaces (extracellular edema resulting in cell compression; Fig. 26B,C,E). Generally, water accumulation within retinal tissue results from an imbalance between the water influx from the blood into the retina and the water clearance from the retinal tissue into the blood (Bringmann et al., 2004). The water flux is driven by hydrostatic and osmotic gradients between the blood and retina (Stefánsson, 2009). There are systemic and retinal factors that contribute to retinal edema. Systemic factors cause an influx of water from the blood into the retinal tissue, either by an increase in the hydrostatic pressure (hypertension and intravascular fluid overload due to vessel dilation after the loss of blood flow regulation) or a decrease of the blood osmotic/oncotic pressure, e.g., in cases of hyponatremia and hypoalbuminemia resulting from renal or hepatic failures (Gardner et al., 2002; Qin et al., 2009a; Stefánsson, 2009). Retinal conditions that contribute to edema development are ischemia-hypoxia leading to mitochondrial dysfunction (Fig. 26A) and oxidative stress, inflammation, and metabolic alterations resulting from enhanced glucose metabolism (Tso, 1982; Bresnick, 1983; Yanoff et al., 1984; Marmor, 1999; Guex-Crosier, 1999; Aiello, 2002; Miyake and Ibaraki, 2002).

Edema in the brain and retina can be vasogenic and/or cellular in origin (Bringmann et al., 2004; Kimelberg, 2005). In the brain, water accumulation in perivascular astrocytes (cytotoxic edema) usually occurs concomitantly with vasogenic edema (Kimelberg, 2005). Retinal edema is thought to be primarily caused by a breakdown of the blood-retinal barrier resulting in increased vascular permeability (vasogenic edema) (Gass et al., 1985; Marmor, 1999; Antcliff and Marshall, 1999; Aiello, 2002; Klaassen et al., 2013). A breakdown of the blood-retinal barrier occurs under conditions of ocular inflammation, ischemia, and trauma, and after detachment of the posterior vitreous from the retina (see 5.11.11.3.). Vascular leakage results in extravasation of serum proteins

(Figs. 21C, 69B) that causes increased interstitial osmotic pressure which pulls water into the retinal tissue (Klaassen et al., 2013). However, it has been shown that an impairment of the fluid clearance from the retinal tissue is an essential step in edema formation. Excess fluid influx may overburden the fluid clearance capacities of retinal glial and pigment epithelial cells (see 5.5.4.), resulting in retinal water accumulation. Cases of macular edema without angiographic vascular leakage (Marmor, 1999; Lobo et al., 2000) underline the importance of systemic factors and the impairment of the fluid clearance function of glial and pigment epithelial cells for the development of edema. Clinically significant diabetic retinal edema develops when, in addition to vascular leakage, the active transport mechanisms of the blood-retinal barrier are dysfunctional (Mori et al., 2002b). Any anomalies in vessel permeability need to be accompanied by ineffective edema-resolving mechanisms to cause chronic edema (Bellhorn, 1984). In the preclinical stage of diabetic retinopathy, there are two types of increased retinal thickness and intraretinal cyst formation that may be or not associated with vascular leakage (Lobo et al., 2000). The ischemic increase in the permeability of the blood-brain barrier can be prevented by inhibition of HIF-1; however, this inhibition does not prevent the ischemic formation of brain edema (Yan et al., 2011), suggesting that cytotoxic mechanisms contribute independently from vasogenic mechanisms to the development of brain edema. In cases of retinal edema without vascular leakage (Marmor, 1999; Lobo et al., 2000), increases of the intraretinal osmotic pressure (or decreases of the blood osmolarity) cannot be effectively compensated by (dysfunctional) glial and pigment epithelial cells. Such osmotic gradients will pull water from the blood into the retina across the unaffected vessel walls, as shown in the brain in models of water intoxication (Manley et al., 2000). In addition to the increased vascular permeability and the dysregulation of the fluid clearance across retinal glial and pigment epithelial cells, osmotic swelling of retinal neurons and glial cells (cytotoxic edema) is one pathogenic factor involved in the development of retinal edema (Bringmann et al., 2004, 2005; Reichenbach et al., 2007).

5.11.9.1 Vasogenic Edema

In diabetic rats, a disruption of the inner blood-retinal barrier is one of the earliest observable event, occurring after two weeks of hyperglycemia (Corbett et al., 1992; Do Carmo et al., 1998), i.e., before Müller cell reactivity is apparent by the increased expression of GFAP (Lieth et al., 1998; Rungger-Brändle et al., 2000). The disruption of the blood-retinal barrier before glial reactivity suggests that glial cells are early targets of vascular hyperpermeability (Rungger-Brändle et al., 2000). Increased vascular permeability is caused by opening of tight junctions between vascular endothelial cells and an increased vesicular transport of serum proteins across the vascular endothelia (Cunha-Vaz and Travassos, 1984; Vinores et al., 1990a; Joussen et al., 2007; Klaassen et al., 2013).

5.11.9.1.1 Glial Regulation of the Blood-Retinal Barrier Retinal capillaries are closely ensheathed by glial cell processes arising from astrocytes and Müller cells. Both astrocytes and Müller cells contribute to endothelial cell differentiation and the formation of the blood-retinal barrier (Chan-Ling and Stone, 1992; Tout et al., 1993; Jiang et al., 1995; Gardner, 1995; Wisniewska-Kruk et al., 2012). Astrocytes and Müller cells secrete factors that increase the barrier function of retinal vascular endothelial cells (Gardner, 1995; Gardner et al., 1997). Müller cells enhance the endothelial cell barrier function under normoxic conditions but impair the barrier function under hypoxic conditions (Tretiach et al., 2005). Glial factors which enhance the barrier function of vascular endothelial cells are, for example, GDNF, neurturin, thrombospondin-1, and PEDF (Igarashi et al., 2000; Eichler et al., 2004a, b; Nishikiori et al., 2007; Liu et al., 2012b). Conditional ablation of Müller cells in transgenic mice results in vascular telangiectasis, breakdown of the blood-retinal barrier, and intraretinal neovascularization (Shen et al., 2012, 2014a; Byrne et al., 2013). In this model, vascular leakage was, at least in part, mediated by the induction of VEGF in pericytes and reduced expression of tight junction proteins in vascular endothelia (Shen et al., 2012). Downregulation of the glutamine synthetase in the rat retina by using siRNA induces glial dysfunction which results in a breakdown of the blood-retinal barrier (Shen et al., 2010a). This suggests that impairment of Müller cell's glutamate metabolism (see 5.5.2.1.12.) results in pathological events that finally disturb the integrity of the blood-retinal barrier. A breakdown of the blood-retinal barrier may occur in the presence of mechanical stress to Müller cells after posterior vitreous detachment (see 5.11.11.3.). Activation of the retinoic acid receptor-α induces upregulation of GDNF and downregulation of VEGF in retinal glial cells (Nishikiori et al., 2007). Both increase the tight junction function of vascular endothelia sufficient for significant reductions of vascular leakage in the diabetic retina (Nishikiori et al., 2007).

In diabetic retinopathy and other ischemic-hypoxic and inflammatory retina diseases, glial malfunction plays an important role in the pathogenesis of vasogenic edema. Diabetic retinopathy is associated with a reduced expression and redistribution of the tight junction protein occludin in retinal vascular endothelial cells (Barber et al., 2000). The major vessel-permeabilizing factor induced by hypoxia is VEGF, the "vascular permeability factor" (Murata et al., 1996; Luna et al., 1997; Schlingemann and van Hinsbergh, 1997; Aiello et al., 1997; Qaum et al., 2001; Caldwell et al., 2003; Zhang et al., 2006b,c; Penn et al., 2008; Huang et al., 2011a; Campochiaro, 2013). VEGF is an important survival factor for vascular endothelial cells, photoreceptors, neurons, and glial cells (see 5.11.1.1.); this prosurvival signaling is apparently the reason for the early upregulation of VEGF in ischemia. In addition to VEGF, other cytokines such as bFGF and IGF-1, inflammatory factors like TNFα, IL-1β, IL-6, and prostaglandins, as well as proteins of the blood coagulation cascade increase the permeability of retinal vessels (Maruo et al., 1992; Claudio et al., 1994;

Luna et al., 1997; Derevjanik et al., 2002; Miyake and Ibaraki, 2002; Huang et al., 2011b). VEGF reduces the expression of tight junctional proteins and increases the number of intercellular gaps in vascular endothelia (Antonetti et al., 1998; Wisniewska-Kruk et al., 2012). Normally, VEGF is expressed in the neuroretina at low level in vascular endothelial cells, all major classes of neurons, and glial cells (Famiglietti et al., 2003; Saint-Geniez et al., 2008). Müller cells, astrocytes, and retinal neurons increasingly express VEGF in non-proliferative diabetic retinopathy, at times when there is no anatomical evidence of retinal malperfusion (Amin et al., 1997; Abu-El-Asrar et al., 2004b; Yang et al., 2009). Conditional disruption of the VEGF expression in Müller cells reduces the depletion of tight junction proteins and vascular leakage in the diabetic retina, suggesting that Müller cell-derived VEGF is essential for the diabetes-induced vascular leakage (Wang et al., 2010b). Further sources of VEGF are vascular cells activated by leukocytes adhering to the endothelium as well as microglial cells (see 3.3.).

The effect of high glucose on the VEGF expression in Müller cells remains unclear. It has been shown that high glucose stimulates the production of VEGF in Müller cells (Mu et al., 2009; Ye et al., 2012) but also that glucose deprivation induces VEGF expression in Müller cells (Aiello et al., 1995; Eichler et al., 2000). High glucose inhibits the hypoxic expression of VEGF in Müller cells and human retinal cells, suggesting that the metabolic effects of hypoxia can be compensated by a surplus of glucose (Eichler et al., 2000; Kennedy and Frank, 2011; Brooks et al., 1998) likely because Müller cells rely mainly on anaerobic glycolysis (see 5.5.7.1.). Apparently, retinal cells increase their VEGF production when their energy supply, either via glucose or oxygen, is reduced (Kennedy and Frank, 2011). High glucose protects retinal cells from mitochondrial oxidative stress and apoptosis (Han et al., 2013), and hyperglycemia improves the retinal function in experimental retinal ischemia and in diabetic patients (Holman et al., 2010; Holfort et al., 2010). It has been suggested that lowering the blood glucose level in patients with diabetic retinopathy, by a tight glucose control regimen, will worsen the disease by stimulation of the VEGF production as a compensatory mechanism (Kennedy and Frank, 2011). The high glucose-induced formation of AGEs in diabetic retinas may contribute to the induction of VEGF (Hirata et al., 1997) via activation of the AGE receptor on Müller cells (see 5.10.13.). In addition, ALEs increase the expression of VEGF, IL-6, and TNFα in Müller cells (Yong et al., 2010).

VEGF and other cytokines released from Müller cells, e.g., TGF-β, bFGF, and TNF, increase the release of MMPs from endothelial cells (Mignatti et al., 1989; Unemori et al., 1992; Lamoreaux et al., 1998; Behzadian et al., 2001; Majka et al., 2002). In addition, Müller cells themselves secrete MMPs, e.g., in response to hypoxia and stimulation of purinergic receptors (Fig. 86) (Milenkovic et al., 2003; Noda et al., 2005). High glucose increases the production of MMPs in retinal cells (Giebel et al., 2005). MMPs impair the barrier function of vascular endothelial cells

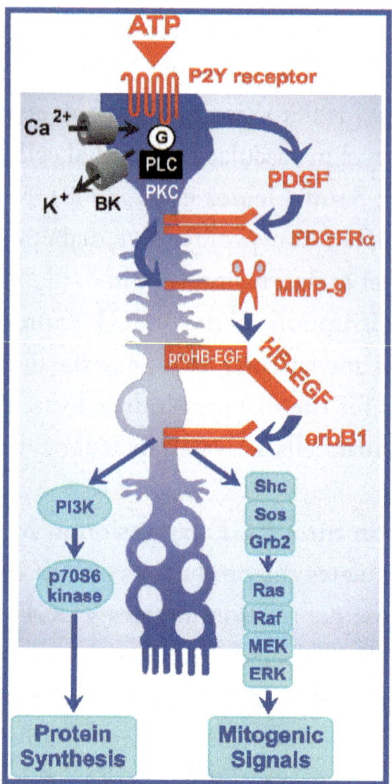

FIGURE 86: Activation of G protein-coupled P2Y receptors by extracellular ATP stimulates the proliferation of Müller cells via calcium signaling and transactivation of growth factor receptor tyrosine kinases. Mechanical stress induced, for example, by retinal detachment or tractional forces resulting from posterior vitreous detachment induces a release of ATP from Müller cells. Activation of P2Y receptors stimulates the activity of the phospholipase C (PLC) resulting in the formation of inositol 1,4,5-trisphosphate (IP$_3$) and diacylglycerol (DAG). IP$_3$ evokes a rapid release of calcium from intracellular stores. Following this initial calcium response, external calcium enters the cell interior through calcium-permeable membrane channels, providing a second and more sustained calcium signal phase. The cytosolic calcium increase results in a opening of calcium-activated, big-conductance potassium (BK) channels. DAG and calcium stimulate the activity of the protein kinase C (PKC). The intracellular calcium response causes a release of platelet-derived growth factor (PDGF) from Müller cells. Activation of the PDGFα receptor tyrosine kinase results in a release of heparin-binding epidermal growth factor-like growth factor (HB-EGF) from the extracellular matrix through shedding of the membrane-bound pro-HB-EGF by the matrix metalloproteinase-9 (MMP-9). HB-EGF activates the EGF receptor tyrosine kinase (erbB1), resulting in activation of the extracellular signal regulated kinases (ERK) that transmit the mitogenic signal into the cell nucleus. In addition, the phosphatidylinositol-3 kinase (PI3K) signaling pathway is implicated in the P2Y receptor-induced proliferation of Müller cells. Modified from Milenkovic et al. (2003).

by the proteolytic degradation of the tight junction protein occludin (Giebel et al., 2005). Glia-mediated autoimmune processes may contribute to the increased vascular permeability in diabetic retinopathy (Teplinskaia et al., 2006).

5.11.9.1.2 Impairment of the Fluid Clearance   In addition to the effect on the integrity of the blood-retinal barrier, glial cells may also contribute to the development of retinal edema by the impairment of the fluid clearance from the edematous retinal tissue (Bringmann et al., 2005, 2006; Reichenbach et al., 2007). Impairment of the fluid clearance is considered to be an essential step in edema formation (Bellhorn, 1984; Mori et al., 2002b), in particular in macular edema without angiographic vascular leakage (Marmor, 1999; Lobo et al., 2000). It has been shown that the water content of the rat retina displays a biphasic elevation in the course of experimental ischemia-reperfusion: during ischemic episodes, the water content progressively increases and falls to near-control level within hours after reperfusion; a second increase occurs after two days of reperfusion (Stefánsson et al., 1987). The resolution of the ischemic edema within hours after reperfusion (Stefánsson et al., 1987) indicates that the water clearance function of Müller cells is not disturbed early after transient ischemia. However, the increase of the retinal water content within two days after reperfusion suggests that there occurs a slowly developing disturbance of the water transport through Müller cells in the postischemic retina (Bringmann et al., 2005). The fluid clearance capacity of retinal glial and pigment epithelial cells can be exceeded when excess blood-derived fluid enters the retina and/or when the cells alter their expression of ion channels, transporters, and AQPs (Bringmann et al., 2004).

When Müller cells become gliotic under various pathological conditions, they downregulate functional Kir4.1 channels (see 5.5.3.5.). This downregulation is a time-dependent process, occurring within days after transient ischemia (Fig. 8F) (Pannicke et al., 2004, 2005a). A functional impairment of rat Müller cells indicated by cellular depolarization is observed two days after ischemia-reperfusion (Fig. 8H) (Pannicke et al., 2004, 2005a) which coincides with the second increase of the retinal water content (Stefánsson et al., 1987). The downregulation of functional Kir4.1 channels will disrupt the spatial buffering potassium currents through Müller cells and the export of potassium into the blood and vitreous. Because the Müller cell-mediated absorption of excess water from the retinal tissue is (at least in part) coupled to the potassium clearance function of the cells (Figs. 40A, 68, 69A, 70, 71; see 5.5.4.), the disruption of the transglial potassium currents will also disturb the transport of water through Müller cells, resulting in an impairment of the dehydration of the inner retina, and should impair the compensation of osmotic gradients between the blood and retina and within the retinal tissue. The downregulation of functional Kir4.1 channels results in an almost fully absence of passive outward potassium currents from Müller cells whereas a significant amount of inward currents remains present (Fig. 7A,B) which are mediated by strongly rectifying Kir channels such as Kir2.1 (Figs. 8C, 12B; see 5.5.3.1.). The uptake of potassium which is not counterbalanced by an efflux will result in an accumulation of potassium in Müller cells as well as in the extracellular space resulting in increased intracellular and extracellular osmotic pressures. The extracellular accumulation of neuron-derived excess potassium will osmotically pull water from the blood and vitreous into the retinal parenchyma resulting in extracellular edema (Figs. 26B,C,E, 70, 71), and the intracellular accumulation of potassium will osmotically pull water into the perivascular and endfeet regions of Müller cells, resulting in Müller cell swelling (Fig. 69B) and edematous Müller cell degeneration (Fig. 54B; see 5.11.5.). Intra- and extracellular edema are observed, for example, after one day of experimental detachment of the porcine retina (Fig. 26A–E); intracellular edema (associated with mitochondrial swelling) is apparent in Müller cells and single neurons in the ganglion cell and inner nuclear layers (Fig. 26A,D) (Jackson et al., 2003; Hollborn et al., 2008). The downregulation of perivascular Kir4.1 under pathological conditions (see 5.5.3.5) results in an uncoupling of the AQP4-mediated water transport from the potassium currents around the deep retinal vessels (Figs. 8C, 15A, B, 19) which facilitates the osmotic water flux across the glio-vascular interface into Müller cells (Bringmann et al., 2004). The assumption that the downregulation of glial Kir4.1 contributes to the development of extracellular retinal edema is supported by the colocalization of the main potassium secretion sites of Müller cells and of intraretinal edematous cysts (Fig. 20C; see 5.11.5.). Because retinal detachment is usually not associated with vascular leakage, the fluid accumulation in the detached retina (Figs. 20A,B, 26A–E, 54A) is suggested to be primarily caused by the dysregulation of the fluid absorption through Müller cells (Wurm et al., 2006a). A disturbance of the Müller cell-mediated water absorption from the retinal tissue, and an osmotic swelling of Müller cells, may underlie the edema formation in the ischemic retina within days after reperfusion. In the ischemic-hypoxic retina, there is a close relationship between the localization of AQP4 and of cystoid spaces in the outer retina (Figs. 19, 20A–C) (Rehak et al., 2009). However, it is unclear whether the water flux through AQP4 contributes to the formation or resolution of edema. Deletion of Dp71 in mice results in a mislocation of Kir4.1 and a downregulation of AQP4, and is asscociated with increased retinal vascular permeability (Sene et al., 2009). In the brain, the water transport through glial AQP4 is implicated in both the development of cytotoxic edema (i.e., astrocyte swelling) and resolution of vasogenic edema (Manley et al., 2000; Papadopoulos et al., 2004).

5.11.9.2 Cytotoxic Edema

The increase of the retinal water content during an ischemic episode is accompanied by a progressive thickening of the inner retina while the photoreceptor layer remains unaffected (Stefánsson et al.,

1987; Szabo et al., 1991). This suggests that the early ischemic edema is caused by over-excitation of glutamatergic synapses resulting in a swelling of inner retinal neurons (see 5.5.1.1.). However, the biphasic elevation of the retinal water content during ischemia-reperfusion (Stefánsson et al., 1987) suggests that different mechanisms are involved in edema formation in early and late phases after reperfusion. It was suggested that the early phase of retinal water accumulation is caused by glutamate-induced swelling of retinal neurons, whereas the late phase of water accumulation is caused by a disturbance of the Müller cell-mediated water homeostasis and water accumulation in glial cells (Bringmann et al., 2005; Reichenbach et al., 2007). This assumption is supported by various experimental and clinical observations. During ischemic episodes of the rabbit retina, both plexiform layers and the cytoplasm of neuronal cells become edematous while the Müller cells appear to be unaffected, whereas in the postischemic tissue, neural elements degenerate and Müller cells become edematous (Johnson, 1974). In diabetic retinopathy, the swelling of ganglion cell bodies and their processes precedes the loss of these cells and the gliosis of the inner retinal layers (Duke-Elder and Dobree, 1967). Although in the retina of hypoxic rats, hypertrophy of astrocytes and Müller cells is observed as early as 3 h after hypoxia, swollen Müller cell processes with a loss of cytoplasmic organelles resulting in vacuolated appearance is seen three days after hypoxic exposure (Kaur et al., 2007).

5.11.9.2.1 Neuronal Cell Swelling   Neuronal degeneration in the ischemic retina is predominantly attributed to the formation of damaging oxygen free radicals (Stefánsson et al., 1987; Block and Schwarz, 1997; Muller et al., 1997; Szabo et al., 1991, 1997) and to the cytotoxicity of excessively released glutamate (Lucas and Newhouse, 1957; Louzada-Junior et al., 1992; Osborne et al., 2004). Intravitreal administration of AMPA/KA or NMDA receptor agonists results in swelling and vacuolization of different retinal layers (Sahel et al., 1991). Metabolic stress and ischemia causes an excessive release of glutamate from overstimulated neurons resulting in sodium, chloride, and water influx into the postsynaptic structures and neuronal cell swelling (Fig. 3C) (Zeevalk and Nicklas, 1997; Izumi et al., 2003; Osborne et al., 2004; Uckermann et al., 2004b). The ischemic neuronal cell swelling results in a thickening of the inner retinal tissue (Fig. 3F). Removal of sodium or blockade of chloride channels fully inhibits the glutamate toxicity in the retina (Olney et al., 1986; Zeevalk et al., 1989). Overstimulation of ionotropic glutamate receptors during an ischemic episode results in long-term depolarization of retinal neurons that causes an opening of voltage-gated calcium channels leading to neuronal calcium overload (Fig. 40C). The long-lasting intracellular calcium overload activates the apoptosis machinery of the cells resulting in neuronal cell death. The swelling of retinal neurons is mainly mediated by a sodium flux through ionotropic glutamate receptors associated with a water flux (see 5.5.1.1.). The ischemic water accumulation in the retinal tissue is induced by oxidative stress (Stefánsson et al., 1987; Szabo et al., 1991). It has been shown that under euglycemic and normoxic conditions, glutamate is not neurotoxic in the retina but causes glial cell swelling (Izumi et al., 2003). However, under ischemic conditions, glutamate produces severe neuronal swelling and neurodegeneration (Izumi et al., 2003).

Further factors may contribute to the osmotic swelling of retinal neurons. Neuronal activity is associated with rapid ion shifts between intra- and extracellular spaces which cause osmotic imbalances in the retinal tissue. Intense neuronal activity in the retina causes a decrease in the osmolarity of the extracellular fluid (see 5.5.1.1.). It has been shown that bipolar cells, but not Müller cells, swell in the presence of a hypoosmotic environment (Vogler et al., 2013a; Garcia et al., 2014). Diabetic retinopathy is characterized by an increased polyol pathway flux of glucose which results in increased intracellular sorbitol levels (Dagher et al., 2004; Obrosova and Kador, 2011). Sorbitol does not diffuse easily through cell membranes and accumulates intracellularly, causing osmotic damage. Inhibition of the sorbitol production decreases the diabetic retinal swelling and prevents the apoptotic death of retinal neurons (Asnaghi et al., 2003; Yeung et al., 2010). The increased glucose flux through the polyol pathway decreases the activity of the sodium-potassium-ATPase. This results from the activation of PKC and the increase of the cytosolic PLA_2 activity which increases the production of arachidonic acid and PGE_2 (Xia et al., 1995), two inhibitors of the sodium-potassium-ATPase (Lees, 1991; Staub et al., 1994; Owada et al., 1999). The net sodium influx which results from the inhibition of the sodium-potassium-ATPase increases the intracellular osmotic pressure. Hypertension, a risk factor of neovascular retinal diseases such as diabetic retinopathy and wet AMD (Bringmann et al., 2014), is associated with an edematous degeneration of retinal neurons. It has been shown that high salt intake, a major cause of hypertension (Bringmann et al., 2014), induces a swelling of retinal ganglion cells (Qin et al., 2009a).

Müller cells contribute to the neuronal cell swelling and degeneration, for example, by the malfunction of the glial glutamate uptake (see 5.5.2.1.6.) and the downregulation of Kir4.1 potassium channels (see 5.5.3.5.) which impair the resolution of osmotic gradients and the spatial buffering of excess potassium resulting in neuronal hyperexcitation. Moreover, a release of glutamate from Müller cells induces a swelling of retinal neurons (Figs. 39B, 74E; see 5.6.1.3.). For osmotical reasons, the ion currents through ionotropic receptors and voltage-gated ion channels are coupled to a water flux. Müller cells may also contribute to the glutamate-induced swelling and degeneration of retinal neurons by providing the water required for the rapid ion flux into activated neurons (see 5.5.4.6.). Because synapses are closely ensheathed by Müller cell membranes, the water that flows into the synapses will be delivered predominantly from the Müller cell interior through AQP4 water channels (Bringmann et al., 2005). An inhibition of the rapid water transport through Müller cells should delay the ion flux into neurons, resulting in lower levels of neuronal cell swelling and apoptosis. Indeed, disruption of the AQP4 gene in mice protects against impaired retinal function and neuronal cell death after retinal ischemia (Da and Verkman, 2004). Thus, neuronal cell swelling and apoptosis in the ischemic retina is suggested to be supported by the Müller cell-mediated water transport (Bringmann et al., 2005). In retinas of hypoxic rats, an increase in the gene and protein expression of AQP4 is observed as early as 3 h after hypoxic exposure (Kaur et al., 2007; but see 5.5.4.4.).

5.11.9.2.2 Glial Cell Swelling

Glutamate-induced rapid ion and water shifts between intra- and extracellular spaces will influence the osmohomeostasis of the tissue; the intracellular osmolarity of Müller cells will increase due to the uptake of potassium ions and neurotransmitter molecules (which is associated with an influx of sodium ions via electrogenic uptake carriers; see 5.5.2.1.3. and 5.5.2.2.1.) and the decreased activity of the sodium-potassium-ATPase under diabetic conditions, for example (see 5.5.2.1.6.). Under normal conditions, an increase of the intracellular osmolarity is balanced by the efflux of potassium ions through Kir4.1 channels into the blood and vitreous fluid. Therefore, functional Kir4.1 channels are one prerequisite for the capability of Müller cells to held their volume constant despite variations in the extra- and intracellular osmolarity (see 5.5.5.1.).

By the transcellular transport of water and osmolytes, in particular potassium, Müller cells also compensate osmotic imbalances within the retinal tissue and across the glio-vascular interface. In animal models of various ischemic-hypoxic and inflammatory retinopathies including retinal ischemia-reperfusion, diabetic retinopathy, retinal vein occlusion, ocular inflammation, retinal detachment, blue light-induced retinal degeneration, and inherited photoreceptor degeneration, as well as in the detached human retina, an alteration of the osmotic swelling properties of Müller cells was observed (see 5.5.5.). While Müller cells in adult healthy retinas held their volume constant for up to 10-15 min when the osmolarity of the extracellular medium is abruptly decreased (Figs. 50A, 57D) (Uckermann et al., 2006; Hirrlinger et al., 2008; Lipp et al., 2009; Wurm et al., 2010; Brückner et al., 2012), Müller cells in diseased retinas promptly swell upon hypoosmotic challenge (Figs. 8I, 12M, 21E, 23F,G, 50A,B, 57F, 61C,E, 73A) (Pannicke et al., 2004, 2005b, 2006; Uckermann et al., 2006; Weuste et al., 2006; Wurm et al., 2006a,b, 2008a,b, 2011a; Iandiev et al., 2006b, 2008a; Kuhrt et al., 2008; Rehak et al., 2009; Krügel et al., 2010, 2011; Neumann et al., 2010; Grosche et al., 2012; Vogler et al., 2013b; Garcia et al., 2014). Apparently, induction of Müller cell swelling is a general phenomenon under conditions associated with osmotic pertubations, oxidative stress, and inflammation. The change in the osmotic swelling characteristics of Müller cells suggests that the transglial water transport driven by osmotic gradients is dysregulated.

Whether an intracellular edema or even a swelling of Müller cells contribute to macular edema remains controversial. Early electron microscopic studies suggested that Müller cell swelling is apparent in cystoid macular edema, in particular in cases without significant angiographic vascular leakage, and that the cysts are formed by swollen and dying Müller cells (Fine and Brucker, 1981; Yanoff et al., 1984). The swelling of Müller cells was suggested to precede the development of extracellular edema (Yanoff et al., 1984). Dominantly inherited cystoid macular edema was suggested to be a primary Müller cell disease because degenerated Müller cells and altered basement membranes were found around virtually intact retinal vascular endothelia (Loeffler et al., 1992). A similar situation was described for the brain where the ischemic edema is characterized by a swelling of perivascular astroglial processes (Kimelberg, 2005). However, later studies disagreed with the assumption that a swelling of Müller cells contributes to the cystic degeneration of the diabetic retina (Gass et al., 1985). On the other hand, it has been shown that experimental diabetic retinopathy is associated with a water accumulation within Müller cells and in the interstitial space of the retina resulting in extended extracellular spaces in the inner and outer nuclear layers and edematous Müller cell endfeet, as well as swollen and degenerated perivascular processes of Müller cells (Kumar et al., 2013b, 2014). A similar water accumulation within Müller cells was found in animal models of retinal hypoxia-ischemia (Stepinac et al., 2005; Kaur et al., 2007). However, Müller cell edema is apparent at the electron microscopical, but not light microscopical level (Kumar et al., 2013b). This is in agreement with a recent study that showed that retinal edema in diabetic rats is recognizable with magnetic resonance imaging but not histologically on sections of fixed and dehydrated retinas (Berkowitz et al., 2012). Retinal light injury is characterized by a degeneration of photoreceptor and pigment epithelial cells, as well as by a swelling and vacuolization of Müller cells (Berler, 1989; Green and Robertson, 1991).

Although intracellular edema of Müller cells caused by water accumulation within the cells was described to occur in animal models of ischemic and diabetic retinopathies (Kaur et al., 2007; Kumar et al., 2013b, 2014), a swelling of Müller cells in the diabetic retina was rarely observed. This may suggest that endogenous mechanisms are present that inhibit the swelling of Müller cells despite the presence of osmotic gradients that favor water influx into the cells. Although the osmotic/mechanical release of ATP is abrogated in Müller cells of diabetic retinas, the receptor ligand-induced inhibition of osmotic swelling is functional (see 5.5.5.3.2.). Many of the receptor ligands which were shown to inhibit osmotic Müller cell swelling (see 5.5.5.3.) including VEGF, HB-EGF, NPY, and natriuretic peptides are upregulated in the ischemic retina (Yoon et al., 2002; Weuste et al., 2006; Kalisch et al., 2006; Rehak et al., 2009). Thus, the receptor ligand-induced inhibition may represent one reason for the fact that Müller cells do not swell despite the presence of intracellular edema.

5.11.9.2.3 Mechanisms of Osmotic Müller cell swelling   Water influx into Müller cells occurs when the intracellular osmotic pressure is increased compared to the osmotic pressure of the extracellular fluid, blood, and vitreous. Under normal conditions, Müller cells are surrounded by a hypoosmotic environment during periods of intense neuronal activity (see 5.5.1.1.). In addition, the uptake of neuron-derived osmolytes such as potassium and sodium-glutamate increases the osmotic pressure of the Müller cell interior relative to the extracellular fluid (Izumi et al., 1996, 1999; Pannicke et al., 2004). Thus, neuronal activity in the retina generates an osmotic gradient that favors water flux from extracellular to intracellular spaces. The osmotic gradients across the Müller cell membrane are exacerbated under pathological conditions which are characterized by glutamate-induced hyperexcitation and an impairment of Müller cells to redistribute osmolytes such as potassium. A decrease of the blood osmolarity, e.g., in cases of hyponatremia and hypoalbuminemia, produces an osmotic gradient across the glio-vascular interface resulting in intracellular edema and a swelling of perivascular glial processes (Manley et al., 2000; Berkowitz et al., 2012). Both, an increase in the osmolarity of the Müller cell interior and a decrease in blood osmolarity pull water from the blood into the perivascular processes of Müller cells, resulting in cytotoxic edema.

Passive potassium currents through Kir4.1 channels are crucially involved in the homeostasis of the Müller cell volume under varying osmotic conditions. Prompt transmembraneous potassium currents through Kir4.1 channels compensate osmotic gradients across the Müller cell membrane and thus prevent cellular swelling (see 5.5.5.1.). In most cases, reactive oxygen radicals and inflammatory lipids which inhibit the sodium-potassium-ATPase are the final mediators of the osmotic Müller cell swelling; inhibition of the sodium-potassium-ATPase results in intracellular sodium overload (see below). A decrease of the activity of the sodium-potassium-ATPase is a characteristic of retinal diseases associated with oxidative stress and inflammation (see 5.5.2.1.6.). Under pathological conditions when the Kir4.1 channels are downregulated or functionally inactivated (see 5.5.3.5.), the intracellular sodium overload cannot be rapidly compensated by a passive potassium efflux through Kir4.1 channels; this results in an increase of the intracellular osmotic pressure which pulls water into the cells. (This situation is aggravated by the abrogation of the purinergic signaling cascade that normally regulates the Müller cell volume under hypoosmotic conditions via opening of potassium and chloride channels; see 5.5.5.3.2.) A long-lasting influx of sodium ions driven by sodium-dependent glutamate transporters contributes to the increase of the intracellular sodium level (Casper et al., 1982; Izumi et al., 1996). Further mechanisms, e.g., endocytosis of serum proteins (Fig. 21C; see 5.11.1.1.) and an increased expression of AQP4 (Rama Rao et al., 2003; Kaur et al., 2007; Zou et al., 2009), may contribute to a water accumulation in Müller cells. Because the retinal glucose uptake and metabolism occurs predominantly in Müller cells (see 5.5.7.1.), accumulation of sorbitol, produced by the polyol pathway, will increase the intracellular osmotic pressure of Müller cells under diabetic conditions. Deficiency of the aldose reductase protects from diabetic retinal swelling which is correlated with a less expression of AQP4 (Yeung et al., 2010). The age-dependent decrease in the potassium conductance of Müller cells (Fig. 45D) (Bringmann et al., 2003c) may contribute to the higher incidence of retinal edema in the elderly.

The final steps in the induction of osmotic Müller cell swelling are mediated by oxidative-nitrosative stress and activation of enzymes that produce inflammatory lipid mediators (Figs. 35C, 69B) (Uckermann et al., 2005c; Pannicke et al., 2006; Wurm et al., 2006a,b, 2008b; Iandiev et al., 2008a; Krügel et al., 2011; Karl et al., 2011). The osmotic swelling of Müller cells is prevented when the activity of PLA_2 (that forms arachidonic acid) or of cyclooxygenases (that forms prostaglandins) are pharmacologically blocked, or when the oxidative stress level is decreased by reducing agents. Conversely, acute administration of arachidonic acid, PGE_2, hydrogen peroxide, or of a NO donor causes osmotic swelling of Müller cells in retinas of healthy adult animals (Uckermann et al., 2005c; Pannicke et al., 2006; Krügel et al., 2011; Vogler et al., 2013b). Arachidonic acid and its metabolites, in particular PGE_2, are major mediators of retinal edema (Guex-Crosier, 1999; Miyake and Ibaraki, 2002). Osmotic stress is known to induce activation of various enzymes that produce reactive oxygen and nitrogen species including xanthine oxidase, NADPH oxidases, and NO synthases (Du et al., 2004; Offer et al., 2005; Bedard and Krause, 2007). Osmotic and oxidative stresses induce an increased activity of PLA_2, resulting in peroxidation of membrane lipids and the release of arachidonic acid (Birkle and Bazan, 1989; Davidge et al., 1995; Lambert et al., 2006; Balboa and Balsinde, 2006). Free radicals, hydroperoxides, NO, and peroxynitrite stimulate also the activities of lipoxygenases and cyclooxygenases (Asano et al., 1987; Landino et al., 1996; Du et al., 2004). Ischemic retinopathies are characterized by an increased arachidonic acid metabolism (Hardy et al., 2005). The retinal expression of the cyclooxygenase-2 increases early under pathological conditions (Fig. 12H), e.g., in diabetic retinopathy (Joussen et al., 2001; Du et al., 2004). Retinal glial cells increase the expression of cyclooxygenase-2 under various conditions including retinal detachment (Fig. 12H-J), retinal ischemia, and diabetes (Ju et al., 2003; Nakamichi et al., 2003; Sennlaub et al., 2003; Wurm et al., 2006a). Arachidonic acid and prostaglandins potently inhibit the sodium-potassium-ATPase which leads to intracellular sodium overload and cellular swelling (Lees, 1991; Staub et al., 1994; Owada et al., 1999). Arachidonic acid also blocks membrane channels such as volume-regulated anion and outwardly rectifying K_A and K_{DR} channels (Lambert, 1991; Sanchez-Olea et al., 1995; Bringmann et al., 1998b) which otherwise mediate a compensatory efflux of osmolytes such as amino acids, chloride, and potassium. Because extracellular sodium-free conditions prevent the osmotic swelling (Uckermann et al., 2006), the intracellular sodium overload induced by arachidonic acid and prostaglandins is a major mechanism of Müller cell swelling.

One consequence of oxidative stress is the activation of the mitochondrial permeability transition that leads to mitochondrial dysfunction, energy failure, and enhanced free radical production. Dysfunctional mitochondria are also a major source of superoxide radicals and hydrogen peroxide.

Mitochondrial dysfunction plays a significant role in the pathogenesis of ischemic-hypoxic retinal diseases, e.g., diabetic retinopathy (Nishikawa et al., 2000; Du et al., 2003; Kowluru and Abbas, 2003; Kowluru, 2005; Brownlee, 2005; Kowluru et al., 2006; Silva et al., 2009). A swelling of Müller cell mitochondria was observed after one day of experimental detachment of the porcine retina (Jackson et al., 2003). A swelling of retinal glial cell mitochondria was also observed after high salt intake which causes hypertension (Qin et al., 2009a). Hyperglycemia increases the mitochondrial superoxide production in the retina; inhibition of superoxides attenuates the glucose-induced mitochondrial dysfunction and the apoptotic death of retinal capillary cells (Du et al., 2003; Kowluru, 2005; Kowluru et al., 2006). Oxidative stress resulting from mitochondrial dysfunction is also a main factor involved in the induction of osmotic Müller cell swelling in animal models of diabetic and hepatic retinopathies (Figs. 35C, 69B) (Krügel et al., 2011; Karl et al., 2011; see 5.5.2.1.14.). Blockade of the mitochondrial free radical formation or of the mitochondrial permeability transition prevent the swelling (Krügel et al., 2011; Karl et al., 2011). In addition, superoxide produced by xanthine oxidases and NADPH oxidases may be implicated in the induction of osmotic Müller cell swelling (Fig. 69B) (Krügel et al., 2011; Vogler et al., 2013b). The barium-induced swelling of Müller cells (see 5.5.5.1.) is also inhibited by the blockade of NO synthases and by peroxynitrite scavengers (Krügel et al., 2011; Karl et al., 2011; Vogler et al., 2013b).

Osteopontin inhibits the hypoosmotic swelling of Müller cells induced by hydrogen peroxide but not by NO and the mitochondrial complex I inhibitor rotenone, suggesting that osteopontin inhibits the cytosolic but not the mitochondrial generation of reactive oxygen species (Wahl et al., 2013). Osteopontin also prevents the barium-induced swelling of Müller cells (Wahl et al., 2013). It has been shown that barium ions do not alter the inner mitochondrial membrane potential in Müller cells (Karl et al., 2011). Because dissipation of this potential is a consequence of mitochondrial oxidative stress, barium ions apparently do not induce generation of reactive oxygen species in the mitochondria. Instead, the barium-induced swelling is (at least in part) mediated by activation of xanthine and NADPH oxidases (Fig. 69B). Activation of NO synthases are also involved in the barium-induced osmotic Müller cell swelling (Krügel et al., 2011; Karl et al., 2011; Vogler et al., 2013b). It may be assumed that osteopontin inhibits the activities of NO synthases (but not the action of NO), xanthine oxidases, and NADPH oxidases.

5.11.9.3 Link between Vasogenic and Cytotoxic Edema

Vasogenic edema usually occurs concomitantly with cytotoxic edema of retinal glial cells (Fine and Brucker, 1981; Yanoff et al., 1984; Stepinac et al., 2005; Bringmann et al., 2005). Hypoxia-reoxygenation induces both vasogenic edema and cytotoxic edema indicated by the swelling of astrocytes and Müller cell processes (Kaur et al., 2007). The relative contribution of vasogenic edema and dysfunction of Müller cells (or even Müller cell swelling) to the formation of retinal edema may vary in dependence on the specific conditions in individual patients. Various soluble factors link vascular leakage and Müller cell swelling. Blood constituents including thrombin and glutamate (a constituent of blood plasma) close Kir channels (see 5.5.3.5.). Increased vascular permeability is associated with extravasation of albumin. Serum albumin is a multifunctional protein with neuro- and vasoprotective properties (Emerson, 1989; Zoellner et al., 1996; Belayev et al., 2001). However, albumin may have also detrimental effects in the neural tissue such as induction of hyperexcitability and epileptiform activity (Ivens et al., 2007). It has been shown that serum albumin induces Müller cell swelling in the presence of osmotic gradients (Löffler et al., 2010). Albumin activates the TGF-ß receptor type II (Fig. 69B); activation of the receptor results in oxidative stress, the production of arachidonic acid and prostaglandins, and intracellular sodium overload (Löffler et al., 2010). Albumin is internalized by Müller cells via receptor-mediated endocytosis (Löffler et al., 2010). Endocytosis is known to be associated with the generation of oxygen radicals and activation of PLA_2 (Lennartz, 1999; Whaley-Connell et al., 2007).

5.11.9.4 Resolution of Edema

Retinal edema is a major cause of neuronal degeneration and visual deterioration (Bresnick, 1983; Rothova et al., 1996; Fong et al., 2004; Larsen et al., 2005; Joussen et al., 2007), and removal of extraneous fluid in retinal edema aids in restoration of vision (Kent et al., 2000). Edema can be resolved by inhibition of vascular leakage and/or stimulation of the fluid clearance from the tissue. Vascular leakage is mainly caused by VEGF and inflammatory mediators (Figs. 69B, 70), and antiinflammatory substances as well as agents that inhibit the formation or action of VEGF are effective in the resolution of edema. However, at present, there is no established neuroprotective treatment that avoids visual disturbance in patients with diabetic retinopathy, for example. Common treatments of diabetic retinopathy include laser photocoagulation to improve tissue oxygenation, intravitreal corticosteroids to reduce inflammation, intravitreal anti-VEGF agents, and vitreoretinal surgery, i.e., the removal of the posterior hyaloid and the inner limiting membrane (Michels, 1978; Gandorfer et al., 2000; Gillies et al., 2006; Eichler et al., 2006; Fraser-Bell et al., 2008; Elman et al., 2011; Witkin and Brown, 2011).

VEGF is the main factor which induces vascular leakage and neovascularization (see 5.11.8. and 5.11.9.1.1.), and intravitreal administration of anti-VEGF agents is one major strategy to resolve retinal edema and choroidal neovascularization (Eichler et al., 2006; Elman et al., 2011). VEGF inhibitors which are clinically administered into the vitreal chamber, e.g., bevacizumab (Avastin), bind VEGF and thus reduce the level of free VEGF in the retina. Ruboxistaurin blocks the activity of PKCβ which is an intracellular mediator involved in mediating the VEGF-induced vascular permeability (Aiello, 2002). However, because VEGF is also a prosurvival factor of vascular endothelial, glial, and neuronal cells (see 5.11.1.1.), trapping of VEGF or inhibition of VEGF signaling might present a risk to neuronal survival (Foxton et al., 2013). Nevertheless, intravitreal bevacizumab, a full-length humanized monoclonal IgG antibody that recognizes all VEGF isoforms, was described to have no effects on the retinal structure and does not induce gliosis or apoptosis in the porcine retina (Iandiev et al., 2011b). Intravitreal bevacizumab decreases the expression of VEGF and increases the expression of Kir4.1 in the porcine retina, suggesting that it might be protective against both vasogenic and cytotoxic edema, and that it may improve the Müller cell-mediated fluid clearance from the retinal tissue (Iandiev et al., 2011b). Because VEGF is a proinflammatory factor, trapping of VEGF might reduce the level of retinal inflammation resulting in increased expression of Kir4.1 and decreased expression of VEGF. Indeed, it was found that anti-VEGF agents strongly reduce the retinal level of IL-1β in a rat model of retinal ischemia (Drechsler et al., 2012). However, bevacizumab was recently shown to cause vein thrombosis and glial cell activation in the retina (Schraermeyer and Julien, 2013).

Antiinflammatory corticosteroids like triamcinolone acetonide (9α-fluoro-16α-hydroxyprednisolone) are clinically used for the rapid resolution of retinal edema (Fraser-Bell et al., 2008). Steroids are effective in preventing vasogenic edema and inflammation. Triamcinolone reduces vascular permeability (Ando et al., 1994; Sakamoto et al., 2002; Edelman et al., 2005; Tamura et al., 2005), the vitreal level of VEGF (Brooks et al., 2004), the expression and secretion of VEGF by vascular smooth muscle cells and retinal cells including Müller cells (Nauck et al., 1998; Matsuda et al., 2005; Sears and Hoppe, 2005; Itakura et al., 2006), the cellular effects of VEGF, for example the VEGF-induced secretion of MMPs (Hollborn et al., 2007), the inflammatory expression of endothelial adhesion molecules (Penfold et al., 2000), and the leukocyte-endothelial interaction in the diabetic retina (Tamura et al., 2005), and increases the retinal level of tight junction proteins (McAllister et al., 2009). Triamcinolone inhibits the overexpression of VEGF without affecting its basal expression in the normal retina (Shen et al., 2014a). Steroids are also effective in the resolution of retinal edema in cases not associated with angiographic vascular leakage, suggesting that they (in addition to the prevention of vasogenic edema) also inhibit cytotoxic edema and/or may improve the fluid clearance from the retinal tissue, e.g., by upregulation of Kir4.1 and AQP4 (Zhao et al., 2010). It has been shown that triamcinolone acetonide induces a rapid reduction of the retinal edema that is evident as early as 1 h after intravitreal administration (Miyamoto et al., 2006; Sonoda et al., 2011). This time pattern cannot be explained by an alteration of the gene expression (which requires several hours) and suggests that nongenomic, receptor-dependent mechanisms are involved in the therapeutic effect of triamcinolone (Miyamoto et al., 2006). It was suggested that triamcinolone reduces the hydrostatic pressure in the capillaries by inducing vasoconstriction (Stefánsson, 2007). Triamcinolone acetonide also prevents the osmotic swelling of Müller cells from diabetic animals, the swelling of Müller cells in animal models of retinal ischemia, hypoxia, and inflammation (Uckermann et al., 2005c; Wurm et al., 2006a, 2008b; Iandiev et al., 2008a), as well as the swelling of Müller cells from control animals induced by oxidative stress, albumin, and the inflammatory lipids arachidonic acid and PGE_2, respectively (Uckermann et al., 2005c; Pannicke et al., 2006; Wurm et al., 2006a; Löffler et al., 2010). In addition, triamcinolone prevents the osmotic swelling of Müller cells from AQP4-deficient mice (Pannicke et al., 2010; see 5.5.5.2.). On the other hand, triamcinolone has no effect on the glutamate-induced swelling of retinal ganglion cells (Uckermann et al., 2005c). Triamcinolone activates the final steps of the swelling-inhibitory glutamatergic-purinergic signaling cascade (see 5.5.5.3.), i.e., it stimulates the nucleoside transporter-mediated release of endogenous adenosine, which in turn activates adenosine A_1 receptors resulting in opening of potassium and chloride channels (Fig. 73B) (Uckermann et al., 2005c; Wurm et al., 2008a, 2009b). In the retina of diabetic animals, the effect of triamcinolone involves the extracellular nucleotide degradation by NTPDase1 (Fig. 73B) (Wurm et al., 2008b). This suggests that triamcinolone also induces a release of ATP in the retina of diabetic animals.

The triamcinolone-induced opening of ion channels may reestablish the ion and water transport through Müller cells under conditions in which Kir4.1 channels are inactivated. (In addition, the antiinflammatory action of triamcinolone may prevent the ischemic downregulation of Kir4.1; Rehak et al., 2011.) This may improve the Müller cell-mediated fluid clearance from the edematous retinal tissue and may also protect the tissue from potassium-induced neuronal hyperexcitation (Reichenbach et al., 2007). *In situ*, the direction of the potassium currents and the associated water flux through Müller cells is determined by the potassium gradient between the tissue and blood (high potassium in the retinal parenchyma, normal potassium in the blood). A similar mechanism has been described for the retinal pigment epithelium. Here, ATP release and autocrine/paracrine stimulation of purinergic $P2Y_2$ receptors stimulates the fluid absorption from the subretinal space (Meyer et al., 2002; Maminishkis et al., 2002; Reigada and Mitchell, 2004). Receptor activation results in an increased rate of ion transport across the pigment epithelium and, thus, of the water absorption from the subretinal space. Because the clinical long-term use of triamcinolone acetonide is associated with numerous adverse side effects (Chung et al., 2007), novel drugs targeting adenosine A_1 receptors or openers of two pore-domain channels (see 5.5.5.3.) may represent promising alternatives for the resolution of retinal edema. Agonists of adenosine A_1 receptors may also more directly prevent neuronal degeneration by inhibiting neuronal hyperexcitation and inflammation (see 5.6.3.4.).

All bioactive agents that inhibit the osmotic swelling of Müller cells (see 5.5.5.3.) should also stimulate the Müller cell-mediated fluid clearance from the edematous retinal tissue. Erythropoietin is a potent neuroprotective factor in the retina (Grimm et al., 2002, 2004; Zhu et al., 2008; McVicar et al., 2011). The ocular erythropoietin level is strikingly increased in diabetic macular edema (Hernández et al., 2006). Erythropoietin has a protective effect in retinal vasogenic edema, as it inhibits vascular cell death and suppresses the permeability of the blood-retinal barrier (Zhang et al., 2008). Because erythropoietin inhibits the osmotic swelling of Müller cells (see 5.5.5.3.), it may also inhibit cytotoxic edema in the retina and might stimulate the Müller cell-mediated fluid clearance from the edematous tissue (Krügel et al., 2010). In the retina, 17β-estradiol and progesterone attenuate ischemia-reperfusion injury (Nonaka et al., 2000; Lu et al., 2008) and protect photoreceptor and ganglion cells from death (O'Steen, 1977; Kaja et al., 2003; Dykens et al., 2004; Zhou et al., 2007; Russo et al., 2008). 17β-Estradiol is a multiactive steroid with antiinflammatory, antiapoptotic, and antioxidant properties (Behl et al., 1997; Ayres et al., 1998; Jover et al., 2002; Prokai et al., 2003), and was shown to prevent vasogenic brain edema (Tomás-Camardiel et al., 2005). Progesterone alleviates brain edema after traumatic injury (Stein, 2001; Grossman et al., 2004). Sex steroids such as 17β-estradiol, estriol, progesterone, and testosterone were shown to inhibit the osmotic swelling of Müller cells in postischemic and diabetic retinal tissues (see 5.10.11.), suggesting that steroids may inhibit cytotoxic edema in the retina *in situ*, and may stimulate the Müller cell-mediated fluid clearance from the edematous tissue; both may contribute to the neuroprotective effects of sex steroids. The inhibitory effects of 17β-estradiol and estriol on the osmotic Müller cell swelling are mediated by receptor-independent mechanisms (Neumann et al., 2010). Because the generation of inflammatory lipids and oxidative stress are involved in the induction of osmotic Müller cell swelling (see 5.11.9.2.3.), the swelling-inhibitory effect of sex steroids may also result from their antiinflammatory and antioxidative action (Behl et al., 1997; Dykens et al., 2004; Kumar et al., 2005). One of the key receptor-independent mechanisms by which estrogens afford neuroprotection occurs through scavenging free radicals, resulting in decreased lipid peroxidation. Estrogens are potent antioxidants; micromolar concentrations of 17β-estradiol attenuate oxidative damage (Ayres et al., 1998). Hydrogen peroxide mimicks the edema-inducing effect of retinal ischemia-reperfusion (Stefánsson et al., 1987). Hydrogen peroxide induces a swelling of Müller cells under hypoosmotic conditions (Uckermann et al., 2005c), and formation of reactive oxygen species is a critical step in the induction of osmotic Müller cell swelling under various conditions (see 5.11.9.2.3.). It is, therefore, conceivable that radical scavengers which inhibit vascular leakage in the ischemic retina (Szabo et al., 1991) also block cytotoxic Müller cell swelling.

The water transport through Müller cells is facilitated by AQP4 water channels and appears to be essential for the swelling and apoptosis of retinal neurons in the ischemic retina (Fig. 40C;

see 5.11.9.2.1.). The death of retinal neurons in the ischemic retina may be inhibited by disruption of the water transport through Müller cells, e.g., by inhibition of AQP4 (Da and Verkman, 2004). However, because water movements through AQP4 is involved also in the resolution of edema (as shown in the brain; Papadopoulos et al., 2004), stimulation of the fluid clearance function of Müller cells via activation of osmolyte extrusion into the blood will be preferable.

The inhibitory effect of triamcinolone on the osmotic swelling of Müller cells from AQP4-deficient mice (Pannicke et al., 2010) suggest that triamcinolone and adenosine may also have protective effects in neuromyelitis optica. Neuromyelitis optica is caused by complement-activating serum antibodies to AQP4 (Lennon et al., 2005; Takahashi et al., 2007a; Roemer et al., 2007) that induce endocytosis of AQP4 in glial cells (Hinson et al., 2008) resulting in glial degeneration and tissue edema, for example, in the optic nerve and the retinal nerve fiber layer (Wingerchuk et al., 2007; Plant, 2008). The particular susceptibility of the retinal nerve fiber layer to anti-AQP4 antibodies could be explained by the enrichment of AQP4 at the inner limiting membrane and within the nerve fiber/ganglion cell layers, and by the particular sensitivity to pathogenic stimuli of glial cells that surround the superficial vessels of the retina (Iandiev et al., 2006a).

5.11.10 MÜLLER CELL PROLIFERATION

Unlike neurons, glial cells have the live-long capability to dedifferentiate und reenter the proliferation cycle. Müller cell proliferation commonly occurs in response to retinal injury (Bringmann et al., 2009b; Jadhav et al., 2009). Under most pathological conditions, Müller cells display a transient short-term and low-level proliferation (Bringmann et al., 2009). However, in proliferative retinopathies, Müller cells display a massive long-term proliferation resulting in the formation of periretinal membranes. Aberrant proliferation of retinal glial cells is a major causative factor for the formation of fibroproliferative tissues associated with PVR and PDR (Laqua and Machemer, 1975; Van Horn et al., 1977; Hiscott et al., 1984; Nork et al., 1986, 1987; Hui et al., 1988; Guerin et al., 1990; Vinores et al., 1990b; Stödtler et al., 1994; Cantó Soler et al., 2002b; Sethi et al., 2005). Periretinal fibroproliferative membranes represent one type of glial scars and protect the retinal tissue from pathogenic factors present in the vitreous and the injured retinal pigment epithelium (Bringmann and Wiedemann, 2009). Contraction of epiretinal membranes results in retinal detachment and aggravation of the disease process (see 5.11.11.). Therefore, inhibition of glial proliferation associated with massive gliosis is a major clinical aim when attempting to prevent blindness. PVR and PDR are commonly treated with vitreoretinal surgery, while an effective pharmacological therapy of PVR is still missing. Approaches with general inhibitors of cellular proliferation and growth factor action (De Souza et al., 1995; Wiedemann et al., 1998) remained unsatisfying. The involvement of a multitude of different cellular and soluble factors in the development of PVR, including growth and inflammatory factors, serum, fibrin, hemoglobin, iron, MMPs, mechanical stress, etc. (Bringmann and Wiedemann, 2009), makes it rather unlikely that pharmacological inhibition of a few growth factors will be effective in preventing PVR.

Most knowledge regarding factors that regulate Müller cell proliferation was obtained in cultured cells (Fig. 83A, B). Results obtained in cultured cells may reflect properties of glial proliferation in reactive gliosis *in situ* (Wakakura and Foulds, 1988). For example, cultured Müller cells and Müller cells from patients with proliferative retinopathies display similar alterations in their plasma membrane characteristics, e.g., decreased Kir currents and cell membrane depolarization (Kuhrt et al., 2008; Wurm et al., 2009b; see 5.11.10.2.). Distinct proteins, e.g., Thy-1, which is normally expressed by retinal ganglion cells, are expressed by Müller cells after ganglion cell death *in situ* and in pure Müller cell cultures (Dabin and Barnstable, 1995). Cultured Müller cells change their morphology from a radial to a flat shape (Fig. 83A). Porcine Müller cells cultured for more than 3 days display a downregulation of proteins involved in specific physiological functions, such as glycolysis, transmitter recycling, carbon dioxide siphoning, visual pigment cycle, and detoxification, while cytoskeletal proteins and proteins involved in motility and proliferation are upregulated (Hauck et al., 2003). Cell separation decreases the glutamine synthetase expression, for example (Oren et al., 1999).

Another similarity between proliferating Müller cells *in situ* and *in vitro* is the transdifferentiation into contractile myofibrocytes (Guidry, 1996, 2005, 2009; see 5.11.11.2.). This transdifferentiation is characterized by a reduction of Müller cell-specific proteins such as GFAP, vimentin, carbonic anhydrase, glutamine synthetase, and CRALBP, while proteins involved in motility and proliferation such as α-smooth muscle actin are upregulated (Hui et al., 1988; Sramek et al., 1989; McGillem et al., 1998; McGillem and Dacheux, 1999; Guidry, 2005; Abrahan et al., 2009). Moreover, Müller cells in culture display a distinct transdifferentiation into neuron-like cells which is also observed under pathological conditions *in situ* (see 5.11.12.).

5.11.10.1 Cellular Signaling Involved in Müller Cell Proliferation

Acute retinal damage induces activation of ERK1/2 and CREB and a transient expression of the immediate early genes c-Fos and Egr1, that are known to be downstream of MAPK signaling, in Müller cells (Fischer et al., 2009b). ERK1/2 are the major MAPKs implicated in the proliferation-stimulatory effects of growth factors, cytokines, and agonists of G protein-coupled receptors (Milenkovic et al., 2003; Hollborn et al., 2004b; Fischer et al., 2009b). After activation of ERK1/2 by phosphorylation of threonine and tyrosine residues through the MAPK/ERK kinase

(MEK)1/2, ERK1/2 are translocated to the cell nucleus where they activate transcription factors involved in the regulation of cell cycle proteins and the production of growth factors (Hauck et al., 2006). Activation of p38 MAPK is predominantly associated with promotion of cell migration, while activation of PI3K, a family of enzymes that phosphorylate phospholipids which engage other enzymes such as Akt, results in stimulation of the protein synthesis at the translational level. The latter pathway is involved in prosurvival signal transduction cascades and the production of growth factors and cytokines such as VEGF (Hollborn et al., 2004a,b). In dependence on the type of growth factor, activation of p38 MAPK and PI3K-Akt pathways can be also involved in the regulation of Müller cell proliferation (Milenkovic et al., 2003; Hollborn et al., 2004b, 2005).

The control of mammalian cell proliferation by extracellular signals occurs largely during the G1 phase of the cell cycle. During this phase, growth-stimulatory and -inhibitory signals transduced from the extracellular environment act on the cell cycle clock operating in the cell nucleus. This clock apparatus, composed of cyclins and their associated cyclin-dependent kinases (CDKs), may respond by directing the cell into an autonomous cell division program that carries the cells through the S, G2, and M phases or, alternatively, by causing the exit from the cell cycle into the quiescent G0 state. Once formed and activated in the G1 phase, complexes of specific cyclins and CDKs trigger the cell cycle progression by the phosphorylation of critical cellular substrate proteins. Cyclin D1 is one of the G1 cyclins which is rapidly induced upon exposure of cells to mitogens and inflammatory factors such as PGE_2 (Wang et al., 2013e). $p27^{Kip1}$ is an inhibitor of the G1 cyclin-CDK protein kinase activity. Degradation of the $p27^{Kip1}$ cyclin kinase inhibitor is required for the cellular transition from the quiescent to the proliferative state (Dyer and Cepko, 2000). In the normal mature retina, $p27^{Kip1}$ is expressed in the nuclei of Müller cells in association with cyclin D3. Following retinal injury, reactive Müller cells downregulate $p27^{Kip1}$ before they reenter the cell cycle (Dyer and Cepko, 2000). Activated ERK1/2 induces the phosphorylation and subsequent degradation of $p27^{Kip1}$, and the expression of cyclin D1 and of the proliferating cell nuclear antigen (PCNA) in the nuclei of reactive Müller cells (Yoshida et al., 2004b; Kase et al., 2006). In cases of non-proliferative gliosis, cyclin D3 is quickly downregulated. The downregulation of cyclin D3 is associated with an exit from mitosis which prevents uncontrolled proliferation of Müller cells (Dyer and Cepko, 2000). In retinas of mice lacking $p27^{Kip1}$, a widespread reactive gliosis is observed in the absence of any injury (Dyer and Cepko, 2000; Levine et al., 2000).

The immediate early gene products c-Jun and c-Fos are components of the AP-1 complex of transcription factors which is involved in the control of genes that regulate cellular proliferation (Angel and Karin, 1991). Müller cells *in situ* display c-Fos gene expression within 30 minutes after retinal injury (Fig. 82A) (Yoshida et al., 1995). Dissociation of the retinal tissue into separated cells results in a rapid increase of the c-Jun expression and stimulation of glial cell proliferation.

In the neural retina, various growth factors such as bFGF, EGF, TGF-α, and NGF stimulate the expression of c-Jun selectively in Müller cells (Sagar et al., 1991; Kruchkova et al., 2001). The cell type-specific activation of the c-Jun-signaling pathway may underlie (at least in part) the fact why differentiated neurons lose the capability to proliferate whereas glial cells do not. Activation of ERK2 is involved in the induction of c-Fos. The inverse relation between Müller cell proliferation and expression of proteins involved in neuron-glia symbiosis is regulated (at least in part) by the level of c-Jun protein (Kruchkova et al., 2001; see 5.5.2.1.11.).

5.11.10.2 Membrane Conductance of Proliferating Müller Cells

Reactive gliosis of Müller cells in proliferative retinopathies is associated with alterations of the ion channel expression and activity which support the proliferation of the cells (Bringmann et al., 2000a, 2009). The most prominent alteration is the almost complete downregulation of Kir channels, in particular Kir4.1 (Tenckhoff et al., 2005). The downregulation of Kir channels results in a loss of the inward potassium currents across the Müller cell membrane (Figs. 46A-D, 56B, 62, 63B) and a shift of the resting membrane potential from about -80 mV to -75 to -35 mV (Figs. 45E, 46A,B,D). A severe decrease of the Kir currents was found in Müller cells of patients suffering from PVR and PDR (Reichelt et al., 1997a; Francke et al., 1997; Bringmann et al., 1999b, 2001, 2002b) and in animal models of PVR (Francke et al., 2001a, 2002). The downregulation of functional Kir channels is a prerequisite for the reentry of gliotic Müller cells into the proliferation cycle (Bringmann et al., 2000a). It causes a switch from the normal stable, very negative resting membrane potential (approximately -80 mV; Figs. 8H, 45E, 46A,B,D) to a membrane condition which is basically depolarized (between -75 and -35 mV) but may become subject of rapid oscillations of the membrane potential due to openings and closures of other types of ion channels. The current pattern with an almost complete absence of Kir currents and a high activity of BK channels is reminiscent to the pattern displayed by non-differentiated glial cells early in the retinal development (Figs. 46A, 62, 63B) (Bringmann et al., 1999a, 2000a). In retinal detachment, the increase of BK currents also results from an increase of BK channel protein expression (Fig. 11A) (Bringmann et al., 2007).

Among the channels which cause rapid fluctuations of the membrane potential are depolarization-activated calcium (see 5.9.1.) and sodium channels (see 5.9.2.), and cation channels such as $P2X_7$ receptor channels (see 5.10.2.2.), which, upon activation, further depolarize the membrane, as well as K_A channels (see 5.5.3.9.) and calcium-activated BK channels (see 5.5.3.6.) which, upon opening, hyperpolarize the membrane. Müller cells of patients with PVR display an increase of the $P2X_7$ receptor currents and decreases of voltage-gated calcium currents (Bringmann et al.,

2000b, 2001). The decreases of functional voltage-gated calcium channels was suggested to be protective for the cells because it may avoid a cytotoxic calcium overload under conditions of sustained membrane depolarization (Bringmann et al., 2000b). Rapid fluctuations of the membrane potential result in increased levels of sodium and calcium in Müller cells which support the proliferation of the cells. Müller cells of patients with PVR and PDR display also a severe increase of the amplitude of voltage-gated sodium currents (Figs. 56A, 67A) compared to cells from donor eyes (Francke et al., 1996; Bringmann et al., 2002b). In cells with large voltage-gated sodium currents, depolarizing voltage steps from very negative potentials can induce action potential-like discharges (Fig. 67C) (Francke et al., 1996), suggesting that the cells transdifferentiate into a neuron-like phenotype (see 5.11.12.). Reactive gliosis is also associated with increases of the incidence and amplitude of K_A currents (Figs. 8G,H, 61B) (Bringmann et al., 1999b; Pannicke et al., 2001, 2005a,b, 2006).

The depolarization of reactive Müller cells increases the activity of BK channels; at the resting membrane potential, the BK channel activity of Müller cells from patients with PVR is ten-fold higher compared to cells from donor eyes (Figs. 60B, 62) (Bringmann et al., 1999b, 2000a). Because these channels are channels with large conductance (Fig. 56C), opening and closure of a few or even single BK channels cause rapid shifts of the actual membrane potential between the resting membrane potential (-75 to -35 mV) and the potassium equilibrium potential (-80 to -90 mV). Alternating opening of cation channels (e.g., $P2X_7$ receptor channels) and BK channels causes large changes of the membrane potential between 0 mV and the potassium equilibrium potential (-80 to -90 mV). Rapid depolarization-hyperpolarization cycles induced by the alternating activity of cation and BK channels allow the opening of voltage-gated sodium, calcium, and potassium (K_A) channels.

Both activation of BK channels and calcium influx through voltage-gated calcium channels are required for the proliferation of Müller cells induced by extracellular nucleotides, growth factors, and high extracellular potassium (Puro et al., 1989; Puro and Mano, 1991; Kodal et al., 2000; Bringmann et al., 2001; Moll et al., 2002; Milenkovic et al., 2003). BK channels act as positive feedback regulators of the calcium influx from the extracellular space through cation and voltage-gated calcium channels (Bringmann et al., 2000a). Opening of BK channels hyperpolarizes the Müller cell membrane that increases the electrochemical driving force of the calcium influx through cation channels. The rapid membrane depolarization induced by the closure of BK channels increases the open probability of voltage-gated calcium channels. The activity of BK channels prolongs the mitogen-induced calcium responses in Müller cells, e.g., calcium responses induced by ATP (Fig. 83C) and EGF (Fig. 83C,D) (Kodal et al., 2000; Moll et al., 2002). This suggests that the BK channel activity is required for the sustained calcium influx from the extracellular space through voltage-gated calcium channels (Fig. 83C,E) (Kodal et al., 2000 ; Moll et al., 2002). The resulting increase of the cytosolic free calcium stimulates the Müller cell proliferation by activation of calcium-dependent enzymes such as PKC and calpains (Moll et al., 2002). There is a correlation between the duration of the ATP-induced calcium response and the basal proliferation rate of Müller cells (Fig. 83F) (Moll et al., 2002). Shortening of the P2Y receptor-mediated intracellular calcium transients results in abrogation of the ATP-induced proliferation (Kodal et al., 2000; Moll et al., 2002). Both suggest that autocrine/paracrine stimulation of P2Y receptors is implicated in the maintenance of Müller cell proliferation.

The alterations in the membrane conductance of Müller cells, in particular the decrease of Kir currents which is associated with a depolarization of the cells, will impair the regular glial-neuronal interaction in the retina and thus may contribute to the degeneration of retinal neurons in PVR and PDR. A closure or downregulation of functional Kir channels impair the electrogenic glutamate uptake (see 5.5.2.1.6.) and the spatial buffering potassium currents which normally flow through Müller cells (see 5.5.3.), and may alter the water transport through the cells which was suggested to be (in part) coupled to the potassium currents (see 5.5.4.). An impairment of the spatial potassium buffering can result in neuronal hyperexcitability (Bringmann et al., 2006; Reichenbach et al., 2007), and an impaired glial water transport may contribute to the development of retinal edema (see 5.11.9.1.2.). An impairment of the water transport through Müller cells in PVR is also suggested by the downregulation of AQP4 Tenckhoff et al., 2005).

5.11.10.3 Purinergic Stimulation of Müller Cell Proliferation

Proliferative retinopathies are associated with an upregulation of functional purinergic receptors in Müller cells (see 5.10.2.5.). A high level of purinergic signaling is implicated in the cellular proliferation of both multipotent progenitor cells in the developing retina (see 5.10.2.4.) and reactive Müller cells in the injured retina of adult animals and man (see 5.10.2.5.). The signaling mediated by calcium-permeable $P2X_7$ receptor channels may play a role in the induction of proliferative gliosis in the human retina, while P2Y receptor-mediated signaling may stimulate the Müller cell proliferation in the retinas of various other mammalian species (Fig. 87) (Bringmann et al., 2000a, 2001; Franke et al., 2001; Moll et al., 2002). ATP and UTP, but not adenosine, stimulate the proliferation of guinea-pig Müller cells (Moll et al., 2002 ; Milenkovic et al., 2003, 2005). Activation of $P2X_7$ receptors increases the proliferation rate of human Müller cells; this effect is reversed by blocking BK channels (Bringmann et al., 2001).

A bidirectional cross-talk between P2Y receptors and growth factor receptor tyrosine kinases is involved in the proliferation-stimulatory effect of ATP in guinea-pig Müller cells. The P2Y receptor-induced proliferation of Müller cells depends upon the transactivation of receptor tyrosine

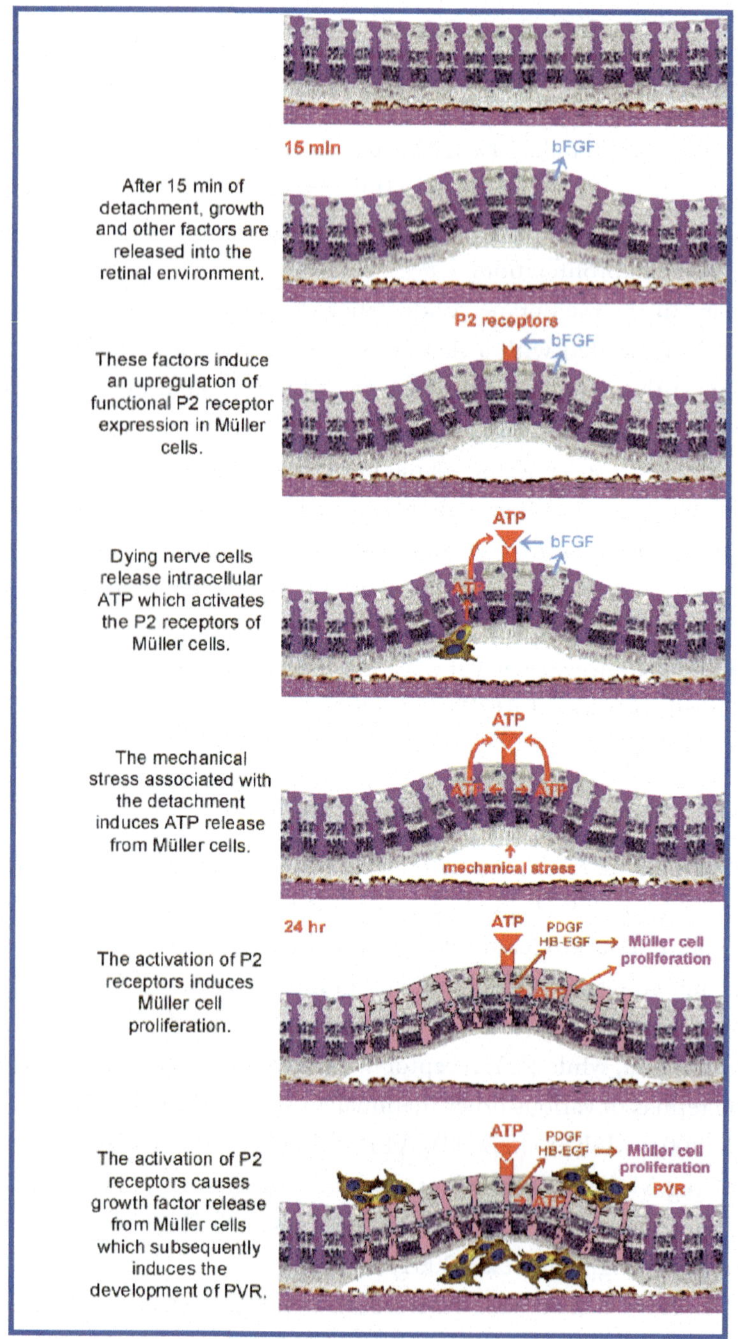

FIGURE 87: Hypothetical scheme of the involvement of the activation of Müller cell's P2 receptors in retinal detachment and PVR.

kinases. Activation of P2Y receptors induces the consecutive release of PDGF and HB-EGF from Müller cells (Fig. 86) (Milenkovic et al., 2003). The proteolytic activity of the MMP-9 is implicated in the transfer of the signal from the PDGF- to the EGF receptor tyrosine kinase (Fig. 86) (Milenkovic et al., 2003). P2Y and growth factor receptors are localized in close proximity on the surface of Müller cells (Milenkovic et al., 2003), probably in lipid rafts or caveolae (Krishnan and Chatterjee, 2013; Gu et al., 2014). The transactivation of the receptor tyrosine kinases results in activation of ERK1/2 and PI3K (Milenkovic et al., 2003). As HB-EGF stimulates the autocrine release of ATP from Müller cells (Weuste et al., 2006), HB-EGF may exert a positive feedback on the mitogenic signaling cascade. The gene expression of HB-EGF is increased in retinas from patients with PVR, and HB-EGF is localized to glial cells in epiretinal fibroproliferative membranes (Hollborn et al., 2005).

While the effects of ATP and EGF on Müller cell proliferation are non-additive, suggesting that these factors share common intracellular signaling pathways, the proliferation-stimulatory effects of ATP and blood serum are additive, indicating that their mitogenic effects are mediated by different intracellular signaling pathways (Moll et al., 2002). This suggests that when proliferation *in situ* is further stimulated by serum after the breakdown of the blood-retinal barrier, other strategies in addition to inhibition of purinergic and/or EGF receptors will also be necessary to inhibit intraocular proliferation (Milenkovic et al., 2003).

A short-term administration of ATP results in a long-term (up to 48 h) desensitization of P2Y receptors in Müller cells, resulting in strongly reduced ATP-induced intracellular calcium responses (Weick et al., 2005). The ATP-induced receptor desensitization is not caused by the depletion of internal calcium stores, and is independent of PKC and PI3K activation (Weick et al., 2005). Various growth factors including PDGF, EGF, and NGF induce a rapid (within min) resensitization of P2Y receptors that were formerly desensitized by ATP (Weick et al., 2005). The growth factors increase both the incidence of responding cells and the amplitude of ATP-induced calcium transients (Weick et al., 2005). The growth factor-induced resensitization of P2Y receptors is dependent on an intact cytoskeleton and the activation of protein phosphatases and PI3K, and independent of PKC, Src kinase, and ERK1/2 activation (Weick et al., 2005).

In experimental PVR, Müller cells exhibit an increase in P2Y receptor-mediated signaling, as indicated by the higher incidence of cells that show ATP-induced intracellular calcium responses (Fig. 63B,C) (Francke et al., 2002). Müller cells of patients with PVR exhibit a greater density of cation currents through $P2X_7$ receptor channels, and greater increases in BK currents upon activation of $P2X_7$ receptors, than cells from donor eyes, suggesting an increase in functional $P2X_7$ receptors (Bringmann et al., 2001). The increase in $P2X_7$ receptor currents is correlated with other alterations in membrane properties such as the reduction in Kir currents; this may imply a causal relationship between $P2X_7$ receptor activation and the strength of gliosis (Bringmann et al., 2001).

Human Müller cells from patients with non-proliferative gliosis (e.g., in the presence of choroidal melanoma) show no increase in $P2X_7$ receptor currents and no decrease in Kir currents, although other signs of gliosis (e.g., cellular hypertrophy) are observed (Bringmann et al., 2001).

The increase of the purinergic calcium responsiveness may facilitate the release of mitogens such as PDGF and HB-EGF which are involved in the purinergic stimulation of Müller cell proliferation (Fig. 86) (Milenkovic et al., 2003). Activation of PDGFα receptors (Fig. 85) and PDGF-induced activation of the PI3K-Akt pathway are key events in the pathogenesis of experimental PVR (Andrews et al., 1999; Ikuno et al., 2000, 2002b; see 5.11.10.4.2.). One effect of growth factor-PI3K signaling is the potentiation of the action of nucleotides as mediators of Müller cell gliosis and proliferation.

Membrane stretching is a major cause of ATP release from Müller cells (see 5.6.3.1.) and is also implicated in the development of epiretinal fibroproliferative membranes in PVR (see 5.11.11.3.). One cause of PVR is the detachment of the neuroretina from the retinal pigment epithelium associated with mechanical deformations of the retina (Bringmann and Wiedemann, 2009). Müller cells sense mechanical deformations of the retina by calcium-dependent mechanisms (see 5.5.1.4.). Stretching of the retinal tissue induces calcium responses, activation of c-Fos and ERK1/2, and upregulation of growth factors like bFGF in Müller cells (Fig. 42B–F) (Lindqvist et al., 2010). Activation of stretch-activated calcium-permeable cation channels of Müller cells (Puro, 1991a) results in an influx of calcium from the extracellular space and activation of BK channels (Puro, 1991a). Calcium influx also stimulates the release of growth factors from Müller cells (Fig. 86). *In situ*, vitreous fibers, which adhere to Müller cell endfeet at sites of vitreo-retinal attachment after partial detachment of the vitreous from the retina, exert tractional forces on the cells (Schubert, 1989; see 5.11.11.). Tractional forces may induce a release of ATP from Müller cells, resulting in autocrine/paracrine activation of the cells, cellular hypertrophy and proliferation, as well as vascular leakage due to the release of factors such as bFGF (Schubert, 1989). The contraction of epiretinal membranes may be stimulated by stretch-induced autocrine ATP signaling in Müller cells (Innocenti et al., 2001) via a decrease in cell volume due to the water efflux that accompanies the potassium efflux (Puro, 1991a; Uckermann et al., 2005c) and the ATP-induced release of factors that promote Müller cell contraction, e.g., PDGF (Guidry, 2005). Thus, inhibition of the purinergic signaling of Müller cells might prevent early and late stages of epiretinal membrane formation, an important cause of blindness in proliferative retinopathies (Bringmann and Wiedemann, 2009).

5.11.10.4 Growth Factor Stimulation of Müller Cell Proliferation

The proliferation and migration of Müller cells is stimulated by numerous growth factors and cytokines derived from retinal and blood cells, and blood serum (Puro, 1995; Burmeister et al., 2009).

5.11.10.4.1 FGFs   The action of bFGF is involved in the pathogenesis of proliferative retinopathies (Hueber et al., 1996; Cassidy et al., 1998; Kon et al., 1999). In cases of disease and injury, FGFs are rapidly released within the retinal tissue. After experimental detachment, bFGF is released within minutes from its storage sites in the retina, as indicated by the phosphorylation of the FGF receptor-1 and activation of ERK1/2 (Geller et al., 2001; see 5.11.5.). In addition to astrocytes, ganglion cells, and pigment epithelial cells, Müller cells are a major source of retinal bFGF (Fig. 33A, B), and are a target of bFGF action (Morimoto et al., 1993; Cao et al., 1997b; Guillonneau et al., 1998; Harada et al., 2000; Blanco et al., 2000; Geller et al., 2001; Walsh et al., 2001; Nakamichi et al., 2003; Fischer et al., 2009a; see 5.11.7.7.). Intravitreal injection of bFGF induces proliferation of retinal glial and vascular cells, but not neurons (Lewis et al., 1992; Fischer et al., 2002, 2009). Subretinal injection of bFGF induces Müller cell expression of GFAP followed by migration of the cells into the subretinal space and membrane formation (Kimura et al., 1999).

bFGF (acting at FGF receptor 1) and FGF9 (acting at FGF receptors 2 and 3) are mitogens of Müller cells (Puro and Mano, 1991; Small et al., 1991; Mascarelli et al., 1991; Hicks and Courtois, 1992; Lewis et al., 1992; Ikeda and Puro, 1995; Meuillet et al., 1996; Heidinger et al., 1998; Cinaroglu et al., 2005). The proliferative effect of bFGF is mediated by activation of ERK1/2, p38 MAPK and CREB, a decrease of the nuclear level of p27^{Kip1}, an increase of cyclin D1, and induction of c-Fos and c-Jun (Cao et al., 1998; Wahlin et al., 2000; Kinkl et al., 2001; Hollborn et al., 2004b; Kase et al., 2006; Fischer et al., 2009b). bFGF also induces a secretion of VEGF and HGF from Müller cells via activation of PI3K (Hollborn et al., 2004b). bFGF increases the currents through L-type voltage-gated calcium channels and the activity of calcium-activated, calcium-permeable cation channels in Müller cells (Puro and Mano, 1991; Puro, 1991b). The mitogenic effect of bFGF is in part mediated by enhanced production of prostaglandins; PGE$_2$ increases the proliferation, dedifferentiation, and stem cell-like properties of Müller cells (Wang et al., 2013e).

5.11.10.4.2 PDGF   Activation of the PDGF receptor-α plays a critical role in the development of proliferative retinopathies (Andrews et al., 1999; Ikuno et al., 2000; Ikuno and Kazlauskas, 2002; Zheng et al., 2003; Cui et al., 2009; Velez et al., 2012, 2013). In PDR, both PDGF and VEGF contribute to the progression of epiretinal membranes (Campochiaro, 1997). Overexpression of PDGF-A in transgenic mice causes a retinopathy similar to PVR (extensive proliferation of glial cells and traction retinal detachment without vascular cell involvement) whereas overexpression of PDGF-B results in a retinopathy similar to PDR (proliferation of vascular, glial, and pigment epithelial cells resulting in the formation of fibrovascular membranes and detachment of the retina) (Seo et al., 2000; Mori et al., 2002a). Cells of both PVR and PDR membranes produce PDGF and have PDGF receptors (Robbins et al., 1994; Cui et al., 2007). Müller cells in PVR retinas, but not in control retinas, express PDGF (Westra et al., 1995).

With vitreous and retinal hemorrhage, retinal cells are exposed to serum-derived PDGF. In human serum, PDGF has a concentration of 50–70 ng/ml (Antoniades and Scher, 1977; Campochiaro and Glaser, 1985) which is greater than the maximally effective concentration of PDGF for the stimulation of Müller cell proliferation (30 ng/ml) (Uchihori and Puro, 1991). PDGF may be also derived from other cells such as pigment epithelial cells, platelets, and invading macrophages. Human platelet suspensions contain PDGF at a concentration of ~80 ng/ml (Castelnovo et al., 2000).

Retinal glial cells express PDGF receptor-α (Fig. 85) and -β (Mudhar et al., 1993; Milenkovic et al., 2003; Cox et al., 2003; Cui et al., 2009; Velez et al., 2012). Increased expression of the PDGF receptor-α in Müller cells results in an increased capability of the cells to induce experimental PVR (Velez et al., 2012). PDGF is an autocrine growth factor of Müller cells that stimulates cell proliferation and that induces chemotaxis and secretion of VEGF (Harvey et al., 1987; De Juan et al., 1988; Uchihori and Puro, 1991; Ikeda and Puro, 1995; Milenkovic et al., 2003; Hollborn et al., 2004b; King and Guidry, 2012). In addition to MAPKs, PI3K is a downstream effector of the PDGF receptor-α involved in elicitation of PVR and of the PDGF-induced cell cycle progression, chemotaxis, contraction, and secretion of growth factors such as VEGF (Rosenkranz et al., 1999; Ikuno et al., 2002b; Milenkovic et al., 2003; Hollborn et al., 2006).

The proliferative effect of PDGF (acting at PDGF receptor-α) is mediated by transactivation of the EGF receptor tyrosine kinase after shedding of HB-EGF from the extracellular matrix and subsequent activation of ERK1/2 and PI3K (Milenkovic et al., 2003; Hollborn et al., 2004b; see 5.11.10.3.). Autocrine release of PDGF and activation of the PDGF receptor-α play a critical role in the transmission of mitogenic signals from G protein-coupled receptors (such as purinergic P2Y and NPY receptors) to the EGF receptor tyrosine kinase (Milenkovic et al., 2003, 2004). Cholesterol depletion of the plasma membrane (which disperses lipid rafts) abolishes the mitogenic effects of PDGF, ATP, and HB-EGF (Milenkovic et al., 2003), suggesting that P2Y receptors, PDGF receptors-α, and EGF receptors are expressed in close spatial proximity in the Müller cell membrane, likely within caveolae or lipid rafts (Krishnan and Chatterjee, 2013; Gu et al., 2014), which facilitates the interaction between these receptors.

5.11.10.4.3 EGF, HB-EGF   The EGF receptor erbB1 (which has various agonists such as EGF, TGF-α, and HB-EGF) is expressed in cultured Müller cells and Müller cells *in situ* (Roque et al., 1992; Milenkovic et al., 2003; Weuste et al., 2006). In the rat retina, EGF receptors are expressed at high level in late progenitor cells and Müller cells during the first two postnatal weeks; the expression declines in parallel with the maturation of the retina (Close et al., 2006). The reduced expression of EGF receptors in Müller cells, along with an increased TGF-β signaling, correlates with the reduced proliferative capacity of Müller cells in the mature mammalian retina (Close et al., 2006). In addition to glial cells, retinal neurons express the EGF receptor and its ligands, suggesting a pleiotropic function (Chen et al., 2007b). In response to retinal injury such as light damage, EGF receptor expression is upregulated in Müller cells to levels close to those in the neonatal retina, resulting in a renewed mitotic response to EGF (Close et al., 2006). The decrease of EGF receptor expression was suggested to be one mechanism by which Müller cells maintain mitotic quiescence in the mature retina (Close et al., 2006). *In situ*, EGF induces expression of c-Fos and c-Jun, and a decrease of the cortisol-induced upregulation of the glutamine synthetase in Müller cells (Sagar et al., 1991; Kruchkova et al., 2001; see 5.5.2.1.11. and 5.5.2.1.13.). HB-EGF is upregulated in the retina during ischemia-reperfusion (Weuste et al., 2006) and in the course of PVR, and is localized to glial cells in fibroproliferative epiretinal membranes of patients with PVR (Hollborn et al., 2005). In the fish retina, HB-EGF is necessary and sufficient to induce Müller cell dedifferentiation and retinal regeneration (Wan et al., 2012).

EGF and HB-EGF stimulate the proliferation of Müller cells (Reichelt et al., 1989; Roque et al., 1992; Arrindell et al., 1992; Hicks and Courtois, 1992; Scherer and Schnitzer, 1994; Ikeda and Puro, 1995; Puro, 1995; Heidinger et al., 1998; Kodal et al., 2000) via activation of erbB1, voltage-gated calcium channels, BK channels, ERK1/2, PI3K, and BMP signaling pathways (Milenkovic et al., 2003; Hollborn et al., 2004b, 2005; Ueki and Reh, 2013). In addition, EGF and HB-EGF stimulate the migration and the secretion of VEGF from Müller cells (Hollborn et al., 2005; Nickerson et al., 2011). MMP-9-mediated shedding of HB-EGF from membrane-bound proHB-EGF is critical for the mediation of mitogenic responses of agonists of purinergic G protein-coupled receptors and PDGF receptor-α (Fig. 86) (Milenkovic et al., 2003, 2004).

5.11.10.4.4 HGF   HGF (also known as scatter factor) induces scattering of retinal cells (which is a precondition for cell migration and cell shape alterations), chemotaxis, and epithelial-to-mesenchymal transformation in cellular phenotype (He et al., 1998; Lashkari et al., 1999; Briggs et al., 2000). HGF is expressed in the inner retina within 24 h of ischemia-reperfusion, likely by Müller cells (Shibuki et al., 2002), suggesting a role of this factor in the early response of the cells to ischemic-hypoxic insults and in neuroprotection (Wong et al., 2014). Neuroretinas of patients with PVR (but not control retinas) express HGF (Hollborn et al., 2004a, 2005). HGF is elevated in the vitreous of patients with PDR (Umeda et al., 2002). In epiretinal membranes of patients with PVR or PDR, HGF and its receptor c-Met are expressed by various cell types including glial and pigment epithelial cells (Hollborn et al., 2004a; Hinton et al., 2002; Cui et al., 2007). HGF stimulates the chemotaxis (but not proliferation) of cultured Müller cells, and promotes the secretion of VEGF (Hollborn et al., 2004a). Blood serum and bFGF increase the secretion of HGF from Müller cells (Hollborn et al., 2004a).

5.11.10.5 Other Proliferative Factors and Conditions

Other growth factors of Müller cells are NGF (Ikeda and Puro, 1994, 1995) and IGF-1 acting at IGF-1 receptors (Charkrabarti et al., 1991; Ikeda and Puro, 1995; Ikeda et al., 1995; Layton et al., 2006; but see King and Guidry, 2012). In the immature neuroretina, IGF-1 is expressed by Müller and ganglion cells (Hansson et al., 1989; Lee et al., 1992). Elevated intravitreal levels of IGF-1 and VEGF were shown to correlate with the neovascular activity in PDR (Paques et al., 1997). It has been suggested that insulin (used to optimize blood glucose levels) acts at IGF-1 receptors and may thus accelerate the progression of PDR by stimulation of the VEGF production and Müller cell proliferation, and inducing vitreoretinal traction forces (Chantelau et al., 2008; Zhang et al., 2009b; Kaya et al., 2013; see 5.11.11.2.).

In addition to extracellular nucleotides and growth factors, there are various other signaling molecules and conditions that stimulate the proliferation of Müller cells. A direct contact between Müller cells promotes the proliferation of the cells (Burke, 1983, 1989). Elevated extracellular potassium increases the proliferation of Müller cells under serum-containing but not serum-free conditions; this effect is mediated by an increase in the activity of BK channels (Reichelt et al., 1989; Kodal et al., 2000). Wnt signaling stimulates Müller cell proliferation, survival, and dedifferentiation to retinal progenitor cells (Liu et al., 2013b; see 5.11.12.3.).

Blood serum is a mitogen and motogen of Müller cells (De Juan et al., 1988; Kodal et al., 2000; Moll et al., 2002; Milenkovic et al., 2003; King and Guidry, 2012). Because glial cells closely ensheath the vessels they are among the first cells exposed to extravasated serum. Serum contains various mitogenic and chemotactic factors including PDGF (Antoniades and Scher, 1977; Campochiaro and Glaser, 1985) and fibronectin (De Juan et al., 1988). Fibronectin stimulates the migration of retinal glial cells (Harvey et al., 1987; Castelnovo et al., 2000). The serum-induced proliferation is not mediated by activation of BK channels (Kodal et al., 2000; Moll et al., 2002) nor by transactivation of growth factor receptor tyrosine kinases, and is not inhibited by cholesterol depletion of the plasma membrane, suggesting that serum and agonists of G protein-coupled and growth factor receptors activate different intracellular signaling pathways and that inhibition of growth factor receptors will be not sufficient to prevent intraocular proliferation when serum enters the retina (Milenkovic et al., 2003). Components of damaged erythrocytes such as hemoglobin and iron also induce proliferation and migration of retinal glial cells (Burke and Smith, 1981).

Thrombin stimulates the proliferation of Müller cells by inducing a release of calcium from internal stores and closure of Kir channels (Puro et al., 1990; Puro and Stuenkel, 1995). Thrombin enters the retinal tissue at sites of hemorrhage. In addition, the retinal tissue express mRNA for prothrombin, the precursor of thrombin, suggesting that this molecule may be endogenous to the retina (Rehak et al., 2009). IL-2 released from activated lymphocytes in inflammatory eye diseases stimulates the proliferation of Müller cells (Small et al., 1991).

NPY has antiproliferative and proliferative effects on Müller cells (see 5.10.10.). Shh is a potent mitogen of Müller cells, and promotes the dedifferentiation of the cells to progenitor cells (see 5.11.12.). Intravitreal administration of AMPA/KA or NMDA receptor agonists induces Müller cell proliferation (Sahel et al., 1991). A prolonged (>3 h) exposure to high concentrations of glutamate induces proliferation of cultured Müller cells via activation of NMDA receptors and an influx of calcium from the extracellular space (Uchihori and Puro, 1993; but see Hyndman, 1984). Normally, the uptake of glutamate by Müller cells (see 5.5.2.1.) prevents sustained, elevated levels of glutamate, and the mitogenic effect is thought to be limited to pathological conditions when the glutamate recycling by Müller cells is disturbed (Uchihori and Puro, 1993; see 5.5.2.1.6.). Subretinal administration of subtoxic levels of glutamate induces Müller cell proliferation and migration *in situ* (Takeda et al., 2008). NMDA receptor agonists also stimulate the proliferation of Müller cell-derived retinal progenitor cells via activation of CREB (Ramírez and Lamas, 2009).

MMPs (in particular MMP-2 and -9) are involved in the development of PVR and PDR (Limb et al., 1997; Kon et al., 1998; Webster et al., 1999; Salzmann et al., 2000; Noda et al., 2003). MMPs mediate the remodeling of the extracellular matrix required for cellular migration and proliferation, and the shedding of matrix-bound growth factors such as VEGF and HB-EGF (Milenkovic et al., 2003). In fibrovascular membranes, MMP-2 and -9 are localized to endothelial and glial cells; MMP-2 is colocalized with MT1-MMP and TIMP-2 which are known activators of MMP-2 (Noda et al., 2003). The expression of MMP-9 in Müller cells can be increased by inflammatory factors such as TNFα (Limb et al., 2002a). Hypoxia stimulates the expression of MT1-MMP in Müller cells; this effect is mediated by VEGF in an autocrine fashion (Noda et al., 2005).

5.11.10.6 Antiproliferative Factors

Normally, glial cells do not proliferate in the mature retina despite the presence of distinct mitogens; endogenous antiproliferative molecules and the downregulation of distinct growth factor receptors may prevent the glial cell proliferation (Ikeda and Puro, 1995; see 5.11.10.4.3.). BMPs and CNTF inhibit the dedifferentiation and proliferation of Müller cells after excitotoxic damage of the chick retina (Fischer et al., 2004a). TGF-β2 released from inner retinal neurons was suggested to be responsible for the developmental decline in the proliferation of retinal precursors (Close et al., 2005). Müller cells express TGF-β receptors and are a source of TGF-β (Anderson et al., 1991; Pfeffer et al., 1994; Ikeda et al., 1998; Close et al., 2005) and thrombospondin-1 (Eichler et al., 2004a), an activator of latent TGF-β (Crawford et al., 1998). TGF-β blocks the mitogenic response of Müller cells to a variety of growth factors that activates tyrosine kinase-linked receptors including bFGF, EGF, PDGF, IGF-I, and NGF (Ikeda and Puro, 1994, 1995). However, in another study, TGF-β was found to slightly stimulate the proliferation of Müller cells (Hollborn et al., 2004b). After experimental retinal detachment, the expression of TGF-β and TGF-β receptor II is increased in Müller cells and in hypertrophied Müller cell processes that form periretinal membranes (Guerin et al., 2001). A downstream mediator of the TGF-β action is CTGF. CTGF was localized to glial cells, pigment epithelial cells, vascular endothelial cells, and myofibrocytes in PVR and PDR membranes (Hinton et al., 2002; Cui et al., 2007; Abu-El-Asrar et al., 2007). The proliferation of Müller cells in the detached retina is also prevented by BDNF (Lewis et al., 1999b).

Although prolonged exposure to glutamate stimulates the proliferation of Müller cells, glutamate acts also as an antiproliferative factor in cultured Müller cells, via activation of mGluRs (Ikeda and Puro, 1995). Activation of mGluRs inhibits the mitogenic effects of growth factors which are also inhibited by TGF-β (Ikeda and Puro, 1994, 1995). The antiproliferative effects of TGF-β and glutamate involve the activation of PKC and subsequent inhibition of growth factor receptor tyrosine kinases (Ikeda and Puro, 1995). However, TGF-β and activation of mGluRs do not inhibit the proliferation induced by thrombin and NMDA receptor activation (Ikeda and Puro, 1995).

LRP1 clears α2-macroglobulin-bound growth factors and proteinases from the extracellular space via receptor-mediated endocytosis which decreases the extracellular availability of the factors (see 5.10.13.). In PVR retinas, the gene expression of LRP1 is increased compared with control retinas (Hollborn et al., 2004c). In retinas of rats with ischemia-induced neovascularization or diabetes, and in the vitreous and retinas of human subjects with neovascular glaucoma or PDR, the expression of LRP1 and α2-macroglobulin is increased (Luna et al., 2003; Gerhardinger et al., 2005; Sánchez et al., 2006 ; Barcelona et al., 2010). Blood-derived α2-macroglobulin may enter the retinal tissue at sites of hemorrhage. The protease-activated form of α2-macroglobulin induces cell migration and proMMP-2 activation in cultured Müller cells which is mediated by a mechanism involving LRP1 and MT1-MMP (Barcelona et al., 2013). The use of α2-macroglobulin was suggested to be a strategy for the inhibition of uncontrolled retinal cell proliferation (Hollborn et al., 2004c). However, α2-macroglobulin inhibits the proliferation induced by agonists of G protein-coupled receptors (ATP, NPY) but has no effect on the proliferation induced by serum and agonists of receptor tyrosine kinases (EGF, PDGF) (Milenkovic et al., 2005). Inhibition of LRP increases the proliferation in the presence of α2-macroglobulin (Milenkovic et al., 2005), likely via a decreased clearance of α2-macroglobulin-bound mitogenic factors and proteinases that prolongs the extracellular availability of these factors.

5.11.11 GLIAL CELL INVOLVEMENT IN EPIRETINAL MEMBRANE FORMATION

Despite advances in surgical management of fibrocontractive retinal disorders, PVR and PDR remain major causes of blindness. PVR is an inflammatory fibrotic disorder which frequently develop after retinal detachment, and is the most common failure of vitreoretinal surgery (Ryan, 1985; Fisher and Anderson, 1994). In PVR, subretinal, intraretinal, and/or epiretinal avascular fibroproliferative membranes are formed; these fibrotic membranes further detach the retina due to the contractile properties of myofibroblasts that are abundantly present in the membranes (Machemer, 1978; Thomas et al., 1982; Wiedemann and Weller, 1988; Hui et al., 1988; Pastor et al., 2002). Long-lasting retinal ischemia in diabetic retinopathy causes an outgrowth of new vessels from superficial veins and venules onto the posterior vitreous cortex. Once retinal neovascularization develops, diabetic retinopathy is classified as proliferative (PDR); the contraction of the fibrovascular membranes threatens the retinal anatomy. Formation of epiretinal membranes can occur also in various other retinal disorders (Bringmann and Wiedemann, 2009) and is an age-related process (McLeod et al., 1987b).

PVR is considered to represent a maladapted retinal wound repair process driven by growth factor- and cytokine-induced overstimulation of proliferation, migration, extracellular matrix production, and contraction of retinal cells (Weller et al., 1990; Wiedemann, 1992; Campochiaro, 1997). The pathogenesis of proliferative retinopathies, in particular the early steps of epiretinal membrane formation, are incompletely understood. Glial cells, in particular Müller cells, in association with blood-derived immune cells and factors within the vitreous are suggested to play a central role (see 5.11.11.3.). Epiretinal membranes develop predominantly at sites where astrocytes and Müller cells proliferate and migrate onto the inner surface of the retina and where hyperthrophied astrocytic and Müller cell processes extend into the vitreous cavity (Laqua, 1975; Foos and Gloor, 1975; Szamier, 1981; Ohsawa and Miki, 1982). Periretinal membranes are focally connected to the retina via hypertrophied processes of Müller cells that rise from the retinal tissue into the membranes (Laqua, 1975; Charteris et al., 2002, 2007; Fisher and Lewis, 2003). The outgrowth of Müller cell processes onto the vitreal surface of the retina was suggested to represent the initial event of epiretinal membrane formation (Fisher and Lewis, 2003).

5.11.11.1 Composition of Epiretinal Membranes

Epiretinal membranes are composed of two main components: extracellular matrix (consisting of collagen, laminin, tenascin, fibronectin, vitronectin, thrombospondin, etc.) and cells of retinal and extra-retinal origin. The membranes contain a wide variety of cell types including glial cells (microglia, Müller cells, fibrous astrocytes), epithelial cells from the retinal pigment epithelium and ciliary body, blood-borne leukocytes (macrophages, lymphocytes, neutrophils), fibrocytes, and myofibrocytes (Laqua, 1975; Laqua and Machemer, 1975; Van Horn et al., 1977; Kampik et al., 1981; Hiscott et al., 1984; Yamashita et al., 1986; Nork et al., 1986, 1987; Sramek et al., 1989; Guerin et al., 1990; Weller et al., 1992; Esser et al., 1993; Fekrat et al., 1995; Sethi et al., 2005; Abu-El-Asrar et al., 2007; Zeng et al., 2008a; Guidry et al., 2009; Oberstein et al., 2011; Feist et al., 2014). The main cells in the preretinal membranes of patients with macular pucker and retinitis pigmentosa are glial cells (Szamier, 1981; Yamashita et al., 1986). Idiopathic macular holes are associated with epiretinal proliferation of glial cells and hyalocytes which transdifferentiate into myofibroblasts (Schumann et al., 2011). In PDR, vascular endothelial cells, pericytes, and astrocytes are involved in the formation of epiretinal vessels (Forrester and Lee, 1981). Müller cells are a source of fibroblast-like cells in PDR membranes (Guidry, 1997; Guidry et al., 2003, 2009).

Macrophages and pigment epithelial cells play important roles in the initiation of preretinal membrane formation in PVR; over time, the proportion of glial cells in PVR membranes increases (Yamashita et al., 1986). In a rabbit model, administration of autologous blood into the vitreous cavity resulted in the formation of epiretinal membranes which were composed of glial cells, macrophages, and erythrocytes (Kono et al., 1995). After six months, macrophages and red blood cells disappeared from the membranes, and the membranes mainly contained glial cells and extracellular matrix (Kono et al., 1995).

5.11.11.2 Transdifferentiation to Myofibrocytes

Within the membranes, glial and pigment epithelial cells transdifferentiate into contractile myofibrocytes (Guidry, 1996, 2005, 2009). The transdifferentiation is, at least in part, induced by macrophages (Jo et al., 2011). Transdifferentiated glial and pigment epithelial cells generate tractional forces through contraction of extracellular matrices in response to growth factors of the vitreous, resulting in traction retinal detachment. The fibroblastic transdifferentiation is characterized by a reduction of cell-specific proteins such as GFAP, carbonic anhydrase, glutamine synthetase, CRALBP, and cytokeratins while proteins involved in motility and proliferation such as α-smooth muscle actin (which is normally not expressed by the cells) are upregulated (Hui et al., 1988; Sramek et al., 1989; McGillem and Dacheux, 1999; Guidry, 2005, 2009; Gao et al., 2013; Feist et al., 2014). α-Smooth muscle actin is essential for the extracellular matrix contraction (Arora and McCulloch, 1994). The GFAP content of epiretinal fibroproliferative tissues correlates inversely with the clinical contractility (Sramek et al., 1989), suggesting that the transdifferentiation to myofibroblasts increases the capacity of glial cells to generate tractional forces (Guidry, 2005). The cellular transdifferentiation may represent one reason for the fact that relatively few glial and pigment epithelial cells can be detected in fibrocellular epiretinal membranes with the commonly used immunocytochemical markers. TGF-β is a major inducer of myofibroblastic differentiation and a contributor to tissue fibrosis, via stimulation of the synthesis of extracellular matrix components and transglutaminases which cross-links extracellular matrix proteins to proteolysis-resistant complexes (Castelnovo et al., 2000; Priglinger et al., 2003; Gamulescu et al., 2006). A downstream mediator of the TGF-β action is CTGF. In fibrovascular membranes, CTGF is localized to glial cells, vascular endothelial cells, and myofibrocytes (Abu-El-Asrar et al., 2007). The number of CTGF-expressing myofibrocytes correlates with the number of blood vessels in PDR membranes (Abu-El-Asrar et al., 2007).

Blood serum and members of the PDGF and IGF protein families cause contraction of the extracellular matrix by Müller cells whereas other growth factors which are mitogens for Müller cells such as bFGF and EGF do not induce a contractile response (Guidry, 1997, 2005; King and Guidry, 2012). Apparently, the IGF and PDGF content of the vitreous account for the majority of biological activity to which myofibroblastic Müller cells respond with a contraction of the extracellular matrix (Hardwick et al., 1997; Guidry et al., 2004; Guidry, 2005). Transdifferentiated retinal pigment epithelial cells and platelets are sources of IGF, PDGF, and TGF-β that promote Müller cell contraction (Mamballikalathil et al., 2000; Burmeister et al., 2009). The TGF-β-induced cell contraction is (at least in part) mediated by PDGF receptor-α (Ikuno and Kazlauskas, 2002). Generation of tractional force by Müller cells involves integrin receptors constituted of α2 and β1 subunits (Guidry et al., 2003). Laminin stimulates the migration of Müller cells by activation of α-dystroglycan, a laminin-1 receptor (Méhes et al., 2005).

5.11.11.3 Pathogenic Mechanisms of Early Epiretinal Membrane Formation

The early steps of the development of proliferative retinopathies are incompletely understood. There are different possible scenarios of early epiretinal membrane formation. In PVR, glial cells undergo mitosis in the retina, and the nuclei of the cells migrate, passing through the inner limiting membrane onto the retinal surface. The vitreo-retinal gradient of chemoattractants and growth factors, which are present at high concentration in the vitreous (El-Ghrably et al., 1999; Guidry, 2005), represents a major factor that direct the process extension and migration of Müller cells. Increases in vitreous growth factor and cytokine activities are suggested to precede the development of PVR and PDR (Wiedemann, 1992; Kon et al., 1999; Guidry, 2005; King et al., 2011). Growth and inflammatory factors released from infiltrating immune cells and platelets, and plasma-derived factors, may activate Müller cells (Roberge et al., 1985; Puro et al., 1989; Kosnosky et al., 1994; Burmeister et al., 2009). Among the various growth factors and cytokines present in significant amounts in fibrocellular membranes and in the vitreous humor of patients with PVR, particularly HGF and PDGF were implicated in the development of the disease (Cassidy et al., 1998; Andrews et al., 1999; Briggs et al., 2000; Mitamura et al., 2000; Ikuno et al., 2000; Mori et al., 2002a). Multiple further factors are involved in the formation and progression of epiretinal membranes via inducing autocrine and paracrine signaling loops. Examples of such signaling loops are the mediation of the ATP-induced Müller cell proliferation by autocrine release of PDGF and EGF (Fig. 86) (see 5.11.10.3.), the mediation of the TGF-β-induced cell contraction by PDGF (Ikuno and Kazlauskas, 2002), and the stimulation of glial VEGF expression by various growth factors and cytokines such as HB-EGF, HGF, and TGF-β (see 5.11.8.).

Vitreous hemorrhage resulting in activation of glial cells was suggested to be a major causative factor of epiretinal membrane formation (Ehrenberg et al., 1984; Kono et al., 1998; Robaszkiewicz et al., 2010). A breakdown of blood-ocular barriers occurs (in addition to conditions of ocular inflammation, ischemia, and trauma) as a result of mechanical stress to Müller cells after detachment of the posterior vitreous from the retina (McLeod et al., 1987b; Schubert, 1989; Pournaras, 1995). Normally, the vitreous body adheres to the retinal tissue at the peripheral retina, the major superficial retinal vessels, the optic disc, and the macula (Schubert, 1989). Pathological processes at the vitreo-retinal junction result in increased adhesiveness of vitreal collagen fibers to the retinal internal limiting membrane (Robaszkiewicz et al., 2010). In the elderly, the basement membrane of the inner limiting membrane becomes thinner at the sites of vitreo-retinal attachment, and vitreous fibers adhere directly to Müller cells. It was suggested that under normal conditions, many vitreous fibers distribute tractional forces evenly to numerous Müller cells (Schubert, 1989). However, in cases of vitreous shrinkage and partial posterior vitreous detachment (as occurring during aging), fewer vitreous fibers and Müller cells endure most of the traction; this results in a chronic mechanical stress for Müller cells and a local release of factors which induce Müller cell gliosis and vascular leakage including ATP (Figs. 54C, 87), bFGF (Fig. 42E,F; see 5.5.1.4.), and MMPs (Wang et al., 2013d). ATP induces activation of MMPs and the release of further growth factors from Müller cells such as PDGF and HB-EGF (Fig. 86; see 5.11.10.3.). Mechanical stretching of Müller cells induces extensive changes in the expression of genes implicated in cell proliferation, tissue remodeling, and vasculogenesis (Wang et al., 2013c). Thus, mechanical stress triggers molecular responses in Müller cells (e.g., activation of ERK1/2 and release of bFGF and MMPs) that prevent neuronal degeneration and that induce vascular permeability and proliferation of endothelial and Müller cells (Fischer et al., 2009a; Bringmann et al., 2009b). This explains why the sites of vitreoretinal junctures are oftenly the sites of age-related cellular proliferation and vascular leakage in pars planitis (McLeod et al., 1987b; Schubert, 1989). Tractional forces onto Müller cells will also increase the calcium influx into the cells through stretch-activated channels (Fig. 42B,C; see 5.5.1.4.) which may result in activation of calcium-dependent potassium channels and stimulation of Müller cell proliferation (see 5.11.10.2.). The calcium-dependent Müller cell responses, which are involved in the release of growth factors and Müller cell proliferation, are facilitated in the elderly because the currents through voltage-gated calcium channels display an age-dependent increase (Fig. 45D; see 5.9.1.). Posterior vitreous detachment with normal adhesions to the retina is frequently found in age-related liquefaction and collapse of the vitreous, while vitreous detachment with abnormal adhesions and shrinkage are observed in association with diabetes, PVR, and inflammation (Schubert, 1989).

After retinal detachment, Müller cells induce and propagate retinal inflammation (see 5.11.5. and 5.11.6.) which contributes to the breakdown of the blood-retinal barrier. In the retina of patients with PVR, genes which support cell proliferation, cell signaling, cell motility, and extracellular matrix remodeling are upregulated (Hollborn et al., 2005). A significant fraction of the genes are associated with inflammatory and immune responses (Hollborn et al., 2005). Local immune and inflammatory responses develop within one day after experimental retinal detachment (Hollborn et al., 2008). The genes upregulated in detached retinas are related to inflammation and immune responses, antioxidants and metal homeostasis, intracellular proteolysis, and blood coagulation/fibrinolysis (Hollborn et al., 2008). Müller cells upregulate genes of proinflammatory factors such as TNF, IL-1β, and MCP-1 after retinal detachment (Nakazawa et al., 2006b; Hollborn et al., 2008).

The presence of serum, growth factors and cytokines, blood-borne leukocytes, and cell debris in the vitreous is thought to trigger Müller cell process extension and proliferation. However, the precise mechanisms how Müller cells respond to vitreous hemorrhage are unclear. After breakdown of the blood-retinal barrier (Ando et al., 1994), blood-borne immune cells immigrate into the vitreous and are attracted to sites of glial cell reactivity in the retina by glia-derived chemotactic factors such as MCP-1 (Nakazawa et al., 2006b, 2007b; Hollborn et al., 2008). In a rabbit model of early PVR, sites of local Müller cell reactivity in the retina (as indicated by the upregulation of GFAP) are associated with microglia activation and adhesion of blood-borne immune cells to the vitreal surface of the retina (Fig. 24) (Francke et al., 2003). In cases of vitreous hemorrhage, holes in the basement membrane of the inner limiting membrane are formed (by MMPs released from leukocytes and/or Müller cells; Zhang et al., 2004b) at sites where red blood cells and macrophages, as well as hemoglobin, are attached to the inner surface of the retina; glial cell processes extrude through these holes onto the retinal surface in order to engulf the debris mainly of red blood cells (Nishizono et al., 1993). The chronic inflammatory response to the long-lasting presence of red blood cells in the vitreous was suggested to be crucial for the subsequent epiretinal membrane formation (Miller et al., 1986; Lean, 1987; Kono et al., 1990). Defects in the inner limiting membrane also occur during aging (Kishi et al., 1986), retinal ischemia (Juarez et al., 1986), and after edematous degeneration of Müller cells (Fig. 54B) (Faude et al., 2001). In addition to vitreous hemorrhage, AGEs localized to the vitreous cavity and internal limiting membrane (Barile et al., 2005) may activate Müller cells to proliferate towards the vitreous.

Hemorrhage are oftenly associated with blood clotting. Plasma-derived proteins such as prothrombin can enter the retina, and activated thrombocytes may release granules that contain procoagulative proteins. Thrombin is generated from prothrombin after contact to extravascular tissue factor, resulting in the formation of fibrin from fibrinogen. Fibrin constitutes a provisional extracellular matrix that serves as scaffold for the subsequent epiretinal membrane formation (Charteris et al., 2002); the fibrin deposition is later replaced by a matrix made of locally synthesized collagen and fibronectin (Wiedemann, 1992). The provisional fibrin matrix supports the invasive growth of cells and blood vessels. Choroidal neovascular membranes formed in wet AMD are oftenly surrounded by a rim of fibrin, and newly formed vessels grow into the fibrin matrix (Schlingemann, 2004).

Vitreous hemorrhage also stimulate the formation of retinal folds that are suggested to be sites where epiretinal membranes develop in the course of PVR (Cantó Soler et al., 2002b). The mechanism of retinal fold formation in the absence of periretinal membranes is unclear and may involve mechanical stress due to contraction of the vitreous body focally attached to Müller cells, a contraction of Müller cells in response to vitreal growth factors and cytokines, and process extension and migration of Müller cells onto the inner surface of the retina towards the vitreal gradient of chemoattractants (Fig. 24) (Hui et al., 1988; Castelnovo et al., 2000). Retinal fold formation was also explained with a loss of Müller cells (Lai and Rana, 1985), and spontaneous reattachment of detached retinas can result in retinal folding (Nour et al., 2003). Once epiretinal membranes are formed, the contraction of the membranes produces further retinal folds (Hui et al., 1988).

5.11.11.4 Peeling of Epiretinal Membranes

Ischemic areas of the retina may obtain a significant portion of oxygen and nutrients from the vitreal fluid. When preretinal membranes or the posterior vitreous body are attached to the retina, the oxygen and nutrient supply from the vitreal humor to the ischemic retina is impaired. Therefore, surgical removal of epiretinal membranes (similar as posterior vitreous detachment or vitrectomy;

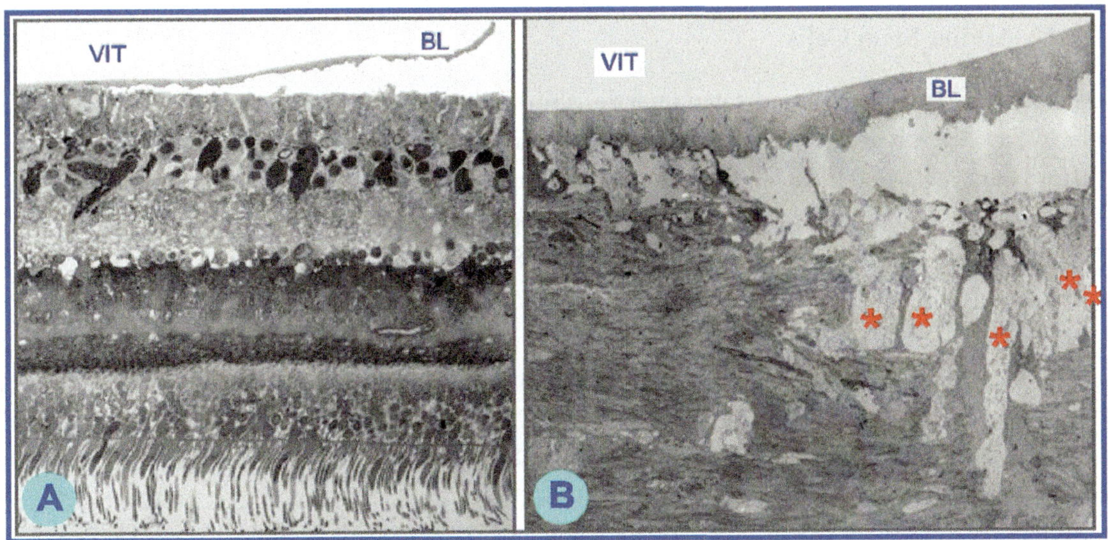

FIGURE 88: Human donor retina, with peeling of the basal lamina shortly after enucleation. **A.** Light microscopy of a semi-thin section. The basal lamina (BL) is still attached to the retina at the *left side*, but detached in the peeled region at the *right side*. The transition zone between the two regions is shown in **B. B.** Electron microscopy of the transition zone between the unpeeled (*left*) and the peeled area (*right*). Note that where the basal lamina got peeled off, many (*asterisks*) but not all Müller cell endfoot structures were severely damaged. VIT, vitreous. Modified from Wolf et al. (2004).

Stefánsson, 2001; Quiram et al., 2007) improves the retinal oxygenation, by allowing oxygen and nutrients to be transported within the vitreous cavity from well oxygenated to ischemic areas of the retina. Peeling of preretinal membranes also eliminates the vitreo-retinal interface pathology (Robaszkiewicz et al., 2010), and removal of the inner limitng membrane attenuates the proliferation of retinal astrocytes (Mittleman et al., 1989). In addition, epiretinal membrane peeling may improve glial homeostatic functions such as potassium buffering across the endfeet of Müller cells. However, it was shown that peeling of the inner limiting membrane may cause retinal detachment and disruption of adhering Müller cell endfeet (Fig. 88A,B) (Mittleman et al., 1989; Wolf et al., 2004; La Heij et al., 2005). This should impair rather than improve the exchange of molecules between the retina and the vitreous and may provoke additional reactive gliosis (Wolf et al., 2004; Robaszkiewicz et al., 2010). Excised epiretinal membranes contain Müller cells, astrocytes, and neuronal elements (Ishida et al., 2000; Sach et al., 2000). The therapeutic value of the inner limiting membrane peeling is thus still a matter of debate (Kuhn, 2002; Hassan and Willliams, 2002).

5.11.12 Müller Stem Cells

Several lines of evidence have indicated a relationship among neural progenitor/stem cells and Müller cells; in fact, late progenitor cells were suggested to be immature Müller cells (Seigel et al., 1996; Walcott and Provis, 2003; Angénieux et al., 2006; Mochizuki et al., 2014) and *vice versa*, a subset of Müller cells in the mature retina was suggested to represent latent neural progenitor/stem cells (Das et al., 2006; Bernardos et al., 2007; Roesch et al., 2008; Jadhav et al., 2009). In the zebrafish, Müller cells express low levels of the multipotent progenitor marker Pax6, and Müller cell-derived progenitors express α1-tubulin and cone-rod homeobox (Crx), and generate photoreceptors and ganglion cells in the postembryonic retina (Fausett and Goldman, 2006; Bernardos et al., 2007; Fimbel et al., 2007; Fausett et al., 2008). Müller cells of the mature rodent retina display a gene expression profile resembling that of progenitor cells (Blackshaw et al., 2004); a subset of Müller cells express progenitor genes such as Car2, Dkk3, Ceh-10 homeodomain-containing homologue (Chx10), Sox9, and Pax6 (Rowan and Cepko, 2004; Roesch et al., 2008; Wang et al., 2013b). Müller cells of the mature murine retina express cell cycle genes such as cyclinD3, Cdc14A, Cdk10, and Spbc25, and genes of the Notch pathway that regulate the reentry of Müller glia into the cell cycle under pathological conditions (Roesch et al., 2008). The promoters of several regeneration-associated genes, including achaete-scute homologue 1 (Ascl1), Lin28, HB-EGF, and insulinoma-associated 1 (Insm1), display a low basal level of methylation in Müller cells of the mature retina (Powell et al., 2013).

In response to retinal injury, Müller cells rapidly dedifferentiate, proliferate, and generate neuronal stem cells that migrate to the damaged retinal layer and differentiate into lost neurons and photoreceptor cells (Fig. 89A–J) (Fischer and Reh, 2001; Ooto et al., 2004). This neurogenic program is fully retained in Müller cells of cold-blooded vertebrates (teleost fish, amphibians), which have the capability of full regeneration following ocular injury (Mensinger and Powers, 1999; Lindsey and Powers, 2007; Sherpa et al., 2008), whereas Müller cells of adult homeothermic vertebrates have only a limited potential of transdifferentiation into photoreceptors and neurons (Fischer and Reh, 2001, 2003; Ooto et al., 2004; Kubota et al., 2006; Bull et al., 2008; Takeda et al., 2008; Joly et al., 2011; Goldman, 2014). Apparently, Müller cells reactivate distinct cellular programs under pathological conditions which are normally used in the ontogenetic retinal development. Cellular dedifferentiation is a precondition for glial cell proliferation and migration, and for regenerative processes in the injured retina.

5.11.12.1 Retinas of Cold-Blooded Vertebrates

The retinas of teleost fish and amphibians display a lifelong growth and have the capability of full regeneration following ocular injury. The progenitor properties of fish Müller cells are vital to the

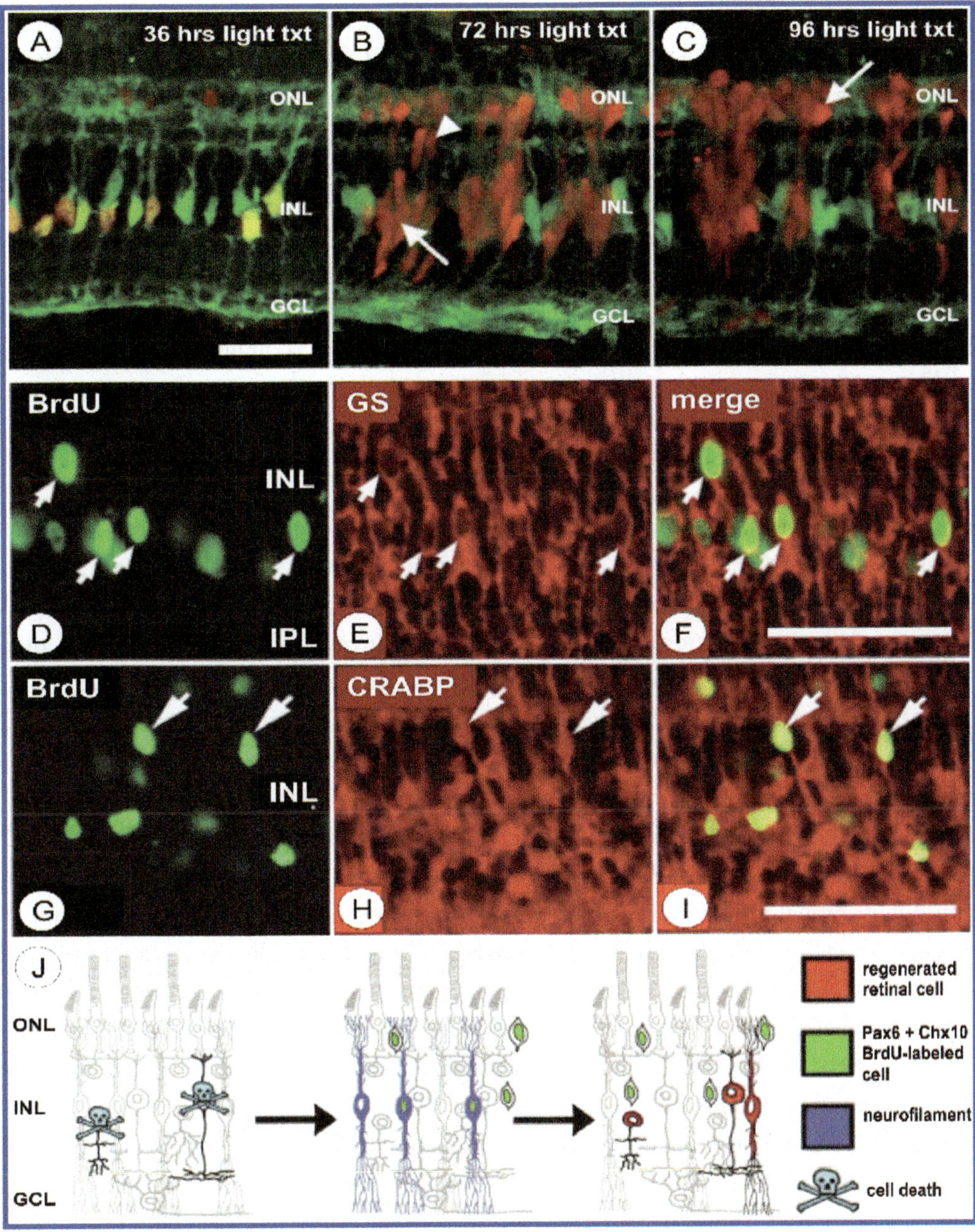

FIGURE 89: Müller cells can act as neuronal progenitor cells in adult ectotherm animals such as fish (**A-C**) and in young birds (**D-J**). In the *Tg(gfap:EGFP)nt11 albino* zebrafish retina, light exposure causes

continued on next page

proliferative activity (indicated by PCNA immunohistochemistry; *red*). After 36 h, many Müller cells (*green* fluorescence) proliferate (**A**) but after 72 (**B**) and 96 h (**C**), most of their daughter cells became EGFP-negative progenitor cells, many of which migrate into the outer nuclear layer (ONL) where they continue to proliferate and generate photoreceptor cells (modified from Thummel et al., 2008). In the young chicken retina (**D–J**) N-methyl-D-aspartate (NMDA)-induced apoptosis of neuronal cells causes the proliferation (i.e., uptake of BrdU; *green*) of many Müller cells expressing glutamine synthetase (GS; *red*) after 2 days (**D–G**). After 14 days, many BrdU-positive cells (*green*) now express the neuronal marker, CRABP (*red*), and can be found outside the sub-layer of the Müller cell nuclei (**G–I**). **J**. Schematic diagram illustrating the response of Müller cells to NMDA-induced damage. Modified from Fischer and Reh (2003). Scale bars, 25 μm (A-C) and 50 μm (D-I); INL, inner nuclear layer; IPL, inner plexiform layer.

---

sustained growth of the retina in adults (Bernardos et al., 2007) and the retinal regeneration after injury (Fausett et al., 2008; Qin et al., 2009c; Ramachandran et al., 2010a; Goldman, 2014). The continuous growth of the fish retina is mediated by passive stretching of the existing tissue (Mack et al., 1998) and the proliferation of Müller cells and stem cells in the circumferential marginal zone; the vast majority of the new retina is added from the margin (Julian et al., 1998; Umino and Saito, 2002; Bernardos et al., 2007; Kassen et al., 2008). During adult growth, the nuclei of Müller cells undergo sporadic, asymmetric, self-renewing mitotic divisions in the inner nuclear layer which generate rod progenitors that migrate along the Müller cell fibers into the outer nuclear layer where these cells proliferate and differentiate into rod photoreceptors (Stenkamp, 2011; Lenkowski and Raymond, 2014). After injury to the mature fish retina, Müller cells dedifferentiate into multipotent retinal progenitors that regenerate all lost retinal cell types including both classes of photoreceptor cells, while the Müller cell-derived rod precursor cells in the outer nuclear layer exclusively regenerate rods; the proliferation of rod precursor cells is stimulated when the proliferation of Müller cell-derived neuronal precursor cells is inhibited (Raymond et al., 2006; Morris et al., 2008; Thummel et al., 2010; Goldman, 2014). The injured amphibian retina may also regenerate via transdifferentiation of the retinal pigment epithelium (Raymond, 1991).

Injury to the mature fish retina induces an increase in the number of proliferating Müller cells in the inner nuclear layer which express stem cell markers, e.g., the proneural gene achaete-scute homolog 1a (Ash1a) which contributes to the transition of the cells into a Notch3-expressing regenerative progenitor (Yurco and Cameron, 2007). The proneural basic helix-loop-helix gene Ascl1 is required to convert quiescent Müller cells into actively dividing neuronal progenitor cells and blocks cell cycle exit (Fausett et al., 2008; Ramachandran et al., 2010b, 2011; Powell et al., 2012; Hufnagel et al., 2013). The generation of neuronal progenitor cells from Müller cells is dependent on global DNA demethylation (for the dedifferentiation of Müller cells) and distinct DNA methylation (for the migration and differentiation of neuronal progenitors), activation of a Lin28–let-7 miRNA signaling loop, Shh and Wnt/β-catenin signaling, interkinetic nuclear migration, and asymmetrical cell division (Ramachandran et al., 2010b, 2011; Meyers et al., 2012; Powell et al., 2012, 2013; Sun et al., 2014). The neuronal progenitor cells migrate in an N-cadherin-dependent manner (Nagashima et al., 2013) along Müller cell processes to different retinal laminas and replenish lost photoreceptors and retinal neurons (Fig. 89A–C) (Hitchcock and Raymond, 1992; Vihtelic and Hyde, 2000; Wu et al., 2001; Hitchcock et al., 2004; Fausett and Goldman, 2006; Fimbel et al., 2007; Fausett et al., 2008; Thummel et al., 2008; Kassen et al., 2008; Ahmad et al., 2011; Ramachandran et al., 2011, 2012; Wan et al., 2012; Lenkowski and Raymond, 2014). Pharmacological activation of the β-catenin signaling pathway by lithium or an inhibitor of the glycogen synthase kinase-3β is sufficient to trigger the generation of neuronal progenitor cells from Müller cells in the uninjured fish retina (Ramachandran et al., 2011). Activation of the the β-catenin signaling pathway induces the expression of Pax6 (Ramachandran et al., 2011) which is necessary for the proliferation of Müller cell-derived neuronal progenitors (Ramachandran et al., 2010b; Thummel et al., 2010; Rajaram et al., 2014). In addition to the activation of pathways that stimulate Müller cell proliferation and progenitor formation, pathways which induce cell differentiation and quiescence (e.g., TGF-β, miRNA let-7-, and Dkk-mediated pathways) are suppressed in Müller cells after injury of the fish retina (Ramachandran et al., 2010b, 2011; Lenkowski et al., 2013; Goldman, 2014).

Secreted factors like HB-EGF, TNFα, a CNTF-like member of the IL-6 family, Wnts, and ADP promote the injury-induced progenitor formation from Müller cells in the fish retina; these factors are produced in Müller cells and (at least in the cases of TNFα and ADP) are additionally released from injured neurons (Faillace et al., 2002; Kassen et al., 2009; Battista et al., 2009; Ramachandran et al., 2011; Wan et al., 2012; Nelson et al., 2013). HB-EGF induces the expression of Ascl1 (Wan et al., 2012) which results in the suppression of genetic programmes that promote cellular differentiation and activation of programmes that promote proliferation. TNFα contributes to the induction of the expression of Ascl1 and STAT3 (Nelson et al., 2013); activation of the JAK/STAT3 signaling pathway is required for the formation of neuronal progenitor cells from Müller cells, among others by the induction of Ascl1 (Kassen et al., 2007; Nelson et al., 2012, 2013). Microglia and other immune cells migrate to the injury site and release factors that influence the proliferation and transdifferentiation of Müller cells (Craig et al., 2008; Goldman, 2014). Furthermore, the phagocytic activity of Müller cells is a precondition of Müller cell proliferation and progenitor formation in the injured fish retina (Bailey et al., 2010). After selective injury to photoreceptors, FGF signaling and the galectin Drgal1-L2 are necessary for the regeneration of rods but not of cones (Craig et al., 2010; Qin et al., 2011). Notch signaling plays a role in restricting the zone of injury-responsive Müller cells (Wan et al., 2012).

The expression of Ascl1 is crucial for the formation of Müller cell-derived neuronal progenitors (Fausett et al., 2008; Ramachandran et al., 2010b, 2011; Goldman, 2014). Ascl1 stimulates the expression of Lin28 which is an RNA-binding protein highly expressed in embryonic stem cells (Shyh-Chang and Daley, 2013). Increased Lin28 levels are associated with decreased levels of let-7 miRNAs that regulate cellular differentiation (Shyh-Chang and Daley, 2013). Ascl1a also inhibits the expression of Dkk-1 (an inhibitor of the Wnt/beta-catenin signaling pathway), activates the expression of Wnt genes, and regulates the expression of Insm1, a transcriptional repressor that is involved in the regulation of Müller cell dedifferentiation and the exit of newly formed progenitor cells from the cell cycle (Ramachandran et al., 2011, 2012).

The factors which determine the differentiation of Müller cell-derived neuronal progenitors into distinct cell types are largely unknown (Goldman, 2014). Notch signaling stimulates the differentiation of photoreceptors (Wan et al., 2012), and Mps1 stimulates the differentiation of progenitor cells into cones (Qin et al., 2009c). N-cadherin is required for the the migration of progenitor cells and thus increases the regeneration of inner retinal neurons (Nagashima et al., 2013).

5.11.12.2 Avian Retina

In the retina of adult warm-blooded vertebrates, neurons have a limited capability to regenerate; only glial cells, quiescent progenitor cells at the ciliary marginal zone, and vascular cells maintain the capability to proliferate. Adult chicken retinas do not regenerate after injury while postnatal chick retinas have a restricted capability of neural regeneration. Injury to the chick retina induces the reentry of Müller cells into the cell cycle. The proliferation of Müller cells is induced by endogenous growth factors, likely bFGF, insulin, and IGF-1 (Fischer and Reh, 2002; Fischer et al., 2002, 2009b; Ritchey et al., 2012), stimulated by Notch signaling (Hayes et al., 2007; Ghai et al., 2010), and mediated by ERK1/2 signaling (Fischer et al., 2009b). Proliferating Müller cells express neurofilaments and transcription factors normally found in embryonic retinal progenitor cells including the neurogenic bHLH transcription factor Cash-1 as well as Pax6, Ascl1, and Chx10 (Fischer and Reh, 2001, 2003; Fischer et al., 2002). A small percentage of newly generated cells differentiate into neurons, a higher percentage differentiate into new Müller cells but most cells remain undifferentiated progenitor cells which continuously express Pax6 and Chx10 (Fischer and Reh, 2001, 2003; Fischer et al., 2002). In response to photoreceptor injury, Müller cells also express Pax6 and translocate their nuclei to outer retinal layers without preceding proliferation (Fischer et al., 2002, 2004a). Müller cells of the chick retina have the potential to regenerate all types of retinal neurons

(Fig. 89D–J) (Fischer and Reh, 2002, 2003). However, the potential of chick Müller cells to be a source of progenitor cells is dependent on the age of the animals. As the animals age, the region in which proliferating Müller cells are found in response to retinal injury becomes increasingly confined to the retinal periphery (Fischer and Reh, 2003); this reflects the centro-peripheral wave of Müller cell differentiation during retinal development (Prada et al., 1991). bFGF stimulates the proliferation and dedifferentiation of Müller cells into progenitor cells (Fischer et al., 2002, 2009a). This effect is in part mediated by microglia and/or infiltrating macrophages activated by components of the complement system and inflammatory cytokines; ablation of microglia/macrophages results in a great reduction of the formation of Müller cell-derived progenitor cells in response to retinal injury or the combination of insulin and bFGF (Fischer et al., 2014).

It is unclear why only a small subpopulation of Müller cells transdifferentiate into neuron-like cells in the injured chick retina. It has been suggested that the local environment, e.g., the presence of glial differentiation factors such as BMPs and CNTF, suppresses Müller cell proliferation and differentiation into progenitors (Fischer et al., 2004a). This assumption is supported by the fact that the injured postnatal chicken retina does also not support the neuronal differentiation of transplanted embryonic retinal progenitor cells (Fischer and Reh, 2003). Another reason may be the persistent activation of the Notch signaling pathway in Müller cells after retinal injury. Notch activity is required for the dedifferentiation and proliferation of Müller cells, and inhibits the differentiation of Müller cell-derived progenitors into neurons (Nelson et al., 2007); thus, persistent Notch activity limits the regeneration of the injured chicken retina (Hayes et al., 2007). Blockade of the Notch pathway after generation of progenitors from Müller cells increases the percentage of newly formed neurons (Hayes et al., 2007). Furthermore, glucocorticoids inhibit the formation of Müller stem cells, at leat in part by antagonizing the bFGF/MAPK signaling in Müller cells (Gallina et al., 2014). Inhibition of the glucocorticoid receptor signaling stimulates the formation of proliferating Müller stem cells in the damaged retina, diminishes the glial differentiation, and enhances the neuronal differentiation of the cells (Gallina et al., 2014). The amount of neurons generated from Müller cells is also increased by overexpression of the neurogenic gene NeuroD (Fischer et al., 2004b). Müller cells of the avian retina have also the capacity to transdifferentiate into lens cells, and to form lentoid bodies in response to retinal injury (Moscona and Degenstein, 1981b; Moscona ct al., 1983; Zeiss and Dubielzig, 2006).

5.11.12.3 Mammalian Retina

Müller cells in retinas of adult mammals have a restricted potential to dedifferentiate into neurogenic progenitor/stem cells. In response to retinal injury, Müller cells of the rodent retina express molecules related to neural progenitors such as brain lipid-binding protein, doublecortin, Sox9, and Crx (Chang et al., 2007; Wang et al., 2013b), may express photoreceptor proteins (Goel and Dhingra, 2012), and some of the cells proliferate through cyclin D1- and D3-related pathways, and produce new neurons and photoreceptors (Ooto et al., 2004; Wan et al., 2008). However, only a very small subpopulation of mammalian Müller cells transdifferentiate to neurons after retinal injury (Karl et al., 2008). Retinoic acid promotes the number of regenerated bipolar cells, while misexpression of basic helix-loop-helix and homeobox genes promotes the induction of amacrine, horizontal, and rod photoreceptor specific phenotypes in Müller cells (Ooto et al., 2004; Ooto, 2006). After subretinal injection of subtoxic levels of glutamate or DL-α-aminoadipic acid (a glutamate analogue which selectively targets glial cells; Pedersen and Karlsen, 1979; Wakakura and Ishikawa, 1982; Karlsen et al., 1982; Ishikawa and Mine, 1983; Pow, 2001a), Müller cells of adult mice dedifferentiate, express progenitor cell markers (nestin and Chx10), proliferate, and migrate to the outer nuclear layer where they can transdifferentiate into photoreceptor cells (Takeda et al., 2008). When these cells are plated in culture, they give rise to almost all types of retinal neurons and glial cells including retinal ganglion, amacrine, bipolar, and photoreceptor cells, as well as astrocytes and Müller cells (Takeda et al., 2008; Nickerson et al., 2008; Zhao et al., 2014b). Cultured murine and monkey Müller cells express a group of proteins related to the dopaminergic phenotype, including tyrosine hydroxylase, and produce dopamine (Kubrusly et al., 2008; Stutz et al., 2014). The potential of differentiation of proliferating Müller cells into retinal neurons was also shown in the injured murine retina *in vivo* (Karl et al., 2008). Adult human retinas contain a small subpopulation of Müller cells that expresses neural progenitor markers including Sox2, Chx10, and Pax6 (Lawrence et al., 2007). The activity of Sox2 also prevents the degeneration of postnatal Müller cells through terminal cell division (Surzenko et al., 2013). Human Müller cell cultures can generate photoreceptors and retinal ganglion cells that have some reparative potential when transplanted into the injured rodent retina (Giannelli et al., 2011; Singhal et al., 2012; Becker et al., 2013; Jayaram et al., 2014).

The mechanisms of activating the dormant stem cell properties in Müller cells in the injured mature mammalian retina involve Wnt/β-catenin, Notch, EGF receptor (see 5.11.10.4.3.), Ascl1-, and possibly TrkB-dependent signaling pathways (Ooto et al., 2004; Das et al., 2006; Jadhav et al., 2006; Osakada et al., 2007; Karl et al., 2008; Takeda et al., 2008; Harada et al., 2011; Wang et al., 2012b; Pollak et al., 2013). Glutamate, GDNF, bFGF, and insulin were described to induce expression of progenitor cell marker genes in Müller cells (Insua et al., 2008; Reyes-Aguirre et al., 2013). Wnt signaling stimulates Müller cell proliferation, survival, the dedifferentiation to retinal progenitor cells, as well as the expression of photoreceptor proteins in Müller cells after retinal injury (Liu et al., 2013b). CNTF induces increased numbers and dispersion of Müller and bipolar cells (Rhee et al., 2007). The expression of cyclin D1 in Müller cells, e.g., after stimulation with bFGF, is induced by PGE$_2$ (Wang et al., 2013e). PGE$_2$ stimulates the proliferation, dedifferentiation, and stem cell-like properties (expression of nestin and Pax6) of Müller cells; the prostaglandin synthesis is highly correlated with the stem cell characteristics of Müller cells (Wang et al., 2013e).

Inactivation of p53 stimulates Müller cells proliferation and enhances the induction of retinal progenitors from Müller cells (Zhao et al., 2014b). Exogenous Wnt3a increases the proliferation of Müller cells in the photoreceptor-damaged retina of adult mice, and retinoic acid or valproic acid induce differentiation of these cells into Crx- and rhodopsin-expressing photoreceptors (Osakada et al., 2007). Overexpression of Ascl1 in combination with EGF treatment stimulates the proliferation of Müller cells and the generation of bipolar neurons in postnatal mouse retinal explants (Pollak et al., 2013). Furthermore, the Shh pathway is an important regulator of the neurogenesis in the mature mammalian retina. Shh is a mitogen for Müller cells and promotes the dedifferentiation of the cells to progenitor cells and subsequent differentiation to rod photoreceptors (Wan et al., 2007). Müller cells of adult mice express patched (ptc), a component of the Shh receptor complex (Jensen and Wallace, 1997). Shh also acts as a mitogen for the persistent progenitor cells in the ciliary marginal zone in chicks and the retinal margin in rodents; Shh induces the differentiation of the cells into retinal neurons (Reh and Fischer, 2001; Moshiri and Reh, 2004; Moshiri et al., 2005). LIF stimulates the proliferation of progenitor cells derived from the adult human retina retina (Carter et al., 2009).

5.11.13 MÜLLER CELLS IN THERAPEUTIC APPROACHES

A proper understanding of the signaling mechanisms implicated in the induction of gliotic responses is essential for the development of efficient therapeutic strategies that increase the supportive/protective and decrease the destructive roles of gliosis. Inhibition of Müller cell hypertrophy and glial scar formation may support the tissue regeneration and the neural integration of retinal transplants (Kinouchi et al., 2003) and may improve the visual recovery after subretinal implantation of electronic devices. It may be conceivable, for example, that suppression of the inhibitory action of gliotic Müller cells on the tissue regeneration may direct the growth of newly formed vessels in PDR into the ischemic retinal tissue rather than into the vitreous. This can be done, for example, by inhibition of the upregulation of intermediate filaments (Hisatomi et al., 2002; Lundkvist et al., 2004) and of the glial secretion of antiangiogenic factors (Eichler et al., 2001, 2004a,b; Yafai et al., 2007; Rivera et al., 2008), or by degradation of inhibitory extracellular matrix molecules with MMPs (see 5.11.2.7.). On the other hand, iatrogenic induction of glial scarring is a therapeutic approach in the treatment of macular holes. Glial cells are involved in the repair of macular holes (Funata et al., 1992; Madreperla et al., 1994). A combination of vitrectomy and administration of autologous serum or platelet suspension (which induces proliferation, migration, and contraction of retinal glial cells; Castelnovo et al., 2000; Burmeister et al., 2009) encourages the closure of retinal breaks, and the holes are plugged by a scar composed of glial cells, pigment epithelial cells, and fibroblasts (Christmas et al., 1995).

Due to their potential of generating neural stem cells, Müller cells have a major impact for future cell-based therapeutic approaches to retinal degenerative diseases (Johnson and Martin, 2013). However, the molecular signals that trigger the neurogenic process remain to be explored to increase the number of newly generated neurons and to stimulate the establishment of regular synaptic connections. One method might be the regeneration of retinal neurons and photoreceptors from cultured Müller stem cells, with the possibility of the simultaneous application of transgenes that guide the direction of differentiation, thus determining specific neuron types which should develop from the cells. Transdifferentiated Müller cells can be obtained from neural stem cell marker-expressing Müller cells of the mature human retina (Mayer et al., 2005; Lawrence et al., 2007; Bhatia et al., 2009, 2011a,b; Giannelli et al., 2011; Johnsen et al., 2012; Singhal et al., 2012; Jayaram et al., 2014) and from immortalized human cell lines (Limb et al., 2002b; Lawrence et al., 2007; Lupien and Salesse, 2007). The latter acquire neural morphology in the presence of extracellular matrix and bFGF or retinoic acid, or by inhibition of Notch1 activity, express neural stem cell markers such as Pax6, Chx10, and Notch1, as well as markers of postmitotic retinal neurons and photoreceptors (Lawrence et al., 2007; Hollborn et al., 2011b; Singhal et al., 2012; Becker et al., 2013). Inhibition of Sox2 activity results in downregulation of neural progenitor and glial markers, and upregulation of markers of retinal neurons; however, it also induces apoptosis of the cells (Bhatia et al., 2011b). The differentiation of retinal progenitors to neuronal or glial cells is also dependent on CNTF, the serum concentration used for culturing, and the glucose/sorbitol ratio in the culture medium (Goureau et al., 2004; Zahir et al., 2006; Bhattacharya et al., 2008; Hu et al., 2013). Subretinal or vitreal transplantation of immortalized human Müller cells results in migration of the cells into the retinal parenchyma and the expression of neuronal cell markers (Lawrence et al., 2007; Bull et al., 2008). Another possible source of Müller stem cells are epiretinal membranes surgically removed from eyes of patients with proliferative retinopathies (Mayer et al., 2003; Johnsen et al., 2012). In the far future, degenerated retinas may be substituted by new autologous retinas generated in culture from Müller stem cells derived from surgically removed epiretinal membranes. The alterations in the membrane properties of Müller cells derived from patients with proliferative retinopathies and in animal models of proliferative retinopathies (with a decrease in Kir currents, increase in K_A currents, increase in BK channel activity, and a membrane potential more positive than that of cells from healthy retinas; Figs. 8F-H, 45E, 46A-D, 56B, 65I) resemble properties of immature radial glial/Müller cells in the early postnatal stage (Figs. 46A,C, 58A, 61A,B, 62, 63B, 67D) (Francke et al., 1997, 2001a, 2002; Bringmann et al., 1999b, 2000a, 2002b; Uhlmann et al., 2003; Pannicke et al., 2004, 2005a,b; Iandiev et al., 2006b; Wurm et al., 2006a, 2009a). The capability of these cells to produce action potential-like discharges upon membrane depolarization (Fig. 67C) (Francke et al., 1996) may reflect a transdifferentiation of the cells into neuron-like cells *in situ*. Other sources of new retinal neurons and glial cells are neural progenitors from the ciliary body, retinal astrocytes and microglial cells, doublecortin-expressing retinal perivascular glial cells which express neural stem cell markers, cells from the iris and retinal pigment epithelium, choroidea, and sclera, as well as (gene-modified) bone marrow- and brain-derived stem cells (Sakaguchi et al., 1997; Tropepe et al., 2000; Ahmad et al., 2000; Nishida et al., 2000; Tomita et al., 2002; Arsenijevic et al., 2003; Coles et al., 2004; Haynes and Del Rio-Tsonis, 2004; Engelhardt et al., 2005; Sun et al., 2006; Tomita et al., 2006; Reh and Fischer, 2006; MacNeil et al., 2007; Boettcher et al., 2008; Bhatia et al., 2010; Zhang and Wang, 2010; Wohl et al., 2012; Goldenberg-Cohen et al., 2012, 2014; Trost et al., 2014). It was also shown that transplantation of stem cells into the subretinal space of RCS rats improves the capability of resident Müller cells to dedifferentiate, proliferate, and transdifferentiate into photoreceptors (Tian et al., 2011). Cultured Müller cells that, among others, produce dopamine, were also suggested to be a tool for the treatment of various other neurodegenerative disorders, e.g., Parkinson's disease (Stutz et al., 2014).

Because Müller cells contact all retinal neurons and show a high resistance against pathogenic stimuli (see 5.11.2.4.), they are well-situated as targets for therapeutic interventions to inhibit neuronal degeneration. It was shown that transcorneal electrical stimulation (that stimulates Müller cell's production of the neuroprotective factor IGF-1) rescues axotomized retinal ganglion cells (Morimoto et al., 2005). An increase of the glutamine synthetase expression in retinal glial cells (via induction of the endogenous gene or supply of purified protein) has been shown to protect against neuronal degeneration in the injured retinal tissue (Gorovits et al., 1997). Another approach for using Müller cells in retinal therapy is somatic gene therapy. Gene transfer of neurotrophic and anti-inflammatory factors to Müller cells may support their protective role (Koeberle et al., 2004). Müller cells are primarily transfected when genes, e.g., for neuroprotective factors such as BDNF, are delivered by adenoviral vector-injections into the vitreous chamber (Isenmann et al., 1998; Sakamoto et al., 1998; Di Polo et al., 1998; Gauthier et al., 2005; Klimczak et al., 2009). A simultaneous transfection of genes for receptors of neurotrophic factors will ensure the protective effect (Cheng et al., 2002). Because Müller cells span the entire thickness of the retina, adenovirus-mediated gene delivery will be useful to modulate the survival of all neuronal cell types in the retina. Stimulation of the supportive function of Müller cells has also the advantage to enhance the survival of retinal neurons and photoreceptors independent of the concrete mutation or pathological condition underlying the neuronal cell death, and may provide a more sustained source of neuroprotection than administration of proteins (Gauthier et al., 2005).

References

Due to the extensive number of references in *Retinal Glia*, the complete reference list has been made available online as a free PDF download. The digital version features hyperlinks to the DOIs of cited sources, allowing you to quickly jump to the primary literature cited by the authors.

To download the free PDF file of References for this book, please visit:

http://www.morganclaypoolpublishers.com/retgliarefs/

If you have any questions or difficulty accessing the pdf file of the references, please contact **info@morganclaypool.com**.

Author Biographies

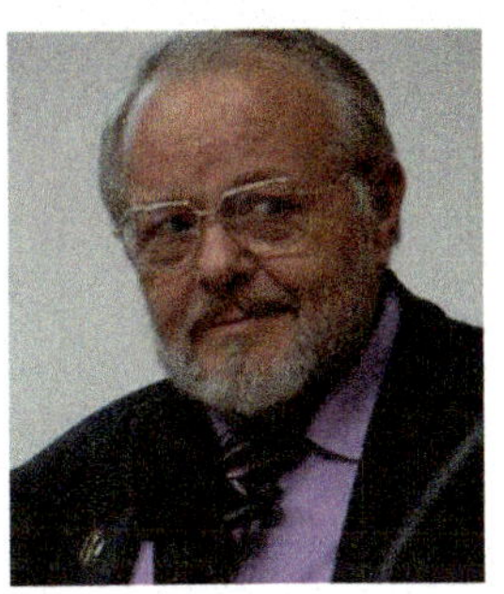

Andreas Reichenbach, Dr. med. habil., started his career as a physiologist. Since 1994 he has been Professor for Neurophysiology and Head of the Department of Pathophysiology of Neuroglia at the Paul Flechsig Institute of Brain Research, Universität Leipzig, Germany. His main fields of research are the development, structure, function, and pathophysiology of the vertebrate retina, and the contribution of neuroglial cells to the functioning and dysfunctions of the retina and brain. In particular, he and his colleagues contributed a great deal to the present knowledge about Müller (radial glial) cells of the mammalian retina. For instance, his group detected that Müller cells guide light to the photoreceptor cells in the inverted vertebrate retina. He has published a total of 400 scientific peer-reviewed papers, reviews, book chapters, and books.

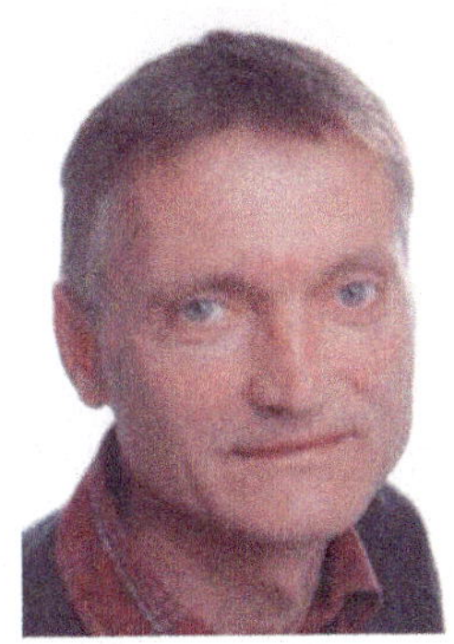

Andreas Bringmann After studying biology, Dr. Andreas Bringmann worked in the field of systemic neurophysiology until he was inspired in 1996 by Andreas Reichenbach to research the most interesting cell, the Müller cell. Since 2002 he has been in the Department of Ophthalmology and Eye Hospital of the University of Leipzig where he is the head of the Basic Research Laboratory.